Developments in
OCCUPATIONAL MEDICINE

DEVELOPMENTS IN Occupational Medicine

Edited by

CARL ZENZ, M.D., Sc.D.

Consultant to Division of Health, State of Wisconsin;
Consultant to National Institute for Occupational Safety and Health, Rockville, Maryland; Associate Professor of Occupational and Environmental Health, University of Illinois, Chicago, Illinois;
Consultant to U.S. Department of Labor, Washington, D.C.

1980

YEAR BOOK MEDICAL PUBLISHERS, INC.
Chicago • London

Printed in the United States of America.

Library of Congress Cataloging in Publication Data
Main entry under title:

Developments in occupational medicine.

Includes index.
1. Medicine, Industrial. I. Zenz, Carl.
[DNLM: 1. Occupational medicine. WA400.3 D489]
RC963 .D45 616.9'803 79-25035
ISBN O-8151-9862-0

Contributors

AXELSON, OLAV, M.D.: Professor, Department of Occupational Medicine and Industrial Ergonomics, University Hospital, Linköping University, Linköping, Sweden

BOND, MARCUS B., M.D.: Corporate Medical Director, American Telephone & Telegraph Company, Basking Ridge, New Jersey

BRIDBORD, KENNETH, M.D.: Director, Office of Extramural Coordination and Special Projects, National Institute of Occupational Safety and Health, Rockville, Maryland

DICKERSON, O. BRUCE, M.D., M.P.H.: Medical director, IBM, White Plains, New York. Formerly Corporate Director, Health and Safety Services, Fairchild Camera & Instrument Corporation, Mountain View, California

HANE, MONICA, Ph.D.: Clinical Psychologist, Department of Occupational Medicine, Regional Hospital, Örebro, Sweden

HERNBERG, SVEN, M.D.: Scientific Director, Institute of Occupational Health, Helsinki, Finland

HOGSTEDT, CHRISTER, M.D.: Associate Physician, Department of Occupational Medicine, Regional Hospital, Örebro, Sweden

KAPLAN, MARSHA, M.S.: Research Consultant, American Health Foundation, New York, New York

KINDWALL, ERIC P., M.D.: Director, Hyperbaric Medicine, St. Luke's Hospital, Milwaukee, Wisconsin.

KNUTSON, SHERI, M.S.: Project Associate, University of Wisconsin School for Workers, Madison, Wisconsin

LaDOU, JOSEPH, M.D.: Medical Director, Peninsula Industrial Medical Clinic, Sunnyvale, California; Assistant Clinical Professor, University of California, San Francisco, School of Medicine

MARGOLIS, IRWIN, M.D.: Associate Director, Section of Pulmonary Diseases, St. Luke's Hospital, Milwaukee, Wisconsin

MESSITE, JACQUELINE, M.D.: Regional Consultant, National Institute of Occupational Safety and Health, New York, New York

METS, JOHANN T., M.D.: Industrial Medical Officer, Volkswagen, Uitenhage/Port Elizabeth, Republic of South Africa

MITCHELL, FRANK L., D.O.: Special Assistant for Medical Criteria, National Institute for Occupational Safety and Health, Rockville, Maryland

NAGLE, GEORGE, M.P.H.: Manager of Industrial Hygiene, Velsicol Chemical Corporation, Chicago, Illinois

OLISHIFSKI, JULIAN B., P.E.: Industrial Hygienist, Alliance of American Insurers, Chicago, Illinois. Formerly Director, Industrial Hygiene, National Safety Council, Chicago, Illinois; Adjunct Assistant Professor of Occupational and Environmental Medicine, University of Illinois, Chicago, Illinois

WINGET, CHARLES M., Ph.D.: Biomedical Research Division, NASA-Ames Research Center, Moffett Field, California

WOODBURY, MARY ANN, M.C.H.: Environmental Epidemiologist, Bureau of Prevention, Division of Health, State of Wisconsin, Madison, Wisconsin

ZENZ, CARL, M.D., Sc.D.: Consultant to Division of Health, State of Wisconsin; Consultant to National Institute for Occupational Safety and Health, Rockville, Maryland; Associate Professor of Occupational and Environmental Health, University of Illinois, Chicago, Illinois; Consultant to U.S. Department of Labor, Washington, D.C.

Preface

SINCE PUBLICATION of *Occupational Medicine: Principles and Practical Applications* in 1975, occupational medicine has seen a massive evolution of special events. Workers have become keenly aware of potential health hazards on their jobs, public interest has developed to the point where articles are appearing on the front pages of newspapers, television specials are shown and business publications regularly describe occupational health problems. Knowledge of increased liver cancer in vinyl chloride workers has become widespread; this workplace crisis was followed by another—the discovery that kepone, a pesticide produced under poor working conditions, caused severe neurologic damage in 28 workers, with 14 men becoming sterile. Shortly thereafter, another alarming occupational health problem was reported among workers manufacturing "DBCP" (dibromochloropropane), a nematocide, which caused reproductive alterations in men ranging from oligospermia to sterility. Additionally, high lead levels in the blood of men reduced sperm counts and produced deformed sperm, underscoring heightened concerns for the health of men and women in the work force. Not only have sterility and fertility become serious grounds for concern but also mutagenesis and teratogenesis, in addition to public anxieties about occupational carcinogens. Paralleling these events were accounts of hazards of "PCBs" (polychlorinated biphenyls) and "PPBs" (polybrominated biphenyls), reports of leukemia in workers in certain rubber factories, and the finding of nitrosamines in cutting fluids.

This book, a continuation of *Occupational Medicine: Principles and Practical Applications*, which has proved successful and well established worldwide, encompasses these recent occupational problems in much detail, along with several other important recognized hazards involving both men and women. The 20 expert contributors explore these and many other factors of concern, stressing control and preservation of the health of all workers. Increasingly, women are entering all types of workplaces, accounting for nearly 50% of some nations' work forces. There may be untold numbers of women workers of childbearing age who are exposed to substances potentially capable of causing birth defects or miscarriages. The National Institute of Occupational Safety and Health (NIOSH) states that about 20 compounds can be linked to such consequences. Benzene, lead, methyl mercury and others known to have caused fetal damage (transplacental transfer) are discussed. The real issue of these occupational hazards is the potential effects on the reproductive systems of both men and women; two chapters are devoted to this. Other chapters describe the subtle central nervous system damage and changes in behavior and performance that result from chronic exposure to solvents, including anesthetic gases. Practical ergonomics, ranging from agricultural fields to electronic assembly lines, clinical laboratory and office work, are noted in detail. The various physical and psychologic stresses imposed on certain working groups, for example, long-distance truck drivers and air traffic controllers—large groups—are documented in a major chapter. The health and safety aspects of the truck drivers correlate with another stress area—"shift" or "rotational" work. Chapter 1 establishes the principles of epidemiology in occupational health.

Joint Occupational Safety and Health Administration (OSHA) and NIOSH standards now incorporate guidelines for informing workers about hazards, monitoring the workplace, developing control measures and hygienic and engineering procedures, setting up medical surveillance and other programs. These features are described in detail in the various chapters, including the important practical medical factors in the use of respirators.

As in *Occupational Medicine: Principles and Practical Applications,* this book is also arranged into major sections, consisting of epidemiology in occupational health, occupational health considerations for women at work, the physical working environment, psychosocial considerations and the chemical working environment.

It is not the intent, nor is it feasible, to describe in detail all chemicals, physical agents or materials potentially encountered in all work places. Those most commonly used or inadvertently produced are described with deliberate grouping of substances, i.e., pesticides, petroleum solvents, metal fumes, solvents, etc., as the most practical method of presentation.

Finally, this book is intended to bring up-to-date information to those involved in occupational health activities for optimal preservation of worker health.

ACKNOWLEDGMENTS

My heartfelt gratitude is given to the contributors for their splendid cooperation and for devoting so much valuable time in the preparation of this book. The greatest credit goes to them. For advice, support and other assistance I give special thanks to Lennart Sundell, M.D., Örebro, Sweden; Gerald W. Grawey, M.D., Peoria, Illinois; Arthur H. Knight, M.D., Phillipsburg, New Jersey; Stuart A. Levy, M.D., Milwaukee, Wisconsin; Lillian S. Nelson, M.D., Milwaukee, Wisconsin; Jane Parker, R.N., M.S., Chicago, Illinois; and Mrs. Magdalene Wos, Medical Librarian, and her staff, St. Luke's Hospital, Milwaukee, Wisconsin.

CARL ZENZ

Contents

PART ONE

Epidemiology—Principles and Practical Examples

1 / Epidemiology in Occupational Health

SVEN HERNBERG, M.D.

EVER SINCE 1775, when Sir Percival Pott described the extraordinarily high occurrence of scrotal cancer among chimney sweeps, who at that time usually were forced to begin work at an early age, epidemiologically oriented thinking has been infiltrating occupational medicine. Yet, with a few brilliant exceptions, most of the investigations published before the middle of this century did not comply with validity criteria and hence sometimes led to erroneous conclusions. Fortunately, the past few decades have shown a favorable development in the quality of epidemiologic studies, but there still is room for improvement. Raising the quality of epidemiologic research essentially involves intensifying the education of research workers—the "producers" of data. This would best be achieved by means of formal training at public health schools or intensive "crash" courses.

There is also another aspect to improvement, however. Not only active research workers but all those who read epidemiologic reports—the "consumers" of data—must be familiar with at least the basic principles of epidemiology. Otherwise, they are unable to form their own critical opinions on the validity of the studies and the justifiability of the conclusions drawn by the authors. This aspect of improvement is becoming more and more important because a substantial part of knowledge in the field of occupational medicine nowadays is derived from epidemiologic studies, especially with respect to work-related diseases with multiple etiologies, mild effects and nonspecific diseases.

This presentation is primarily addressed to the "consumers"; for the "producers" it will be too superficial and fragmentary. For example, data analysis is not even discussed. But, although this is an elementary presentation, comprehension of many essential points will be easier if the reader is at least somewhat familiar with epidemiologic concepts, terminology and study designs. On the other hand, this basic discussion may urge some readers to penetrate deeper into the fascinating science of epidemiology. These people then should acquaint themselves with a textbook on epidemiology. Some good ones now are available; for example, *Epidemiology, Principles and Methods* by B. MacMahon and E. Pugh[15] and *Foundations of Epidemiology* by A. M. Lilienfeld.[13]

1. EPIDEMIOLOGIC RESEARCH AND ITS APPLICATIONS IN OCCUPATIONAL HEALTH—AN OVERVIEW

Definition

Epidemiology can be defined as the *science or discipline of the occurrence of illness in human populations*. This definition has three important components. First, epidemiology is a *science* (or, when practiced, a discipline), not merely a method. Second, it deals with the occurrence of *illness* (= disease + vitium), not health or social behavior or any other phenomenon. This definition, in fact, excludes all topics that are unrelated to the occurrence of illness. The concept "occurrence" delineates epidemiology from other sciences occupied with illness; e.g., pathology, which concerns the nature of illness, and clinical medicine, which deals with the diagnosis and treatment of illness. Third, epidemiology is concerned with *human* illness, not with the morbidity of animals or plants, for which there are other sciences.

It is important to keep this definition in mind, because the term "epidemiologic" has become a fashionable label for a variety of activities. A science always should be defined according to the *category of phenomenon* it concerns, not the methods it uses. Hence, although other sciences may apply methods similar to those used in epidemiologic research, they cannot be labeled "epidemiologic."

Experimental vs Nonexperimental Research

Epidemiologic research is *nonexperimental* whereas experiments and clinical trials represent *experimental* research. The main distinction between experimental and nonexperimental research is that in experiments investigators actively manipulate the conditions. They *decide* what individuals (usually animals) will be exposed or unexposed; furthermore, they determine the exposure level. In a nonexperimental setting, investigators have no control of these factors, and this is a pertinent distinction when causal relationships between two phenomena are being sought, in this case between a disease and some exposure.

Only experimental research can provide definite proof for a cause-effect relationship, because only under experimental conditions is there the opportunity to allocate the animals—rarely humans—into exposed and unexposed categories randomly and thereby eliminate systematic errors (biases). Also, other factors can be strictly controlled. For example, exposure can be dosed exactly, as already mentioned. In addition, other concurrent exposures do not occur, and the effects can be measured systematically and accurately under standardized laboratory conditions.

In nonexperimental (epidemiologic) research, on the contrary, the possibilities of ensuring unbiased conditions are not so good. In particular, the fact that randomization usually cannot be utilized causes uncertainties regarding the presence or absence of systematic errors; hence, the interpretation of the results also becomes more conditional. What these uncertainties are and how they can be minimized are discussed in Section 5. Because perfection rarely, if ever, is achieved, the cause-effect inferences drawn from epidemiologic studies must be viewed in terms of probabilities only; they never are definite. Some guidelines for judging the probability of whether an association is causal or not are given in Section 6.

Although experimental evidence is more definite than nonexperimental results, the latter type of research has its own important role in medicine. Many of the reasons are self-evident, the most central one being, of course, that the study of human illness is best carried out on the human species. Extrapolation of data from animal experiments to human beings always is difficult. On the other hand, experimentation on human beings seldom is ethical, and this aspect generally rules out the experimental approach. Besides, since many environmental factors require a relatively long time to produce their effect, human experiments, even if ethically acceptable, would not be practically possible for the study of many problems.

Different Levels of Epidemiologic Research

Epidemiologic research can be classified into three categories, namely: (1) descriptive epidemiology, (2) etiologic epidemiology and (3) interventive epidemiology.

Descriptive epidemiology observes the occurrence of illness in different categories of people under different circumstances. One may, for example, compare the occurrence of lung cancer in various countries or in different age categories. Descriptive epidemiologic research finds its main use in the planning of health care, but it may also serve as a source of useful hypotheses about the etiology of certain illnesses. These hypotheses then can be tested by means of etiologic research, both experimental and epidemiologic.

Etiologic epidemiology concerns the study of causal connections between diseases and various genetic and environmental factors. Such connections are not directly observable—they must be inferred, and inferences fall in the sphere of abstractions. The research sometimes may focus on one cause and one disease; however, more often several concomitant factors are studied. Sometimes even quantitative estimates of the relative etiologic importance of each of them can be made. For example, epidemiologic research on the etiology of coronary artery disease has revealed a great number of risk indicators, e.g., cigarette smoking, elevated serum cholesterol, high blood pressure, diabetes and physical inactivity, and many studies have also quantitatively estimated the impact of each of them.

Interventive epidemiology studies changes in the occurrence of some illness after a change in exposure (in a broad sense) conditions. For example, once cardiovascular disease has been associated with a number of risk indicators, the question becomes one of what happens to the morbidity if one or more of these indicators are changed in a study population; i.e., what happens when people give up smoking, increase their physical activity, change their dietary habits, etc. The answer is useful in two ways. First, a reduction in morbidity supports the scientific hypothesis according to which the risk indicators indeed cause cardiovascular disease. Second, a successful outcome would be important for health authorities, because it would indicate that changing the habits of the whole population would be worthwhile. Lack of success, of course, would restrain the authorities from such operations.

In the occupational health setting, the first aspect, i.e., the strengthening—or refutation—of the hypothesis, is important. The second one, however, usually is rather self-evident; i.e., lowering the level of exposure to toxic substances cannot be anything but beneficial. In this instance, the question is rather one of how much reduction decreases morbidity how much and, ultimately, one of "cost-benefit."

Epidemiology and Occupational Health—General Aspects

Epidemiologic methods can be, and are today, widely applied to solve occupational health problems—usually not as a single approach but together with other methods. The following presentation is intended to illustrate the main categories of problems that can best be studied with an epidemiologic approach.

OBSERVATION OF THE OCCURRENCE OF ILLNESS IN DIFFERENT CATEGORIES OF WORKERS.—In occupational health care, the procedure of observing the occurrence of illness involves periodically examining the workers; e.g., in conjunction with annual checkups and systematically registering the results by age, department, type of work, length of employment, etc. The examinations are more effective if they are directed toward certain diseases or syndromes relevant for the occupation in question. Alternatively, well-planned, systematic registration of absenteeism (and its reasons) may serve the same purpose. Although not allowing any definite conclusions, this "in-plant epidemiology" may provide useful warning signals of occupational hazards that have passed unrecognized.

In addition, occupational mortality can be registered nationwide, as is being done, for example, in the United Kingdom. Or regional figures for mortality and morbidity can be registered and the differences observed, as is being done for cancer mortality, for example, in the United States. However, as is discussed in Sections 3 and 5, this type of comparison is vulnerable to systematic errors and does not allow cause-effect inferences. At best, clues for further investigations are produced. On the other hand, such observations are important for health administrative purposes. National mortality and morbidity statistics can reveal changes in the pattern of disease when followed over the years. For example, mortality statistics have shown that the occurrence of gastric cancer has decreased in most Western countries during the past few decades whereas colonic cancer has increased concomitantly. However, the reasons for these changes are not clear from such data alone.

OBSERVATION OF CHANGES IN THE OCCURRENCE OF ILLNESS.—Revealing changes in the occurrence of illness is a task for descriptive epidemiology. The preceding example concerning gastric and colonic cancers also illustrated the use of national vital statistics for this purpose. At the occupational health service level, following the morbidity of workers over time sometimes may provide the first clue of a deterioration of work conditions or of the introduction of "new" toxic agents. Of course, such matters should, in principle, be controlled by means of monitoring the workplace, not the workers, but in real life this system does not always succeed. The utilization of the files kept by occupational health services for this purpose requires strict adherence to standardized methods of observation and systematic record keeping. The plant physician should also have an open mind and make the effort to go through his files regularly, preferably with the aid of a computer. As is mentioned later, the effect of preventive measures sometimes can be evaluated in the same way.

COMPLETING THE CLINICAL PICTURE.—One of the most central tasks for etiologic epidemiologic research is to complete the clinical picture. Many occupational diseases are not adequately presented in textbooks, in regard to either breadth or depth. A thorough discussion of this defect of medicine in general can be found in J. N. Morris' book *Uses of Epidemiology*[25]; in this context, only a few illustrative examples from occupational medicine will be given.

Let us first consider completion in *breadth*. Arsenic is a good example. The clinical picture of arsenic poisoning has been known for centuries, partly due to the liberal use of the trioxide for homicidal purposes, partly because of the medical use of arsenicals and partly from observations of patients with occupational poisoning. It is characterized by gastrointestinal colic, diarrhea, hepatic degeneration, polyneuritis, palmar hyperkeratosis and pigmentation of the skin. This is about as far as clinical experience goes. But epidemiologic studies have shown that arsenic also causes skin cancer, bronchial carcinoma and probably also a variety of other tumors (for a review, see reference 7). Recently it was found that smelter workers exposed to arsenic also show an excess of deaths due to coronary artery disease.[2] Epidemiologic research thus has broadened the spectrum of known toxic effects of arsenic by adding information that clinical medicine could not provide.

Completing the picture in *depth* requires, to use an old expression, revealing those parts of the "iceberg" that are under the surface. Formerly, occupational medicine was mainly concerned with clinically manifest disease, but today subclinical changes caused by occupational factors also are considered unacceptable. This requirement, together with the development of sensitive test methods, has focused interest on the "gray" area between health and disease. But many early changes are nonspecific—they can be due to a variety of causes—and, consequently, valid epidemiologic study designs are needed to determine whether or not they are associated with certain exposures.

Consider, for example, carbon disulfide. Clinically, the poisoning is characterized by psychoses, polyneuropathy, extrapyramidal symptoms, hemiplegia, neurasthenia and gastrointestinal disturbances. Such severe cases rarely, if ever, are seen today, but milder forms still persist. Epidemiologic studies have shown that subclinical, nonspecific dysfunctions of both the central and the peripheral nervous systems are prevalent among clinically healthy workers exposed to carbon disulfide.[6, 29, 32] In other words, the present levels are not completely harmless. They produce subclinical poisoning, and epidemiologic studies have identified at least some of the characteristics. The picture of carbon disulfide poisoning thus has been given more depth.

MULTIPLE CAUSES.—Most diseases have more than one cause, although one sometimes is dominant; for example, an infectious agent (bacteria, viruses, etc.) when infections are concerned or a chemical agent in the case of occupational poisonings. Yet, even when one cause dominates, the other contributing factors, such as poor nutritional conditions, other concomitant diseases or genetic susceptibility, may explain why some persons contract disease and others do not. If the intensity of the main cause is weak, the relative importance of the contributing causes increases. For example, exposure to chemical agents at intensities moderately exceeding the hygienic standard causes disease only in some of the workers. Why some become ill and others remain healthy often is not known, but it may be postulated that one or more contributing causes have increased the sensitivity of those who contract overt illness (or, alternatively, some preventive cause has increased the resistance of others).

However, the etiology of most chronic diseases is much more complex. Perhaps the best illustration is coronary artery disease, which indeed has a multifactorial etiology. Other common diseases with several known causes are chronic bronchitis, emphysema, peptic ulcer, hepatic cirrhosis, osteoarthritis, many malignant tumors and a number of other diseases. Some of the causes may be occupational in origin.

Epidemiologic investigations provide possibilities to search for the different causes of such diseases and to evaluate the relative importance of each (the etiologic fraction) in a study population. Alternatively, the investigator may approach a particular exposure by studying what different types of diseases it causes, provokes or aggravates. It may turn out that disease A is associated with factors K, L, M and O and that factor M is associated with diseases A, B, C and D. The common feature is that in both instances there is an association between disease A and factor M. As one illustration from occupational medicine, consider coronary artery disease and carbon disulfide. Coronary artery disease is promoted by cigarette smoking, hypertension, a diet rich in saturated fat, diabetes, etc. *and by* exposure to carbon disulfide, arsenic and nitroglycol. On the other hand, exposure to carbon disulfide causes psychotic symptoms, neurologic disorders, gastritis, etc. *and also* coronary artery disease. Needless to say, almost all this knowledge has been derived from epidemiologic studies.

STUDY OF DISEASES FOR WHICH ANIMAL MODELS DO NOT EXIST.—Apart from the problems of extrapolating data from animal experiments to human beings there are some instances when the problem at issue cannot be studied in animals at all. This is the case for the association between subjective symptoms and occupational exposures. Also, personality changes and deterioration of higher nervous function are difficult or impossible to study in animals. (Behavioral animal toxicology does not solve these problems.) The causes of lumbar disease are not easily studied in animals either, because of the almost unique upright position of mankind. And, to give a specific example, arsenic has not induced cancer in any animal species. Hence, the only option left in such cases is to study the disease in man, preferably by epidemiologic methods. One could find many more examples, but since a comprehensive list is outside the scope of this section, it may suffice to mention finally that the study of industrial accidents represents a large field for which no animal models exist.

EXPOSURE-EFFECT AND EXPOSURE-RESPONSE RELATIONSHIPS.—Once a causal connection has been established, the next question is a quantitative one: How much exposure causes how much disease? This problem is best studied through observation of people exposed to various levels of the agent in question and by the recording of their different manifestations of ill health. This type of research aims at the construction of *dose-effect* and *dose-response* curves; an important pragmatic goal, pertinent for a standard setting, is the definition of the noneffect level. Because the dose usually is not known in an occupational health setting, it is more appropriate to speak in terms of exposure, which can be measured better. The difference between effect and response is that an *effect* is a *biologic change* caused by an exposure whereas a *response* denotes the *proportion* of a population that demonstrates a specific effect. The effect sometimes can be measured on a graded scale of severity. When data are available for the graded effect, their relationship to the exposure is called the *exposure-effect relationship*. A typical example is the relationship between the lead concentration in blood and the concentration of delta-aminolevulinic acid in urine samples of workers.

Any point on an exposure-effect curve may be used (by agreement, for example) to indicate that the effect is "present." The response then is expressed by the proportion of individuals showing the particular effect, and the *exposure-response curve* shows the various proportions at different exposure levels. For example, in the case of blood lead and urinary aminolevulinic acid excretion, the exposure-response curve is constructed from the proportions of workers having an aminolevulinic acid concentration in excess of, for example, 20 mg/l urine at different blood lead levels. Similarly, in the case of an all-or-none effect, e.g., lung cancer, the exposure-response curve will be constructed from the proportion of cases occurring at different exposure levels (provided that the levels have indeed been measured in the past, which unfortunately rarely is the case).

Many exposure-effect and exposure-response data have been derived from animal experiments. But, since human data are more relevant from the point of view of the human species, epidemiologic research is needed for constructing such curves, especially when the curves are used for standard setting. In fact, there still is an almost unlimited field left to investigate in this respect, as everyone who has looked for documentation of threshold limit values certainly has realized.

MEASUREMENT OF THE EFFECT OF PREVENTION.—As already discussed in connection with interventive epidemiology, the effects of some preventive effort, such as the reduction of exposure levels, sometimes can be measured from changes in the health state of the exposed population.

HEALTH CARE EVALUATION.—Because more and more of national incomes are being used for health care, the evaluation of existing systems and methods is becoming increasingly important. In the sphere of public health, questions such as "Does the use of oral antidiabetic drugs improve the prognosis of diabetes or not (or does it, in fact, worsen it?)" and "Are periodic health examinations of any benefit at all and, if so, what type of examinations are best?" become important. In the occupational health setting there are many similar issues, partly because many companies conduct extensive (public) health care programs. Yet, a specific feature is that it usually is self-evident that a reduction of high exposure levels improves health. The question is to define when the costs increase out of proportion to the benefits, as mentioned before.

CONCLUDING REMARKS.—This short review represents an attempt to bring into focus some of the many tasks of epidemiologic research in the field of occupational medicine and occupational health. Next is a short presentation of the most important principles for the conduction of such research.

2. SOME BASIC EPIDEMIOLOGIC MEASURES

Before a discussion of study types and validity problems can be fruitful, some basic epidemiologic terms and concepts must be clear. Only those essential to this presentation are introduced here; the rest can be found in textbooks on epidemiology.

Rates

Because epidemiology is concerned with the study of the occurrence of illness, a central event is the transition of individuals from the state of being healthy to that of being ill. When this occurs in a population, it is referred to as the *incidence* of the particular disease. Hence, incidence is a measure of *new* cases occurring in a population during a certain period of time. By contrast, *prevalence* is a measure of all *existing* cases in the population at some point in time.

Incidence rate (IR) can be expressed as follows:

$$\mathrm{IR} = \frac{\text{number of new cases occurring during a period of time}}{\text{average size of the population during the same time period}}$$

Similarly, *prevalence rate* (PR) denotes the proportion of people affected with the illness, and it can be expressed as:

$$\mathrm{PR} = \frac{\text{number of existing cases}}{\text{size of the population}}$$

The incidence rate can be expressed in two ways. The most common expression is *incidence density* (ID), which measures the number of new cases occurring in a population during a given period of time, as explained above. However, quite often the population is not stationary; i.e., its size varies over the years. Consider, for example, the occurrence of lung cancer among workers in an iron foundry. Suppose the period of follow-up began in 1950 and that the foundry employed 1000 workers in that year. In 1957, the foundry expanded and hired, say, another 500 workers. In addition, normal turnover accounted for, e.g., 500 new employees during 1950–1970, hired at irregular intervals throughout that period. Such a situation—which is common indeed—complicates the process of defining the average population. This difficulty can be overcome, however, if every worker is given a score denoting the number of years he has been in the study, i.e., number of years "at risk." If the study spans 1951 through 1975, a worker employed at the beginning of the follow-up in 1951 has a score of 25 and another who was hired in 1961 has one of 15. These scores are called *person-years*. The person-years for all workers are added and the sum replaces the average size of the population during the time interval studied in the computation of the incidence density. Consequently, ID can also be expressed as follows:

$$\mathrm{ID} = \frac{\text{number of new cases}}{\text{total number of person-years}}$$

Incidence density is an abstract measure, and sometimes its meaning may be difficult to conceptualize. Another, more easily understandable measure of incidence is the *cu-*

mulative incidence rate (CIR). The CIR can be defined as the *proportion* of the population that has become ill during a given period of time. The CIR dimension usually is expressed in per cent. For example, if 70 persons out of 1000 incur lung cancer in 20 years, the CIR_{20} is approximately 7%.

A rate is a characteristic of a population, not its members. In contrast, *risk* characterizes the *individual*. The risk is the probability of an individual developing a particular illness. Being a probability measure, risk is not observable, but it can be calculated for each individual sharing the characteristics of a population for which the CIR is known.

Two rates obtained from different populations, be they prevalence rate, incidence density or the cumulative incidence rate, can be compared if the rate of the "exposed" group is divided by that of the reference group. Hence, the *rate ratio* (RR) (synonyms: risk ratio, relative risk) can be defined as the rate of the exposed group over the rate of the reference category, or

$$RR = R/R_r$$

If the RR is greater than 1, the risk of contracting a particular disease is greater in the exposed group; if it is lower than 1, the risk is lower. Provided that the study is valid (see Section 5), exposure can be inferred to cause disease in the first case and prevent it in the second. The RR as such is a *point estimate* and subject to random variation (i.e., if the study were to be repeated, the RR would vary due to chance). Hence, *confidence limits* should also be given that indicate the probability (e.g., 95% or 99% probability) of the "true" RR being within these limits. If the lower confidence limit is greater than 1, statistically the RR is significantly greater than 1.

The difference between two rates, the rate difference (RD), can be computed if the rate of the reference group is subtracted from that of the exosed group, i.e.,

$$RD = R - R_r$$

The RR and the RD are discussed further in Section 4 in conjunction with different study designs.

ADJUSTED MEASURES.—The morbidity measures that have been discussed are dependent to a great extent on some basic characteristics of the population(s) being studied, e.g., the age and sex distributions. *Crude rates* are computed irrespective of the properties of the population. They are obtained simply by dividing the number of prevalent or incident cases by the size of the population. *Crude rate ratios* and *rate differences* are computed in a similar manner. A meaningful comparison of crude rates presupposes that the populations concerned have a similar distribution of basic characteristics such as age, sex, geographic area, etc.

If the basic characteristics are not similar, the rates must be *adjusted*. An adjusted rate can be obtained if the age, sex, etc. distributions of the population under study are changed artificially to correspond with those of some other population. For example, the age distribution of the reference category can be weighted so as to correspond to that of the exposed group, or vice versa.

Standardization is a method by which the rates of two or more populations are adjusted to correspond with a common distribution—the standard. The most well-known standardized measure is the *Standardized Mortality Ratio*, the SMR. This measure often is used when the mortality of an "exposed" group is compared to "expected values" derived from the general population. The expected values are obtained from the actual mortality rates of the general population, but its age structure is adjusted to correspond with that of the exposed group. Consequently, the actual rates in each age category become weighted so as to describe the mortality of a hypothetic general population with the *same age structure* as that of the exposed group.

Because this procedure has to be accomplished separately for each exposed group with its age distribution as the standard, two or more SMRs cannot be directly compared. They are not, in fact, mutually standardized, since the expected figures in each case depend on the age structure of the exposed group in question.[21,30]

The SMR, obtained by dividing observed rates with the expected ones, customarily is multiplied by 100. Hence, an SMR greater than 100 denotes increased risk in the exposed group. SMRs of less than 100 are more difficult to interpret because of a number of factors leading to a better-than-expected mortality experience in occupationally active populations. This so-called healthy worker effect is discussed in Section 7.

Precurrence Period

There often is a silent, asymptomatic period between the onset of exposure and the manifestation of disease. Miettinen[23] calls it the *precurrence period* whereas others have named it the *induction period* or *latency period*. These terms are not exact synonyms, however. Precurrence period is a general term for the waiting time until illness occurs whereas the latency period is defined as the time from the first *exposure* to the appearance of clinical disease. The induction period, on the other hand, stands for the time between the *initiation* of, for example, cancer to the appearance of the disease. Hence, latency time is the sum of the preinduction period and the induction period.

The precurrence period should be taken into account, if known, in the computation of person-years at risk. If its exact length is not known, one or two periods of tentative duration may be tried. In practice, then, the person-years during the precurrence period are not accounted for; i.e., the person in question is not yet "at risk" because not enough time has passed for him to incur the illness. For example, if a worker was employed as an insulator (exposed to asbestos) in 1940, and if the mean latency period is 20 years, the computation of person-years should not start earlier than 1950, which represents half that time. By 1978, he will have accrued 28 person-years instead of 38. The effect of this technique is that the expected figure becomes smaller (fewer cases are expected to occur in 28 years than in 38). Of course, the observed figure also becomes smaller, but if there is indeed an occupational factor causing cancer, the effect on that figure is not so marked, since the "occupational" cases will appear after the end of the latency period.

It should be stressed that allowing for a latency period does *not* bring about an artificial "manipulation" of the data, since this concept is based on a true biologic phenomenon (see also the example under retrospective follow-up studies in Section 4, reference 26).

Risk Indicators

During the precurrence period, the risk of contracting a particular disease sometimes can be evaluated with the aid of certain *risk indicators* (or risk factors) known to be associated with the disease. A noncausal risk indicator is associated with the disease without having any etiologic impact (e.g., use of antihypertensive drugs is associated with the occurrence of stroke) whereas a causal risk indicator is a true determinant of it (e.g., blood pressure is a determinant of stroke). A determinant thus is some characteristic that is believed to cause—alone or together with other characteristics—the disease in question.

3. SOURCES OF INFORMATION

Many countries, among them the Nordic ones, have excellent central and local registers that greatly facilitate the obtaining of data for epidemiologic research, but many other countries are not so privileged. The registers can, broadly speaking, be classified into *vital records* and *exposure registers*.

Vital Records

Vital records, the two main types of which are death and morbidity registers, are essential for epidemiologic research. Yet, their shortcomings must be realized. Death registration is more or less complete in the United States, Canada, Europe and Japan, but this is certainly not the case in many other parts of the world. As a rule, death registers are central, national ones, but local registers also exist, e.g., parish registers. Morbidity registers may also be national, e.g., the National Health Care registers and cancer registers of the Nordic countries, or local. For example, coronary registers exist in several counties and cities around the world.

Although the fact of death can be accepted as a certainty, the registered cause is less reliable. The reliability of death registers is to some extent related to the frequency of autopsies in a country—but not always, because a death certificate may be completed before the autopsy and not amended to include later findings.[15] Furthermore, different diseases are recorded in different proportions. For example, cancer usually appears in a high proportion of death certificates whereas other diseases, such as diabetes, hypertension and pneumonia, are not recorded to the same extent even if present at the time of death.[15] Multiple causes of death further confuse the picture. Although two or more diagnoses appear on more than half of the death certificates listed in most registers, only one usually is taken into account in mortality statistics.

The use of death statistics in the study of causal relations between disease and occupation is also hampered by the fact that the occupation almost invariably is deficiently noted on the certificate. There are two main reasons. First, no satisfactory system for coding occupations for investigative purposes exists. Second, the recorded occupation seldom yields relevant information about the entire exposure history of a person. Most workers have been employed in several jobs during their lifetime, and their last employment often is without any significance with respect to possible occupational risks. Therefore, crude death registers alone are of little or no value for the establishment of causal connections between occupation and disease. Morbidity statistics are even less useful for this purpose because of diagnostic uncertainties and reporting defects, and therefore they are useless as such for the study of causal connections.

Vital statistics are useful in other ways, however. First, they are the basis for the computation of expected figures. Second, they provide relevant data once the population group or disease under study has been defined from other sources. For example, it is possible to form a cohort fulfilling certain exposure or other criteria from, say, a paper mill and then to note the number and causes of death from the register during a follow-up period. From population or Social Security registers it is also possible in many countries to trace subjects who have "disappeared" or at least check whether they are dead or alive or have emigrated. For example, in a case-referent study, one may select from the cancer register all those who have died of a certain form of neoplasm during a given period of time, whereafter exposure data can be obtained from relatives and employers.

Exposure Registers

If an exposure is broadly defined, exposure registers include employee rolls, registers of occupational groups (e.g., physicians, dentists, divers, bricklayers), military records, etc. In some countries, sales and customs records are kept on toxic compounds. Moreover, by January of 1978, the ILO*

*International Labor Organization.

convention concerning prevention and control of occupational hazards caused by carcinogens had been ratified by the German Federal Republic, Finland, Hungary, Sweden, Switzerland and Yugoslavia. These countries have thereby committed themselves to set up registers of workers exposed to carcinogens. Registers of this type may aid the defining of exposed groups, and they may help locate scattered and rare exposures. But their quality will vary from case to case and from country to country—and, accordingly, their usefulness. Therefore, one must become familiar with such registers before starting a survey.

In epidemiologic studies on occupational medicine, *population registers* are mainly used merely for tracing persons who have "disappeared" during a follow-up. The situation is somewhat different in public health research, which utilizes such registers for several other purposes.

Linkage

The easy availability of computers has raised a specific problem: namely, that of linking vital records with exposure registers. In principle, this procedure is a good one. But the quality control of large amounts of data always is more difficult than that of more limited amounts, and no register can be more reliable than the data fed into it. Furthermore, since register data usually are compiled for some purpose other than the actual study, they do not take into account the special needs of the latter. Many of the inaccuracies may be unsystematic. Hence, they do not lead to false positive conclusions but may mask true positive findings. On the other hand, many systematic errors may be involved, such as regional overreporting of some disease, different nomenclature for cause of illness or of occupations and over classification or underclassification of workers exposed to, say, carcinogens. Since statistically significant p values are yielded from small differences in large series, such flaws may result in grossly erroneous conclusions if record linkage is (mis)used uncritically. Finally, in practice, the utilization of linkage usually becomes expensive due to the vast amount of irrelevant data it produces (with respect to a particular problem). All these circumstances greatly impair the reliability of crude register data, and mechanical linkage of registers exposes the uncritical user to the danger of drawing too far-going or completely erroneous conclusions. Hence, even a small, well-planned and controlled ad hoc study is preferable to the linkage of large registers. This is a well-known fact among experienced epidemiologists, but it is hard to comprehend for those less familiar with scientific epidemiologic research.

Privacy

The increasing public demand for privacy is a problem that is progressively restricting the use of registers, especially vital records, in research work. In some countries—for example, Sweden—legislation already prohibits registries from delivering individual data to "outsiders," among them research workers. Of course, personal integrity must be protected, but regulations that are too strict make the use of registers impossible for research purposes.

Ad Hoc Registers

If there are no useful basic registers, which unfortunately often is the case, information regarding the study population must be found in another way. The first task then is to define the problem in terms of the quality, minimal duration and intensity of exposure, the age, sex and geographic area of the exposed population, etc. Subsequently, employee rolls form the basis for an ad hoc register of all persons complying with the established criteria. After examining the size of the exposed population and the nature of the problem, the researcher may either select a suitable group from his compiled register or include all persons in the study. Of course, no register can be established if employee rolls are lacking or insufficient. In such a situation, the study cannot utilize retrospective data, and the only option becomes a prospective follow-up.

Similarly, in case-referent studies, autopsy records, hospital records and industrial health service registers can be used in the absence of basic morbidity registers. However, the use of such sources exposes the investigator to several possible uncertainties—for example, doubt about representativeness of the cases, the accuracy of the diagnoses, etc.

Measures of Exposure

Measures of any particular exposure include quality, intensity, duration, fluctuations and other concomitant exposures. All these data usually can be obtained during a survey. But they rarely are available retrospectively or, when available, they can be highly defective. In addition, data obtained during an investigation seldom can be used as such a basis for estimating past exposure. When faced with the problem of defective retrospective exposure data, the investigator has two options; namely, that of giving up the whole study or making the best of the situation. The latter alternative often is preferable, but the uncertainties must be understood. When comparison of current and past conditions is the method chosen, old workers, foremen and safety personnel can be interviewed for their opinions as to how much conditions have changed. In addition, the time of major improvements, such as the installation of exhaust ventilation, usually is listed in company records. The result will be a coarse classification into, for example, heavy, medium, light and no exposure, but this procedure often is quite enough for cause-effect inferences, although many times insufficient for exposure-response ones (see the example given under case-referent studies, reference 2). A time factor also can be combined with the intensity dimension. Simulation of past conditions is a more accurate method, but for practical reasons rarely is possible.

Measures of Effect

Some occupational diseases are characterized by typical symptoms and signs. For example, lead causes certain well-defined disturbances of the heme synthesis, measurable, for example, as increased excretion of delta-aminolevulinic acid and coproporphyrin in the urine. Asbestos exposure causes typical radiologic findings, characterized by fibrosis and pleural calcifications, aromatic amines cause methemoglobinemia and organophosphorus pesticides inhibit the activities of serum and erythrocyte cholinesterase. On the other hand, symptoms and signs that are by no means "typical" belong to the picture of many occupational diseases. Several organic solvents, for example, cause nonspecific neurologic disorders, i.e., peripheral neuropathy and central nervous system damage, brought about by many other causes also, such as systemic diseases, infections, nutritional deficiencies, medicines and alcohol abuse. Moreover, occupational carcinogens cause cancers that usually do not differ from cancers with other origins. In addition, some exposures, such as to carbon disulfide, arsenic and nitroglycol, increase the occurrence of coronary artery disease, but individual patients are indistinguishable from "natural" cases of that disease.

The measures of effects belonging to the first category can be termed *specific* measures and those belonging to the second are *nonspecific*. In etiologic research, specific measures are not as useful in cause-effect inferences, the causal connection already being known. Instead, they provide a fuller picture of what happens at different intensities of exposure; i.e., they aid in the search for exposure-effect and exposure-response relationships.

On the other hand, nonspecific effects, such as changes in "natural" mortality and morbidity, are important in the search for causal connections. In addition, they can be used in exposure-response-oriented research as well. Etiologic epidemiology is predominantly occupied with nonspecific effects.

As indicators of morbidity, an investigator may use either mortality or morbidity statistics, Social Security benefit registers, long sickness absences (but rarely short ones, since they may reflect causes other than illness), objective measurements of different manifestations of disease and subjective opinions expressed by the workers themselves. In this context, the terms "hard" and "soft" parameters often are used, death being the hardest and subjective opinions the softest.

When selecting parameters for a study, a researcher always should consider the optimal "hardness." In general, the harder the parameter the more reliable the information. As mentioned before, the event of death is subject to no ambiguity, but the cause of death already is less reliable. The softer the parameter the greater the possibility for error. Questionnaires, for instance, may give highly misleading data, and their use requires careful standardization of the method and critical interpretation of the results. Yet, it does not necessarily follow that hard parameters always should be preferred. Death is such a crude measure that mortality statistics can reveal only the most severe health hazards. In addition, quite a few ailments, such as disorders of the musculoskeletal system, mental disease and eczema, do not appear in mortality statistics at all, and when milder health effects, such as fatigue, headache, nervousness, irritation symptoms, etc., are being studied, no better methods than interviews or questionnaires are available for their evaluation. Thus, the ideal hardness of a parameter depends on the problem in question, i.e., on the anticipated effect of exposure. Sometimes the ideal is the simultaneous use of several parameters differing in hardness.

4. DIFFERENT STUDY TYPES AND THEIR APPLICATIONS IN OCCUPATIONAL HEALTH RESEARCH

Epidemiologic studies are either cross-sectional or longitudinal. In a cross-sectional study, the observation of both the cause and the effect relates to a single point in time whereas in longitudinal studies their measurement is separated by a time interval, even though the collection of data may take place simultaneously.

Cross-sectional studies are prevalence studies, often "descriptive," and their main use is in health administration (e.g., the prevalence of diabetics needing regular control, say, among plant personnel). Etiologic research, on the other hand, usually requires a longitudinal study design, although a cross-sectional approach often may be tempting because of its relative simplicity and low cost. The latter is useful in etiologic research in very few situations; namely, when the effect is immediately time-related to the exposure (e.g., acute effects of irritant gases) or when exposure is relatively permanent in relation to the effect (e.g., steady lead exposure and neurophysiologic abnormalities) or when the effect is of long duration and its selective force is negligible (e.g., the prevalence of noise-induced hearing loss in various types of work). In most other instances longitudinal studies provide the only possible nonexperimental way of deriving cause-effect inferences.

Since training in epidemiologic methods often has been rather diffuse among practitioners of occupational health, a brief presentation of the different epidemiologic study designs may be appropriate. It is hoped that it will supplement the discussion of their uses (and misuses) in occupational health research, which appears later.

Epidemiologic Study Designs—Basic Features

Cross-sectional studies measure the case (exposure) and the effect at the same point in time. There are two types. The first compares the rates of diseases or symptoms of an exposed and a nonexposed group; for example, the frequency of symptoms of bronchial irritation among pulp workers exposed to chlorine and among nonexposed referents. The second type compares differences in exposure rates between persons with and without disease. Now, the question becomes whether or not pulp workers are overrepresented among patients complaining of bronchial irritation as compared with other patients. In occupational health research, the former type is more common, since workers generally are viewed in categories of occupation and exposure or both, rather than being classified according to disease, as in clinical medicine. Yet, in both instances, a cross-sectional study always estimates the prevalence of a disease or an exposure at the time of the investigation.

Purely descriptive cross-sectional surveys, made for health administrative purposes, do not require measurements of exposure (e.g., mere estimation of the prevalence of diabetes in a group of employees). However, as soon as etiologic aspects become involved, some measure of the exposure suspected to be causative of the disease—even if it is as broad as the district of habitation—must be included. Since, by definition, the exposure status is considered at the time the effects are measured, there must be a biologic rationale before a temporal relation between the two measures can be assumed. In other words, unless the current exposure intensity or, alternatively, past exposure *as reflected by* the current level theoretically could be responsible for the effects under scrutiny, the relationship is meaningless. For example, the prevalence of silicosis in a foundry has little to do with current dust concentrations. But current exposure to lead, measured from the lead concentration in blood or urine, can easily be related to the current urinary excretion of delta-aminolevulinic acid; hence, a cross-sectional study of the interrelationship between these parameters is valid. Similarly, provided that no major changes in exposure have taken place over the years, but only then, the current concentration of lead in blood can be (etiologically) related to a slowing of conduction velocities in peripheral nerves. If variations in the intensity of exposure have occurred, some other parameter, e.g., the time-weighted average concentration of lead in blood, is more representative, and a purely cross-sectional design is invalid.

Longitudinal studies are divided into *follow-up studies, case-referent studies* and *intervention studies*. In a *follow-up study* (synonyms: cohort study, prospective study), the groups under scrutiny—the exposed and nonexposed cohorts—are defined on the basis of exposure status. In this sense, the situation is the same as in an experiment, where the investigator randomly exposes animals or leaves them unexposed. The basic distinction is that the epidemiologist, unlike the experimentalist, cannot *decide* to which category he or she will allocate the persons; the decisions already have been made, e.g., when the workers were hired.

When selected into the exposed cohort, the subject must fulfill certain criteria, set up in advance (e.g., with respect to age, sex, minimal exposure). Then the cohort is followed over a period of time, or its members are traced at the end of the period, and all new cases (= incidence) of the disease(s) under study are recorded. The morbidity rate of the exposed cohort may be contrasted to "expected" figures computed from the experience of the general population and adjusted for age, sex and calendar time. Preferably, the incidence is compared to that of a nonexposed cohort that is similar in as many relevant ways as possible except for the exposure (Fig 1–1). Because the cohorts are formed on the basis of exposure or its absence, only one exposure can be considered at a time. On the other hand, this de-

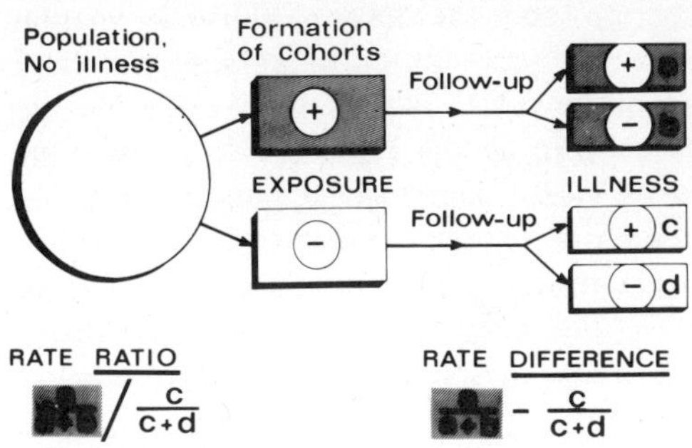

Fig 1–1.—General outline of a follow-up study.

sign permits the study of several different diseases simultaneously.

Traditionally, a *fixed* cohort design is preferred. In this setting, all those who enter the cohort, when formed, must be traced irrespective of the exposure status at the end of the follow-up, and their health state must be recorded. Strictly speaking, no new members should enter the cohort during the follow-up, but, in practice, this constraint seldom is rigidly obeyed, at least not in retrospective follow-up studies. In contrast, a *dynamic* population accepts new entries throughout the investigation, and those who drop out are not accounted for and, accordingly, need not be traced. Unfortunately, this effort-saving design rarely can be utilized in occupational health research because of turnover due to health selection. However, in public health studies, a dynamic population design often is appropriate.

A follow-up study may be *retrospective* (historical) or *prospective* (concurrent). In both cases, the scientific logic is the same, the principal differences being timing and methodology. In a retrospective follow-up study, the cohorts are defined at a suitable point in time in the past, e.g., 20–30 years earlier. The members then are *traced* over time, usually to the present (or, for practical reasons, to 1 or 2 years before the present—for example, to ensure accumulation of pertinent morbidity data in the registers). Retrospective follow-up studies usually focus on mortality, since other reliable retrospective data seldom are available. Prospective follow-up cohorts are defined in the present and *followed* for a number of years. This design permits the recording of a variety of morbidity data, not only deaths.

As explained in Section 2, the various measures of disease occurrence are computed as rates, i.e., the proportion of diseased in the exposed and nonexposed cohorts (Table 1–1). When two rates are compared, the rate ratio (risk ratio, relative risk, RR) is computed in the following way (for symbols, see Table 1–1):

TABLE 1–1.—GENERAL OUTLINE FOR DATA FROM FOLLOW-UP STUDIES

	DISEASE PRESENT	DISEASE ABSENT	TOTAL
Exposed	a	b	a + b
Nonexposed	c	d	c + d
TOTAL	a + c	b + d	N = a + b + c + d

$$RR = a/(a + b)/c/(c + d)$$

An RR of 1 denotes no observed difference between the cohorts. If it is greater, there is more disease and, if lower, less disease in the exposed cohort. When no referent cohort is available (e.g., for economic reasons), the over-all and cause-specific mortality (rarely morbidity) experiences of the exposed cohort can be contrasted with those of the general population, adjusted for age, sex and calendar time. In this case, the rate ratio is called the standardized mortality ratio, or the SMR. An SMR in excess of 100% denotes an increased risk in the exposed cohort and one below 100% a decreased risk (but note the discussion of "healthy worker effect" in Section 7).

Whereas the RR gives a proportional estimate of the risk, the *rate or risk difference* (RD) yields an absolute measure of it. The RD is computed as follows:

$$RD = a/(a + b) - c/(c + d)$$

Figure 1–2 shows the difference in the in-

	"COMMON"		"RARE"	
	Obs.	Exp.	Obs.	Exp.
INCIDENCE DENSITY (cases / 10,000 person-years)	150	100	2	0.01
RATE RATIO	150/100 = 1.5		2/0.01 = 200	
RATE DIFFERENCE	150 - 100 = 50		2 - 0.01 = 1.99	

Fig 1–2.—Computation of rate ratio and rate difference from a follow-up study. Comparison between these measures in the case of a "common" and a "rare" disease.

formation obtained with the RR and the RD. The former is a measure of the *strength* of the association, i.e., the biologic effect, the latter of the severity of the problem in terms of *number* of excess cases. Self-evidently, all comparisons between the exposed cohort and the reference population should be subjected to statistical testing, but, as is discussed later (see Section 6), scientific inferences cannot be drawn merely from p values.

Computation of person-years at risk sometimes is difficult or even impossible, for example, when personnel records are deficient or lacking. Then an increase in the *cause-specific* mortality can be shown by means of *proportional mortality* figures indicating what proportions of all deaths are due to the particular causes. These percentages then can be contrasted with the "expected" ones, obtained from national figures. However, this procedure yields less reliable results than those obtained from absolute figures, since an excess of or a defect in the other causes of death changes the proportion attributable to the cause in question. For example, the proportion of violent deaths is greater than the average among blue-collar workers and results in a correspondingly lower proportion of natural causes. This bias can be avoided if the distribution of natural causes of death is studied separately.

Proportional mortality data, despite a more difficult interpretation, often offer the first clue of an occupational factor that increases the cause-specific mortality of some disease. For example, in 1967, our research team found that 52% of the workers in a viscose rayon factory had died of coronary artery disease, the expected mortality figure being only 32%.[8] Subsequently, a follow-up study revealed 14 coronary deaths between 1967 and 1972 among the exposed cohort (343 men) in contrast to only 3 corresponding deaths in an equal-sized matched reference cohort selected from local paper mill workers. The RR of 4.7 was statistically significant.[33]

In *case-referent studies* (synonyms: case-control study, case-history study, retrospective study), the groups are defined on the basis of *disease* (cases) or its *absence* (referents). In a density-type case-referent study, the cases, which are collected during a certain period of time, are compared in regard to past exposure(s) with referents drawn from a suitable population (Fig 1–3).

The referents often are matched to the cases with respect to some important parameters (see Section 5). For each case, 1 or more referents can be used; their number depends on how easily available they are. However, more than 4 referents for each case increases only slightly the statistical efficiency of the study.[19] Similarly, for unmatched series, a balanced design (i.e., equal-sized groups) is optimal.

A general outline for data from a case-referent study is shown in Table 1–2. Similar tables can be constructed for each exposure studied.

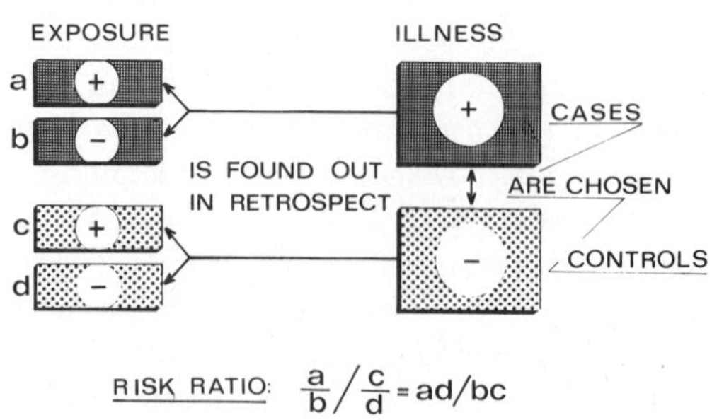

Fig 1–3.—General outline of a case-referent study.

TABLE 1–2.—GENERAL OUTLINE FOR DATA FROM CASE-REFERENT STUDIES (UNMATCHED SERIES)

	EXPOSURE PRESENT	EXPOSURE ABSENT	TOTAL
Cases	a	b	a + b
Referents	c	d	c + d
TOTAL	a + c	b + d	N = a + b + c + d

Since the study groups are defined on the basis of presence or absence of a given disease, only one disease can be studied at a time. In contrast, many exposures can be studied simultaneously (cf. follow-up studies, where the circumstances are reversed). Exposure data in a case-referent study usually are collected by means of interviews and questionnaires. The methodologic problems involved are discussed in Section 5.

Most, if not all, textbooks on epidemiology state that the RR (for the disease, not the exposure) cannot be computed in case-referent studies unless the disease is "rare." However, Miettinen[24] recently proved this assumption to be erroneous insofar as density-type studies are concerned. According to him, the RR can be computed as follows without any rare disease assumption (for explanation of symbols, see Table 1–2):

$$RR = (a/b) / (c/d) = ad/bc$$

In some instances it may be feasible to combine a follow-up and a case-referent approach; i.e., to "nest" a case-referent study in a cohort. This approach is discussed later.

The *intervention study* comes rather close to being an experiment, and the term "experimental epidemiology" often is used as a synonym. It resembles an experimental study in that the investigator actively manipulates the conditions—for example, by lowering the exposure level or by removing workers from exposure. But it differs from an experiment in that randomization rarely, if ever, is possible.

An intervention study can well be performed with a small group of workers, such as when changes in morbidity are observed after exposure to some toxic substance has been lowered. Large-scale projects are also feasible. For example, a study of the effects of changing the diet, smoking habits, etc. on coronary morbidity has involved a whole county, i.e., Northern Carelia in eastern Finland in the mid-1970s.[35]

In an intervention study, changes in morbidity can be compared both with the situation in the same population before the intervention and with that of a similar group not subjected to intervention. It should be repeated in this context that positive results strongly argue in favor of a causal connection between exposure and effects.

Study Designs in Occupational Health Research—Options, Advantages and Limitations

No single study type is, in principle, superior to all others. Yet, longitudinal designs are to be preferred in etiologic research. The choice of the approach depends on several factors, and quite often the same, scientifically "true" result can be obtained in different ways.

Since the limitations of cross-sectional studies already have been discussed and since longitudinal studies are by far the most important sources of epidemiologic knowledge in occupational medicine, only longitudinal designs are reviewed here.

PROSPECTIVE OR RETROSPECTIVE TIMING? The fact that *timing* and *design* differ conceptually may be difficult to understand, but the distinction must be kept clear. Prospective follow-up studies always—and intervention studies usually—are timed prospectively; i.e., they start at the present and move forward. In contrast, both retrospective follow-up studies and case-referent studies are timed retrospectively; i.e., they deal with past events. Even so, the *design* of a retrospective follow-up study is prospective whereas a case-referent study is retrospective in this regard also.

Retrospective studies offer the advantage

that the results become available rather quickly, usually within a few years. In a retrospective follow-up study, the starting point of which lies in the past, the cases, in fact, already have occurred. The problem is to trace and find the cohort members, both the exposed and nonexposed, rather than to wait for the development of disease. Also, in a case-referent study, the cases already are at hand. Still, a disadvantage of retrospective timing is that past exposure data usually are scanty, unreliable or even nonexistent. The same usually is true for data on other risk indicators, such as blood chemistry and blood pressure. Another restraint is that a retrospective follow-up study must be confined to hard indicators of disease, usually death, since data on softer indicators rarely are available or, if recorded, often are unreliable. This limitation does not concern a case-referent study, however, which can well be based on morbidity, provided that the diagnostic criteria are valid (see Section 3).

The following example illustrates typical features of a retrospective follow-up study. Ott and his co-workers[26] were interested in whether or not occupational exposure to benzene results in excess mortality, especially from leukemia. To study this problem, they designed a retrospective follow-up study of the mortality of employees who had been employed in three different plants and exposed to benzene.

In this investigation, the fact that only mortality data could be used probably did not distort the results because of the severe prognosis of leukemia. But had the problem been one of, for example, colonic cancer with a curability of about 35%, the observed differences in mortality figures could have been affected by systematic differences in early diagnosis and treatment, not necessarily by an occupational factor.

The investigators identified the exposed workers from annual census lists for 1938–1970. (Such a procedure usually is possible, however, only in large companies with well-kept records.) They abstracted job histories from personnel records, coded them according to a standardized system and assigned 1 month as the minimal exposure time for entry into the cohort. This, of course, was an arbitrary decision. Stricter criteria would have resulted in loss of material, but, on the other hand, also in an accentuation of the risk.

Because of job mobility within the units, most employees had been exposed at more than one intensity. Some workers also had been exposed to other chemicals. Both of these circumstances are typical for epidemiologic studies in occupational medicine, irrespective of study type, and they are discussed in another context in Section 7.

Measurements of exposure levels had been performed in the past, but, since they were occasional, extrapolations had to be made for a rough classification of the average exposure intensity. Assessment of exposure is difficult, especially in retrospective studies, and Ott and his collaborators were fortunate to have accessibility to better than average data.

The mortality analysis covered those hired between 1940 and 1974. In this respect, a usual—and sometimes practical—deviation from the strictly fixed cohort design was made; namely, they accepted entries until the end of 1973. However, in this case, a dilution of the possible effect arose from the liberal admissibility criteria, since a latent period is involved in the development of environmental cancers. Although the exact length of the latency time is not known, some allowance should be made for it. New entries should not be accepted and person-years for earlier entries should not be calculated during the latency period. Whenever the length of the latency time is not known for certain, the results can be computed with the use of two or more different tentative latencies. In this case (based on experiences from radiation-induced leukemia), 5 and 10 years could have been tried. But Ott and his collaborators did not publish such data for leukemia, although they gave results for some major disease groups, analyzed in subcategories of different intervals since the beginning of exposure.

Through the Social Security Administration, the authors traced those who had left the company; they estimated the results to be 94% successful. The difficulty in tracing resigned and retired employees varies from one country to another, but the aim should be a success of at least 95%.

The expected number of deaths was calculated indirectly from U.S. white male mortality statistics for 7 representative years between 1940 and 1970, and the SMRs were computed from the obtained figures. The over-all mortality of the exposed cohort showed no excess, but 3 fatal cases of leukemia were found against the 0.8 expected. Statistically, the difference was almost significant ($p < 0.047$), but the expected figure would have been considerably lower had a latency time been allowed for when the person-years were calculated and had the minimal exposure criteria been stricter (e.g., at least 1 year). Hence, a very conservative estimate was obtained.

Prospective studies offer the following advantages: (a) the study can be better designed to meet the investigator's requirements, (b) exposure data can be systematically collected, (c) several indicators of the disease can be measured, (d) the measurements can be repeated over time if needed, (e) the methodology can be standardized and its validity checked and, finally, (f) an intervention can be combined with the follow-up. The main inconvenience of prospective timing is the long period sometimes required before the results are at hand. In the study of chronic diseases, such as occupational cancer, this period may be 20–40 years.

High expenses often are said to be an obstacle to prospective follow-up studies, but this is not strictly true in terms of *cost per amount of information*. Because a prospective follow-up, in contrast to a retrospective one, allows the collection of a variety of both exposure and morbidity data, the absolute costs will, of course, be higher. But since much more information is gained, the costs in relative terms do not necessarily differ considerably. The key to cost reduction in this respect is to confine the collection of data to the most relevant items. This comparison relates to follow-up studies only; case-referent studies usually are less expensive.

Prospective follow-up studies are rather rare in the literature on occupational medicine, and therefore pedagogically suitable examples are difficult to find. The following study was chosen to illustrate the difference as markedly as possible between this type of study and a retrospective mortality study (a prospective mortality study would be rather similar); it furthermore demonstrates that prospective studies can indeed be both quick and simple.

Tola and his co-workers[31] were interested in the time sequence of the appearance of lead-induced hematologic abnormalities. They studied 33 lead workers who had no prior occupational exposure to toxic agents. Freedom from disease at entry (in this case lead-induced disease) was ascertained in a pre-employment examination. The following parameters were measured: blood and urinary lead, hemoglobin, hematocrit, erythrocyte delta-aminolevulinic acid (ALA), dehydratase activity and urinary ALA and coproporphyrin. The methods were strictly standardized and continually controlled. The original study plan involved starting the sampling before the beginning of exposure (day 0). Subsequent samples then would be taken on the second, fourth and sixth days of exposure, followed by weekly samplings until the end of the third month, and two additional samplings at 2-week intervals during the fourth month.

In this study, some of the benefits of a prospective design become evident, namely repeated measurements, inclusion of several parameters of disease, precise exposure data (repeated blood and urinary lead concentrations) and method control. Yet, some practical difficulties arose. First, the planned sampling scheme could not be followed rigorously because of weekends, sick leaves and public holidays. Second, dropouts reduced the cohort so that only 18 persons remained in the study for more than 70 days. In 2 cases, the blood lead level rapidly increased above the recommended value, and the exposure had to be interrupted.

Subjects dropping out before the minimal exposure criteria are met probably is the most difficult complication of a prospective follow-up because it causes waste of time and money. Later dropouts are not a loss in the same sense, but tracing them is necessary and may be costly. The other problem illustrated by this example is an ethical one. The investigator must not allow his examinees to be dangerously exposed; hence, there may arise a conflict between ethical and study-efficiency aspects.

The results of this study showed that depression of ALA dehydratase occurred without a time lag whereas the increase of ALA and coproporphyrin excretion in urine had a latency period of some 2–3 weeks. The ALA and coproporphyrin values concomitant to the blood lead values corresponded well with those found in cross-sectional studies. The establishment of the time sequence for these effects was the major benefit obtained by the prospective design utilized.

The major inconvenience of a prospective follow-up study, namely, a long waiting time for the results, was no problem in this example because a rather quick phenomenon was studied. But whenever the problem involves a long latency period (e.g., occupational cancer), it is understandable that the investigator prefers a retrospective approach. However, it seems appropriate to advise research institutes and companies to initiate long-spanned prospective follow-up studies for future benefit by defining risk groups and by monitoring their exposure systematically. Similarly, the routine use of continual health monitoring of the personnel of a company could be effected by the standardization of test methods and "computer-minded" record keeping. These procedures would help overcome many of the difficulties faced today in the study of diseases with long latency times.

FOLLOW-UP OR CASE-REFERENT DESIGN? Problems related to timing may also affect the decision of whether to use a follow-up or case-referent study, but they will not be discussed further. Instead, questions pertinent to options between different types of *designs* will be dealt with. First of all, both a follow-up and a case-referent design often are equally valid in solving a problem, and feasibility aspects determine the choice. For example, the first evidence in favor of the causal connection between cigarette smoking and bronchial cancer came from case-referent studies. Later, the same conclusion was reached in numerous follow-up studies, and still later it was confirmed by intervention studies.

One of the major differences between the two options is that in a follow-up study only one exposure but several diseases can be studied at the same time whereas in a case-referent study only one disease but several exposures can be investigated. Therefore, the latter is more suitable when the hypothesis as to the etiologies of a disease is weak or nonexistent and when one wishes a simultaneous comparison of etiologic fractions for several exposures. For example, in a case-referent study on bladder cancer, the effect of various chemical exposures, cigarette smoking and the use of medicines can be evaluated simultaneously. But if one would, say, suspect vinyl chloride to cause not only angiosarcoma of the liver but also a variety of other malignant tumors, a follow-up study would be the method of choice.

Another distinction is that a case-referent

study is the only sensible one when the *disease* is rare whereas follow-up studies must be preferred when *exposure* is rare. (Otherwise, enormous amounts of material would be required.) However, the reverse is *not* necessarily true, i.e., that case-referent studies would be unsuitable for common diseases and follow-up studies for common exposures. The major advantage of a case-referent study over a follow-up is its relative simplicity and its low costs. In a follow-up, most cohort members do not incur the disease in question, but, despite that, they must be followed or traced and their exposure history must be recorded. For example, Ott and his co-workers[26] traced and followed 594 workers, of whom only 3 died from leukemia. Yet, the occupational history had to be recorded for everybody, although 591 of the workers provided data only for the person-year calculations (insofar as leukemia was concerned) needed for the computation of the "expected" value, which turned out to be 0.8. But suppose a hypothetical case-referent study revealed that of 100 patients with leukemia 11 had had some contact with benzene (in this plant and elsewhere) but only 3 of 100 referents. Then approximately the same rate ratio (3.75 vs 4.0) could be obtained with considerably less effort. In this case, detailed exposure histories would have been required from 14 patients only and less-detailed histories from another 186 (less-detailed because many of them would have had no industrial exposure whatsoever). The crucial questions now, of course, are whether these histories would have been available outside the plant actually studied by Ott and co-workers and whether the 3 cases in a case-referent approach would have been included in the sample of 100, the exposure to benzene being rare in the general population. On consideration, the follow-up approach chosen in this case seems to be the best solution despite the effort involved.

A good example of a multiple case-referent study was published recently by Axelson and his colleagues.[2] The authors investigated the connection between exposure to arsenic and lung cancer in a large Swedish copper smelter and, using separate series of cases, also some other diseases. Both the cases and the referents were drawn from the register of deaths and burials in the local parish. The cases pertinent to this example had died from malignant lung tumors (the other diseases were "other cancers" and cardiovascular diseases) and the referents were all those subjects who had died of any of the remaining causes. One of the problems in this study was that, since arsenic may also cause several other diseases, liberal admission criteria for the referents would dilute the results. The investigators overcame this difficulty by having separate series of cases for all these diseases and by using the remaining diagnoses for the referent group. As always in retrospective studies, the assessment of exposure was a problem. The authors requested an experienced safety engineer to classify the probable exposure intensity into three categories: (a) one considerably below the previous threshold limit value of 0.5 mg/m^3, (b) one close to it and (c) one exceeding it (see Section 3). Unlike Ott and his colleagues,[26] the Swedish authors allowed for a latency period for the development of lung cancer. They applied a median latency period of 34–36 years, and in the exposure classifications only exposures occurring before half the median latency period, i.e., 17 years, were considered. In short, a 4.6-fold increase was observed in the mortality from lung cancer for workers employed in the smelter.

The obstacle of rare exposures can be avoided if the cases and referents are drawn from a geographic area where the particular exposure is much more common than in the country, state, county or city at large. This was exactly how Axelson and his co-workers[2] proceeded in their study.

"Nesting" a case-referent study into a cohort[23] is even more effective. In this setting, one exposed and another nonexposed cohort are formed and pooled, whereafter both the cases and the referents are selected from this pooled population. However, the nesting is effective only when the disease is common enough to yield a sufficient number of cases. In addition to the exposure now being common within the *study material,* the advantage over a "pure" design is that one can neglect the histories of all those who are neither cases nor referents, and therefore a lot of effort is saved. This idea is so new that very few studies have utilized the "nesting" technique so far.

There are several other aspects that help determine optimal study design, but, as validity aspects are involved, they are discussed in the next section.

5. PROBLEMS RELATED TO THE VALIDITY OF EPIDEMIOLOGIC STUDIES

Validity means the lack of systematic error or bias. A systematic error is one that distorts the results of a study in such a way that hypothetical replications of it would produce the same results under the same premises, so that a false conclusion is reached. There are two dimensions of validity, *internal* and *external.*[3] The former refers to how "true" the results of a study are with respect to the study itself. The latter stands for the generalizability of the results beyond time and place, i.e., to other similar situations and, finally, to the sphere of scientific theories.

Internal Validity

Miettinen[23] classifies the components of internal validity in the following manner:

1. Validity of selection.
2. Validity of information.
3. Validity of comparison.
   a) Validity of reference entity.
   b) Unconfoundedness of comparison.

VALIDITY OF SELECTION.—Validity of selection means that the probability of a subject being nominated for the study must not depend in a systematic way on the disease or exposure under study.

The effect of selection bias in *cross-sectional studies* can be illustrated by the following example. Let the problem be: Does physically strenuous work cause low-back disease? In a cross-sectional study, the groups are chosen according to current occupation. Suppose the investigator compares the prevalence of lumbar disease (using some fixed criteria) among foundry workers with that of car assembly workers. In this design, the selection is invalid because, first, workers who already have back problems, knowing that foundry work is strenuous, may prefer other types of jobs. Second, some of those who develop back trouble during foundry work may have to quit. And, third, since foundry work is heavier than car assembly, the same severity of lumbar disease may cause more sickness absence in a foundry than in a car assembly plant at the time of the survey. Then, because of selection, sick persons are underrepresented among foundry workers and the possible effect of foundry work may totally or partly escape discovery (negative bias). By contrast, the inverse effects of selection may cause overrepresentation of lumbar disease in certain light occupations (positive bias). These examples are pertinent because the knowledge of the effects of work on lumbar disease is predominantly based on prevalence studies (for a review, see reference 34). Most of them, despite the inherent negative bias, show that lumbar degeneration is associated with heavy work. Hence, the true effect must be even greater than what is revealed by cross-sectional data.

In a *case-referent study,* a selection bias may arise in the following way. Suppose that there is a hospital specializing in occupational medicine where a physician wishes to study the effects of various environmental factors, among them occupational exposures, on the occurrence of gastritis. Patients with this disease (according to preset criteria) are defined as cases, and patients with, for example, lumbar disease as referents. A surprisingly high frequency of lead exposure among the cases probably will emerge. The result is an overestimate of the role of lead exposure in the etiology of gastritis *in general* (positive bias). Of course, there is no doubt that overexposure to lead causes a gastritis-like syndrome. But workers exposed to lead and having epigastric pain are more likely to be admitted to this specialized clinic because plant physicians usually suspect lead poisoning in such a situation. In this hypothetical example, the reasons for selection bias were (a) there was a hospital specializing in occupational medicine and (b) the connection between lead exposure and epigastric pain was known in advance. Had there been no specialized hospital and had the local physicians been unaware of the connection between gastric symptoms and lead exposure, a selection bias of this kind would have been unlikely.

Selection bias seldom is a problem in *follow-up studies* in general. But in occupational medicine one of the most difficult factors is the assessment of self-selection into an occupation or trade. Its effects are insignificant for diseases with long, silent latency times, but they are important whenever symptoms of the disease under study are provoked or worsened by the work in question. For example, persons with chronic bronchitis are not attracted to jobs known to be dusty and those with previous back pain avoid physically heavy jobs. Preemployment examinations tend to strengthen this type of selection even further. However, it should be emphasized that a true selection bias arises only when the *disease under study* is responsible for the selection. If other, concomitant diseases (e.g., bronchial asthma in a study of coronary artery disease) cause "selection," the type of the bias, in fact, is negative confounding (see Section 7).

Later health-biased selection, occurring after the worker has become "exposed," can be methodologically controlled by means of tracing all those who change employment or retire and by considering them to be exposed. However, from an exposure-response point of view, such selection causes dilution and leaves those classified as having ill health with short exposure times (because the disease forces them to interrupt the exposure earlier than those not affected).

Selection bias must be avoided at the *planning stage* of a survey, since there exists no method to control it during data handling. If it cannot be completely avoided, its effects should be assessed and considered when conclusions are drawn. A slight selection bias does not invalidate a study, provided that its direction and magnitude are known. Effective handling of selection bias requires a thorough knowledge of the selective forces operating in every specific occupation, hospitalization process and the scientific problem in general.

VALIDITY OF INFORMATION.—Validity of information means that the inaccuracy of the information gathered from both the cases and the referents, or from both the exposed and the nonexposed, is similar. Inaccuracy in itself does not necessarily affect validity, provided that it is symmetric; i.e., only asymmetric inaccuracy causes bias. By contrast, the *sensitivity* (the power to detect a causal association, if present) of the study suffers from symmetrically inaccurate information. Information bias may affect all types of epidemiologic investigations, but the problem is the worst in case-referent studies.

In *case-referent studies* deriving information from questionnaires and interviews rather than from measurements, the greatest problem is how to ensure comparability between the histories obtained from the cases and the referents (or their relatives). Consider, for example, a case-referent study of congenital malformations in which the cases are mothers of malformed children and the referents are mothers of healthy babies. Data on possible deleterious exposures during pregnancy would be collected by means of interviews. Such exposures would be use of medicines, past infections, occupational exposures, radiologic examinations, traumas, etc. It is a well-known fact that mothers of malformed babies often feel guilty and brood about why such a disaster has happened. Hence, they remember and report all possible exposures in detail (provided that a feeling of guilt does not force them to hide some facts). However, mothers of healthy babies have no reason to dwell on such matters and therefore give a less detailed history. Consequently, the information causes a positive bias by being asymmetrically inaccurate. Insofar as occupational exposures are concerned, this bias can be overcome if other sources of information are utilized—namely, employers. But for some other exposures—for example, alcohol, tobacco and medicines—there is no such possibility.

Retrospective follow-up studies are also subject to information bias because there is a general tendency to observe "exposed" populations more thoroughly than "nonexposed" ones, by means of periodic health examinations, for example. By contrast, the design of a *prospective follow-up* can avoid information bias if, for example, the investigator is "blinded" and a similar quality of data is obtained from both the exposed and the nonexposed cohorts. Special care should be taken to ensure a minimal loss of subjects from follow-up, since lost (unknown) information may be asymmetric and hence affect validity even more than inaccurate information.

The requirement of information validity sometimes determines the study design. For example, if it is judged that unbiased retrospective exposure data cannot be obtained by means of interviews in a case-referent design, the remaining option is a prospective follow-up study.

VALIDITY OF COMPARISON.—As already mentioned, the validity of comparison has two components: validity of the reference group and unconfoundedness of comparison.

The *validity of the reference entity* must be ensured irrespective of study type. An ideal reference group should share all characteristics of the study group relevant to the problem at issue, save for the property that defines the groups, namely, the exposure in a follow-up study and the disease in a case-referent study. If this goal cannot be completely achieved, emphasis should be put on those factors that most affect the particular problem under study in the light of prior knowledge. For example, in the aforementioned study on the effect of exposure to carbon disulfide on the occurrence of coronary artery disease,[8, 33] the exposed cohort was formed from workers in a viscose rayon plant and the reference cohort from paper mill workers. The assumption was that the two types of occupations had the same effect on the occurrence of coronary artery disease apart from the effect of carbon disulfide. Next, comparability had to be ensured with regard to as many known risk factors of coronary artery disease as possible. Table 1–3 summarizes the procedure followed.

The groups were intentionally not equalized with respect to blood lipids, blood pressure and blood glucose concentration because the literature indicated that these risk factors may represent the mechanisms through which carbon disulfide causes coronary artery disease. Matching should be avoided on the intermediate steps in the etiologic sequence from exposure to disease, since such a procedure is known to mask a true effect.

Attention may also be drawn to the fact that the birth district had to be taken into account. This is a specific Finnish problem. Eastern Finland has a considerably higher coronary mortality than western Finland, and a preliminary screening showed that 40% of the viscose rayon workers were born

TABLE 1–3.—EXAMPLE SHOWING THE ACHIEVEMENT OF COMPARABILITY BETWEEN THE EXPOSED AND THE REFERENCE GROUP IN A STUDY ON THE EFFECT OF CARBON DISULFIDE EXPOSURE ON THE INCIDENCE OF CORONARY ARTERY DISEASE*

CHARACTERISTIC	SIMILARITY	METHOD
Age	Same	Pair-matching
Birth district	Same	Pair-matching
Type of work	Same	Pair-matching
Social structure	Same	Result of matching
District of habitation	Same	Questionnaire
Cigarette consumption	No major differences	Questionnaire
Leisure-time physical activity	No major differences	Questionnaire
Physical work capacity	No major differences	Ergometry
Relative body weight	Same	Measurement
Drug therapy	No major differences	Questionnaire
Diet	No major differences	Judgment

*See reference 8.

in eastern Finland against 25% of the paper mill workers. This is a good illustration of the importance of knowing the substance of the problem under study when the reference group is defined.

Another example may illustrate the situation in a case-referent design, where the referent group should represent a condition that is neither caused nor prevented by the exposure at issue. Consider a study on occupational factors in the etiology of nasal cancer. The cases are, of course, selected from patients with that disease. If the referents are patients with some other type of cancer, the symmetry of the data will best be ensured, since healthy people probably would not give similarly accurate histories. However, the referents must have a type of cancer with an etiology completely unrelated to any occupation. Self-evidently, no respiratory cancer fulfills this requirement, and the use of several other cancers would also be doubtful. However, gastrointestinal cancer is considered to be predominantly nonoccupational in origin and therefore patients with colonic cancer could be used as referents. The ideal design for complete validity of reference entity would include two separate series of referents, one with colonic cancer and another without cancer of any type. Kolonel,[10] in fact, used such an approach in a study on renal tumors and cadmium exposure. He used patients with kidney tumors as cases. One series of referents was composed of patients with colonic cancer and another of healthy individuals. As it turned out, the result of the study was the same, irrespective of which reference group was used for comparison; i.e., cadmium exposure was more prevalent among the cases.

Unconfoundedness of comparison is the last dimension of internal validity. Miettinen[22] defines a confounder as an extraneous factor that is intermixed with a scientific problem. Because of this intermixing, the confounder disturbs the assessment of the effect under study. To have this confounding effect, the factor (a) must be a determinant of the illness (see Section 2) and (b) it must be associated with the exposure. More specifically, the confounder must be a causal risk indicator of the illness and not associated with it by chance in a particular study. In contrast, its association with the exposure can either be systematic ("always occurring") or it can be a chance association, occurring only in a particular study.

Age is a good example of a confounder. Consider, for example, the effect of cigarette smoking on respiratory cancer. The incidence of lung cancer increases with age, which thus is a risk indicator of lung cancer. Age is also associated with smoking, because old people usually have smoked longer and more than young persons. Hence, age complies with both requirements for a confounder; i.e., it is a determinant of the disease (lung cancer) and it is associated with the exposure (smoking).

Consider next the aforementioned study on the connection between exposure to carbon disulfide and coronary artery disease. The question arises as to whether cigarette smoking should be considered a confounder in this instance. It is well known that smoking is a risk factor for coronary artery disease; hence, it fulfills the first requirement for a confounder. To fulfill the other, it should be associated with the exposure in the particular study; i.e., the viscose rayon workers should smoke more than the reference category. If the cigarette consumption is not known in advance, the smoking histories must be obtained, usually by means of a questionnaire. If smoking turns out to be more prevalent in the exposed group, it is a confounder. If not, it does not fulfill the second requirement for a confounder and, contrary to what most people think, *need not be controlled* in that particular study.

The effect of a confounder may be "positive," producing a false association, or "negative," masking a true association. Had smoking in the preceding example been more common among the exposed subjects, positive confounding would have arisen; had it been less common, negative confounding may have masked the excess of coronary artery disease in the exposed cohort.

In occupational medicine, confounding usually is a less severe problem than selection. Insofar as smoking is concerned, Axelson[1] calculated the effect of various hypothetical smoking distributions on the rate ratio of lung cancer. As can be seen from Table 1–4, the asymmetry must be rather extreme to produce serious bias. More specifically, the effects of differences in smoking habits between common categories of

TABLE 1–4.—ESTIMATED CRUDE RATE RATIOS IN RELATION TO FRACTION OF SMOKERS IN VARIOUS HYPOTHETIC POPULATIONS. TWO DIFFERENT RISK LEVELS ARE ASSUMED FOR SMOKERS, I.E., 10 TIMES AND 20 TIMES THAT OF NONSMOKERS FOR "MODERATE" AND "HEAVY" SMOKERS, RESPECTIVELY*

POPULATION FRACTION (%)			
NONSMOKERS (1×)	MODERATE SMOKERS (10×)	HEAVY SMOKERS (20×)	RATE RATIO
100	—	—	0.15
80	20	—	0.43
70	30	—	0.57
60	35	5	0.78
50†	40†	10†	1.00†
40	45	15	1.22
30	50	20	1.43
20	22	25	1.65
10	60	30	1.86
—	65	35	2.08
—	25	75	2.69
—	—	100	3.08

*From Axelson.[1]

†Reference population (similar to the general population in countries such as Sweden). Smoking habits in various industrial populations rarely diverge outside the dashed lines.

workers only slightly affect the rate ratio for lung cancer. In practice, then, the control of smoking in a study becomes relevant when the rate ratio is at the order of 3 or less. The share of confounding caused by smoking becomes insignificant whenever the rate ratio exceeds 3, which often is the situation in research on occupational lung cancer.

Confounding can be controlled in a study either at the planning stage or during data analysis (in contrast to selection, which always must be controlled at the planning stage). The most effective means of controlling confounding is random allocation into the exposed and nonexposed categories, which is the method used in experiments. However, epidemiologic studies rarely, if ever, can utilize randomization; instead, they use the following procedures:

1. Restriction.
2. Matching.
3. Stratification.
4. Modeling (multivariate analysis).

1. *Restriction* means that the study focuses on a certain category only, such as persons over 40 years of age, males, normotensives or "heavily" exposed subjects. Apart from improving the symmetry of the series, restriction makes a study more effective, since persons with a low risk of contracting the particular disease can be excluded. For example, a study on occupational lung cancer becomes more efficient if only persons over 50 years of age are included. Restriction can be used alone or in combination with other methods.

2. *Matching* refers to the equalization of cases (or exposed subjects) and referents, for example, with respect to age, sex, occupation. Matching is used most often in case-referent studies; it ensures that the distribution of the matched property becomes equal among the cases and referents. A series can be matched on one or more factors. The more factors that are matched the harder it becomes, however, to find suitable referents. Hence, unnecessary matching must be avoided. Under no circumstances is matching allowed on some intermediate step in the causal sequence of events (cf. preceding example on p. 28) because such "overmatching" creates a negative bias.[20] Matching may be combined with other methods of controlling confounding also; i.e., only some properties are matched whereas others are controlled using alternative methods. The question of how many referents there should be for each case is discussed in Section 4.

3. *Stratification* is commonplace in follow-up studies. It represents a means of controlling confounding in connection with data analysis. Hence, it is especially suitable when restriction or matching has not been utilized. Stratification is performed by dividing the groups examined into *strata* according to such factors as age, sex, smoking habits and body weight. The comparisons then are performed within the strata and biases caused by primarily asymmetric distributions thereby are eliminated. However, the more asymmetric the primary total series are, the more loss of material results from stratification, since each end of the distribution will contain enough subjects from only one series (Table 1–5).

Stratification according to several variables requires large series; otherwise, the strata run out of numbers. Therefore, the investigator should consider at the planning

TABLE 1–5.—HYPOTHETICAL RESULT OF STRATIFICATION ACCORDING TO AGE. BECAUSE OF ASYMMETRIC AGE DISTRIBUTION, COMPARISONS CAN BE MADE FOR AGE CATEGORIES 30–59 YEARS ONLY

	NUMBER OF SUBJECTS	
AGE STRATUM	EXPOSED (N = 485)	REFERENTS (N = 388)
19	1	28
20–29	6	77
30–39	82	94
40–49	143	128
50–59	116	56
60–69	86	4
70	51	1

stage the extent to which stratification will be used.

4. *Modeling* or multivariate analysis is used when many variables must be controlled at the data analysis stage. Consequently, this method is an alternative to stratification, especially when the strata run out of numbers. Modeling is a complicated procedure that requires a skilled statistician and a computer.

Another method to improve validity is the use of *multiple referent* series. Of course, this design has the same requirements of validity as the use of one referent series only. However, in practice, costs increase considerably if several referent series are used; hence, one rarely has an opportunity to use such a design.

External Validity

External validity can be defined as the generalizability of the results beyond the data. Thus, it refers to scientific inference. First, the data of the study should be generalizable to other (larger) populations having the same characteristics (e.g., intensity of exposure, age distribution, type of work). Next, there should be "scientific truth"; for example, the excess occurrence of coronary artery disease among viscose rayon workers indicates that exposure to carbon disulfide (of a certain intensity and duration) *in general* causes or accelerates the development of coronary artery disease. If there is reason to formulate such an assumption, a scientific theory has arisen from the data.

However, quite often, plant physicians can apply epidemiologic methods in the study of employees in their plant without aiming at generalizability, and the results still can have practical importance. Thus, there indeed are situations in which external validity is not so significant.

The question of external validity must be considered at the planning stage of a study, and the study population and the reference category must be defined accordingly. Then the results can be generalized. This kind of generalization differs from the statistical sample-to-population generalization in the sense that specific categories of events are more interesting than the extrapolation of the finding to people at large. In other words, if one finds that spray painters show neurologic abnormalities, it is more interesting to formulate the hypothesis that solvent exposure *causes neuropathy* than to postulate that, say, 10% of *all spray painters* have this disorder.

Assessment of external validity is very much a matter of judgment, but one absolute requirement is good internal validity.

6. SOME GUIDELINES FOR INTERPRETING EPIDEMIOLOGIC STUDIES

The interpretation of an epidemiologic study also is very much a matter of judgment. Unfortunately, readers cannot always assume that the author's evaluation is correct. They must be able to examine the data presented in a critical way and form their own opinions. In addition to sufficient knowledge of the subject in question, they must have some insight into epidemiology before this is possible. The preceding sections have illustrated questions related to the planning and execution of epidemiologic studies; this one gives some elementary guidelines for critically evaluating them. It focuses on general methodologic aspects because the diverse areas of occupational medicine cannot be covered in this context.

Checking the Validity

Readers can estimate the validity of a study only if enough details of the design, materials and methods are given in the report. Articles with superficial, incomplete or otherwise defective methods sections easily make the authors seem nonchalant or ignorant of how to ensure validity. Even worse, one may suspect that the authors avoid going into particulars on purpose because they know that the study is biased. Irrespective of the reason for the lack of detail, such papers must be regarded as noninformative.

When the ingredients for evaluating validity are present, readers will profit if they check the article systematically with respect to each of its components. They first should consider to what extent the study fulfills the criteria of valid design in general (such as "correct" study type and "sufficient" material). Next, they should turn their attention toward the components of internal validity and look for selection bias, information bias, validity of the reference group and, finally, confounding. The last issue may be subtle indeed and even impossible to judge without thorough knowledge of the subject matter. If systematic errors are detected, their direction and, if possible, their magnitude should be estimated. Minor ones do not necessarily invalidate a study, provided that their effects are known. In fact, sometimes the authors themselves point out a bias and discuss its effects.

External validity should not be neglected, either. Readers should consider whether or not the results can be generalized. Do they allow the formulation of new hypotheses or do they support or challenge existing ones?

Finally, readers should critically weigh the conclusions of the authors against their own opinions. This process brings into play the general principles of scientific inference. Since these principles may be unfamiliar to those not actively engaged in research, some simple guidelines follow.

Supporting Evidence for Cause-Effect Inferences

It may once more be repeated that definite cause-effect conclusions cannot be derived from nonexperimental research. Causality, therefore, can be viewed in terms of *probability* only. The following circumstances support the causality of a relationship.

1. Self-evidently, the exposure must *precede* the illness. When latency periods are involved, the exposure must have commenced early enough, i.e., at least earlier than half the mean latency period. (Since the exact length rarely is known, this, too, becomes a matter of judgment.)

2. The *stronger the association* (meaning that the rate ratio is high) the greater the probability of a causal association. An exception is "small" series (say, smaller than 30–40), because their rate ratios are subject to substantial random variation. Hence, unless the lower 99% confidence limit is greater than 1 (or, using another expression, $p < 0.01$), the results are noninformative. Some persons may require even stricter criteria, for example, $p < 0.001$, before they believe in results from small series. How strict the criteria one requires is a matter of judgment; there are no fixed rules. But if a moderately large or a large series yields a high rate ratio, the probability of a causal relationship is great. It should be added that the confidence limits for rate ratios from large series are narrow; therefore, statistical significance is easily obtained even for rather low rate ratios in such instances. Under these premises, mere statistical significance is not enough evidence for a causal relationship, since rather small, uncontrolled systematic errors may be responsible for the difference found. But such errors do not have enough "power" to distort the statistical significance of moderate-sized series, which require higher rate ratios to yield "significant" differences. Consider, for example, Table 1-4, which shows the confounding effect of various smoking distributions on the rate ratio. If a series is large, a ratio of about 1.4 may be statistically significant (e.g., $p = 0.01$). But the confounding effect of even a moderate asym-

metry of smoking habits can produce a rate ratio of 1.4. On the other hand, if a moderate-sized series yields a rate ratio of, for example, 6, and the p value again is 0.01, not even maximally extreme (unrealistic) smoking asymmetry can be the only responsible factor. Consequently, it is likely that the exposure, not the confounding, has produced the effect. In summary, one should look for the rate ratio of a large series and the p value of a small series. A "very small" series is noninformative.

3. The presence of an *exposure-response relationship* supports the causality of an association. However, it should be noted that a confounding factor sometimes may be so intermixed with the exposure that the effects of the two cannot be separated. Concomitant exposure to a variety of metals in many smelters is a typical example. In this case, the carcinogenic effect of one metal cannot be separated from the possible effects of the others, and the exposure-response relationship becomes confounded and cannot be considered to support a causal connection between the disease in question and a particular exposure.

4. The credibility of results in the light of *prior knowledge* usually supports causality. For example, if animal experiments have shown an agent to be carcinogenic, epidemiologic evidence of excess cancer among exposed workers becomes more credible. However, conformity with prior knowledge cannot always be required, since it would inhibit the creation of new ideas.

5. Known or possible explanatory *biologic mechanisms* speak strongly in favor of the causality of an association. In contrast, it is difficult to place much confidence in associations that have no explanation. Remember, by definition, 1 in 20 associations is statistically significant at a level of 0.05, and 1 in 100 at a level of 0.01, without having any meaning at all. The availability of computers has greatly increased the production of such nonsense associations.

6. Perhaps the most conclusive evidence of causality is provided when a *change in the exposure brings about a change in the illness*. This type of evidence is obtained in interventive epidemiologic studies, and its strength of evidence is connected with the similarities between intervention and experiment that already have been discussed. The intervention may be arranged by the investigator or exposure may be changed for other reasons. For example, suppose that the concentration of raw cotton dust in the air of a cotton mill decreases due to the installation of an exhaust ventilation system. The symptoms of Monday morning asthma among the workers then diminish. However, suppose that more machines are installed in the same space without the ventilation system being changed. The dust concentrations again increase and more symptoms occur. The ventilation once more may be improved and the symptoms subside. Such a sequence must be regarded as strong evidence in favor of a causal relationship between a particular exposure and an illness, but the possibility of confounding by some other concomitant exposure cannot be completely ruled out.

Studies Yielding Negative Results

The definition of safe work conditions is the main goal of research in occupational health and therefore studies showing the absence of effect are as important as positive findings. However, in order to be meaningful, negative studies must fulfill certain requirements.

First, since proving the negative theoretically requires an infinite number of observations, a negative study must be *large*. Negative results from small studies are completely noninformative.

Second, the study must be *sensitive*. This requirement has to do both with random errors and with the choice of measuring methods. Random errors may arise, for example, from the use of poorly calibrated instruments, and they tend to mask true associations. In other words, random errors weaken the power of the study to detect the effects of some exposures. If they occur in a study, one cannot be sure whether the results are true negative ones or masked positive ones. Similarly, if the measurements are crude, early manifestations of the disease may pass undetected and the negative results will be false.

Third, since true negative studies are essential for the setting of standards, it is important that they report the exposure level that, according to the study, has not produced an effect.

In summary, to be meaningful, a negative study must be large, sensitive and provide accurate exposure data. Otherwise, the result is not negative but "nonpositive," which is the same as noninformative.

Epidemiologic Findings and Individual Diagnosis

When epidemiologic studies reveal increased morbidity, it always is at the group level. A typical study outcome would be, for example, that lung cancer was 4 times more frequent in an exposed group than in a reference group. In such an instance, 3 of 4 cases would be "occupational" and 1 "natural." Such an outcome indicates the presence of a carcinogen that should be identified and eliminated from the work environment, and, so far, the matter is simple. But, because compensation claims often become involved, identification of those cases with an "occupational" etiology would be helpful.

However, single "occupational" cases *never* can be identified on a scientific basis. The only possibility of resolving this problem is *by agreement* (or legislation based on agreement). For example, it may be agreed that *all cases* complying with certain criteria such as "enough" exposure, "long enough" latency time or absence of "other evident" causes (although cigarette smoking would be very problematic in the case of lung cancer) would receive compensation or, alternatively, that all cases occurring in certain occupations would be compensated. The higher the rate ratios usually found in epidemiologic studies the easier it would be to reach such an agreement. The real problems arise when the disease is a common "general" one and the rate ratio is rather low. But no scientific advice can be given for this dilemma—its solution is entirely a matter of policy.

Another typical problem arises when an epidemiologic study reveals some subclinical, nonspecific effect among clinically healthy workers. Slowing of nerve conduction velocities provides a good example. At the group level, this phenomenon has been found to occur in exposure to several solvents, lead and vibration.[28] Although statistically significant group differences occur, it does not directly follow that individual workers have contracted an occupational disease. What can be said is that an "environmental diagnosis" has been made that indicates that a certain exposure causes some functional changes. If these changes are considered unacceptable (which is a matter of combined scientific and political agreement), work conditions should be improved and the hygienic standards revised. But individual diagnosis needs more specific and definite manifestations; it cannot be based solely on a single, sensitive test.

7. SPECIAL PROBLEMS OF EPIDEMIOLOGIC RESEARCH IN OCCUPATIONAL MEDICINE

Epidemiologic research in occupational medicine faces the same general problem as any other branch of medicine, and the methods used to overcome them are similar. Some peculiarities characterize this field, however, and they are discussed in this section.

The Healthy Worker Effect

One of the prerequisites for being employable is a relatively good state of health. The more physically demanding the job the higher the health requirements. Those who are not fit will not be hired, and those already employed will not remain so once their health deteriorates below a certain level. This selective process, enforced by pre-employment examinations, periodic checkups and other activities of occupational health services, results in lower death rates than in the general population for occupationally active groups—provided that no life-shortening hazards occur in the work environment. It has become commonplace to call this phenomenon the "healthy worker effect."

From the methodologic point of view, this effect presents some problems for epidemiologic studies. Occupational cohorts often are contrasted with the general population in mortality studies because economic or other feasibility circumstances do not permit the use of a more appropriate reference entity. Usually the standardized mortality ratio (SMR) obtained in such a manner is well below 100. In fact, figures on the order of 60–90 have been reported often;[16] for example, 87 for rubber workers in the 40–64 age range,[18] 82 for steel workers,[14] 89 for talc miners,[27] 65 for workers in a communications company[17] and 90 for foundry workers.[11] These figures obviously are underestimates of the "true" mortality, partly because of health selection, usually leading to negative confounding, and partly because of the use of an inappropriate reference category, i.e., the general population. According to the scheme presented in Section 5, the healthy worker effect is caused by (1) invalidity of the reference entity and (2) negative confounding; i.e., "good health" is associated with the exposure under study because of "health selection" and is (often) a determinant of a favorable vital prognosis. Astonishingly, the healthy worker effect is *not a true selection bias* in spite of the "health selection" (resulting in confounding). The only exception is when the *disease under study* (and not some associated condition) causes selective turnover.

Overcoming the bias caused by the healthy worker effect and interpreting the data if it cannot be overcome require knowledge of the nature of this effect. Some information is available, but much more still is needed.

Goldsmith[5] has discussed the impact of the healthy worker effect on total mortality. The main reason for the better-than-expected mortality experience of occupational groups lies in the fact that the general population also includes unemployable and unemployed persons. Among them are those in institutions, those with congenital anomalies, those handicapped during childhood, those otherwise ill at the time job seeking commences and those unemployed or with unstable employment. All these groups have a higher mortality than the active population. Kitagawa and Hauser[9] reported that those U.S. white males unemployed in 1950 or later (4.3% of the population) had an SMR of 204. An additional 4% with no occupation showed an SMR of 125. Since occupational cohorts often contain a relatively high number of elderly workers and since the inactive part of the population increases in the older age categories, a general population adjusted to correspond to the age distribution of such cohorts may comprise up to 10% of those with exceptionally high mortality. Hence, in such a comparison, any SMR exceeding, say, 85 or 90 would indicate elevated mortality. A corresponding correction coefficient could be used to yield a "true" SMR, as has been proposed by Goldsmith.[5] However, this procedure would be an oversimplification.

It has been shown that the healthy worker effect is not constant but varies, depending on a number of circumstances. The following five factors are especially important in this respect.

1. The healthy worker effect is more marked in *younger age groups*.[16] Its influence declines with age until it no longer is significant in the postretirement age range. For example, McMichael[16] found an SMR of 81 for male rubber workers in the age range of 50–54 whereas the age group 55–64 had an SMR of 89. In the postretirement years, the SMR was 95 for those 65–74 years of age and 113 in the oldest age group (75–84 years).

2. The *passage of time* since the beginning of employment or, alternatively, the identification of the cohort decreases the healthy worker effect (provided that dropouts are traced and accounted for). This is so because the selective effect of many major diseases that present subjective symptoms—for example, most cardiovascular and pulmonary diseases—is strong at the time a job is sought. Hence, the workers are at their "healthiest" as employment begins. In addition, if a cohort is formed from active workers only, irrespective of when hired, the health status of its members will be higher than the average simply because they are active. As the years pass, different diseases develop, and the health status of workers begins to approach that of the general population. For example, Enterline[4] found that asbestos product workers had an SMR of 83 for diseases other than cancer during the first 5-year period after cohort identification. During the second period it increased to 100 and during the third it reached 106.

3. The healthy worker effect is greater for *nonwhites than for whites* in countries with a mixed labor force.[16] The explanation probably lies in the fact that more nonwhites than whites are unemployed in the general population. However, the health requirements set by employers may also be stricter for nonwhites. Thus, the reference bases for employed whites and nonwhites are different. Whites are being compared to the national average middle-class white population whereas nonwhites are being contrasted to a nonwhite population that represents a national average of lower social level.[16]

4. The healthy worker effect *is not uniform for each cause of death*. In general, diseases with silent early stages and a rapid, fatal course do not cause a healthy worker effect (except for the first 1 or 2 years after cohort identification). Cancer is a typical example. The symptoms appear late, the early diagnosis of asymptomatic cancers is not well developed and there are no means to predict it before symptoms or signs appear. Hence, even medical examinations are not selective in this respect, except in cases of cancers that would have manifested themselves anyway within a short time. In contrast, a high risk for death due to coronary artery disease can be established in advance by means of early diagnosis of the disease or identification of its risk factors. Furthermore, self-selection occurs because of symptoms or earlier warnings from physicians to avoid demanding jobs. For example, McMichael[16] cites a study on carpenters and joiners whose SMRs for cancer were close to 100 in all age groups whereas those for ischemic heart disease were around 60 in the younger age groups and between 70 and 80 in the older age categories.

5. In addition to these general modifiers of the healthy worker effect there are others with a more "local" character. For example, if there is a labor shortage, the health criteria for hiring workers will be loose. The reverse is true during periods of underemployment. Furthermore, different companies may have different policies in general, particularly in times of underemployment. In addition, the healthy worker effect is stronger for physically demanding jobs, as already mentioned, and local variations in the supply of workers with certain occupational qualifications may confuse the picture. All these circumstances, most of which are unquantifiable, complicate the

evaluation of the strength of the healthy worker effect.

Once all these aspects are taken into consideration, it is evident that the healthy worker effect poses a serious methodologic problem when occupational groups are compared with the general population. Whenever possible, a more appropriate reference entity should be used. But if an ad hoc reference group cannot be utilized for practical or economic reasons, the *active* general population would form a better reference entity than the total general population. In some countries there are statistical data on this population, too. The healthy worker effect can be further decreased if the calculation of person-years does not start immediately at the time of cohort identification but, say, 5 or 10 years later. Alternatively, a separate comparison can be made at different intervals after the identification. The mortality rates also should be compared separately for different causes and within different age groups. Finally, whenever possible, comparisons should be made within the cohort itself between different categories of exposure intensity. These procedures often reduce the healthy worker effect; however, many uncertainties still will be left to the intuitive judgment of both the author and the reader of a report.

Turnover

Turnover of workers may impair the validity of epidemiologic studies; in addition, it causes practical problems. It occurs for a variety of reasons, but turnover due to health is the most troublesome from the methodologic point of view. Such turnover contributes to the healthy worker effect, but it also has other consequences that must be realized.

Turnover is most pronounced in demanding or otherwise "unpleasant" jobs. A study made of Finnish foundry workers[12] provides a good example. Active foundry workers and those who had left foundry work for one reason or another were asked on a questionnaire with a rating scale of 0–10 to compare their current physical fitness with the best state they had ever experienced. A score of 0–4 was classified as indicative of a substantial deterioration of the fitness. Figure 1–4 shows the proportion of active and former foundry workers reporting such deterioration. There were fewer scores of 0–4 among active foundry workers than among former ones and the difference became more accentuated with advancing age. The results indicate that deteriorating health is a common reason for changing occupation.

Selective turnover invalidates cross-sectional studies and may distort longitudinal ones, despite the fact that dropouts are traced and accounted for and an appropriate reference group has been used. The problem occurs when the exposure under study causes symptoms that force the worker to seek other employment; the most affected persons, therefore, will have short exposure times. This negative bias distorts the exposure-response relationship.

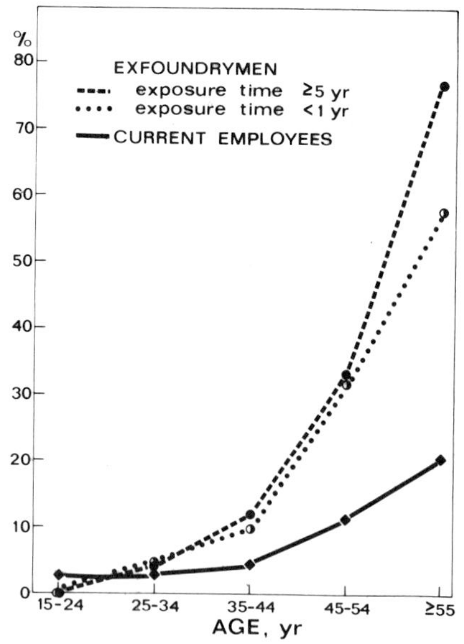

Fig 1–4.—Percentages of current and former foundrymen who considered that their work capacity was poor (0–4 points on a 10-point scale).

Turnover also causes practical problems. In retrospective follow-up studies, the cohort size must be large to provide enough experience, and therefore both costs and effort increase. Also, the costs of tracing dropouts become higher. A prospective study may fail completely if the turnover is underestimated when the cohort is defined, because too few persons complying with the minimal exposure criteria are left at the end of the follow-up.

Multiple Exposure and Several Jobs

Often workers hold several different jobs during their lifetime, and they may have been exposed to many different hazards. In such a situation it may be difficult to judge which of the hazardous exposures is responsible for a disease manifesting itself in older workers. Furthermore, workers may be exposed to many hazards concomitantly. For example, foundry workers are exposed to silica dust, carbon monoxide, noise, heat radiation, metal fumes, polycyclic hydrocarbons, etc. Under these circumstances, relating excess morbidity to one specific exposure is also extremely difficult. It can only be said that the work environment in general is hazardous; specific cause-effect inferences must be left to "cleaner" studies.

Lack of Quantitative Exposure Data

It has been pointed out many times that past exposure data often are unavailable or deficient. Usually the investigator cannot be blamed. But, unfortunately, the exposure data given in a report may be deficient even though there might have been an opportunity to obtain them. Research in occupational health almost always is a multidisciplinary enterprise, and if epidemiologists fail to appreciate this fact, they can not perform their job well. Broad categories of factory departments or occupations are not a good substitute for exact, quantitative measurements of the exposure in question. In order to be of good quality, therefore, an epidemiologic survey usually requires the aid of an experienced occupational hygienist. In multidisciplinary institutes, the need for such teamwork constitutes no problem, but practical difficulties may arise in medical schools.

The most difficult obstacle, of course, is the refusal of companies to collaborate. Such a situation is extremely rare in the Nordic countries but is said to be more common elsewhere. It is indeed a pity if an investigator cannot obtain access to existing exposure data, because an otherwise good study may fail completely.

Whenever exposure data can be gathered, the investigator should do everything possible to ensure that they are detailed enough and of good quality. Being able to relate a few pertinent effects to accurate exposure data is much more important (and rare) than overloading the medical protocol with a great number of examinations (which may be irrelevant or useless anyway if concurrent exposure levels are not known).

Disease with a Long Latency Period

One of the most central concerns in occupational health care is whether or not the current level of exposure to a toxic agent is safe for workers. Unless the exposure-response curve is known, the answer can only be an educated guess. As long as the effects are immediate, an ad hoc study may yield useful information within a reasonable time. But late effects—or rather their relationship to current exposure levels—simply cannot be quickly elucidated by means of ad hoc studies.

At present, two types of late effects are primary sources of concern. One is degeneration of the central nervous system and the other is cytogenetic damage that possibly results in malignant growth, malformed offspring or genetic impairment. Both questions are problematic, because the literature rarely, if ever, provides a basis for exposure-response considerations.

Suppose one wants to know if continual exposure to, for example, 1 ppm of benzene is safe, or if this low level increases the occurrence of leukemia. The literature will be of no help because most reports on leukemia in connection with benzene exposure are clinical observations and the few epidemiologic studies published deal with high exposure levels. The only reasonably quick way to gather the information needed would be a retrospective follow-up study. But, since past exposure data seldom have been recorded (and, even if they exist, they may not be released by the companies concerned), such a study would face many practical difficulties. Even a valid study would cause dispute, however. A "positive" result would have critics arguing that unrecognized exposure peaks exceeding the critical level by many times may have occurred and a "negative" one would have others claiming that the study material was too scanty or the observation period too short or the tracing of dropouts unsuccessful. In other words, critics representing particular interests would try to invalidate the results in any case. A whole bulk of evidence, requiring years to attain, probably would be necessary before the matter would become clarified. Meanwhile, nothing would happen to the current standard. It is sad indeed that such pessimistic views must be expressed in a textbook such as this one, but the violent arguing, in public hearings and in print, that has occurred over a number of intended standard changes based on new epidemiologic data has not been constructive.

However, as long as there is doubt as to what is safe and what is not, the only ethically defendable attitude of personnel in charge of occupational health care is one of cautiousness. In other words, a possible error in judgment should be in the overprotective direction. What society ultimately decides is an acceptable risk is another matter. In this decision, factors other than health also become involved.

Another typical situation related to the one just presented occurs when a survey reveals that the frequency of cancer is indeed higher than it should be among workers in some type of industry. Let us suppose that the study is valid and that consequently there is a "proved" cancer risk. What, then, is the impact of such a finding on the occupational health care in plants where the agent in question is being used?

One must realize that studies dealing with current cancer rates always are retrospective and that the excess disease found reflects exposure levels that prevailed decades ago. During the past 20 years or so, hygienic conditions have improved substantially in most industries. Hence, the results by no means prove that present conditions would impose the same degree of risk as the one found in the survey in question. But, on the other hand, there are no guarantees that the conditions are completely safe either. Their effect should be studied by means of a prospective follow-up. However, this procedure would take some decades and the results would be unrepresentative of the conditions prevailing then. Therefore, one can see that defining conditions of safety at present is difficult indeed, and the situation outlined in the preceding example is created.

These are merely some illustrations of the difficulties arising from the profound ignorance of exposure-response relationships for long-term effects that characterize occupational medicine. There are indeed unlimited tasks for objective, competent research workers, and it may once again be stressed that valid *negative* studies are extremely pertinent for the characterization of safe work conditions.

ACKNOWLEDGMENTS

The methodologic sections of this presentation are based to a great extent on the international courses in epidemiology taught by Prof. Olli S. Miettinen, Harvard School of Public Health, and arranged by the Institute of Occupational Health, Helsinki, in 1972–1978. Sakari Tola, M.D., Matti Tolonen, M.D., and Markku Nurminen, L.Pol.Sc., have revised the manuscript. I wish to thank them for their constructive criticism.

REFERENCES

1. Axelson, O.: Letter to the Editor: Aspects on confounding in occupational health epidemiology, Scand. J. Work Environ. Health 4:98, 1978.
2. Axelson, O., Dahlgren, E., Jansson, C-D., and Rehnlund, S. O.: Arsenic exposure and mortality: A case-referent study from a Swedish copper smelter, Br. J. Ind. Med. 35:8, 1978.
3. Campbell, D. T.: Factors relevant to the validity of experiments in social setting, Psychol. Bull. 54:297, 1957.
4. Enterline, P. E.: Mortality among asbestos products workers in the United States, Ann. N. Y. Acad. Sci. 132:156, 1965.
5. Goldsmith, J.: What do we expect from an occupational cohort?, J. Occup. Med. 17:126, 1975.
6. Hänninen, H., Nurminen, M., Tolonen, M., and Martelin, T.: Psychological tests as indicators of excessive exposure to carbon disulfide, Scand. J. Psychol. 19:163, 1978.
7. Hernberg, S.: Incidence of Cancer in Populations with Exceptional Exposure to Metals, in Hiatt, H. H., Watson, J. D., and Winsten, J. A. (eds.), *Origins of Human Cancer. Book A, Incidence of Cancers in Humans* (Cold Spring Harbor, N.Y.: Cold Spring Harbor Conferences on Cell Proliferation, 1977), Vol. 4, p. 147.
8. Hernberg, S., Partanen, T., Nordman, C-H., and Sumari, P.: Coronary heart disease among workers exposed to carbon disulphide, Br. J. Ind. Med. 27:313, 1970.
9. Kitagawa, E. M., and Hauser, P. M.: *Differential Mortality in the United States* (Cambridge, Mass.: Harvard University Press, 1973).
10. Kolonel, L. N.: Association of cadmium with renal cancer, Cancer 37:1782, 1978.
11. Koskela, R. S., Hernberg, S., Kärävä, R., Järvinen, E., and Nurminen, M.: A mortality study of foundry workers, Scand. J. Work Environ. Health 2(Supp. 1):73, 1976.
12. Koskela, R. S., Luoma, K., and Hernberg, S.: Turnover and health selection among foundry workers, Scand. J. Work Environ. Health 2(Supp. 1):1, 1976.
13. Lilienfeld, A. M.: *Foundations of Epidemiology* (New York: Oxford University Press, 1976).
14. Lloyd, J. W., and Ciocco, A.: Long-term mortality study of steelworkers. I. Methodology, J. Occup. Med. 11:299, 1969.
15. MacMahon, B., and Pugh, E.: *Epidemiology, Principles and Methods* (Boston: Little, Brown and Company, 1970).
16. McMichael, A. J.: Standardized mortality ratios and the "healthy worker effect." Scratching beneath the surface, J. Occup. Med. 18:165, 1976.
17. McMichael, A. J., Haynes, S. G., and Tyroler, H. A.: Observations on the evaluation of occupational mortality data, J. Occup. Med. 17:128, 1975.
18. McMichael, A. J., Spirtas, R., and Kupper, L. L.: An epidemiologic study of mortality within a cohort of rubber workers, 1964–72, J. Occup. Med. 16:458, 1974.
19. Miettinen, O. S.: Individual matching with multiple controls in the case of an all-or-none response, Biometrics 25:339, 1969.
20. Miettinen, O. S.: Matching and design efficiency in retrospective studies, Am. J. Epidemiol. 91:111, 1970.
21. Miettinen, O. S.: Standardization of risk ratios, Am. J. Epidemiol. 96:383, 1973.
22. Miettinen, O. S.: Confounding and effect-modification, Am. J. Epidemiol. 100:350, 1974.
23. Miettinen, O. S.: Notes for the WHO course in scientific research methods of the epidemiology of industrial intoxications, Helsinki, October, 1975. World Health Organization, Regional Office for Europe, Copenhagen, 1975 (Mimeo).
24. Miettinen, O. S.: Estimability and estimation in case-referent studies, Am. J. Epidemiol. 103:226, 1976.
25. Morris, J. N.: *Uses of Epidemiology* (Edinburgh: Livingstone, 1970).
26. Ott, M. G., Townsend, J. C., Fishbeck, W. A., and Langner, R. A.: Mortality among individuals occupationally exposed to benzene, Arch. Environ. Health 33:3, 1978.
27. Rubino, G. F., Scansetti, Q., Piolatto, G., and Romano, C. A.: Mortality study of talc miners and millers, J. Occup. Med. 18:186, 1976.
28. Seppäläinen, A. M.: Applications of neurophysiological methods. A review, Scand. J. Work Environ. Health 1:1, 1975.

29. Seppäläinen, A. M., and Tolonen, M.: Neurotoxicity of long-term exposure to carbon disulfide in the viscose rayon industry: A neurophysiological study, Work Environ. Health 11:145, 1974.
30. Silcock, H.: The comparison of occupational mortality rates, Population Studies 13:183, 1959.
31. Tola, S., Hernberg, S., and Nikkanen, J.: Parameters indicative of absorption and biological effect in new lead exposure: A prospective study, Br. J. Ind. Med. 30:134, 1973.
32. Tolonen, M.: Chronic subclinical carbon disulfide poisoning, Work Environ. Health 11:154, 1974.
33. Tolonen, M., Hernberg, S., Nurminen, M., and Tiitola, K.: A follow-up study of coronary heart disease in viscose rayon workers exposed to carbon disulphide, Br. J. Ind. Med. 32:1, 1975.
34. Wickström, G.: Effect of work on degenerative back diseases. A review, Scand. J. Work Environ. Health 4(Supp. 1):1, 1978.
35. World Health Organization: Methodology of multifactor preventive trials in ischaemic heart disease. WHO Euro 8202 (6), Copenhagen, 1973.

PART TWO

WOMEN AT WORK

2 / Occupational Health Considerations for Women at Work

JACQUELINE MESSITE, M.D., and MARCUS B. BOND, M.D.

GENERAL

THREE INTERRELATED FACTORS justify the need for separate chapters devoted to the medical interests of women at work: (1) women, *on the average*, are of smaller stature and have less physical strength than most men, (2) the woman's unique reproductive function of pregnancy means that a pregnant woman must carry her embryo and later her fetus with her into the workplace, thus possibly exposing the fetus to her occupational environment, and (3) the increased number of women at work makes them as important a component as men for consideration in occupational medicine.

In addition, major pieces of United States legislation during the past decade and a half mandate consideration of the woman at work. Among these are the Occupational Safety and Health Act of 1970 and Title VII of the Civil Rights Act of 1964 with the guidelines adopted thereunder by the Equal Employment Opportunity Commission (EEOC). The Occupational Safety and Health Act has, as its charge, the provision of a safe and healthful workplace for every worker, male or female, in this nation, and the preservation of our human resources. Title VII of the Civil Rights Act bars discriminatory practices for any reason, including sex, in the hiring of employees. Basic to the provisions of the federal regulations is the inherent assumption that tolerance to industrial stresses, susceptibilities to toxic materials and performance capabilities are similar in all workers so that permissible levels of industrial hazards that will not endanger the health and life expectancy of any worker can be set.[22] Furthermore, "the preservation of our human resources" implies not only the protection of the health of our working men and women but also the preservation of their reproductive capacity and the products of such capacity, who will make up the human resources of the future. In order to ensure proper implementation of these pieces of landmark legislation, and to eliminate the often-stated contention that these laws have opposing goals in regard to women workers, it is meaningful to take an in-depth look at the facts concerning industrial exposures and their effects on women. Furthermore, the implementation of the guidelines of the EEOC signals a potential for substantial increases in employment of women in traditionally male jobs.

These facts are important to physicians for a proper perception of this subject. Because there may be an increasing number of women requesting placement in physically stressful and other nontraditional jobs, physicians are being asked for recommendations about placement—is it safe?—what are the differences in susceptibility to occupational stresses between men and women?—what are the potential effects of the job on pregnancy and the fetus, etc., etc.? The medical profession does not have good data on many of these questions, but the questions are currently pertinent and the best scientific responses must be found and offered. Myths and realities about greater susceptibility of women than men to exposures to chemical and physical agents must be separated in order to make the best judgment possible in occupational placement of female workers.

An important premise is that there is no job for which some woman, somewhere in the pool of available women workers, would not be as qualified, as competent and of no greater susceptibility to harmful effects than any man. Fitting the individual woman to the specific job, as in the case with men, should be the primary consideration. Differences do exist between men and women in certain work capacities and physiologic responses, but these differences are, for the most part, based on averages of female and male populations and should not serve as the basis for placement recommendations for any one particular person.

TRENDS

Since about 1950, the sex composition of the civilian labor force in the United States has undergone a marked change. The proportion of the labor force made up of women 16 years of age and over rose from 29% in 1950 to 40% in 1975, a percentage point increase almost equal to that of the preceding 60 years.[46] In 1970, of all women in the United States 16 years of age and over, 43% participated in the civilian labor force. As seen in Table 2–1, by 1975 there were 37

TABLE 2–1.—CIVILIAN NONINSTITUTIONAL POPULATION, LABOR FORCE (% CHANGE) AND LABOR FORCE PARTICIPATION RATE BY AGE AND SEX, ACTUAL 1975 AND PROJECTED 1990. (NUMBERS IN THOUSANDS)

SEX AND AGE	CIVILIAN POPULATION 1975 (ACTUAL)	CIVILIAN POPULATION 1990 (PROJECTED)	CIVILIAN LABOR FORCE 1975	CIVILIAN LABOR FORCE 1990	% CHANGE 1975–1990	CIVILIAN LABOR FORCE PARTICIPATION RATE 1975	CIVILIAN LABOR FORCE PARTICIPATION RATE 1990
TOTAL							
16 years and over							
Women	79,921	94,588	36,998	48,619	(+ 31.4)	46.3	51.4
Men	71,468	84,379	55,615	65,220	(+ 17.3)	77.8	77.3
16–19 years							
Women	8225	6612	4038	3649	(− 9.6)	49.1	55.2
Men	8049	6485	4760	3976	(− 16.5)	59.1	61.3
20–24 years							
Women	9486	8852	6069	6656	(+ 9.7)	64.0	75.2
Men	8769	8129	7398	6671	(− 9.8)	84.4	82.1
25–34 years							
Women	15,514	20,582	8456	13,077	(+ 54.6)	54.5	63.5
Men	14,566	19,590	13,854	18,545	(+ 33.9)	95.1	94.7
35–44 years							
Women	11,618	18,525	6493	11,678	(+ 79.9)	55.9	63.0
Men	10,745	17,471	10,288	16,571	(+ 61.1)	95.7	94.8
45–54 years							
Women	12,206	12,885	6665	7795	(+ 17.0)	54.6	60.3
Men	11,330	12,085	10,426	10,901	(+ 4.6)	92.0	90.2
55–64 years							
Women	10,349	10,671	4244	4514	(+ 6.4)	41.0	42.3
Men	9221	9592	6982	6704	(− 4.0)	75.7	69.9
65 years and over							
Women	12,521	16,461	1033	1250	(+ 21.0)	8.2	7.6
Men	8784	11,027	1906	1852	(− 2.8)	21.7	16.8

Source: Fullerton, H. N., and Flaim, P. O. (1976), New Labor Force Projections to 1990, U.S. Department of Labor, Bureau of Labor Statistics, Special Labor Force Report No. 197, page 5.

million women workers, representing a 46.3% participation. The projected numbers and rate for 1990 are 48.6 million and 51.4% (see Table 2–1). Comparable percentages for male participation in the labor force are 79.3% for 1970, 77.8% for 1975 and 77.3% projected for 1990. The percentage increase in the civilian labor force participation by sex, projected for 1990 from the 1975 data, is 31.4% for women and only 17.3% for men.

Among the factors underlying this trend is an increasing proportion of young women who are unmarried, a decline in the number of children women are bearing and a growing participation in the labor force of women with children—even young children.[16, 26] Table 2–2 illustrates the changing percentages of women in various occupational groups from 1962 to 1974.[15] At present, women are largely employed in service industries, in white-collar clerical jobs and as semiskilled operatives in manufacturing industries. In the trade industry, women

TABLE 2–2.—OCCUPATIONAL PARTICIPATION RATES: WOMEN AS A PERCENTAGE OF THE TOTAL EMPLOYED WORKERS, 1962–74

OCCUPATIONAL GROUP	1962	1974	OCCUPATIONAL GROUP	1962	1974
TOTAL EMPLOYED	33.9	38.9	TOTAL EMPLOYED	33.9	38.9
Professional	35.9	40.5	Storekeepers and stock clerks	17.4	25.2
Accountants	18.7	23.7	Telephone operators	96.3	93.8
Lawyers and judges	2.8	7.0	Ticket and station agents	21.1	38.0
Librarians	85.7	81.7	Typists	94.8	96.2
Chemists	8.6	14.0	Office machine operators	72.9	71.3
Personnel and labor relations	27.4	34.9	*Craft workers*	2.5	4.5
Pharmacists	10.4	16.5	Bakers	18.3	41.1
Physicians (including osteopaths)	5.5	9.8	Compositors and typesetters	6.3	19.9
Registered nurses	98.5	98.0	Decorators and window dressers	50.0	62.4
Psychologists	41.7	41.4	Painters, construction and maintenance	2.5	2.6
Social workers	60.2	61.3			
Teachers, college and university	19.2	30.9	*Operatives*	25.9	31.1
Elementary school teachers	86.5	84.3	Checkers, inspectors	45.4	50.6
Drafting technicians	4.1	7.7	Gas station attendants	1.5	5.3
Designers	26.3	24.0	Graders and sorters	54.8	75.0
Editors and reporters	37.8	43.6	Packers and wrappers, except meat	60.3	63.1
Painters and sculptors	40.7	41.6	Photo process workers	41.2	47.0
Public relations	20.0	28.8	Weavers	44.8	59.5
Managers	15.3	18.5	Welders	6.0	5.0
Purchasing agents	10.7	17.9	Bus drivers	11.9	37.4
Salesworkers	39.2	41.8	Delivery workers	1.6	4.4
Hucksters and peddlers	65.9	75.1	Taxicab drivers	3.7	11.5
Insurance agents	10.1	13.3	*Laborers, except farm*	2.6	8.1
News vendors	3.2	25.3	*Farmers and farm managers*	5.1	6.0
Real estate agents	28.5	38.3	Owners and tenants	5.2	6.0
Clerical workers	68.8	77.6	*Farm laborers and supervisors*	32.0	27.4
Bank tellers	71.5	91.5	Farm laborers (wage workers)	16.8	14.6
Bookkeepers	85.4	89.2	Farm laborers (unpaid family)	56.9	63.6
Cashiers	82.5	87.7	*Service workers, except private household*	53.5	58.7
Collectors, bill and account	21.2	46.0			
Dispatchers, vehicle	9.1	24.2	Bartenders	11.5	32.6
Insurance adjusters	9.4	45.6	Cooks	63.6	58.8
Mail carriers	2.9	7.5	Food counter workers	67.5	85.2
Messengers	14.9	23.7	Waiters	87.4	91.8
Payroll timekeepers	61.5	77.4	Attendants, recreation	14.9	35.9
Postal clerks	14.7	28.0	Hairdressers	88.1	92.4
Secretaries	98.5	99.2	Guards and watchers	5.0	6.1
Shipping and receiving clerks	7.6	15.9	Nursing aides	75.2	86.9

Source: Garfinkle, S. H., Occupations of women and black workers, 1962–74, Monthly Review, U.S. Department of Labor, Bureau of Labor Statistics, p. 29, November, 1975.[15]

are found in the retail trades whereas men predominate in the wholesale field. In education, women are primarily the precollege teachers whereas men predominate in the faculties of colleges and universities, particularly at the higher levels. Manufacturing employs the largest share of the male work force.[48]

In the past 10–15 years there have been appreciable changes in attitudes and expectations of women at work. A high proportion of women currently expect gainful employment to be a major part of their lives' activities. This is consistent with, and a part of, the women's movement, which strives to increase the variety and importance of women's roles in our society. Included is a desire by many women to acquire and achieve success in jobs traditionally held by men.

Inroads are beginning to be made in some typically masculine jobs such as bartending and bus driving, although most female bus drivers work only part-time operating school buses.[48] There has been some progress in the professions. From 1962 to 1974, the proportion of physicians and surgeons who were women rose from 6% to 10% and that

TABLE 2–3.—EXAMPLES OF POSSIBLE EXPOSURES RELATED TO VARIOUS OCCUPATIONS

OCCUPATION	POTENTIAL EXPOSURES
1. Agriculture ("Migrant" workers' wives work in fields while pregnant and sustain work as long as able)	Multitude of substances and conditions, including physical and biologic. Excessive work hours; intermittent and prolonged heavy work. Chemicals, especially pesticides, herbicides, insecticides, solvents, dusts, fumes, gases, heat and high humidity, infections (bacterial, viral, rickettsial) and vibration (see Chapter 13)
2. Chemical and pharmaceutical production workers	
a. Concomitant exposures and physical stressors and possible synergistic effects are factors to be considered	See text
b. Ergonomic/biomechanic deficiencies (see Chapters 5 and 6)	See text
3. Cleaning personnel	
a. Launderers	Contaminated clothing, detergents, enzymes, soaps, heat, humidity
b. Dry cleaners	Contaminated clothing, heat, perchloroethylene, Stoddard solvent, naphtha, benzene, trichloroethylene and others
4. Clerical personnel	Carbon tetrachloride and various other cleaners, physical stresses, poor illumination, ergonomic deficiencies (see Chapters, 3, 4, 5 and 6)
5. Domestic workers (homes, hotels, motels, office buildings)	Alkalies, bleaches, detergents, heat, cold (physiologic factors), shift work, at times hard work, and various solvents in cleaning agents
6. Electronics assemblers	Antimony, epoxy resins, lead, methyl ethyl ketone, methylene chloride, tin, trichloroethylene and visual stresses and strain (see Chapter 6)
7. Hairdressers and cosmetologists	Acetone, aerosol propellents (freons), benzyl alcohol, ethyl alcohol, hair dyes, hair spray resins (polyvinylpyrrolidone), halogenated hydrocarbons and other solvents of a wide variety
8. Hospital/health personnel	
a. Registered nurses, aides, orderlies, physicians, students, patients	Alcohol, anesthetic gases, ethylene oxide, infectious diseases (bacterial and viral), puncture wounds and x-ray radiation.
b. Dental hygienists	Anesthetic gases, infectious diseases (bacterial and viral), mercury, puncture wounds, ultrasonic noise, vibration, and x-ray radiation

of lawyers and judges rose from 3% to 7%.[15] Given opportunities for training at all levels from apprenticeships in industry to education in the higher professions, it is expected that women will be moving into areas for the most part previously closed to them. With growth of child-care facilities there will be continued increasing participation in the labor force by women in the childbearing age groups.

Table 2–3 includes examples of occupations and their exposures in which significant numbers of women presently are represented in the work force.[17] No attempt will be made in this chapter to cover hazards associated with industries where the work force has been predominantly female but in which males can be expected to respond in similar ways, if similarly exposed. Most of the hazards associated with such industries—e.g., textile manufacture, laundries, food services, health services, and office workers—are covered elsewhere in this volume as well as in *Occupational Medicine: Principles and Practical Applications*, Carl Zenz (ed.) (Chicago: Year Book Medical Publishers, 1975).

This chapter will consider sex-related dif-

TABLE 2–3.—*Continued*

OCCUPATION	POTENTIAL EXPOSURES
c. Laboratory workers (clinical and research)	Infectious diseases (bacterial and viral), puncture wounds, wide variety of toxic chemicals, including carcinogens, mutagens and teratogens; and x-ray radiation. Many workers are subject to shift rotation (see Chapter 10)
9. Opticians and lens grinders	Coal tar, pitch, volatiles, hydrocarbons, iron oxide, other polishing and grinding dusts and solvents
10. Photographic processors	Bromides, caustics, iodides, iron salts, mercuric chloride, pyrogallic acid and silver nitrate
11. Plastic fabricators	Acids, acrylonitrile, alkalies, hexamethylenetetramine, peroxide, phenol formaldehydes, styrene, urea formaldehydes, vinyl chloride and vinylidene chloride. High heat and humidity
12. Printing operatives	Benzene, carbon tetrachloride, ink mists, lead, methanol, methylene chloride, microwave, 2-nitropropane, pigments, trace metals, toluene, and various solvents, including trichloroethylene; ultraviolet, microwave and other radiation sources. Noise and vibration
13. Sign painters and letterers	Epichlorohydrin, lead chromate pigments, lead oxide, toluene, trace metals and xylene. A wide diversity of other chemicals as solvents and strippers
14. Textile and related operatives	
a. Textile operatives	Asbestos, dyes, flame retardants, formaldehyde, heat, noise, raw cotton dust, synthetic fiber dusts
b. Sewers and stitchers	Asbestos, cotton and synthetic fiber dusts, flame retardants, formaldehyde, noise and organic solvents
c. Upholsterers	Same as above
(Some specific chemicals encountered in the above occupations are benzene, carbon disulfide, chloroprene, perchloroethylene, styrene, toluene and trichloroethylene)	
15. Transportation	
a. Bus, taxi, truck and other vehicle drivers b. Airlines	Carbon monoxide, polynuclear aromatics, lead and other combustion products of gasoline and jet fuels; circadian dysfunctions; heat; physical stresses; shift changes; and vibration (ultrasonic, noise and hypersonic) (see Chapters 7 and 10)

Adapted from Guidelines on Pregnancy and Work, Amer. College of Ob-Gyn, 1977.[17]

ferences between females and males in work capacities, responses to adverse conditions or substances in the work environment and the effects of exposure to chemical and physical agents on the pregnant woman and the fetus. The reproductive effects of chemicals on male workers also will be discussed where pertinent.

RESPONSE TO CHEMICALS

There have been a number of reports that women have a greater susceptibility than men to the effects of exposure to toxic substances in the work area. Among the specific exposures most often mentioned are lead and organic solvents. There is a dearth of information concerning studies of men and women with comparable occupational exposures to chemicals. This can be partially explained by the difficulty in obtaining adequate cohorts for study of women in jobs similar to those of men in industries where significant chemical and physical hazards exist. However, even where such working populations have existed, there has been little interest to stimulate such studies. Oliver's report[33] on women exposed to lead in the white lead industries and Hamilton's report[21] on women exposed to lead in the pottery and tile manufacturing industries are well known. One of the earliest reports of the hematologic effects of benzene exposure was made by Selling in 1916 on three young Maryland females exposed to a commercial grade of benzene used as a rubber solvent in sealing tin cans.[41] During World War II there were a considerable number of women in the work force who had significant toxic exposures, but these populations have never been investigated adequately.

In acute toxicity studies in mice and rats with oral administration of more than 200 chemical compounds, Krasovskij[27] concluded that differences in susceptibility between males and females are not very great. If the susceptibility of males were taken as unity, average values of the ratios were found to be 0.92 ± 0.058 and 0.88 ± 0.036 for female mice and rats, respectively. In some cases, males were more susceptible to the poisons tested. Studies with organophosphorus pesticides indicate the female rats to be more susceptible to some organophosphorus compounds whereas male rats are more susceptible to others.[12]

Of further interest is the report that male mice of certain strains are much more susceptible to the effects of chloroform than are female mice of the same strain.[50] The female mice show virtually no effect from chloroform exposure that is lethal to the males. Castration and administration of estrogens to the males will reduce the effect whereas administration of androgens to the females increases susceptibility.[12]

Ferguson,[12] in commenting on a review by Weston Hurst of some chemicals that have been found to be more toxic in females than in males, observes that in many of the examples, the effect occurs in a single species, and often in a particular strain of that species. He proposes that where differences in susceptibility have been suggested there is some correlation with the rate of metabolism by liver microsomal enzymes of the parent compounds and the relative toxicity of the parent substance and its metabolites. He believes that the most likely explanation for any sex-related differences in toxicity, if any exists, is that the enzymatic biotransformation of the toxicant is influenced by sex hormones. When the metabolites of chemicals are more toxic than their parent compounds, the male sex, with a more rapid rate of liver metabolism, is likely to be more susceptible. On the other hand, when the parent compound is more toxic than its metabolites, the male sex is likely to be more resistant. Since estrogens have a relatively lesser stimulating effect on liver metabolism than androgens, the female of the species might be expected, in general, to be more susceptible than males to those chemicals detoxified by such metabolism. As an example of this, Ferguson[12] cites the report by Hirakawa[23] of greater sensitivity of female rabbits than males to the effects of benzene, and the reduction of the relative resistance of males after castration.

In general, the animal data are limited, often conflicting and are difficult to relate to differences in susceptibility between men and women. Baetjer,[5] in 1946, made a critical review of the data on which conclusions were based that women were more susceptible than men to chemical exposures. She found that most of the statements were made on the basis of studies of small numbers of cases or on poorly designed studies without consideration being given to the extent and duration of exposure between men and women or, at times, by simple repeated quoting in the literature of statements made by one or two industrial health authorities. Sometimes statements were simply personal opinions. She found no significant basis for a conclusion that nonpregnant women were more susceptible than men to the effects of chemical exposure. It is noteworthy that very little new information has been added to the literature since her review.

LEAD.—Sir Thomas Oliver,[32] in the late nineteenth century, was a leading proponent for the abolition of female labor in the white beds, stoves and dusty processes of white lead manufacture in England. In discussing lead poisoning in that industry, he noted that "employers cannot be too frequently reminded that the susceptibility of females to lead poisoning is greater than that of males, and that the symptoms are usually of a graver character." He indicated that women are most likely to develop poisoning between the ages of 18 and 23 years, earlier than men and after shorter exposure. He described a greater number of cases of lead poisoning in women than in men admitted to the Royal Infirmary, Newcastle upon Tyne. When Baetjer[5] compared her data to the number of males and females employed in the lead industry in the particular town during the same periods, she did not find any differences in the incidence of severe lead poisoning in the two sexes. Of note is that Oliver went on to say that "apart from the influence of sex, women's wages are smaller, and they are therefore less able, if fighting the battle alone, to obtain proper food, which is a protection to some extent against plumbism." In addition, he added that "there is not the least doubt that females had been employed in larger numbers than males in the dangerous processes."[32] From the information presented by Oliver himself, factors other than possible differences in susceptibility between the sexes, such as socioeconomic status and degree of exposure, should be considered for possible explanations for any excess in the number of cases of lead poisoning that might have existed in women in the white lead industry in England at the time of his report. After women were eliminated from the heavy exposure, the incidence of lead intoxication decreased in females and increased in males. The exclusion of women in that industry is a classic example of the emphasis for reducing occupational diseases being placed on a specific group of workers rather than on control of the environment.

Oliver[33] also reported that there was a greater incidence of lead "encephalopathy" in women with severe lead poisoning than in men. A similar finding was reported by Prendergast[36] in his review of workers with severe lead poisoning, where he found an incidence of 34.9% "encephalopathy" in women as compared to 15.0% in men. Blindness was also more common in women and "paralysis" was present in 30% of females and 59% of males. In 1975, Seppäläinen et al.[42] reported more abnormal values in the sensory conduction velocities of the ulnar and median nerves, with lower blood lead values in female than in male lead storage battery workers, although the number of female subjects was too small to be conclusive.

In Baetjer's review[5] of the U. S. Public Health Service Study of the pottery industry, she found that where there were adequate numbers of men and women workers with similar exposures, the women had a slightly lower rate of presumptive cases of lead poisoning. Hamilton's study[21] of the pottery industry showed varying results, depending on socioeconomic status. In whiteware potteries, where women had a much lower socioeconomic status than men, the rate of lead poisoning was 4.9% for men and 19.3% for women. In the tile workers, where men and women were of equal socioeconomic status, the male rate was 15.8% and the female was 11.5%. Regardless, Hamilton believed that women were more susceptible to lead than were men.

TABLE 2–4.—BLOOD LEAD LEVELS IN ADULT MEN AND WOMEN WITH SIMILAR EXPOSURES

BLOOD LEAD LEVEL (μg/100 gm)		PERCENTAGE INCREASE IN MALE COMPARED TO FEMALE BLOOD LEAD LEVEL
Male	*Female*	
17.2	14.9	15%
19.9	12.4	60%
24.0	18.0	33%
19.0	15.0	27%
16.6	10.6	57%
16.6	12.9	29%
18.5	14.7	26%
11.8	9.1	30%
13.0	9.3	40%
14.4	10.9	24%
19.0	14.9	28%
23.7	19.2	23%
22.7	16.7	36%
16.0	9.9	62%
17.0	12.7	34%
20.6	12.7	62%
40.9	30.4	35%

Source: Bridbord, K.: Occupational lead exposure and women, Prev. Med. 7:311, 1978.

Several reports indicate that, with comparable exposure, women have lower blood and urine lead levels than do men. Table 2–4 shows the mean blood lead levels by sex of varying populations exposed to similar environmental conditions. In the reports, all blood leads of males were higher than those of females, averaging more than 30% higher. Although these studies do not generally include comprehensive assessments of exposure that could explain some of the differences, nevertheless, the consistent pattern in Table 2–4 is of interest. Similarly, Table 2–5 indicates mean urine and blood lead levels by sex with varying degrees of exposure. At any level of exposure, the mean lead levels in both blood and urine were lower in females than in males. Explanations for these differences were not offered. Roels et al.[38] studied the responses of various biologic parameters of the heme synthesis pathway in a group of male and female workers moderately exposed to inorganic lead with the identical range of blood lead levels in both groups. The women exhibited a larger increase in free erythrocyte protoporphyrin (FEP) and in delta-aminolevulinic acid than did men. Also, Stuik and Zielhuis[45] reported on male and female volunteers who ingested 20 mg lead acetate daily for 3 weeks. The increase in protoporphyrin IX in the erythrocytes of women was significant as compared with men whereas the blood lead level was consistently lower in women (30 μg/100 ml) than in men (40μg/100 ml).

The differences in clinical response in the presence of lower blood and urine lead levels in women suggest that women may have a different distribution of lead in the body and perhaps even different target organs for lead effects than do men. However, the interpretation of these findings is not clear at this time, and it is difficult to relate them to clinically significant effects at the lower levels of exposure in the current OSHA lead standards.[9]

ORGANIC SOLVENTS.—Reports that women are more susceptible than men to the effects of organic solvents, particularly benzene (benzol), are conflicting and often

ber[19] found a greater incidence of lung cancer in men than in women among nonsmokers. These authors suggest that the sex difference in incidence of lung cancer probably is due to a steroidal factor rather than the amount of intake of carcinogen. Occupational exposure to carcinogens in jobs traditionally held by men may also contribute to the difference in lung cancer rates between men and women.

In summary, there is little evidence to suggest that the nonpregnant woman is more sensitive to the effects of toxic chemicals than is her male counterpart. While physiologic distinctions exist that could account for differences in susceptibility between males and females to certain exposures, there is no available evidence to suggest that the differences in susceptibility between the male and the nonpregnant female worker are sufficient at existing or proposed levels of exposure to be a present consideration in the occupational placement of women workers. Nonetheless, well-controlled, well-designed epidemiologic studies of cohorts of male and female populations equally exposed to low levels of toxic chemicals and physical agents should be a priority in order to provide the data to make this conclusion a certainty for the benefit of all workers.

TOLERANCE TO HEAT

Women are considered to tolerate heat less well than do men. In the 1972 NIOSH Criteria Document on working in hot environments, the proposed work standards included a lower maximal permissible environmental heat stress for unacclimatized women than for men, i.e., 79°F WBGT for men and 76°F WBGT for women (25.5°C and 24.4°C).[8]

As reported in the Criteria Document, some rest-in-heat and work-in-heat studies have indicated that women do not adjust to heat extremes as well as do men. Based on the usual methods of measuring physiologic stress from heat, women showed higher skin temperatures and pulse rates and lower sweating rates than did men exposed to the same environmental stresses. But other reports have not agreed with these findings. Weinman et al.[49] stated that their studies on men and women using treadmills in a hot environment revealed higher sweat rates in males but lower pulse rates and core temperatures in females who were physically fitter than the men. Wyndham et al.[51] tested women and men who were unacclimatized to work in a hot, moist environment. Females tolerated the heat less well than did the males and showed higher core temperatures and pulse rates but less sweating. Morimoto et al.[30] found no differences in sweat rates of men and women working in a hot, dry environment, but when relative humidity was increased to 80%, the sweat rate in women increased significantly less than in the men but core and skin temperatures remained equal.

Physiologic differences between the sexes in response to heat stress is suggested, but the evidence so far is not conclusive. Both men and women develop acclimatization to heat stress approximately well.[11] Fitness of individuals appears to play an equally important role. The important factor after acclimatization and fitness is the proportion of maximal capacity that a particular work load has for a particular individual, whether male or female. A person of relatively small work capacity obviously will be using more reserve capacity at a given work load than will a larger and stronger person, and will show appropriate physiologic response to such stresses—pulse, temperature, ventilation, cardiac output. If there are basic physiologic differences in heat response between the sexes, such differences probably are small and may not be sufficient to affect medical recommendations about job placement. Fortunately, there are relatively few jobs in our society that involve both strenuous physical stress and high thermal stress. Whether male or female, to be successful in such jobs, a person will have to achieve acclimatization to heat and have above-average maximal aerobic work capacity, which is based mainly on height, weight, and fitness.

AEROBIC CAPACITY AND PHYSICAL STRENGTH

Reports in the scientific literature on physical strength comparisons of men and women indicate that, on the average, women have about two-thirds the physical strength of men[6, 44] (Fig. 2–1).

This is of interest to those who work in job and equipment design, especially for jobs that are likely to be filled predominantly by one sex. However, the same reports indicate an appreciable overlap in individual measurements, and there are some women who have more physical strength

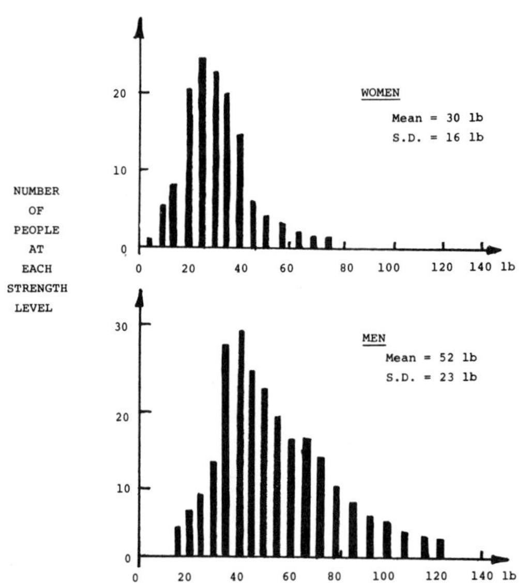

Fig 2–1.—Lifting strengths demonstrated by employees in standard position strength testing. (From Chaffin, D. B., Biomechanics of Manual Materials Handling and Low-Back Pain, in Zenz, C. [ed.], *Occupational Medicine: Principles and Practical Applications* [Chicago: Year Book Medical Publishers, 1975], p. 462.)

than do some men. This is of interest to occupational health practitioners, who must evaluate *individuals* for jobs.

Asmussen and Heeboll-Nielsen[2] reported studies that showed that isometric strength of 25 different muscle groups were maximal in women at about age 20 and in men at about age 30. There was a gradual but slow decrease in strength with increasing age, with a more rapid decrease in women than in men after age 40. Aerobic capacity also decreased with age in both sexes. Absolute values for women averaged about two-thirds those of men at all ages tested. Similar results were reported by Åstrand,[4] who measured maximal aerobic capacity in liters O_2/min using a bicycle ergometer and correlated this with heart rate. The correlations were good and both were highest at about age 20 and declined gradually with increasing age. Mean oxygen uptake was 3.6 l/min for men and 2.7 for women. Fitness and size of the individual were responsible for most of the variation. Measurements of work production at normal jobs and usual pace of work revealed that construction workers worked at about 40% of maximal aerobic capacity and any increase above this level resulted in unacceptable fatigue.

Work capacity during various phases of the menstrual cycle in women with dysmenorrhea was tested by Gamberale et al.[14] by use of bicycle ergometers and a number of mental ability tests. Differences were minimal or none. There were no differences sufficient to affect medical recommendations about job placement. Of course, such tests are not the same as productive work at actual jobs, but rather are tests of physiologic and psychologic capacity for short periods of time in well-motivated women.

Guzman and Caplan[18] studied 8 healthy pregnant women monthly to term for cardiorespiratory response to bicycle exercise. Control studies were done 3 months post partum. They found oxygen consumption for a given work load to be similar at each stage of pregnancy and in the control period. But at each work load, ventilation, heart rate, cardiac output and stroke volume were all higher and AV oxygen differences lower during pregnancy. The rate of increase of these parameters per unit increase in work was the same in the pregnant and nonpregnant states. Also, the increases in cardiovascular dynamics were well established by the end of the first trimester and did not change appreciably during the remaining pregnancy. This latter is in contrast to the belief that blood volume increases gradually throughout pregnancy.

Pernoll et al.[34,35] studied oxygen consumption and ventilation in 12 normal women during and after pregnancy, using a bicycle ergometer for exercise so as to minimize the differences in weight in the pregnant state. Oxygen consumption at rest and exercise was greater during pregnancy than 3 months post partum, the increase being gradual throughout pregnancy. Ventilation also showed a gradual increase throughout pregnancy due to a greater tidal volume. Oxygen debt was greater from exercise during pregnancy than 3 months post partum. The reports by Pernoll et al. thus are different from those by Guzman and Caplan in regard to oxygen consumption during various stages of pregnancy. Pernoll et al. concluded that there is a slightly decreased efficiency of muscular exercise during pregnancy, but were unable to offer an explanation.

All of the physiologic studies were made under laboratory conditions that differed from actual work situations. The differences between individuals appear to be of greater importance than the differences between the sexes. But the averages of strength and aerobic capacity cannot be totally ignored. At work with moderate or greater physical strength requirements, there probably will be a greater proportion of women than men who lack the physical capacities required. The data quoted above indicate that an individual might be expected to perform satisfactorily if placed at a job in which the physical work requirements were about 40% or less of his/her maximal aerobic capacity. Measuring the physical work requirements of jobs and expressing them in kilocalories/minute, kilopondmeters (kpm) or other units is not easy, but can be done. An approximation might be satisfactory after measuring certain tasks for job components common to several jobs. Measuring the maximal aerobic capacity also is not easy but can be done. Much experience has been accumulated in estimating the maximal aerobic work capacity, and this is less difficult. Maximal aerobic capacity often is estimated by utilizing submaximal exercise and relating heart rate to amount of work done, with results expressed in ml O_2/kg body weight/minute. These units are a measure of fitness but do not represent the actual physical capacity, as the latter varies directly with body weight and height. Therefore, l/min O_2 uptake may be a better method to express the physical work capacity of an individual.

The work measurements and tests referred to generally have been limited to the laboratory. One of the reasons for this is that such measurements are expensive and time-consuming and require highly trained individuals to carry them out. Another practical reason is that work performance in most jobs may depend more on motivation and learning ability than on physical strength, plus many other quite subtle factors that are nearly impossible to measure. Improved mechanization of work tasks has taken away much of the sustained heavy work, but there remain many jobs requiring intermittent heavy exertion. This is discussed further in the chapter on preplacement examinations and recommendations (Chapter 4). Certain occupational ergonomic deficiencies are discussed in Chapter 5.

REFERENCES

1. Altman, P. L., and Dittmer, D. S. (eds.): Biology Data Book, Vol. III, Section XI, 2d ed., p. 1528 (Bethesda, Md.: Federation of American Societies for Experimental Biology, 1974) (cited in Ferguson[12]).
2. Asmussen, E., and Heeboll-Nielsen, K.: Isometric muscle strength in relation to age in men and women, Ergonomics 5:167, 1962.
3. Åstrand, I.: Aerobic work capacity—its relation to age, sex, and other factors, Circ. Res., Supp. I, Vol. XX, March, 1967.
4. Åstrand, I.: Aerobic work capacity in men and women with special reference to age, Acta Physiol. Scand. 49(Supp. 169):1, 1969.
5. Baetjer, A.: *Women in Industry, Their Health and Efficiency* (Philadelphia: W. B. Saunders Company, 1946), pp. 145–156.
6. Chaffin, D. B.: Human strength capability and low back pain, J. Occup. Med. 16:248, 1974.
7. Chaffin, D. B., et al.: Pre-employment strength testing in selecting workers for material handling jobs, University of Michigan NIOSH (CDC–74–62) 1976.
8. Criteria for a recommended standard . . . occupational exposure to hot environments, DHEW, PHS, NIOSH 72-10269, 1972.
9. Occupational Safety and Health Admin., U.S. Dept. of Labor: Occupational exposure to lead, final standard, U.S. Fed. Reg. 43:52952, Nov. 14, 1978.
10. Doll, R., Payne, P., and Waterhouse, J.: In *Cancer, Incidence in Five Continents* (Berlin and New York: Springer-Verlag, 1966) (cited in Ferguson[12]).
11. Drinkwater, B. L.: Physiological Responses of Women to Exercise, in Wilmore, J. H. (ed.), *Exercise and Sport Sciences Reviews* (New York: Academic Press, 1973).
12. Ferguson, D. M.: Toxicological Problems Related to the Employment of Women, in *Health of Women at Work,* Proceedings of Symposium of Society of Occupational Medicine Research Panel, R. Soc. Med., London, England, pp. 41–52, 1976.
13. Firminger, H. I., and Reuber, M. D.: Influence of adrenocortical, androgenic, and anabolic hormones on the development of carcinoma and cirrhosis of the liver in AXC rats fed N–2–fluorenyldiacetamide, J. Natl. Cancer Inst. 27:559, 1961 (cited in Toh[47]).
14. Gamberale, F., Strindberg, L., and Wahlberg, I.: Female work capacity during the menstrual cycle, Scand. J. Work Environ. Health 1:120, 1975.
15. Garfinkle, S. H.: Occupations of women and black workers, 1962–74, Monthly Labor Review, U. S. Dept. of Labor, Bureau of Labor Statistics, p. 29, 1975.
16. Grossman, A. S.: Women in the labor force: The early years, Monthly Labor Review, U.S. Dept. of Labor, Bureau of Labor Statistics, pp. 3–9, 1975.
17. Guidelines on Pregnancy and Work, American College of Ob-Gyn., Chicago, 1977.
18. Guzman, C. A., and Caplan, R.: Cardiorespiratory response to exercise during pregnancy, Am. J. Obstet. Gynecol. 108:600, 1970.
19. Haenszel, W., and Taeuber, K. E.: Lung cancer mortality as related to residence and smoking histories. II. White females, J. Natl. Cancer Inst. 32:803, 1968 (cited in Toh[47]).
20. Hamilton, A.: *Industrial Toxicology* (New York: Haifer & Bros. Publ., 1934), p. xv.
21. Hamilton, A.: Lead poisoning in potteries and tile works, U. S. Dept. of Labor, Bureau of Labor Statistics, Bull. #104, 1912.
22. Henschel, A.: Women in Industry—The Difference, Transactions of the 33d Meeting of the American Conference of Governmental Industrial Hygienists, Toronto, Canada, pp. 73–76, 1971.
23. Hirakawa, T.: Some observations on benzene poisoning, Arch. Mal. Prof. 21:46, 1960 (cited in Browning, E., *Toxicity and Metabolism of Industrial Solvents* [London: Elsevier Publishing Co., 1965]).
24. Hirakawa, T.: Studies on poisoning by benzol and its homologues, Jpn. J. Med. Sci. Biol. 8:275, 1955 (cited in Browning, E., *Toxicity and Metabolism of Industrial Solvents* [London: Elsevier Publishing Co., 1965]).
25. Hunter, T.: Chronic exposure to benzene (benzol). II. The clinical effects, J. Ind. Hyg. Toxicol. 21:331, 1939.
26. Klein, D. P.: Women in the labor force: The middle years, Monthly Labor Review, U. S. Dept. of Labor, Bureau of Labor Statistics, pp. 10–16, 1975.
27. Krasovskij, G. N.: Species and Sex Differences in Sensitivity to Toxic Substances, in Methods Used in the USSR for Establishing Biologically Safe Levels of Toxic Substances, WHO, Geneva, Switzerland, pp. 109–125, 1975.

28. Lee, S. H., and Ts'o, T. O. T.: Histological typing of lung cancers in Hong Kong, Br. J. Cancer 17:37, 1963 (cited in Toh[47]).
29. Leuchtenberger, C., et al.: Cytological and cytochemical alterations in the respiratory tract of mice after exposure to cigarette smoke, influenza, virus, and both, Cancer Res. 23:555, 1963 (cited in Toh[47]).
30. Morimoto, T., Slabachova, Z., Naman, R. K., and Sargent, F.: Sex differences in physiological reactions to thermal stress, J. Appl. Physiol. 22:526, 1967.
31. Morris, H. P., and Firminger, H. I.: Influence of sex and sex hormones on development of hepatomas and other hepatic lesions in strain AXC rats ingesting 2-diacetylaminofluoramide, J. Natl. Cancer Inst. 16:927, 1956 (cited in Toh[47]).
32. Oliver, T.: *Diseases of Occupation* (New York: E. P. Dutton Co., 1908).
33. Oliver, T.: Lead poisoning and the racer, Br. Med. J. 1:1096, 1911.
34. Pernoll, M. L., et al.: Ventilation during rest and exercise during pregnancy and postpartum, Respir. Physiol. 25:295, 1975.
35. Pernoll, M. L., et al.: Oxygen consumption at rest and during exercise in pregnancy, Respir. Physiol. 25:285, 1975.
36. Prendergast, W. D.: The classification of the symptoms of lead poisoning, Br. Med. J. 1:1164, 1910.
37. Purchase, I. F. H., and Steyn, M.: The metabolism of aflatoxin B in rats, Br. J. Cancer 23:800, 1969 (cited in Toh[47]).
38. Roels, H. A., Lauwerys, R. R., Buchet, J. P., and Vrelust, M-Th.: Response of free erythrocyte porphyrin and urinary delta-aminolevulinic acid in men and women moderately exposed to lead, Int. Arch. Arbeitsmed. 34:97, 1975.
39. Sato, A., Nakajima, T., Fujiwara, T., and Hirosawa, K.: Pharmacokinetics of benzene and toluene, Int. Arch. Arbeitsmed. 33:169, 1974 (cited in Ferguson[12]).
40. Savilahti, M.: More than 100 cases of benzene poisoning in a shoe factory, Arch. Gerwerbepathol. Gewerbehyg. 15:145, 1956 (translation).
41. Selling, L.: Benzol as a leucotoxin—studies on the degeneration and regeneration of the blood and hematopoietic organs, Johns Hopkins Hosp. Rep. 17:83, 1916.
42. Seppäläinen, A. M., Tola, S., Hernberg, S., and Koch, B.: Subclinical neuropathy at "safe" levels of lead exposure, Arch. Environ. Health 30:180, 1975.
43. Shinton, N. K.: Differences in biological characteristics of various histological types of lower respiratory tract tumours, Br. J. Cancer 17:222, 1963 (cited in Toh[47]).
44. Snook, S. H., and Ciriello, V. M.: Maximum weights and work loads acceptable to female workers, J. Occup. Med. 16:527, 1974. 1974.
45. Stuik, E. J., and Zielhuis, R. L.: Increased Susceptibility of Females to Inorganic Lead, in Recent Advances in the Assessment of the Health Effects of Environmental Pollution, Commission of the European Communities, Luxembourg, pp. 537–541, 1975.
46. Sum, A. M.: Female labor force participation: Why projections have been too low, Monthly Labor Review, U. S. Dept. of Labor, Bureau of Labor Statistics, pp. 18–24, 1977.
47. Toh, Y.C.: Physiological and biochemical reviews of sex differences and carcinogenesis with particular reference to the liver, Adv. Cancer Res. 18:209, 1973.
48. Waldman, E., and McEaddy, B. J.: Where women work—an analysis by industry and occupation, Monthly Labor Review, U. S. Dept. of Labor, Bureau of Labor Statistics, pp. 3–13, 1974.
49. Weinman, K. P., et al.: Reactions of men and women to repeated exposure to humid heat, J. Appl. Physiol. 22:533, 1967.
50. Weston Hurst, E.: Sexual Difference in the Toxicity and Therapeutic Amount of Chemical Substances, in Walpole, A. L., and Spinks, A. (eds.), *Symposium on the Evaluation of Drug Toxicity* (London: J. & A. Churchill, Ltd., 1958), pp. 12–25 (cited in Ferguson[12]).
51. Wyndham, C. H., Morrison, J. F., and Williams, C. G.: Heat reactions of male and female Caucasians, J. Appl. Physiol. 20:357, 1965.

3 / Reproductive Toxicology and Occupational Exposure

JACQUELINE MESSITE, M.D., and MARCUS B. BOND, M.D.

RESEARCH in occupational safety and health has not adequately focused attention on the effect of occupational exposure to chemical and physical agents on the reproductive system of either men or women.[7] This has resulted in a dearth of information to assist the occupational physician and the obstetrician in advising workers and management of the potentially deleterious effects of various agents on reproduction. Furthermore, the existing data base on the reproductive effects of occupational toxins is inadequate to serve as a guideline for the establishment of occupational health standards. With few exceptions, current standards for occupational exposures to chemical and physical agents in the work environment do not consider the reproductive effects, including mutagenesis, teratogenesis and transplacental carcinogenesis.

The reproductive concerns, when addressed, have for the most part focused attention only on the woman's reproductive capacity and on the developmental effects in offspring solely from maternal exposures. Such a limited view fails to recognize that there are a large number of female workers of reproductive capacity who are not pregnant or currently planning pregnancy, and, in addition, it does not consider the role of paternal exposure to such agents in the causation of reproductive abnormalities.

The reproductive capacity of women workers generally is in the age range of 15–45 years. During this century, most childbearing ends by the age of 35,[12] and there are many years of work outside the home for women still of childbearing capacity. According to the National Center of Health Statistics,[7] of about 3,034,000 women who had a live birth during a 12-month period in 1972–1973, an estimated 1,260,000 women (41.5%) worked during their pregnancy. This 41.5%, however, represented only about 8.8% of the estimated 14,357,000 ever-married women of reproductive age in the labor force at the time.[7] Even if another 30% are added to include women workers whose pregnancies may not result in live births, it is clear that the number of women of childbearing age who are pregnant or who are planning pregnancies at any one time is relatively small in comparison to the total number of such women available for participation in the work force. Any sweeping policy excluding women of childbearing capacity from any particular employment is not only discriminatory but does not allow for the participation by women workers, in cooperation with the occupational physicians, in the decision-making process concerning their employment, and also needlessly eliminates from consideration a large number of productive employees.

Many women now are employed in jobs that present no greater potential hazards than those normally encountered at home or in the community. However, a sizable number of women are presently employed in positions with significant exposures in work environments that often are not appreciated as being hazardous; e.g., laboratories and health services, electronics industry and dry-cleaning establishments. In addition, there is the potential that many more women may seek employment in nontraditional, hazardous jobs and, as such, they require special consideration.

A second area that needs to be emphasized is that concern for healthy offspring must include concern for paternal as well as maternal exposure. The role of paternal exposure in producing adverse effects on reproduction has been highlighted recently in studies of worker populations exposed to such substances as vinyl chloride and dibromochloropropane (discussed later in this chapter). Further studies may well disclose other similarly noxious agents in the work environment to which males are susceptible.

Table 3-1 is a graphic representation of some highlights to be considered in a brief review of the dynamics of reproductive toxicology pertinent to this subject.

PRECONCEPTION (GAMETOGENESIS AND FERTILIZATION).—A chemical substance or physical agent may act directly on the germ cells so that fertilization does not take place or it may cause such severe anomalies in the zygote as to result in an early unrecognized abortion. There are only a few reports of parental exposures related to either outcome, although the risk is recognized.[13] It is during this preconception period that paternal exposure to mutagenic agents must be considered along with maternal exposure, for both, collectively or independently, may result in the inhibition of fertilization, impaired placental implantations, spontaneous abortion or the production of abnormal embryos.

An unpublished NIOSH Interagency Report of a Work Group on Occupational Mutagenesis, Teratogenesis and Transplacental Carcinogenesis, in November, 1976,[10] reported that, "it is difficult to anticipate the relative sensitivity to germinal mutagenic events in men compared to non-pregnant women. Depending on the action of a particular chemical, the expected effects will differ depending on the sex of the exposed individual. Spermatogenesis involves a con-

TABLE 3–1.—DYNAMICS OF REPRODUCTIVE TOXICOLOGY

	STAGES OF PREGNANCY			
	PRECONCEPTION	INTRAUTERINE DEVELOPMENT		PERINATAL PERIOD
Stages of development	Gametes (sperm, ova)	1st trimester Embryo	2d trimester 3d trimester Fetus	Infant
Vulnerable areas	Spermatogenesis Oogenesis Fertilization	Organogenesis (primarily 1st trimester)	Central nervous system late	Lactation
Major developmental effects (nature of exposure)	Mutagenesis (acute or chronic)	Teratogenesis (primarily 1st trimester) (Acute)	Transplacental carcinogenesis (chronic primarily)	
Adverse manifestations	Sterility Decreased fertility Chromosomal aberrations	Implantation defects Spontaneous abortion	Premature delivery	Stillbirth Structural, behavioral or functional alterations
Parental source of exposure	Maternal and paternal		Maternal	Maternal (lactation) Paternal and maternal (home contamination)

tinuously replicating cell population with billions of cells; oogenesis is a prenatal event in mammals, and the female germ cell population is finite at birth with no further replication. Therefore, chemicals whose mechanisms of toxicity depend upon cell division would have their greatest effects in the adult on the male germ cells; chemicals affecting non-replicating cells might have their greatest effect on the limited oocyte population. Chemical exposure which decreases the total number of germ cells would also have a more prominent effect on the female since damaged cells are not replaced as in a male." Unfortunately, our state of knowledge generally is inadequate to define the mechanism of chemical mutagenesis as it relates to male and female cells. Thus both sexes must be considered at risk from mutagenic hazards.

Most anomalous conceptions, including 95% of those with chromosomal abnormalities, rarely go to term and therefore are concentrated among spontaneous abortions. Anomalies are about 60–100 times more frequent in spontaneous abortions than in live births.[5] Errors during early intrauterine development have variously been estimated to produce a pregnancy loss in the human from 15% to 40%.[9,11,14] Serious defects can be detected in about 3% of newborn babies, but the number gradually rises to about 8%, including children during the first 10 years of age.[9,11] Up to 6% of these birth defects are due to known environmental agents, and at least 20–30% have a major genetic etiology.[9] The remaining birth defects are of unknown causes and, therefore, future research into environmental components may further our awareness of these components as causes for such occurrences and in suggesting preventive measures. Some of the causes undoubtedly will be found in the occupational environment.

POSTCONCEPTION—MATERNAL ORGANISM.—The maternal organism, in some ways, may be more vulnerable during pregnancy. There are alterations in detoxification mechanisms and metabolic pathways and also there may be unusual dietary habits.[8] In addition, there are physiologic changes in blood volumes and composition, as well as alterations in lung function, the nature of which could result in increased absorption of air contaminants, particularly those that follow the inhalation route.[4]

As noted in Chapter 2, there is a progressive increase in ventilation during pregnancy due mostly to an increase in tidal volume. There is also a decrease in arteriovenous oxygen differences, as reported by Guzman and Caplan.[3] This could mean that a pregnant woman uses a portion of respiratory and cardiovascular reserve in the pregnancy itself and, therefore, could have a reduced capacity for additional stresses. Physical factors of shift in center of gravity and resulting alterations in posture and progressively increasing weight could contribute to reduced abilities to perform physically demanding tasks. However, the Guidelines on Pregnancy and Work, quoted in Chapter 4, indicated that women usually have no problems continuing with work that is usual for them but may have problems adjusting to different or increased physical tasks.

In regard to increased ventilation and possible increased absorption of air contaminants, there is inadequate information on which to draw any firm conclusions. Existing Standards (TLV) should have sufficient margin of safety so that this is not a problem.

EMBRYO.—During the first week following fertilization, even before placental implantation, embryotoxic agents absorbed by the mother can reach the free-lying blastocyst very rapidly, and the clearance rate from the blastocyst of maternally transmitted agents is lower than their elimination rate from the maternal peripheral fluids.[15]

The 1st trimester, particularly the first 8-week period of embryonic organogenesis, is the time of greatest susceptibility to environmental influences, and the majority of teratologic effects are induced during this period. The drug thalidomide is a well-documented example of a substance that produces its effects only during this critical period.[6] In almost every case, the embryo is more sensitive to toxins than is the maternal organism. This is attributed to more rapid cell turnover by the embryo and fetus, their relative lack of detoxification mechanisms and their immature biologic barriers.

FETUS.—From 8 weeks to term, the fetus, generally considered less vulnerable than the embryo but more susceptible than the child or adult, is subject to adverse influences that possibly could lead to physical growth retardation and postnatal behavioral and functional abnormalities. Battaglia[1] notes that the 2d trimester is a time of rapid fetal growth, when the placental blood flow reaches its maximum and the delivery of substances to the fetus can be very high. In general, susceptibility to teratogens decreases with gestational age whereas susceptibility of the fetus to transplacental carcinogenesis tends to increase. As for agents requiring metabolic transformation before exerting carcinogenic effects, the fetus appears to be most vulnerable to them just prior to term.[2]

PERINATAL PERIOD—INFANT.—Certain developmental processes are not completed until after birth (e.g., physical growth, structural and physiologic maturation of the central nervous system and some of the endocrine glands) and may be adversely affected by environmental exposures during this period.[7] In addition, immediately following delivery, the immature metabolic system of the infant may be unable to cope with some environmental agents, thus making the infant more susceptible to their effects.

Furthermore, exposure of the infant during this period may occur from contamination of the home by the working father or mother, or from contamination of the milk in lactation. Maternal exposure to chemicals may alter the amount of lactation and the quality of the milk. Also, some chemicals may be excreted in the milk, resulting in direct exposure of the infant to potentially dangerous substances (e.g., lead, mercury, polychlorinated biphenyls) (see discussion of specific substances).

REFERENCES

1. Battaglia, F. C.: The susceptibility of the fetus and child to chemical pollutants. Perinatal effects of chemical pollutants: Suggested studies, Pediatrics 53:838, 1974.
2. Bridbord, K.: Occupational safety and health and the reproductive process: Oral presentation at Meeting of Organization Research Counselors, Arlington, Va., May 2, 1978.
3. Guzman, C. A., and Caplan, R.: Cardiorespiratory response to exercise during pregnancy, Am. J. Obstet. Gynecol. 108:600, 1970.
4. Hunt, V.: Pregnancy. Occupational Safety and Health Symposia, 1976, NIOSH Publication #77-179, July, 1977.
5. Kline, J., et al.: Surveillance of spontaneous abortions, Am. J. Epidemiol. 106:345, 1977.
6. Lenz, W., and Knapp, K.: Fetal malformations due to thalidomide, Ger. Med. Mon. 7:253, 1962 (cited in Strobino et al.[13])
7. National Center for Health Statistics, U.S. Dept. of HEW: Statistics needed for determining the effects of the environment on health, HRA 77:1457, July, 1977.
8. National Center for Health Statistics, U.S. Dept. of HEW: Advance Data, Pregnant Workers in the U.S., Sept. 15, 1977.
9. NIH, U.S. Dept. of HEW, PHS: Human Health and the Environment—Some Research Needs—2nd Task Force for Research Planning in Environmental Health Science, Publication #NIH 77-1277, 1977.
10. NIOSH Interagency Report of Work Group on Occupational Mutagenesis, Teratogenesis, Transplacental Carcinogenesis, 1977 (unpublished).
11. Shepard, T. H., and Miller, J. R.: Methods for detecting teratogenic agents in man, Environ. Health Perspect. 13:141, 1976.
12. Stellman, J.: *Women's Work, Women's Health, Myths and Realities* (New York: Pantheon Books, 1977).
13. Strobino, B. R., Kline, J., and Stein, Z.:

Chemical and Physical Exposures of Parents: Effects on Human Reproduction and Offspring. Early Human Development. (Amsterdam: Elsevier-North-Holland Biomedical Press, 1978).
14. Manson, J. M.: Human and laboratory animal test systems available for detection of reproductive failure, Prev. Med. 7:322, 1978.
15. Lutwak-Mann, C.: Drugs and the Blastocyst, in Boréus, L. (ed.), *Fetal Pharmacology* (New York: Raven Press, 1973).

REPRODUCTIVE EFFECTS FROM SELECTED OCCUPATIONAL EXPOSURES

Table 3–2 is a list of some of the reproductive toxins that can be found in the work environment. The substances listed are those reported to have significant reproductive effects in animals and/or humans. It is predictable that more substances will be added as further research in this area is performed. Additional information on mutagenesis, teratogenesis and carcinogenesis useful for the occupational health physician can be found in the NIOSH Registry of Toxic Effects of Chemical Substances, NIOSH Criteria Documents and in NIOSH Current Intelligence Bulletins. Substances that have been found to be mutagenic only in microbiologic systems and/or in DNA studies have not been included in this chapter. Although such findings are helpful in screening for carcinogens (which probably are related to mutagens), the findings solely in these screening tests can be regarded as suspicious, but at this time do not provide sufficient information to serve as a basis for judging the safety of occupational exposures or in predicting reproductive effects from the occupational environment.

The discussion in this chapter is essentially limited to the reproductive effects of these agents. Information on their general toxicity may be found elsewhere in this volume as well as in *Occupational Medicine: Principles and Practical Applications*, Carl Zenz (ed.) (Chicago: Year Book Medical Publishers, 1975).

Lead

FEW SUBSTANCES have received as much attention in regard to reproductive effects as has lead. Lead has long been known as an abortifacient[18, 19] and, more recently, lead has been associated with premature deliveries and premature rupture of the membranes, even at relatively low maternal and fetal blood lead levels.[9] The reaction to the early reports of the effects on reproduction essentially ignored effects on men. In England, women were not permitted employment in the English potteries and white lead industries. The response to more recent reports of the adverse reproductive effects on both men and women workers continues to focus on the women lead workers, and the inadequate data have resulted in conflicting opinions as to the placement of women workers in lead operations. Greater cognizance and concern for the reproductive effects of lead exposure in male workers must be set forth and this aspect of the problem clarified.

Lead compounds readily pass the placental barrier and levels of lead in the fetal tissues correlate well with that of the mother. Some studies indicate fetal blood levels lower than that of the mother, but this is not a consistent finding.[3, 9–11] Regardless, embryonic and other rapidly growing tissues are more vulnerable to lead than are adult tissues and, therefore, levels of lead producing adverse effects in the embryo probably are lower than those producing adverse effects in adults.

Lead is known to be present in milk of lactating mothers who have been exposed, so further exposure to newborns is possible

TABLE 3–2.—Reproductive Effects—A Summary

Agent	Systemic Effects*: Neurologic	Hepatic	Renal	Hematologic	Cardiovascular	Pulmonary	Other Special Effects	Suggested Biologic Testing	Carcinogenesis	Parental Exposure	Decreased Fertility (Includes Decreased Spermatogenesis)†	Mutagenesis (Chromosomal Aberration)	Spontaneous Abortion	Low Birth Weight (Premature)
Heavy Metals Lead (inorganic)	+		+					Blood lead Blood zinc protoporphyrins Urine ALA Urine coproporphyrins		Maternal	+1 +4	+7	+1 +2 +8	+
										Paternal	+1 +5 +10	+7	+1 +8	+ + +
Cadmium		+	+	+	+	+		Urine cadmium Low molecular weight proteins in urine	? Prostate	Maternal	+1 +3 −8	+9 −10 −11	−8	+ + +
										Paternal	+1 (testicular damage) −2	−12		
Mercury	+		+					Blood mercury Urine mercury		Maternal	?2	microbiologic +5, +6		+
										Paternal	−7 −8 ?11 ?12			
Organic Solvents Benzene	+			+				CBC Urine phenols	+ Leukemia	Maternal	−1 +5	−1 +2 +3 +4		
Halogenated Hydrocarbons 2-Chlorobutadiene (chloroprene)	+	+	+	+		+		Liver function tests	? Skin Liver	Maternal	+1	microbiologic +4, −5, +6	?3	?
										Paternal	+1 −2 +3		?3	
Dibromochloropropane		+	+				Azoospermia, oligospermia	Sperm count Serum testosterone	? Gastric, mammary in female rats	Maternal	+4	microbiologic ?5		
Epichlorohydrin		+	+			+		Liver function tests	? Skin	Paternal	+2 +3 −4 (single dose)	microbiologic +1		

?Variable or questionable data.
*Plus signs indicate positive data; minus signs, negative data.
†Numbers throughout refer to authors listed in table.

LLBIRTH AND ONATAL EATHS	CONGENITAL ANOMALIES	BEHAVIORAL OR DEVELOPMENTAL DISABILITIES	OTHER RELATED REPRODUCTIVE EFFECTS	REFERENCES FOR REPRODUCTIVE EFFECTS (SEE TEXT)	WORKPLACE AIR STANDARDS: OSHA: EXISTING	NIOSH: RECOMMENDED	NIOSH: REPRODUCTIVE CONSIDERATION
+1 +4 +8 +1		+4 +6 +8 +9		1. Oliver 2. Pindborg 3. Fahim 4. Rom (review) 5. Lancranjan 6. Carson 7. Infante (review) 8. Bridbord (review) 9. Palmisano 10. Hilderbrand	50 $\mu g/m^3$ air 40 $\mu g/100$ ml blood (Nov. 14, 1978)	40 $\mu g/m^3$ air blood lead 60 $\mu g/100$ ml (May, 1978)	Women of reproductive age Blood Pb < 30 $\mu g/100$ ml
+4	+4 ?5 +7 +6 ?8	+13	Zinc protective action +3 +7	1. Parisek 2. Nordberg 3. Kar 4. Chernoff 5. Barr 6. Ishizu 7. Ferm 8. Tsvetkova 9. Shiraishe 10. Bui 11. Epstein 12. Galiavod 13. Webster	*Fume* 0.1 mg/m^3 (ceiling—0.3 mg/m^3) *Dust* 0.2 mg/m^3 (ceiling—0.6 mg/m^3)	40 $\mu g/m^3$	?
+5 +10	+3 +9 +10	+1 +3 +4 +10		1. Harada (1968) 2. Bakir 3. Amin-Zaki 4. Pierce, Snyder 5. Ramel 6. Fahmy 7. WHO (Firman) 8. Harada (1971) 9. Oharazawa 10. Spyker 11. Suter 12. Lee	Inorganic 0.1 mg/m^3 Organic 0.01 mg/m^3	Inorganic 0.05 mg/m^3	*WHO recom* Org. mercury none Koos and Longo review recommends elem. Hg 10 $\mu g/m^3$ Inorg. and phenyl 20 $\mu g/m^3$ Org. none
	+6			1. Forni 2. Vigliani 3. Tough 4. Wurster-Hill 5. Gofmekler 6. Watanabe	1 ppm	1 ppm	?
	?3 −2			1. von Oettingen 2. Culik 3. Sanotskii 4. Bartsch 5. Litton Biometics 6. Vogel	25 ppm	1 ppm	Probably
				1. Torkelson 2. Rakhmatulayeve 3. Faydysh 4. Reznick 5. Rosencranz	10 ppb (emerg. std.)	10 ppb	Yes
(single ose)				1. NIOSH Review 2. Hahn 3. Cooper 4. Epstein	1 ppm	1 ppm	?

TABLE 3–2.—*(cont.)*

AGENT	SYSTEMIC EFFECTS*							SUGGESTED BIOLOGIC TESTING	CARCINOGENESIS	PARENTAL EXPOSURE	DECREASED FERTILITY (INCLUDES DECREASED SPERMATOGENESIS)†	MUTAGENESIS (CHROMOSOMAL ABERRATION)	SPONTANEOUS ABORTION	LOW BIRTH WEIGHT (PREMATURE)
	NEUROLOGIC	HEPATIC	RENAL	HEMATOLOGIC	CARDIOVASCULAR	PULMONARY	OTHER SPECIAL EFFECTS							
Ethylene dibromide		+	+			+			+	Maternal Paternal	+3 (avian) +1 +2	microbiologic +3		
Tetrachloroethlene (Perchloroethylene)	+		+			+			?	Maternal	−2 ?1			?1
Polychlorinated biphenyls (PCBs)		+		+			Chloracne, swollen eyelids, hyperpigmentation of skin	Blood analysis Adipose tissue analysis Serum triglycerides	? + liver in animals	Maternal Paternal	+1 +6 +7 +4	microbiologic (weak) ?9 −8	+7	+1 +2
Vinyl Chloride	+	+			+		Acroosteolysis	Liver function tests	+ Angiosarcoma liver	Maternal Paternal	+4	microbiologic +1, +2, +3 +6	+4	
Hypoxia Carbon monoxide	+			+	+			Carboxyhemoglobin		Maternal Paternal	+8		Absorption of fetal rats +6	+ + +
Anesthetic Gases Halogenated gases, e.g., halothane methoxyfluorane	+	+							? Leukemia, lymphatic system	Maternal Paternal	−5		?2 +3 +4 +5 +7 +9 +12 +3 −5 +7 +8 −9 −12	? ? + −
Pesticides Carbaryl	+									Maternal ? Paternal	(only high doses) +10 ?6 (high doses) (lower doses) −6 +10 +11	microbiologic −1, −2, −3, ?4, ?6	−8	

?Variable or questionable data.
*Plus signs indicate positive data; minus signs, negative data.
†Numbers throughout refer to authors listed in table.

LBIRTH AND ONATAL EATHS	CONGENITAL ANOMALIES	BEHAVIORAL OR DEVELOPMENTAL DISABILITIES	OTHER RELATED REPRODUCTIVE EFFECTS	REFERENCES FOR REPRODUCTIVE EFFECTS (SEE TEXT)	WORKPLACE AIR STANDARDS: OSHA: EXISTING	WORKPLACE AIR STANDARDS: NIOSH: RECOMMENDED	WORKPLACE AIR STANDARDS: NIOSH: REPRODUCTIVE CONSIDERATION
	+4			1. Amir 2. Edwards 3. NIOSH Review 4. Short	20 ppm	1 mg/m^3	?
?1	?1			1. Schwetz 2. Carpenter	100 ppm	50 ppm	No
7 1	+1 −5	−2 −5	Menstrual alteration +3, +7	1. NIOSH Review 2. Funatsu 3. Kusuda 4. Schwartz 5. Inoue 6. Allen 7. Barsotti 8. Green 9. Wyndham	42% chlorine 1 mg/m^3 54% chlorine— 0.5 mg/m^3	1 $\mu g/m^3$	Yes
+4	+4, −5			1. Bartsch 2. Magnussen 3. Huberman 4. Infante 5. Edmonds 6. Ducatman	1 ppm	1 ppm	?
orted hu- ans, imals	Neurologic sequelae; brain damage	+5 +2, +4, +5, +6	Decreased litter size Decreased survival Decreased libido (hypoxic)	1. Astrup 2. Ginsberg 3. Grahn 4. Leway 5. Longo 6. Wells 7. Williams 8. Kamet	50 ppm	35 ppm	No
	?2 −3 ?5 +6 +7 +9 +10 +11 +12 −5 (major) +5 (minor) +7 +8 +12			2. Vaisman 3. Askrog 4. Cohen 5. Knill Jones 6. Corbett 7,8. ASA 9. Garska 10. Chang 11. Schwetz 12. Spence	Not specified	Halogenated anesthetics 2 ppm based on weight of special gas sampled not >1 hr	?
8	−5 −6 ?7 −8 +9			1. Epstein 2. Achiyama 3. Elespuru 4. Brazeskij 5. Benson 6. Weil, 1972, 1973 7. Robens 8. Dougherty 9. Smalley 10. Shtenberg 11. Whorton	5 mg/m^3	5 mg/m^3	Probably

TABLE 3–2.—*(cont.)*

AGENT	SYSTEMIC EFFECTS*: NEUROLOGIC	HEPATIC	RENAL	HEMATOLOGIC	CARDIOVASCULAR	PULMONARY	OTHER SPECIAL EFFECTS	SUGGESTED BIOLOGIC TESTING	CARCINOGENESIS	PARENTAL EXPOSURE	DECREASED FERTILITY (INCLUDES DECREASED SPERMATO-GENESIS)†	MUTAGENESIS (CHROMOSOMAL ABERRATION)	SPONTA-NEOUS ABORTION	L BI WE (PR TU
Chlorinated Hydrocarbons, e.g., Chlordane				+				Fat biopsy		Maternal and childhood				
Chlordecone (Kepone)	+	+					Pleuritic and joint pains; visual disturbance	Blood analysis	? Liver	Maternal Paternal	+3 +1 +2 +3			
Estrogenic Compounds Diethylstilbestrol (DES)					+		Women—intermenstrual Men—gynecomastia	Blood analysis	+ Vaginal adenocarcinoma; ? breast	Maternal Paternal	+5 +2 +5 highest dose only +7			
Ionizing Radiation X-ray and gamma rays				+			Gastrointestinal disorder	Personal film badge or pocket dosimetry; thermoluminescent dosimetry	Blood +	Maternal	+2	+1 +2		+
Microwaves	+						Cataract eyes			Maternal Paternal	+1 −2	?5	+4 (Miscarriages)	
Miscellaneous Substances Carbon disulfide	+			+	+		Retinopathy	Urine iodine—azide test		Maternal Paternal	?1 −2 −3 +5 −7 limited exposure +3 +4	−9	?1 −2 +6	+
Ethylene oxide				+		+	Headache; eye irritation; respiratory irritation	CBC		Maternal Paternal	+1 ?3 ?3	+ microbiologic +4 +2		
Ethylene thiourea							Thyroid depressant		+ Liver, thyroid	Maternal				
Glycidyl ethers	+						Skin—strong irritant and sensitizer			Paternal	Mice +4	?2		

?Variable or questionable data.
*Plus signs indicate positive data; minus signs, negative data.
†Numbers throughout refer to authors listed in table.

TILLBIRTH AND EONATAL DEATHS	CONGENITAL ANOMALIES	BEHAVIORAL OR DEVELOPMENTAL DISABILITIES	OTHER RELATED REPRODUCTIVE EFFECTS	REFERENCES FOR REPRODUCTIVE EFFECTS (SEE TEXT)	WORKPLACE AIR STANDARDS: OSHA EXISTING	WORKPLACE AIR STANDARDS: NIOSH RECOMMENDED	NIOSH REPRODUCTIVE CONSIDERATION
			? Neuroblastoma ? Blood dyscrasias	1. Infante review	0.5 mg/m^3		Insufficient data
				1. NIOSH review 2. Good 3. Huber			
		?3 −2 +1 +5 ?3 −2	Adenosis +1, +5 Adenocarcinoma Urinary tract (males) +4	1. Herbst 1971, 1975 2. Gill 3. Lanier 4. Welch 5. McLachlan 6. Coron. Drug Project 7. Harrington 8. Greenwald	Not specified	Not specified	Insufficient data
+1	+1	+1		1. NCRP (Report No. 53) 1977 2. Voelz *(Occupational Medicine)*			NCRP Recommendation Pregnancy 0.5 rem/full pregnancy
	+3 +4		Menstrual alterations +4	1. Lancranjan 2. Siekierzynski 3. Menicke 4. Marha 5. Sigler	10 mw/cm^2		FDA/Bur. of Rad. Health recommends 1 mw/cm^2 max for pregnant women
	−2 ?8 ?8		Increased menstrual bleeding +1 +5	1. Erhardt 2. Finkova 3. Jindrichova 4. Lancranjan 5. Vasilyeva 6. Petrov 7. Wakasuki 8. Barilyak 9. NIOSH	20 ppm	1 ppm (3 mg/m^3)	?
				1. Loveless 2. Emhee 3. NIOSH Review 4. Ehrenberg	50 ppm	50 ppm ceiling not >75 ppm (15 min)	Inadequate data
	+1 +2			1. Stula 2. Khera	No standard (minimize exposure)	No standard (minimize exposure)	
			Testicular degeneration + 2,3,4	1. Pullin 2. NIOSH Criteria Document 3. Hine 4. Shimkin	45 mg/m^3 AGE 270 mg/m^3 BGE 2.8 mg/m^3 DGE 240 mg/m^3 IGE 60 mg/m^3 PGE	(mg/m^3) 45 AGE 30 BGE 1 DGE 240 IGE 5 PGE (all ceiling— 15 min)	?

by this route. In addition, exposure to the infant can occur from contamination of the home by the mother or father who works with lead[2] and brings the lead-containing dust into the home on work clothing and shoes.

Several excellent reviews of the effects of lead on reproduction have been published.[1,4,12,15,20] These reviews refer to human studies that have shown lead to be associated with sterility (male and female), abnormal spermatogenesis, spontaneous abortions, stillbirths, increased infant mortality, decreased infant birth weights, slow infant development and mental retardation. Animal studies corroborating all of the above have also been reported and emphasize the association of lead with impotency, sterility, mutagenesis and decreased learning ability in the offspring following lead exposure of the parent.[6,23]

It is recognized that women are more prolonged direct sources of exposure to the products of conception than are men and lead exposure from the maternal source can continue beyond delivery through lactation; nonetheless, alterations in fertility have been reported in both males and females and genetic changes can be transmitted by either sex.[16,18,22]

Lancranjan et al.[16] studied 150 lead storage battery workers (men) and found that at mean blood levels of 52.8 ± 21.0 μg/100 ml blood, a significant alteration from the controls was noted in spermatogenesis, namely, asthenospermia, hypospermia and teratospermia, and they reported a decrease in libido and orgasm and an increase in "pathologic erections and ejaculations." Even in workers with slightly increased lead absorption (mean of 41 ± 12.0 μg/100 ml blood), significant differences in asthenospermia and hypospermia were found as well as alterations in the sexual dynamics noted previously. Unfortunately, the authors were not able to obtain reliable information on reproductive performance of the subjects with respect to the number of normal pregnancies per couple, the frequency of miscarriages, spontaneous abortions or abnormal births. Alterations in reproductive capabilities in males have been noted in animal studies. Hildebrand et al.[14] reported on the effects of lead acetate ingestion on reproduction in male rats. With blood leads of 30 μg/100 ml blood, they found a 70% reduction in testicular weight, impotency and reduced sperm motility.

OSHA's recently promulgated occupational air standard is 50 μg lead/m^3 of air and biologic standard of 40 μg/100 ml blood (Federal Register 10-13-78). A realistic question is whether these proposed environmental and biologic standards provide an adequate margin of safety for occupational exposure of pregnant women. To consider this question, cognizance must be taken of the greater susceptibility of the fetus than the adult to toxic effects of lead with particular regard to the subtle and, at times, delayed behavioral and neurologic effects and the early alterations in porphyrin metabolism associated with heme synthesis.

Lead is well recognized as a neurotoxin with effects on both the central and peripheral nervous systems. Furthermore, it is generally agreed that the developing immature nervous system, especially in the embryo and fetus, is more sensitive to lead's neurotoxic action than is the nervous system in adults or even in older children.

Lead interferes with the biosynthesis of heme at several enzymatic steps, with the utilization of iron and with globin synthesis in erythrocytes, and an early manifestation of lead exposure in man is associated with lead's interference in heme biosynthesis. Table 3–3 summarizes the no-detected levels for various lead effects by blood leads (μg of lead/100 ml blood).[24] It is likely that a level of exposure that will prevent any significant alterations in the heme biosynthesis pathways will prevent the clinical and subclinical neurologic manifestations and prob-

TABLE 3–3.—NO-DETECTED EFFECT LEVELS IN TERMS OF PB-B (μG OF LEAD PER 100 ML OF BLOOD)

NO-DETECTED EFFECT LEVEL	EFFECT	POPULATION
<10	Erythrocyte ALAD inhibition	Adults, children
20–25	FEP	Children
20–30	FEP	Adult, female
25–35	FEP	Adult, male
30–40	Erythrocyte ATPase inhibition	General
40	ALA excretion in urine	Adults, children
40	CP excretion in urine	Adults
40	Anemia	Children
40–50	Peripheral neuropathy	Adults
50	Anemia	Adults
50–60	Minimal brain dysfunction	Children
60–70	Minimal brain dysfunction	Adults
60–70	Encephalopathy	Children
>80	Encephalopathy	Adults

Source: WHO Environmental Health Criteria.[24]

ably the reproductive effects in both men and women.[24]

The earliest physiologic alteration from lead absorption is a decrease in aminolevulinic acid dehydratase (ALAD) activity, which may be found with blood lead levels as low as 10 μg/100 ml. However, hemesynthesis probably is not significantly affected even if the ALAD is markedly depressed.[25] Zielhuis reports the no-effect level for 70% ALAD inhibition to be 25–30 μg lead/100 ml blood in adults and 20–25 μg/100 ml in children.[25] After ALAD inhibition, elevations of free erythrocyte porphyrins (FEP), inhibition of erythrocyte ATPase and elevations of aminolevulinic acid in urine (ALAU) and coproporphyrin in urine (CPU) follow in order.[24]

According to the Center for Disease Control, "the statistical likelihood of childhood symptoms and permanent damage increases at least arithmetically with confirmed blood lead values above 30 μg/100 ml and EP values above 60 μg/ml."[26] Since the embryo and fetus may be more susceptible than the child, it would be prudent to maintain the exposure to lead of the products of conception in utero so that the fetal blood lead is at least below 30 μg/100 ml. To do so would require blood lead levels in the working woman to be at or below that concentration.

How can this be translated into an acceptable exposure level for airborne lead for pregnant women? As a result of an extensive review of epidemiologic studies on lead exposures wherein environmental and biologic data were included, Bridbord[4] estimated for adult men that occupational exposures to 50 μg lead/m^3 of air would be associated with blood leads ranging from 35 to 45 μg lead/100 ml blood. This level probably is protective for men. Since women at low levels of exposure have been noted to have lower blood lead levels than do men, to keep the blood lead level of women workers at or below 30 μg/100 ml blood would require an occupational exposure to lead of no greater than 50 μg/m^3 of air and no additional lead exposure from any other sources, e.g., eating or smoking in the work area, poor personal hygiene, home hobbies, etc.

For a general overview, as well as detailed aspects of occupational exposure to lead compounds and specific pathophysiology, see Chapter 30 (Hernberg) in *Occupational Medicine: Principles and Practical Applications*, Carl Zenz (ed.) (Chicago: Year Book Medical Publishers, 1975).

REFERENCES

Lead

1. Baetjer, A.: *Women in Industry, Their Health and Efficiency* (Philadelphia: W. B. Saunders Company, 1946), pp. 145–156.
2. Baker, E. L., et al.: Lead poisoning in children of lead workers: Home contamination with industrial dust, N. Engl. J. Med. 296:260, 1977.
3. Barltrop, D.: Transfer of Lead to the Human Fetus, in Barltrop, D., and Burland, W. L. (eds.), *Mineral Metabolism in Pediatrics* (Philadelphia: F. A. Davis Company, 1969), pp. 135–151.
4. Bridbord, K.: Review of lead toxicity, Conference on Women and the Workplace. Soc. of Occup. & Environ. Hygiene, June 17–19, 1976, pp. 227–231.
5. Bridbord, K.: Lead exposure and women: Medical aspects, Prevention (Prev. Med. 7:311, 1978.).
6. Carson, T. L., et al.: Slowed learning in lambs prenatally exposed to lead, Arch. Environ. Health 29:154, 1974.
7. Center for Disease Control, U.S. Dept of HEW: Morbidity and Mortality Weekly Report: Increased lead absorption in children of lead workers—Vermont, February 25, 1977.
8. Center for Disease Control, Atlanta, Georgia: Lead poisoning in children of battery plant employees—North Carolina, Epidemiologic Notes and Reports, September 30, 1977, Vol. 26, No. 29.
9. Fahim, M. S., Fahim, Z., and Hall, D. G.: Effects of subtoxic lead levels on pregnant women in the state of Missouri. Presented at Int. Conf. on Heavy Metals in the Environment, Toronto, Canada, October, 1975.
10. Gershanik, J. J., Brooks, G. G., and Little, J. A.: Blood lead values in pregnant women and their offspring, Am. J. Obstet. Gynecol. 119:408, 1975.
11. Haas, T., et al.: Untersuchunge über die okologische bleibelastung im kindesalter (in German—English summary), in Int. Symp. Environ. Health Aspects of Lead, USEPA, October, 1972.
12. Hardy, H. L.: Editorial: What is the status of knowledge of the toxic effect of lead on identifiable groups in the population?, Clin. Pharmacol. Ther. 7:713, 1966.
13. Hernberg, S.: Lead, in Zenz, C. (ed.), *Occupational Medicine: Principles and Practical Applications* (Chicago: Year Book Medical Publishers, 1975), pp. 715–769.
14. Hildebrand, D., et al.: Effect of lead acetate on reproduction, Am. J. Obstet. Gynecol. 115:1058, 1973.
15. Infante, P. F., and Wagoner, J. R.: The effects of lead on reproduction, in Proceedings of Conference on Women and the Workplace. Soc. of Occup. & Environ. Hyg., June 17–19, Washington, D.C., 1976.
16. Lancranjan, I., et al.: Reproductive ability of workmen occupationally exposed to lead, Arch. Environ. Health 30:396, 1975.
17. Oliver, T.: *Diseases of Occupation* (New York: E. P. Dutton, 1908).
18. Oliver, T.: Lead poisoning and the racer, Br. Med. J. 1:1096, 1911.
19. Pindborg, S.: Om solveroglodforgiftning i Danmark, Ugeskr. Laeger 107:1, 1945 (cited in Rom[20]).
20. Rom, W. N.: Effects of lead on the female and reproduction: A review, Mt. Sinai J. Med. N.Y. 43:542, 1976.
21. Suspected Carcinogens, A Subfile of the Registry of Toxic Effects of Chemical Substances, 2d ed., 1977, USDHEW, PHS, CDC, NIOSH, Rockville, Maryland.
22. Torelli, G.: L'influenza cell avvelena mento cronico caprombo sulla discendexza, Med. Lav. 21:110, 1930 (cited in Hamilton, A., and Hardy, H., *Industrial Toxicology* [2d ed.; New York: Paul B. Hoeber, Inc., 1949], pp. 119–121).
23. Varma, M. M., Joshi, S. R., and Adeyimi, A. O.: Mutagenicity and infertility following administration of lead sub-acetate to Swiss male mice, Experientia 30:486, 1974.
24. WHO: Environmental Health Criteria 3: Lead, Geneva, 1977.
25. Zielhuis, R. L.: Dose response relationships for inorganic lead. I. Biochemical and hematological responses. II. Subjective and functional responses. Chr. sequelae. No response levels. Int. Arch. Occup. Environ. Health 35:1–18, 19–35, 1975.
26. Center for Disease Control, U.S. Dept. of HEW: Increased lead absorption and lead poisoning in young children, March, 1975.

Benzene (Benzol)

BENZENE is an organic solvent. It is present in such industries as gas and coke manufacturing and has enormous usage in others: chemical, printing and lithography, paint, rubber, dry cleaning, adhesives, petroleum and coatings. It is used chiefly as an intermediate in producing other organic chemicals such as phenol, cyclohexane, styrene toluene and in the manufacture of certain detergents and pesticides, and small amounts are present in paint removers.[7] Large quantities are used in chemical laboratories and in pharmaceutical making as a solvent, extractant or reactant. It is present in gasoline (in the United States, 0.3–2%; in Europe, 5–16%) and in numerous hydrocarbon mixtures. In the United States, in 1976, benzene production was estimated to be 5 billion kilograms, and this vast production suggests potential widespread worker contact. NIOSH[7] estimates that about 2 million persons in the U.S. work force are potentially exposed to benzene.

Benzene is well known for its deleterious effects on the hematopoietic system, the most prominent effect, in earlier reports, being depression of single or multiple elements of the blood, including anemia, thrombocytopenia and/or leukopenia to aplastic anemia.[1,4] More recently, emphasis has been placed on the role of exposure to benzene in the etiology of leukemia, particularly acute myelogenous leukemia, and lymphatic and erythroleukemia. According to Vigliani and Saita,[12] the risk of death from leukemia in subjects exposed to benzene is 20-fold that of the general population. Vigliani and Forni[11] have noted from their studies in Italy that there are more cases of leukemia than of pancytopenia, which has led to the belief that the latter cases may, in fact, be examples of aleukemic or hemocytoblastic leukopenic leukemia.[10]

Studies evaluating the reproductive toxicity of male or female workers exposed to benzene have not been reported. One interesting case involving pregnancy was noted by Forni et al.,[2] in which a patient, while severely pancytopenic following exposure to benzene during the prior year and with severe hemorrhagic problems, delivered an apparently normal boy. Chromosome studies in the patient showed an increased rate of chromosome aberrations; however, a cytogenetic study of the peripheral blood performed on the newborn boy did not show chromosomal abnormalities. Subsequently, the patient had another pregnancy and delivered a normal daughter.

Chromosomal aberrations in peripheral blood lymphocytes and in bone marrow cells have been found in benzene workers with or without signs of benzene toxicity.[8,11,14] Vigliani and Forni,[11] in commenting on the results of cytogenic studies in subjects, including some who have, or have recovered from, benzene hemopathy as well as a number who had exposure but no toxic manifestations, noted that the rate of chromosome changes in the peripheral blood lymphocytes of workers exposed to benzene was higher than in the controls. For those with benzene hemopathy, the chromosomal aberrations were noted in the peripheral blood lymphocytes and in bone marrow cells, and the changes persisted several years after exposure ceased. No such changes were found in toluene and xylene workers as compared with controls and no further cases of aplastic anemia were noted in the workers when these solvents replaced benzene as solvents of the inks and glues. Several investigators[11,14] have suggested from their observations in cases of leukemia associated with benzene exposure that these workers may have a genetic predisposition for such effect.

There have been very few studies in animals on the reproductive effects of benzene. In a critical evaluation of benzene toxicity edited by Laskin and Goldstein,[5] one study is described involving groups of female rats exposed continually (24 hours) to 670, 63.3, 56.6, 20.4, 5.6 and 1 mg/m^3 of benzene vapor (209.7, 19.8, 17.7, 6.4, 1.8 and 0.3 ppm) for 10–15 days before impregnation. At the highest concentration (209.7 ppm) there was complete absence of pregnancy and at 19.8 ppm, resorption of embryos was observed in 1 of the 10 treated dams. The number of offspring per female was inversely related to the benzene concentration.[3] The authors note further that there has been only one reported animal study of teratogenicity and benzene exposure. In this experiment, groups of pregnant mice were given a single subcutaneous injection of 3 ml of benzene per kilogram body weight on the 11th–15th day of gestation, respectively, and the fetuses were delivered by cesarean section of the mother on the 19th gestation day. Malformed fetuses occurred more frequently in the group treated on the 13th day of pregnancy than in other groups, and the anomalies included cleft palate, agnathia and micrognathia. The decrease in the maternal white cell count and the increase in body weight in the mother after benzene administration during pregnancy were similar in mice with or without malformed fetuses.[13]

A Litton Bionetics Company report prepared for the EPA in 1977 revealed a study that demonstrated fetotoxic effects in rats exposed to 10 ppm of benzene during the middle trimester of gestation, the lowest dose reported for this effect. At about the same time, the Exxon Corporation submitted a notice under the Toxic Substances Control Act to the EPA that stated that benzene showed weak toxic effects in pregnant females and fetuses of experimental animals at 50 ppm, weak teratogenic effects at 500 ppm, gonadal effects in 50 male animals at a concentration of 80 ppm and fetotoxic effects in rats at a concentration of 10 ppm. The submission reviewed two studies by Exxon and several new references. The Exxon studies concentrated on the reproductive effects of benzene inhalation in female experimental animals, apparently because Exxon's literature search failed to identify sufficient information on the reproductive effects of benzene in females. EPA stated that the Exxon summary indicated that benzene exposure in females could lead to acquired blood dyscrasias, abnormal uterine bleeding and possibly sterility (due to ovarian disturbances), mutagenesis and/or teratogenesis (due to benzene-induced malformed embryos that subsequently are aborted spontaneously).[9]

NIOSH, in its revised recommendation for a benzene standard,[6] has concluded that benzene is leukemogenic and, because it causes progressive malignant disease of the blood-forming organs, should be regulated as a carcinogen. As a result, the recommendation is that exposure to benzene be kept to a minimum and not to exceed 1 ppm (3.5 mg/m^3) for a 2-hour period. OSHA has promulgated this standard. The effectiveness of this standard for the pregnant worker needs to be evaluated.

REFERENCES

Benzene (Benzol)

1. Erf, L. A., and Rhoads, C. P.: The hematological effects of benzene (benzol) poisoning, J. Ind. Hyg. Toxicol. 21:421, 1939.
2. Forni, A., Cappelini, A., Pacifico, E., and Vigliani, E.: Chromosome changes and evolution in subjects with past exposure to benzene, Arch. Environ. Health 23:385, 1971.
3. Gofmekler, V. A.: Effect on embryonic development of benzene and formaldehyde in inhalation treatments, Hyg. Sanit. 33:327, 1968.
4. Greenburg, L., Mayers, M. R., Goldwater, L., and Smith, A. R.: Benzene (benzol) poisoning in the rotogravure printing industry in New York City, J. Ind. Hyg. Toxicol. 21:395, 1939.
5. Laskin, S., and Goldstein, D. B. (eds.): Benzene toxicity—a critical evaluation, J.

Toxicol. Environ. Health, Supp. ll, pp. 1–148, 1977.
6. National Institute for Occupational Safety and Health: Revised recommendation for an occupational exposure standard for benzene, NIOSH, DHEW, 1976.
7. National Institute for Occupational Safety and Health: Criteria for a recommended standard: Occupational exposure to benzene, DHEW, PHS, NIOSH, 74–137, 1974.
8. Tough, I. M., and Court Brown, W. M.: Chromosome aberrations and exposure to ambient benzene, Lancet 1:684, 1965.
9. U.S. Occupational Safety and Health Reporter (BNA), Washington, D.C., Dec. 28, 1978.
10. Vigliani, E. C.: Leukemia associated with benzene exposure, Ann. N.Y. Acad. Sci. 271:143, 1976.
11. Vigliani, E. C., and Forni, A.: Benzene, chromosome changes and leukemia, J. Occup. Med. 11:148, 1969.
12. Vigliani, E. C., and Saita, G.: Benzene and leukemia, N. Engl. J. Med. 271:872, 1964.
13. Watanabe, GI, and Yoshida, S.: The teratogenic effect of benzene in pregnant mice, Acta Med. Biol. 17:285, 1970.
14. Wurster-Hill, D. H., Cornwell, G. G., and McIntyre, O. R.: Chromosomal aberrations and neoplasm—a family study, Cancer 33:72, 1974.
15. Zenz, C.: Benzene—attempts to establish a lower exposure standard in the United States. A review, Scand. J. Work Environ. Health 4:103, 1978.

Cadmium

CADMIUM is found in the sulfide ores of zinc, lead and copper and exposure to cadmium may occur during the smelting and refining processes of these ores. Work production is estimated to be in excess of 16 million kg annually, with the main use for electroplating—from 45% to 60% of the annual amount. Other major uses of cadmium compounds are for stabilizers in plastics, in pigments and as alloying agents, especially in brazing compounds ("silver solders" often contain 20% cadmium). Cadmium dusts, fumes and mists commonly are present in some smelting processes involving zinc, copper and lead, as well as in certain processes for extracting cadmium. NIOSH estimates that 100,000 workers in the United States have a potential occupational exposure to cadmium.[14]

Growth retardation and anemia have been found in young animals following chronic cadmium poisoning whereas in adult animals hypochromic microcytic anemia is characteristic. Webster[22] exposed mice to 10, 20 or 40 ppm cadmium in their drinking water throughout pregnancy. The offspring were obviously much smaller than normal and very anemic. This study confirms the extreme sensitivity of fetal growth to cadmium concentrations as low as 10 ppm. The fact that the fetuses were not only smaller than normal but were also severely anemic suggests that the two are related, the anemia perhaps being the cause of the growth retardation. Observations made during this study indicate that exposure of the nursing mother to cadmium severely limits growth of her litter. In this respect, it is interesting that in the cadmium-treated mice, the anemia seen in the fetuses is very severe as compared with the relatively mild anemia of the mother. This suggests that cadmium might well be interfering with growth and blood formation of the fetus.

Studies in experimental animals indicate that cadmium can have destructive effects on the gonads. Necrotic effects of cadmium on testicular tissue in male rats injected subcutaneously with 1 ml of 0.03 M solution of cadmium chloride have been reported.[16,18] Zinc acetate in large doses prevented testicular damage. Protective effects of zinc and selenium against testicular injury to rats from cadmium have also been reported.[12,13,21] After administering cadmium chloride subcutaneously 2.2–4.5 mg Cd/kg body weight into the interscapular region of rats and mice, Parizek[16] reported hyperemia and interstitial edema in the testes within a few hours after injection, and after 48 hours there was destruction of tubular epithelium and the interstitial tissue was hemorrhagic. A dose-response relationship was noted by Mason et al.[13] for injuries to the seminiferous tubules. Subcutaneous injection in rats of a dose of 0.57 mg/kg produced no effect whereas a dose of 0.85 mg/kg resulted in ischemic necrosis of seminiferous tubules in 32% of the rats. At 1.1 mg/kg there was a 90% incidence and at 1.4 mg/kg 100% of rats showed these injuries. In mice and rabbits, Nordberg[15] found no testicular damage with repeated administration of cadmium at dose levels that caused slight or no kidney malfunction, suggesting that the effect of cadmium on the kidney is an earlier finding in these species.

The effect of cadmium on male gonads stimulated the study of possible effects on ovaries. Kar et al.[11] found a marked change in the rate of follicular atresia in prepubertal rats following administration of cadmium chloride subcutaneously at 10 mg/kg. After 48 hours, all follicles were destroyed and response of the ovaries to exogenous gonadotropin was inhibited. Parizek et al.[17] injected 5-day-old female rats with either testosterone or 19-nortestosterone and after 3–6 months, the rats had a persistent estrus. They then were injected subcutaneously with cadmium chloride or acetate at 0.02–0.04 mmole/kg. All ovaries showed massive hemorrhages accompanied by necrosis. Kar et al.[12] found that simultaneous injection of zinc acetate or selenium oxide with cadmium chloride protected the ovaries from damage produced by cadmium chloride alone.

The animal studies indicating gonadal changes were all acute studies involving high levels of cadmium. Comparable doses in man would represent unusually high exposure, which might even be lethal.[14]

There have been several studies of the teratogenicity of cadmium in animals. Chernoff[3] administered 4–12 mg/kg cadmium chloride to CD-strain rats subcutaneously on 4 consecutive days, beginning on day 13, 14, 15 or 16 of gestation. There was a dose-related increase in fetal deaths, decrease in fetal weight and an increase in the rate of anomalies, which included micrognathia, cleft palate, clubfoot and small lungs. Barr[1] found that cadmium chloride 16 μmol Cd/kg was not teratogenic when administered subcutaneously to two different stocks of Wistar rats on days 9, 10 and 11 of gestation but was when administered intraperitoneally. Among the anomalies found were anophthalmia or microphthalmia, dysplastic or absent ears, hydrocephaly, encephalocele, exencephaly, thin abdominal wall, undescended testes, renal agenesis, diaphragmatic hernia, anal atresia, dysplastic or absent tails, hydronephrosis and a small rate of dysplastic forelimbs. The authors suggested that some of the changes might be due to cadmium interference with zinc metabolism. Teratogenic effects have also been reported in mice[10] and hamsters.[7] The protective effect of zinc for the teratogenic effects of cadmium have also been studied. Ferm and Carpenter[7,8] found that simultaneous intravenous administration of zinc sulfate at 0.45 mg Zn/kg and cadmium sulfate at 0.88 mg Cd/kg reduced embryonic resorption and anomalies to control levels. Gradual delay of zinc injection after cadmium injection reduced the protective effect, and where the delay was 12 hours or greater there was no protective effect.

There have been very few studies on reproductive effects in humans exposed to cadmium. Favino and co-workers[6] found 1 worker with impotence associated with low testosterone blood levels among 10 cadmium workers studied. Tsvetkova[20] investigated effects on reproduction among 106 women workers exposed to cadmium, aged 18–48 with 2–16 years' exposure, some to cadmium oxide at concentrations of 0.1–25 mg/m^3, some to soluble cadmium salts at

0.16–25 mg/m^3. She found no significant changes in the menstrual cycle. Courses and times of pregnancies were normal. Children born weighed less than children of control workers. Four of the children born to cadmium-exposed women had signs of rickets, 1 had retarded eruption of teeth and 2 had dental disease. These conditions were not present in children of control workers, but there were only 20 controls. No mention was made of conditions such as prenatal nutrition, maternal illnesses, maternal weight, smoking habits and other factors that might have had a bearing on the weight of the offspring and on the other findings.[14]

Studies of the possible mutagenic effects of cadmium have been inadequate and conflicting. Shiraishi and Yosida[19] found an excess of chromosomal aberrations in cultured leucocytes among Itai-Itai patients, but these findings were not confirmed in another study of Itai-Itai patients conducted by Bui et al.[2] Itai-Itai (ouch-ouch) disease is the name given to a painful form of osteomalacia in Japan attributed to the pollution of water and crops by industrial cadmium wastes.[14] Bui et al.[2] also reported that Swedish workers exposed to cadmium were found to have a lower incidence of chromosomal changes in cultured lymphocytes than did controls. DeKnudt and Leonard[4] found chromosomal anomalies in leucocytes in workers exposed to cadmium who were also exposed to lead and some to zinc in addition. Studies of dominant lethal mutations in mice by Epstein et al.[5] and by Gilliavod and Leonard[9] revealed that cadmium was not mutagenic, and they found no aberrations in spermocytic chromosomes in male mice and their male first-generation offspring.

Further studies on the effects of cadmium on reproduction are indicated. Damaging effects on human gonads have not been investigated adequately. Although animal studies undertaken at high doses of cadmium have produced harmful effects on ovaries and testes and resulted in fetal abnormalities, there is need for further studies at lower dose levels of cadmium. Furthermore, the role of zinc and selenium in affording protection against injury by cadmium deserves attention.

The present OSHA standard for cadmium is 0.1 mg Cd/m^3 TWA with a 0.3 ceiling for cadmium fume and 0.2 mg Cd/m^3 TWA (0.6 ceiling) for dust. NIOSH has proposed for all cadmium compounds an occupational environmental limit of 40 μg Cd/m^3 of air as a time-weighted average exposure up to a 10-hour workday, 40-hour week and a ceiling concentration of 200 μg Cd/m^3 for any 15-minute sampling period.

There is need for epidemiologic investigation and medical surveillance of cadmium worker populations, male and female, in order to obtain meaningful data relative to the effects of cadmium on reproduction, particularly at the levels of occupational exposure currently recommended as standards.

REFERENCES

Cadmium

1. Barr, M., Jr.: The teratogenicity of cadmium chloride in two stocks of Wistar rats, Teratology, 7:237, 1973.
2. Bui, T-H, Lindsten, J., and Nordberg, G. F.: Chromosome analysis of lymphocytes from cadmium workers and Itai-Itai patients, Environ. Res. 9:187, 1975.
3. Chernoff, N.: Teratogenic effects of cadmium in rats, Teratology 8:29, 1973.
4. DeKnudt, G., and Leonard, A.: Cytogenetic investigations on leucocytes of workers from a cadmium plant, Environ. Physiol. Biochem. 5:319, 1975.
5. Epstein, S. S., Arnold, E., Andrea, J., Bass, W., and Bishop, Y.: Detection of chemical mutagens by the dominant lethal assay in the mouse, Toxicol. Appl. Pharmacol. 23:288, 1972.
6. Favino, A., Candura, F., Chiappino, G., and Cavalleri, A.: Study on the androgen function of men exposed to cadmium, Med. Lav. 59:105, 1968.

7. Ferm, V. H., and Carpenter, S. J.: The relationship of cadmium and zinc in experimental mammalian teratogenesis, Lab. Invest. 18:429, 1968.
8. Ferm, V. H., and Carpenter, S. J.: Teratogenic effect of cadmium and its inhibition by zinc, Nature 216:1123, 1967.
9. Gilliavod, N., and Leonard, A.: Mutagenicity tests with cadmium in the mouse, Toxicology 5:43, 1975.
10. Ishizu, S., et al.: An experimental study of teratogenic effect of cadmium, Ind. Health 11:127, 1973.
11. Kar, A. B., Das, R. P., and Karkun, J. N.: Ovarian changes in prepubertal rats after treatment with cadmium chloride, Acta Biol. Med. Ger. 3:372, 1959.
12. Kar, A. B., Das, R. P., and Mukerji, F. N. I.: Prevention of cadmium induced changes in the gonads of rats by zinc and selenium—a study in antagonism between metals in the biological system, Proc. Natl. Inst. Sci. India 26B (supp.):40, 1960.
13. Mason, K. E., Brown, J. A., Young, J. O., and Nesbit, R. R.: Cadmium-induced injury of the rat testis, Anat. Rec. 149:135, 1964.
14. National Institute for Occupational Safety and Health: Criteria for a recommended standard . . . occupational exposure to cadmium, DHEW, PHS, NIOSH, 76–192, August, 1976.
15. Nordberg, G. F.: Effects of acute and chronic cadmium exposure on the testicles of mice—with special reference to protective effects of metallothionein, Environ. Physiol. 1:171, 1971.
16. Parizek, J.: The destructive effect of cadmium ion on testicular tissue and its prevention by zinc, J. Endocrinol. 15:56, 1957.
17. Parizek, J., Ostadalova, I., Benes, L., and Pitha, J.: The effect of a subcutaneous injection of cadmium salts on the ovaries of adult rats in persistent oestrus, J. Reprod. Fertil. 17:559, 1968.
18. Parizek, J., and Zahor, Z.: Effect of cadmium salts on testicular tissue, Nature 177:1036, 1956.
19. Shiraishi, Y., and Yosida, T. H.: Chromosomal abnormalities in cultured leucocyte cells from Itai-Itai disease patients, Proc. Jpn. Acad. 48:248, 1972.
20. Tsvetkova, R. B.: Materials concerning an investigation of the effect of cadmium compounds on the generative function, Gig. Tr. Prof. Zabol. 12:31, 1970 (Russian) (cited in NIOSH Criteria Document[14]).
21. Webb, M.: Protection by zinc against cadmium toxicity, Biochem. Pharmacol. 21:2767, 1972.
22. Webster, W. S.: Cadmium-induced fetal growth retardation in the mouse, Arch. Environ. Health 33:36, 1978.

Carbaryl

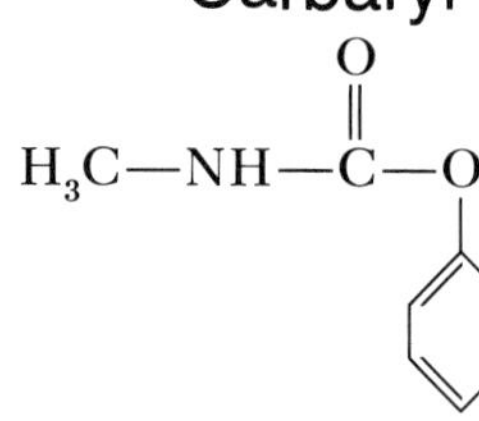

CARBARYL is one of the carbamate insecticides that produce most of their biologic effects by inhibiting cholinesterase enzymes. This inhibition leads to the accumulation of endogenous acetylcholine, the principal choline ester that has demonstrated physiologic significance in humans. Production in the United States was about 24 million kg (53 million lb) in 1972. Of the total produced in 1972, approximately 12 million kg were exported. In the United States, 8.6 million kg were used for agricultural purposes, 1.6 million kg in homes and gardens, 680,000 kg by government and 454,000 kg for industrial and commercial purposes. Slightly more than half the carbaryl used nationwide in 1972 was used in the Southeast and the North Central states (about 3.6 million and 2.3 million kg, respectively). An estimated 40% of the carbaryl used throughout the world is applied in the production of cotton.[9] Occupational exposure to carbaryl may occur in the development, manufacture, distribution and mixing of insecticides, as well as in agricultural use (crops), in plant nursery operations, in spraying and dusting operations, particularly aerial spraying, soil fumigation and extermination. Carbaryl products are widely marketed under the trade name Sevin. NIOSH estimates that 100,000 workers are potentially exposed to carbaryl in the United States.[9]

There is limited information available concerning the effects of carbaryl on human reproduction, and reports of adverse reproductive effects in animals from this substance are limited and, at times, conflicting. Whorton et al.[16] reported on a study of 101 male carbaryl production workers, 47 of whom provided satisfactory semen samples for analysis while 36 of the 47 provided blood for hormone assay (testosterone, follicle-stimulating hormone [FSH] and luteinizing hormone [LH]).

The authors summarized their findings as follows: "No apparent relationships were found between sperm count and exposure category or years worked in classifications based on carbaryl exposure. Also, no relationship was found between fathering children and exposure to carbaryl. When the sperm count distribution of the carbaryl-exposed workers was compared with a distribution of sperm counts representing a non-exposed (control) population, no overall differences were observed that could be related to carbaryl exposure. There was a small excess in the number of sperm counts less than 20 million/ml[3] amoung carbaryl-exposed men, but the excess was not significant (p 0.05)."

All values of the hormone immunoassays were within established laboratory normal ranges except for 4 elevated FSH values and the latter did not correlate with the sperm counts.

Mutagenesis testing of carbaryl in mice[8] and bacteria[7,13] has shown negative results. In Drosophila,[3] carbaryl has been found to be only a weak mutagen. It has been noted, however, that the nitroso compounds of the carbamates are much more strongly mutagenic in bacterial studies, and the possibility exists that nitrosation could occur from the nitrites in human saliva mixing with carbaryl in the acid medium of the stomach.[9] Since occupational exposure is more likely to be from inhalation and skin absorption rather than by ingestion, this factor is not of major occupational health concern.

Studies on the teratogenicity of carbaryl have been made in a number of animal species. Carbaryl has not been found to be teratogenic in the mouse,[2] rat,[15] rabbit,[10] hamster[10] and monkey.[5,6] In beagles, terata were produced.[12] In a study of 55 beagles fed carbaryl in their diets in 5 dosage groups ranging from 3.1 mg/kg to 50 mg/kg, the percentage of pups born alive at all dosages was fewer than the controls, with no live births at the highest dose (50 mg/kg). Of the total number of pregnant beagles from all carbaryl doses, 21% had pups showing embryotoxicity, but there were no abnormal pups in the lowest dose group (3.1 mg/kg) or in the controls. It is to be noted, however, that the dog metabolizes carbaryl differently than man; i.e., the dog does not excrete 1-naphthol or hydroxylate carbaryl and, therefore, the effects found in this animal may not be relatable to man.[9]

In the guinea pig, Robens[10] reported skeletal defects (mostly of the cervical vertebra) with oral intubation of carbaryl at 300 mg/kg (a near-lethal dose) on days 11–20 of gestation. Fetal mortality was 17.5% in the litter of surviving treated dams as compared with 9.5% in the control litters. On the other hand, in another study of guinea pigs comparing carbaryl dosing by gastric intubation and dietary feeding, Weil et al.[14] concluded that a carbaryl dose of 300 mg/kg by diet or 200 mg/kg by intubation did not produce teratogenic effects.

In view of the apparent differences in carbaryl metabolism between man and dogs and the lack of substantial evidence of teratogenicity in rats and guinea pigs, which have carbaryl metabolism similar to man, no significant data associating carbaryl with teratogenicity has been established at this time.

In the consideration of general reproductive effects of carbaryl, of particular interest is a study by Dougherty and Coulston[6] on the rhesus monkey. In their study, including 79 female monkeys divided into 3 groups of 16 each given carbaryl in gelatin capsules at 0.2, 2.0 or 20 mg/kg from days 20 through 38 of gestation, 1 group of 16 given empty gelatin capsules and an untreated control group of 15 animals, the authors reported that carbaryl was not associated with the production of terata, abortion, stillbirths or any other adverse effects on reproduction.

In a multigenerational study in rats utilizing doses as low as 2 and 5 mg/kg by gastric intubation, Shtenberg and Ozhovan[11] noted abnormal reproductive effects, including decreased spermatogenesis, decreased sperm motility, an increase in duration of estrus, a decrease in fertility of females and a decrease in the survival of pups during the first month of life. These findings should be contrasted with those of a 3-generational study by Weil et al.[14] with rats utilizing varying dosages up to 100 mg/kg by oral intubation and 200 mg/kg by dietary feeding. Weil et al. concluded, "The severe effects on reproduction reported by Shtenberg and Ozhovan,[11] following repeated oral intubation (OI) at 2 mg/kg to rats were not encountered in this concurrent study even at the maximum OI level of 100 mg/kg." They suggest that the differences in the findings may be related to the identity and purity of the carbaryl used. The signs of cholinesterase inhibition, the mortality and the reproductive effects these authors found occurred only at the maximal oral intubation dose of 100 mg/kg. The effects included a decrease in the percentage of females that littered (FO → F1b only), an increase in the number of days after first mating to birth of litter (FO → F1b only), a decrease in the number of pups born alive (F1a → F2a; F2a → F3a), a decrease in the number of fetuses and live fetuses (F2a → F3a) and an increase in the percentage of litters with resorption sites (F2a → F3b). These effects did not occur at 25 mg/kg by oral intubation or at the maximal dietary feeding level of 200 mg/kg. For the latter, the authors reported only a decrease in body weight before mating and an increase in the number of days between mating and birth of litter (F1a → F2a only).

In a comparison of mean sperm counts of 47 carbaryl workers and 90 nonexposed control workers, Avashia[1] found no evidence that carbaryl exposure impaired sperm production. Median sperm count in the workers was 92 million/ml and the median for the nonexposed 81 million/ml. Forty of 47 carbaryl workers had counts greater than 20 million/ml and 85 of 90 of the nonexposed had counts above 20 million/ml. Six workers had sperm counts below 20 million/ml and 3 nonexposed were below 20 million/ml, and both groups had 2% azoospermics. Carbaryl exposure levels were not reported.

The present OSHA standard for occupational exposure to carbaryl is an 8-hour time-weighted average of 5 mg/m^3 of air. NIOSH recommends this same TWA concentration for up to a 10-hour day, 40-hour workweek. NIOSH suggests that "if humans and lower animals do not differ significantly in their susceptibility to inhaled carbaryl, the results of inhalation studies in several animal species[4,17] would indicate that 16 mg/m^3 can be considered the no-adverse-effect level with respect to toxic manifestations of cholinesterase inhibition in humans." For such effect, therefore, the proposed standard should provide an adequate margin of safety, and, with the available data, it would appear that the proposed standard should have some margin of safety for the reproductive effects as well, provided that additional exposure through the skin and by ingestion through contaminated hands, etc., is prevented.

REFERENCES

Carbaryl

1. Avashia, B. H.: Testicular function among carbaryl exposed employees. Conference on Pesticides and Human Health, Society for Occupational and Environmental Health, Washington, D.C., Dec. 10–13, 1978.
2. Benson, B. W., Scott, W. J., and Beliles, R. P.: Sevin—Safety Evaluation by Teratological Study in the Mouse. Unpublished report submitted to Union Carbide Corp., 1967, 19 pp (cited in NIOSH Criteria Document[9]).
3. Breskij, V. V., and Vaskov, V. I.: Studies on mutation and calculation of fertility in Drosophila melanogaster under the effect of carbaryl, Angew. Parasitol. 13:23, 1971 (German) (cited in NIOSH Criteria Document[9]).
4. Carpenter, C. P., Weil, S. C., Palm, P. E., Woodside, M. W., Nair, J. H., III, and Smyth, H. F., Jr.: Mammalian toxicity of 1-naphthyl-N-methylcarbamate (Sevin insecticide), J. Agric. Food Chem. 9:30, 1961 (cited in NIOSH Criteria Document[9]).
5. Coulston, F.: *The Effect of Carbaryl on Reproduction in the Rhesus Monkey* (Albany, N.Y.: Albany Medical College, Institute of Experimental Pathology & Toxicology, 1971), 18 pp.
6. Dougherty, W. J., and Coulston, F.: Teratogenic evaluation of carbaryl in the rhesus monkey (Macaca mulatta). Unpublished report submitted to Union Carbide Corp., June 6, 1975.
7. Elespuru, R., Lijinsky, W., and Setlow, J. K.: Nitrosocarbaryl as a potent mutagen of environmental significance, Nature 247:386, 1974 (cited in NIOSH Criteria Document[9]).
8. Epstein, S. S., Arnold, E., Andrea, J., Bass, W., and Bishop, Y.: Detection of chemical mutagens by the dominant lethal assay in the mouse, Toxicol. Appl. Pharmacol. 23:288, 1972 (cited in NIOSH Criteria Document[9]).
9. National Institute for Occupational Safety and Health: Criteria for a recommended standard . . . occupational exposure to carbaryl, DHEW, PHS, NIOSH 77–107, 1976.
10. Robens, J. F.: Teratologic studies of carbaryl, diazinon, norea, disulfram, and thiram in small laboratory animals, Toxicol. Appl. Pharmacol. 15:152, 1969.
11. Shtenberg, A. I., and Ozhovan, M. V.: The effect of low Sevin doses on the reproductive function of animals in a number of generations, Vopr. Pitan. 30:42, 1971 (Russian) (cited in NIOSH Criteria Document[9]).
12. Smalley, H. E., Curtis, J. M., and Earl, F. L.: Teratogenic action of carbaryl in beagle dogs, Toxicol. Appl. Pharmacol. 13:392, 1968.
13. Uchiyama, M., Tadeda, M., Suzuki, T., and Yoshikawa, K.: Mutagenicity of nitroso derivatives of N-methylcarbamate insecticides in microbiological method, Bull. Environ. Contam. Toxicol. 14:389, 1975 (cited in NIOSH Criteria Document[9]).
14. Weil, C. S., Woodside, M. D., Bernard, J. B., Condra, N. I., King, J. M., and Carpenter, C. P.: Comparative effect of carbaryl on rat reproduction and guinea pig teratology when fed either in the diet or by stomach intubation, Toxicol. Appl. Pharmacol. 26:621, 1973.
15. Weil, C. S., Woodside, M. D., Carpenter, C. P., and Smyth, H. F., Jr.: Current status of tests of carbaryl for reproductive and teratogenic effect, Toxicol. Appl. Pharmacol. 21:390, 1972 (cited in NIOSH Criteria Document[9]).
16. Whorton, D. M., Milby, T. H., and Stubbs, H. A.: Testicular function among carbaryl-exposed employees, J. Tox. and Environ. Health 5:929, 1979.
17. Yakim, V. S.: The maximum permissible concentration of Sevin in the air of the work zone, Gig. Sanit. 32:29, 1968 (Russian) (cited in NIOSH Criteria Document[9]).

Carbon Disulfide

CARBON DISULFIDE (CS_2) is a colorless, volatile and extremely flammable liquid at room temperature. Annually, more than 350 million kg (782 million lb) of CS_2 are produced in the United States. Approximately half the carbon disulfide produced in the early 1970s was used in the production of regenerated cellulose (viscose rayon and cellophane) and approximately a quarter was used in the manufacture of carbon tetrachloride. Carbon disulfide is also used in vulcanizing rubber, fumigating grain, chemical analysis, degreasing, dry cleaning and oil extraction. The NIOSH estimates that 20,000 employees are potentially exposed to carbon disulfide in the United States.[2]

Most of the studies of occupational exposure to carbon disulfide involve workers in the viscose industry, where there is concomitant exposure to hydrogen sulfide. The ratio of the concentration of evolved carbon disulfide to hydrogen sulfide is estimated at from 2:1 to 10:1. Several studies have revealed reproductive effects, including threatened abortion, spontaneous abortion and infertility in women and spermatic disorders in men. These studies have appeared primarily in the foreign literature and are reviewed in the NIOSH Criteria Document. The following is a summary of some of the material in the Criteria Document pertinent to reproduction. For further details, the reader is referred to the Document itself.[2]

Vigliani[10] reported on occupational carbon disulfide poisoning in Italy during 1940 and 1941. Factories operated at wartime peaks and employees were exposed 10–12 hours per day at concentrations that were as high as 800 ppm (2.50 mg/liter) with a mean concentration of 144–321 ppm (0.45–1.0 mg/liter). Of the 100 workers examined, 16% complained of "sexual weakness."

Erhardt[3] reported on a viscose rayon factory in the German Democratic Republic that first employed women in 1950 but barred their employment 6 months later because of increased menstrual bleeding. The author reported that by 1966, when the maximal allowable concentration (MAC) of 17 ppm (53 mg/m^3) was not exceeded, there were no identified instances of spontaneous abortions, amenorrhea, sterility or genital organ dysfunction. He suggests that it is not necessary to prohibit all women from exposure but that he would not expose pregnant women to carbon disulfide.

Finkova et al.[4] reported on 35 women exposed to carbon disulfide in a viscose rayon factory who were studied for possible gynecologic abnormalities during 1967–1969. Gynecologic examinations included inspection, palpation and cytologic smear tests. There were no abnormalities found, nor was there any evidence of irregular menstrual function, malformed fetuses, spontaneous abortions, hormonal disorders or altered sexual habits. The NIOSH notes that the report lacks information on methodology, quantitative data, extent of exposure, and there is no statistical analysis of results.

Jindrichova[5] studied workers in a cord-fiber factory who were exposed to carbon disulfide at a mean concentration of 64 ppm (200 mg/m^3). There were 160 men and 23 women included in the study, and it was reported that 99 men and 11 women had symptoms of carbon disulfide "poisoning." Among the symptoms most frequently reported among the men was loss of potency. There were no specific gynecologic conditions or disturbances encountered among the women.

Lancranjan et al.[7] studied young male workers in an artificial-fiber factory who had been exposed to carbon disulfide at an average concentration of 13–26 ppm (40–80 mg/m^3), with peaks of up to 250 ppm (780 mg/m^3). There were 33 workers with a mean age of 22 years and a mean length of exposure of 21 months who were diagnosed as chronically poisoned by carbon disulfide. The controls consisted of 31 males with a mean age of 25.9 years. Seventy-eight percent of the exposed workers showed disturbances of "sexual dynamics," decreased libido in 66% and erection difficulty in 51% being the most common problems. Semen analysis revealed that the poisoned workers had higher frequencies of asthenospermia, hypospermia and teratospermia than did the controls, and the excretion of total neutral 17-ketosteroids was lower in the exposed workers. The authors suggest that carbon disulfide may act on both the hypothalamus and directly on the gonads. In 1972, Lancranjan[6] used the same methods and examined 133 chronically poisoned male viscose workers and 50 controls, both with an average age of 30 years, for spermatic disorders. Again, significantly greater frequencies of hypospermia, teratospermia and asthenospermia were found in exposed workers than in the controls. Vasilyeva[9] studied 3 different groups of female viscose rayon workers that included 500 workers in the spinning department, where the concentrations of carbon disulfide sometimes exceeded 6 ppm (20 mg/m^3) and hydrogen sulfide concentrations never were more than 7 ppm (10 mg/m^3), 209 workers in the trimming department, where the concentration of neither carbon disulfide nor hydrogen sulfide exceeded 3 ppm (10 mg/m^3), and 429 workers in the rewinding-sorting department not exposed to either substance (controls). Among the workers of both the spinning and trimming departments there were increased numbers of women with menstrual flow of more than 5 days, abundant and painful menstruation and abnormal cellular composition of vaginal smears. The data suggest that exposure to carbon disulfide, even at concentrations below 3 ppm (10 mg/m^3), may affect ovarian hormone production in women and that the effect is increased in a dose-response relationship.

Petrov[8] compared a group of 189 women employed in the viscose industry who were exposed to carbon disulfide at levels of 9 ppm (28 mg/m^3) before and during pregnancy with a control group of 191 women who worked in the industry and had had no exposure to carbon disulfide. Adjustments were made for differences in age and job longevity. It was found that the exposed workers had significantly more difficulty than did controls from increased threatened abortions, spontaneous abortions and premature births.

Wakasuki and Higashikawa[11] exposed mature male and female rabbits to carbon disulfide at 300 ppm (930 mg/m^3) 30 minutes per day for 120 consecutive days or to hydrogen sulfide at 100 ppm (140 mg/m^3) or to both substances on the same exposure schedule. The animals were killed and examined 140 days after exposure. There were no significant testicular changes in the carbon disulfide group; seminiferous tubular atrophy leading to diminished spermatogenesis was found in the hydrogen sulfide group and there was complete absence of spermatogenesis in rabbits exposed to both gases. No impairment of ovaries was found among the female rabbits. The authors believed that where there were no observable abnormalities, it was due to the fact that exposure time had been limited to 30 minutes per day or to the period of 140 days that followed exposure, which could have permitted recovery. Damage caused by the combination of vapors was not reversible during this period and suggests toxic synergism when both carbon disulfide and hydrogen sulfide are present.

Barilyak et al.[1] studied the effects of a combination of carbon disulfide and hydrogen sulfide on reproduction in rats. Groups were studied where both parents were exposed, where either the male or female was exposed prior to conception, where females were exposed for up to 20 days of gestation and where females were not exposed during gestation. The authors found that exposure to carbon disulfide and hydrogen sulfide showed definite embryotoxicity and a weak teratogenic effect compared to controls.

Reports on mutagenesis resulting from exposure to carbon disulfide or to the combination of carbon disulfide and hydrogen sulfide have not been found.

Carbon disulfide is toxic when the vapor is inhaled or when there is repeated skin contact with the liquid. Toxic effects other than on the reproductive system are discussed in *Occupational Medicine: Principles and Practical Applications*.* Exposure in combination with hydrogen sulfide may cause toxic effects that are additive or possibly synergistic.

*Carl Zenz (ed.) (Chicago: Year Book Medical Publishers, 1975).

There is a need for additional epidemiologic studies with accurate measurements of exposure to carbon disulfide and to hydrogen sulfide in the viscose industry as well as in other industries where exposure to carbon disulfide may affect the health of the worker. Well-controlled animal experiments at exposures similar to those in the workplace of carbon disulfide and hydrogen sulfide alone and in combination should be conducted. Since some studies have shown reproductive system disorders and a possible teratogenic effect on exposure, it is important that careful records be kept on reproductive problems and offspring abnormalities in both male and female industrially exposed populations.

The current federal standard for carbon disulfide specifies an 8-hour TWA value of 20 ppm (62 mg/m^3), with an acceptable ceiling concentration of 30 ppm (93 mg/m^3) for an 8-hour day, 5-day workweek and an acceptable maximal peak of 100 ppm (311 mg/m^3) for 30 minutes during an 8-hour work shift.

On the basis of reported studies, the NIOSH[2] recommends that the carbon disulfide in the work environment should be controlled so that the concentration does not exceed 1 ppm (3 mg/m^3) as a TWA concentration for up to a 10-hour work shift in a 40-hour workweek and also does not exceed 10 ppm (30 mg/m^3) as a ceiling concentration for any 15-minute period. Compliance with the recommended carbon disulfide standard should also reduce exposure to hydrogen sulfide.

REFERENCES

Carbon Disulfide

1. Barilyak, I. D., Vasilyeva, I. A., and Kalinovskaya, L. I.: Effects of small concentrations of carbon disulfide and hydrogen sulfide on intrauterine development in rats, Arkh. Anat. Gistol. Embriol. 68:77, 1975 (Russian) (cited in NIOSH Criteria Document[2]).
2. National Institute for Occupational Safety and Health: Criteria for a recommended standard . . . occupational exposure to carbon disulfide, DHEW, PHS, NIOSH 77–156, 1977.
3. Erhardt, W.: Experiences with the Employment of Women Exposed to Carbon Disulfide, in Brieger, H., Teisinger, J. (eds.), *Toxicology of Carbon Disulphide* (Amsterdam: Excerpta Medica Foundation, 1967), p. 240 (cited in NIOSH Criteria Document[2]).
4. Finkova, A., Simko, A., Jindrichova, J., Kovarik, J., Preiningerova, O., Klimova, A., and Koriski, F.: Gynecologic problems of women working in an environment contaminated with carbon disulfide, Cesk. Gynekol. 38:535, 1973 (Czech) (cited in NIOSH Criteria Document[2]).
5. Jindrichova, J.: Health status of workers in the cord fiber industry, Prac. Lek. 9:10, 1957 (Czech translation).
6. Lancranjan, I.: Alterations of spermatic liquid in patients chronically poisoned by carbon disulphide, Med. Lav. 63:29, 1972 (cited in NIOSH Criteria Document[2]).
7. Lancranjan, I., Popescu, H. I., and Klepsch, I.: Changes of the gonadic function in chronic carbon disulphide poisoning, Med. Lav. 60:566, 1969 (cited in NIOSH Criteria Document[2]).
8. Petrov, M. V.: Some data on the course and termination of pregnancy in female workers of the viscose industry, Pediatr. Akush. Ginekol. 3:50, 1969 (Russian) (cited in NIOSH Criteria Document[2]).
9. Vasilyeva, I. A.: Effect of low concentrations of carbon disulfide and hydrogen sulfide on the menstrual function of women and the estrual cycle in an experiment, Gig. Sanit. 7:24, 1973 (Russian) (cited in NIOSH Criteria Document[2]).
10. Vigliani, E. C.: Carbon disulphide poisoning in viscose rayon factories, Br. J. Ind. Med. 11:235, 1954 (cited in NIOSH Criteria Document[2]).
11. Wakasuki, T., and Higashikawa, H.: Experimental studies on CS_2 and H_2S poisoning—the histological changes in hematopoietic organs and other main internal organs, Shikoku. Igaku, Zasshi, 14:549, 1959 (Japanese) (cited in NIOSH Criteria Document[2]).

Carbon Monoxide

ERIC P. KINDWALL, M.D., and CARL ZENZ, M.D.

THIS SECTION will not consider details of acute or chronic occupational exposures to carbon monoxide or its pathophysiology and treatment. (For these specific aspects, see Kindwall, in *Occupational Medicine: Principles and Practical Applications*.[22]) Certain aspects pertinent to both men and women working with potential exposure to CO will be emphasized.

The classic explanation for the toxicity of carbon monoxide, which was taught for many years, is that carboxyhemoglobin is incapable of carrying oxygen. This means that even if a person breathes 100% oxygen after exposure to carbon monoxide, the tissues will not be adequately oxygenated for some time. At any given level of carbon monoxide in the air breathed, the rate at which blood becomes saturated with carbon monoxide is directly proportional to cardiac output. Thus, a person working vigorously will note the onset of symptoms and signs much more quickly than will one who is sedentary or at rest. From a practical standpoint, a worker driving a fork-lift truck (a job commonly assigned to women) will have a much lower level of carbon monoxide in the bloodstream than will one who is loading heavy barrels onto a pallet in the same environment. A person running around in a building seeking an escape route from a fire will be overcome more quickly than will someone quietly asleep.

Over the years, however, further research has shown that formation of carboxyhemoglobin is not the main mechanism of carbon monoxide toxicity. In 1975, Goldbaum et al.[15] produced a definitive paper demonstrating that carboxyhemoglobinemia was of only minor or secondary importance in carbon monoxide poisoning. In their experiments at the Armed Forces Institute of Pathology, they used 3 groups of 5 dogs each. Group I was given 13% carbon monoxide by inhalation. Group II was bled to an anemic state, reducing the hemoglobin content of the blood by an average of 68% and then had blood volumes restored to normal with saline and dextran. Group III was bled to the same anemic state as Group II but then transfused with packed red cells that contained 80% carboxyhemoglobin. All the dogs in Group I died within an hour with carboxyhemoglobin levels ranging between 54% and 90%. Group II dogs survived indefinitely. Most important was that Group III dogs survived indefinitely with determined carboxyhemoglobin levels of 60% (57–64%).

From the foregoing it is clear that even extensive combination of the hemoglobin with carbon monoxide is not very dangerous. Other workers[3, 6, 19] have demonstrated that the true site of toxicity is the cytochrome A_3 oxidase in the mitochondria. The clinical condition of the patient, therefore, is determined by the amount of cytochrome A_3 oxidase that is blocked. This is the same enzyme that is affected in cyanide poisoning and hydrogen sulfide poisoning. Fortunately, oxygen competes with carbon monoxide for binding to cytochrome oxidase and, therefore, oxygen treatment is effective. Because it is not clinically possible to measure the level of impairment of the cytochrome system, our only laboratory index is the carboxyhemoglobin. It must be borne in mind that all of the published literature relates various degrees of incapacitation to the carboxyhemoglobin level. These must be interpreted as averages, depending on whether the exposure is acute, chronic or prolonged. The actual clinical status of patients varies widely with any given level of carboxyhemoglobin.

When the tissues of the body become hypoxic due to cytochrome blockade, the heart must supply more blood by increasing both its rate and its output. Thus, the coronary arteries must supply more oxygen to the heart. Normally, the myocardium extracts 75% of the oxygen supplied to it via the coronary arteries. This is much more than the brain uses. Therefore, anyone with coronary heart disease soon will suffer from hypoxia of the myocardium and the heart should be considered the first target organ in carbon monoxide poisoning because of the necessity for increased cardiac output. Normally, the myocardium extracts pyruvate and lactate from the coronary circulation for oxidation. When the carboxyhemoglobin reaches a mean of 8.7%, the myocardium fails to extract either of these two substances and actually produces both.[2] An 8.7% anemia obviously is not the cause, but the mitochondrial cytochrome failure is the explanation.

Chronic exposure to levels of carbon monoxide of various concentrations, but not immediately lethal, has produced extremely variable changes in animals, both behavioral and histologic. On the basis of these findings and the work from a number of investigators, presently it is impossible to state what levels of CO in the blood will produce permanent pathologic changes in humans. However, one investigator found that dogs exposed to 100 ppm CO for 5¾ hours a day, 6 days a week, for 11 weeks showed no electroencephalographic changes but did show psychomotor disturbances and cerebrocortical damage that tended to follow the course of the blood vessels. This same investigator also found that in one experiment a diminished cardiac output was associated with more damage to the brain.

Brain damage can consist of infarction of the cerebral cortex, degenerative changes, formation of cysts, gliosis, paravascular infiltration, loss of myelin and softening of the white matter. The basal ganglia show the most severe damage, with loss of cells and demyelination.[23]

In summary, carbon monoxide produces tissue hypoxia and, along with it, the expected changes in function and, if prolonged and severe, histopathologic changes that are associated with hypoxia.

Insufficient knowledge exists about the biologic effects of CO during intrauterine development and on the newborn; several studies have revealed decreased birth weights and increased mortality in the progeny of animals exposed to relatively high carbon monoxide concentrations, but few studies have reported on subtle effects of low concentrations. There is no information implicating CO effects on the fetus from occupational exposures, but there is much information on such effects from maternal smoking. This section is intended to offer a brief overview of the potential problems involving the developing embryo, fetus and newborn infant to CO exposures not associated with tobacco smoking.

The carboxyhemoglobin concentration in the blood of normal nonsmoking pregnant women varies from 0.5% to 1%.[1] In addition to those factors affecting carboxyhemoglobin in the nonpregnant person,[5] maternal carboxyhemoglobin concentration (HbCOm) reflects the endogenous carbon monoxide production by the fetus and its rate of exchange across the placenta.[25] Fetal endogenous carbon monoxide production accounts for about 3% of the total carboxyhemoglobin present in the blood of a normal pregnant woman.

In 1949, Sjöstrand,[38] utilizing improved methods of measurements, demonstrated that the human body was a net producer of carbon monoxide, identifying the source as the alpha-methene bridge between the four porphyrin units in the heme molecule. During the "recycling" of the heme molecule reclaiming iron, four molecules of carbon monoxide are released for every molecule of heme catabolized.

Not only must endogenous carbon monoxide formation in the human body be considered but other external contaminants may further compound the carbon monoxide problem. Most commonly encountered, both within industry as well as outside industry, especially the smaller working establishments and in homes, is exposure to paint removers containing a variety of hydrocarbon ingredients, a major one being methylene chloride (dichloromethane, CH_2Cl_2), which has been shown to be rapidly metabolized to carbon monoxide.[35] Under conditions of poor ventilation, such as insufficient air movement in a home garage, basement or small workplace, concentrations of methylene chloride vapors can quickly accumulate and be readily inspired. Stewart and Hake[39] have shown that the use of such paint remover for a period of 3 hours can easily produce carboxyhemoglobin saturation of 5–10% in man. It is not possible to determine the extent of use of paint removers in the private sector of the United States, and perhaps equally difficult to determine is occupational exposure to methylene chloride in the thousands of workplaces where solvents are in daily use. From the viewpoint of potential worker exposure, it is noteworthy that methylene chloride, although not the most hazardous chlorinated hydrocarbon compound, is unique in the context of a carbon monoxide source. In addition to its common use as a paint or varnish "stripper" (remover), it is widely used in degreasing, as an aerosol propellant, as a solvent for paint, plastics and textile making, in producing photo films and in preparing certain oils and waxes. (Not to be forgotten, it has been used as a general anesthetic.) The NIOSH estimate of exposure in the United States is about 70,000 workers, excluding home use.[12]

Studies have shown that even relatively low levels of carbon monoxide as blood carboxyhemoglobin concentrations of 4–5% result in subtle alterations in mental ability and the performance of certain functions in normal adults. Additional evidence from several extensive studies with long-term follow-up of the infants of smoking mothers demonstrates retardation of mental abilities. The pregnant woman, her fetus and the newborn infant have been identified as subjects particularly vulnerable to the effects of low concentrations of carbon monoxide.

The relationship of carboxyhemoglobin concentrations to inspired carbon monoxide concentrations in adult humans has been experimentally determined in several studies. Recently, Longo and Hill[28] studied these relationships in pregnant sheep with catheters chronically implanted in maternal and fetal blood vessels. They exposed ewes to inspired carbon monoxide concentrations of up to 300 ppm. At 30 ppm, maternal carboxyhemoglobin concentrations increased over a period of 8–10 hours, equilibrating at about 4.6 ± 0.3% (SEM). The fetal carboxyhemoglobin concentration increased more slowly, equilibrating in 36–48 hours at about 7.4 ± 0.5%. At 50 ppm, the time courses were similar, with maternal and fetal steady-state values of 7.2 ± 0.5% and 11.3 ± 1.1%, respectively. At 100 ppm, maternal and fetal steady-state values were 12.2 ± 1.2% and 19.8 ± 1.4%, respectively. For all concentrations, the half-times for carbon monoxide uptake by maternal and fetal blood were about 2 and 6 hours, respectively.

For ethical and technical reasons, such experiments cannot be carried out with humans. The same investigators[28] examined the experimental data and theorized a mathematical model of the interrelationships of human fetal and maternal carboxyhemoglobin concentrations. The predicted changes in the carboxyhemoglobin concentrations as a function of the time of exposure to inspired carbon monoxide ranged from 30 to 300 ppm. Several points of interest are: The equilibration for fetal carboxyhemoglobin was not achieved for about 30–36 hours, the half-time of the increase in fetal carboxyhemoglobin concentration was about 7.5 hours for all concentrations, the time for fetal carboxyhemoglobin to equal the maternal value varied from 12 to 15 hours and, finally, under steady-state conditions, fetal carboxyhemoglobin concentration was about 15% greater than the maternal. The theoretic relationships in humans and the experimental data in sheep are in reasonably good agreement.

Studies have revealed the effects of carbon monoxide on fetal growth. Wells[41] exposed pregnant rats to 1.5% (15,000 ppm) carbon monoxide for from 5 to 8 minutes 10 times on alternate days during their 21-day pregnancy. This resulted in maternal unconsciousness and abortion or absorption of most fetuses. The surviving newborns did not grow normally. Similar exposure to 5900 ppm affected only a small percentage of animals. Williams and Smith[42] exposed rats to 0.34% (3400 ppm) carbon monoxide for 1 hour daily for 3 months, demonstrating peak carboxyhemoglobin concentrations in these animals of from 60% to 70%, and the number of pregnancies known to occur among those 7 exposed animals was half the number in the controls. The number of rats born per litter decreased, and only 2 of 13 newborns survived to weaning age. There were no pregnancies in the 5 females exposed for 150 days to this concentration.

Astrup et al.[1] reported quantitative data on fetal weights of 2 groups of pregnant rabbits exposed to carbon monoxide continually for 30 days. Exposure to 90 ppm yielded maternal carboxyhemoglobin concentrations of 9–10% from a control value of 4.5%. Mortality of the young rabbits during the following 21 days increased to 25% from a control value of 13%. Doubling the concentration of carbon monoxide to 180 ppm resulted in maternal carboxyhemoglobin concentrations of 16–18%, birth weights decreased 20% from 53.7 to 44.7 gm and neonatal mortality was 35% compared with 1% for the controls. Mortality during the following 21 days was the same value as for the controls, 27%.

Williams and Smith[42] studied the effects of carbon monoxide on newborn survival in animals. They exposed rats to mixtures of illuminating gas in air, with inspired carbon monoxide concentrations of 0.43%. In 22 newborn rats 12–48 hours old exposed to carbon monoxide, the average survival time was about 196 minutes, in contrast to an average survival of about 36 minutes in mature animals. McGrath and Jaeger[31] also noted that 50% of newly hatched chicks could withstand exposure to 1% (10,000 ppm) carbon monoxide concentrations for about 32 minutes. This survival time decreased to about 10 minutes; by day 4 it was 6 minutes and by day 8 it was 4 minutes, where it remained for all subsequent days tested up to 21 days. Subsequently, Jaeger and McGrath[20] showed that decreasing the body temperature increased the time to last gasp from a mean value of 9.8 ± 0.5 minutes at 40° C to 20.7 ± 0.1 minute at 30° C. They noted that hypothermia caused markedly reduced heart and respiratory rates and suggested that its major benefit was a reduction in energy-requiring functions.

In 1977, Fechter and Annau[13] demonstrated reduced birth weight and decreased weight gain in rat offspring, using rats prenatally exposed to concentrations of 150 ppm of carbon monoxide. Neurobehavioral and biochemical testing of these offspring revealed lower behavioral activity levels through the preweaning period, altered central catecholamine activity and reduction in total brain protein at birth. They suggested that the potentially more serious consequences of altered central nervous system function and biochemistry early in life or, perhaps, permanently are only now beginning to be discovered by the use of animal models.

Several mechanisms probably account for the effects of carbon monoxide on developing tissue. As described earlier (Kindwall [22]), undoubtedly the most important of these is the interference with tissue oxygenation. Carbon monoxide also interferes with oxygen transport by displacing oxygen from the hemoglobin in arterial blood, thus decreasing the blood oxygen capacity. For the pregnant woman, these effects on blood oxygenation pose a special threat. Not only is her oxygen consumption increased 15–25% during pregnancy[27] but her blood oxygen capacity is decreased 20–30% or more due to the decreased concentration of hemoglobin.[15] The woman with a significant anemia faces even more severe compromise of her oxygen delivery.

The oxygen affinity of fetal blood is greater than that of maternal blood; hence, its oxyhemoglobin saturation curve is shifted to the left. In addition, human fetal blood contains more hemoglobin than does maternal blood (16.3 vs 12 gm/100 ml); therefore, it has a greater oxygen capacity.[15] Under normal circumstances, maternal arterial oxygen tension is about 100 mm Hg and its oxygen content equals 16.1 ml/100 ml of blood. The placental exchange of oxygen extracts about 5 ml O_2/100 ml of blood, producing a uterine mixed venous oxygen tension of about 34 mm Hg. When the maternal blood contains carboxyhemoglobin, the oxygen capacity is decreased and the oxyhemoglobin curve shifts to the left. Whereas arterial oxygen tension remains essentially the same as under normal conditions, the oxygen content is reduced to 14.5 ml/100 ml. With the same placental oxygen transfer of 5 ml/100 ml of blood, the venous oxygen tension would be about 27 mm Hg, a decrease from normal of about 7 mm Hg.

Ginsberg and Myers[14] studied the effects of carbon monoxide exposure on near-term pregnant monkeys and their fetuses. The anesthetized animals were acutely exposed to 0.1–0.3% carbon monoxide, resulting in maternal carboxyhemoglobin levels of about 60%. These 1–3-hour studies showed the following: fetal blood oxygen content (pH less than 7.05), hypercapnia (P_{CO_2} = 70 mm Hg or greater), hypotension and electrocardiographic changes such as T wave flattening and inversion.[14]

Longo and Hill[28] studied changes in oxygen tension in response to various carboxyhemoglobin concentrations in sheep in which catheters were implanted in maternal and fetal vessels. About 1 week following recovery from anesthesia and surgery, the ewes were exposed to various concentrations of carbon monoxide. Fifty-seven percent of the sheep fetuses in this study died when fetal carboxyhemoglobin values were greater than 15% for 30 minutes or longer (5 of 11 died at 100 ppm and 3 of 3 died at 300 ppm). These deaths were attributed to hypoxia of vital tissues. Hypoxia from carbon monoxide may interfere with tissue oxygenation by increasing the concentration of carboxymyoglobin (MbCO), in relation to carboxyhemoglobin, which is additive to the cytochrome A_3 derangement.

Coburn et al.[7] showed that when arterial oxygen tension decreases to 40 mm Hg or lower, the ratio of carboxymyoglobin to carboxyhemoglobin increases from a normal value of 1.0 to about 2.5 in the resting dog skeletal muscle and myocardium of dogs.[8] Assuming that a similar relationship exists in the fetus, where arterial blood P_{O_2} is normally 30 mm Hg or less, carboxymyoglobin concentrations would be 12.5% when the carboxyhemoglobin is 5%. This degree of carboxymyoglobin saturation may be of importance to fetal myocardial cells.

In a hog-raising building, gas-heated carbon monoxide was emitted because of improper heater function in concentrations ranging from 2.4 to 3 times the allowable 50 ppm. Although the hogs raised in these affected areas displayed no signs of carbon monoxide poisoning, those sows that were placed there a few days before farrowing gave birth to an unusually high proportion of dead piglets; in some cases, 100% were born dead. After the heating system was repaired, the loss of newborn piglets ceased immediately, according to Keller.[21]

The relationship between altitude and birth weight has been noted by Grahn and

Kratchman,[16] who showed that the proportion of low birth weights increased with increasing elevation. The number of infants weighing less than 2500 gm increased to 10.1% at 1500–1580 m (4900—5190 ft) from a control value of 6.6% at sea level. At 2760 m (9055 ft), the number of such newborns further increased to 16.6%. A given carboxyhemoglobin concentration may cause a more profound effect on tissue oxygenation at high altitudes than at sea level. Persons at higher altitudes would be expected to be more sensitive to the effects of carbon monoxide, and this would be especially true of a pregnant mother, whose oxygen demand is greater than when not pregnant, as well as for the newborn infant.

In the United States, approximately 2.2 million people live at altitudes at or above 1525 m (5000 ft), the majority of high-altitude residents living at elevations between 1500 and 2000 m. There are no available data concerning numbers of workers who may be exposed to carbon monoxide at work or away from work living at higher altitudes nor are there figures available for the changes of population due to tourist fluctuations with seasonal factors. A point to consider is that more and more families are using trailers and mobile homes for both living and vacationing purposes, and not all units are safely heated, which means that considerable potential for carbon monoxide exposures exists in the nonoccupational setting for these groups of people.

Longo[27] prepared an intensive review of the biologic effects of carbon monoxide on the pregnant woman, fetus and newborn infant, describing physiologic and biochemical bases and their clinical implications, pointing out significant alterations of certain physiologic functions resulting from relatively low blood carboxyhemoglobin concentrations in pregnant women, fetuses and newborn infants, who are particularly susceptible to carbon monoxide effects. In cases reviewed in his report, mothers exposed to high concentrations of carbon monoxide showed classic signs and symptoms of carbon monoxide poisoning and, in many of these, surviving infants subsequently developed neurologic sequelae. Infants who died at a later date showed brain damage at autopsy.[26, 29, 30] The lesions described resulted from fetal cerebral anoxia during pregnancy, labor and delivery and also during the immediate newborn period.[4]

Longo reiterated that the pregnant woman probably is more susceptible to the effects of carbon monoxide than is the nonpregnant woman. Clearly, then, pregnant working mothers, their embryos and newborn infants certainly constitute a population group at risk from the effects of carbon monoxide. With the increasing numbers of women entering various workplaces, occupational health physicians as well as obstetricians, pediatricians and family practitioners and allied health personnel must recognize these new potential hazards of inadvertent exposure of the fetus and the neonate to carbon monoxide as well as other potential environmental hazards. There are no established guidelines or standards to allow for safe placement of the potentially pregnant woman worker who may be exposed to carbon monoxide concentrations to make any valid predictions to ensure the future well-being of her unborn child.[27] Rational recommendations for "safe upper limits" to exposure in the workplace to carbon monoxide will be developed to protect the unborn child. For the present, appropriate hygienic measures must not be overlooked, and adherence to the TLV for carbon monoxide of 35 ppm is recommended. Of note is that different work loads and energy expenditure were not considered in establishing the present standard (50 ppm) or the recommended one (35 ppm).

The final and most critical point is that we have no solid data regarding transport of unbound CO across the placenta and the importance of its effect on the fetal cytochrome system.

REFERENCES

Carbon Monoxide

1. Astrup, P., Olsen, H. M., Trolle, D., and Kjelken, J.: Effects of moderate carbon monoxide exposure on fetal development, Lancet 2:1220, 1972.
2. Ayres, S. M., et al.: Systemic and myocardial hemodynamic responses to relatively small concentrations of carboxyhemoglobin (COHB), Arch. Environ. Health 18:699, 1969.
3. Ball, E. G., Strittmalter, C. F., and Cooper, O.: The reaction to carbon monoxide, J. Biol. Chem. 193:635, 1951.
4. Bernard, C.: *Lecons sur les Effets des Substances Toxiques et Meticamenteuses* (Paris: J. B. Baillière et Fils, 1957).
5. Caton, W. L., et al.: The circulating red cell volume and body hematocrit in normal pregnancy and the puerperium; by direct measurement, using radioactive red cells, Am. J. Obstet. Gynecol. 61:1207, 1951.
6. Chance, B., Erecinska, M., and Wagner, M.: Mitochondrial responses to CO toxicity, Ann. N.Y. Acad. Sci. 174:193, 1970.
7. Coburn, R. F., Forster, R. E., and Kane, P. B.: Considerations of the physiological variables that determine the blood carboxyhemoglobin concentration in man, J. Clin. Invest. 44:1899, 1965.
8. Coburn, R. F., and Mayers, L. B.: Myoglobin O_2 tension determined from measurements of carboxyhemoglobin in skeletal muscle, Am. J. Physiol. 222:66, 1971.
9. Coburn, R. F., Ploegmakers, F., Gondrie, P., and Abboud, F.: Myocardial myoglobin oxygen tension, Am. J. Physiol. 224:870, 1973.
10. Courville, C. B.: *Contributions to the Study of Cerebral Anoxia. Some Observations on Its History, Its Pathogenesis and Structural Characteristics, the Importance of Its Circulatory Component and Its Significance in the Evaluation of Certain Chronic Diseases of the Brain of Infancy and Early Childhood* (Los Angeles: San Lucas Press, 1953), pp. 155–216.
11. National Institute for Occupational Safety and Health: Criteria document for a recommended standard: Occupational exposure to carbon monoxide, USDHEW, PHS, NIOSH (HSM 73–11000), 1972.
12. National Institute for Occupational Safety and Health: Criteria document for a recommended standard: Occupational exposure to methylene chloride, USDHEW, PHS, NIOSH 76–138, 1976.
13. Fechter, L. D., and Annau, Z.: Toxicity of mild prenatal carbon monoxide exposure, Science 197:680, 1977.
14. Ginsberg, M. D., and Myers, R. E.: Fetal brain injury after maternal carbon monoxide intoxication: Clinical and neuropathologic aspects, Neurology 26:15, 1976.
15. Goldbaum, L. R., Ramierez, R. G., and Absalon, K. B.: What is the mechanism of carbon monoxide toxicity?, Aviat. Space Environ. Med. 46:1289, 1975.
16. Grahn, D., and Kratchman, J.: Variations in neonatal death rate and birth weight in the United States and possible relations to environmental radiation, geology and altitude, Am. J. Hum. Genet. 15:329, 1963.
17. Hellman, L. M., and Pritchard, J. A.: *Williams Obstetrics* (14th ed.; New York: Appleton-Century-Crofts, 1971).
18. Hill, E. P., Hill, J. R., Power, G. G., and Longo, L. D.: Carbon monoxide exchanged between the human fetus and mother: A mathematical model, Am. J. Physiol. 232:H311, 1977.
19. Ingenito, A. J., Fiedler, P. C., and Procita, L.: Negative inotropic action of carbon monoxide on the isolated isovolumic heart with a hemoglobin-free perfusate, Fed. Proc. 33:502, 1974.
20. Jaeger, J. J., and McGrath, J. J.: Effects of hypothermia on heart and respiratory responses of chick to carbon monoxide, J. Appl. Physiol. 34:564, 1973.
21. Keller, H.: Hoher kohlemonoxydgehalt der stalluft als ursache von totgeburten beim schwein, Schweiz. Arch. Tierheilkd. 118:424, 1976.
22. Kindwall, E. P.: Carbon Monoxide, in Zenz, C. (ed.), *Occupational Medicine: Principles and Practical Applications* (Chicago: Year Book Medical Publishers, 1975), pp. 605–612.
23. Lewey, F. H., and Drabkin, D. L.: Experimental chronic carbon monoxide poisoning in dogs, Am. J. Med. Sci. 208:502, 1944.
24. Linderholm, H., and Lundstrom, P.: Endogenous carbon monoxide production and blood loss at delivery, Acta Obstet. Gynecol. Scand. 48:362, 1969.
25. Longo, L. D.: Carbon monoxide: Effects on oxygenation of the fetus in utero, Science 194:523, 1976.
26. Longo, L. D.: Carbon monoxide in the pregnant mother and fetus and its exchange

across the placenta, Ann. N.Y. Acad. Sci. 174:313, 1970.
27. Longo, L. D.: The biologic effects of carbon monoxide on the pregnant woman, the fetus and newborn infant, Am. J. Obstet. Gynecol. 129:69, 1977.
28. Longo, L. D., and Hill, E. P.: Carbon monoxide uptake and elimination in fetal and maternal sheep, Am. J. Physiol. 232:H324, 1977.
29. Longo, L. D., Power, G. G., and Forster, R. E.: II: Respiratory function of the placenta as determined with carbon monoxide in sheep and dogs, J. Clin. Invest. 46:812, 1967.
30. Maresch, R.: Über einen Fall von Kohlenoxydgasschadigung des Kindes in der Gebarmutter, Wien. Med. Wochenschr. 79:454, 1929.
31. McGrath, J. J., and Jaeger, J.: Effect of iodoacetate on the carbon monoxide tolerance of the chick, Respir. Physiol. 12:71, 1971.
32. National Academy of Sciences: Carbon Monoxide, Medical & Biological Effects of Environmental Pollutants, Washington, D.C., 1977.
33. Neuburger, F.: Fall einer intrauterinen Hirnschadigung nach einer Leuchtgasvergiftung der Mutter, Beitr. Gerichtl. Med. 13:85, 1935.
34. Pernoll, M. L., et al.: Oxygen consumption at rest and during exercise in pregnancy, Respir. Physiol. 25:285, 1975.
35. Ratney, R. S., Wegman, D. H., and Elkins, H. B.: In vivo conversion of methylene chloride to carbon monoxide, Arch. Environ. Health 28:223, 1974.
36. Ringold, A., et al.: Estimating recent carbon monoxide exposures: A rapid method, Arch. Environ. Health 5:308, 1962.
37. Schwedenberg, T. H.: Leukoencephalopathy following carbon monoxide asphyxia, J. Neuropathol. Exp. Neurol. 18:597, 1959.
38. Sjöstrand, T.: Endogenous formation of carbon monoxide in man under normal and pathological conditions, Scand. J. Clin. Lab. Invest. 1:201, 1949.
39. Stewart, R. D., and Hake, C. L.: Paint-remover hazard, JAMA 235:398, 1976.
40. U.S. Environmental Protection Agency: Guidelines for Air Quality Maintenance Planning and Analysis. Vol. 9. Evaluating Indirect Sources. EPA 450/4–75–001. Research Triangle Park, N.C.: U.S. Environ. Prot. Agency, Office of Air Quality, Planning and Standards, 557 pp., 1975.
41. Wells, L. L.: The prenatal effect of carbon monoxide on albino rats and the resulting neuropathy, Biologist 15:80, 1933.
42. Williams, I. R., and Smith, E.: Blood picture, reproduction and general condition during daily exposure to illuminating gas, Am. J. Physiol. 110:611, 1935.

Chlordane and Heptachlor

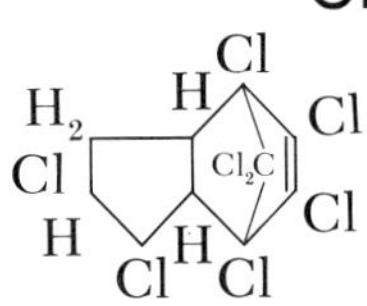

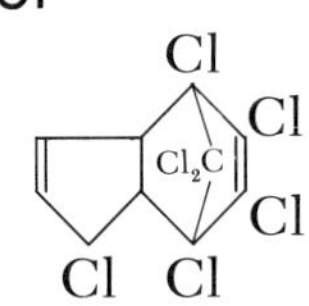

THESE TWO INSECTICIDES are members of the cyclodiene group of chlorinated insecticides, which includes aldrin, dieldrin, endrin and DDT. (See Chapter 13, showing chemical structures and their similarities.) Chlordane, first introduced in 1945, is one of the most widely used pesticides for household and garden applications. In the United States, more than 9.5 million kg are used per year, about 70% applied for termite control and the remainder in agricultural applications. Both chlordane and heptachlor are relatively persistent in the environment, with half-lives of 1 year (chlordane) and 0.8 year for heptachlor when used in agricultural applications. Chlordane and heptachlor have been tested under the carcinogenesis program of the National Cancer Institute, selected by the NCI for bioassay because of known biologic effects of low doses of either compound over extended periods, because of the persistence of both compounds in the environment and the known probability of continued human exposure. In December, 1975, the Environmental Protection Agency ordered a suspension of the use of chlordane and heptachlor, which became effective in August, 1976. There were a number of specific exemptions and use still is permitted for pest control on pineapples, use against root-destroying insects on strawberries, Florida citrus crops and other pest-control programs within specified state areas. The major current use is against termites, which is exempted from the EPA order.[9] Although there was a reduction of use of these compounds from approximately 7.0 million kg, current usage for permitted purposes still amounts to about 3.0 million kg per year in the United States.

Exposure to chlordane and absorption into the body can occur through the intact skin, by inhalation of dust or sprays and by ingestion. Human intoxication, along with fatalities, has been reported from both dermal and oral exposures to chlordane.[1,4,5,8] There are only a few reports concerning occupational exposure to chlordane, these being mainly reports in the manufacturing and handling of these substances. These reports present little data, chiefly because of the small number of workers involved or studied and for apparent high turnover in the working groups reported.[1]

Chlordane is less toxic than other cyclodiene pesticides, but acute exposure has the effect of stimulating the central nervous system. The compound metabolizes to its epoxide, oxychlordane, in which form it may be stored in body fat. It is said to be absorbable through the gastrointestinal tract, respiratory tract and directly through the skin. Both chlordane and heptachlor have been found to be mutagenic when tested in experimental organisms.

Trace amounts of heptachlor epoxide have been found in human fat tissues in most countries. The compound has been found in the blood, fat tissues, heart, adrenal gland and liver of stillborn infants, indicating that it can cross the placenta.[3] It has been found in human milk.[11] In other tests, concentrations of heptachlor epoxide in fat, liver and brain were not found to be significantly different between cancer patients and cancer-free persons.

Under test conditions, chlordane and heptachlor both were found to be carcinogenic for the liver in mice and possibly were causes of thyroid tumors in rats.[10]

Infante et al.[6] reviewed certain blood dyscrasias and childhood tumors suspected from the histories to be related to chlordane and heptachlor. Reports of 5 cases of neuroblastoma related to a history of possible exposure to chlordane during prenatal and postnatal development were identified, as were 3 cases of aplastic anemia and 3 cases of acute leukemia. These authors indicated that the children with neuroblastoma were diagnosed at a single pediatric hospital between December, 1974, and February, 1976. During this period, a total of 14 patients with neuroblastoma were admitted. History of exposure to toxic agents indicated that 5 patients had prior exposure to chlordane formulations. Noteworthy in one case is that the mother took two Valium tablets in early pregnancy and also had received a general anesthetic for a tonsillectomy during the first month of pregnancy and that the general anesthesia was induced with sodium thiopental and was maintained with halothane and nitrous oxide. Infante et al. noted that in the 9 additional cases of neuroblastoma, a history of exposure to chlordane was not known. Their report included, in addition to the cases mentioned, a review of other cases in the literature suspected to have had exposure to chlordane or heptachlor, either alone or in combination with other drugs. Infante et al. clearly indicated that in the absence of epidemiologic studies, the statistical demonstration that any chemical or drug has an etiologic relationship to blood dyscrasias is difficult to make. Reports of "associated with exposure to" from history only and lacking credible quantifying exposure data must be considered speculative.

Chlordane and heptachlor and their metabolites are persistent in the environment and their affinity for lipids makes them subject to possible bioaccumulation and transfer in the food chain, and components of technical-grade chlordane and its metabolites have been found commonly in dairy, meat, fish and poultry components of the diet. As has been the case with other chlorinated hydrocarbon pesticides, metabolites of chlordane and heptachlor may accumulate in man, and the oxychlordane and heptachlor epoxide residues have been detected in the adipose tissue in more than 90% of large samples of hospital patients studied in 1970–1972.[7]

Heptachlor epoxide residues have been detected in the organs of stillborn infants and also in samples of human milk. Because of environmental accumulation, humans may be exposed from time of conception on throughout adult life. There is a need for epidemiologic studies to further evaluate short-term and long-term health risks associated with chlordane in home use and in the agricultural setting.

The World Health Organization in 1967 established a maximal daily intake for heptachlor and its epoxide of 0.005 mg/kg of body weight. Measurement of average U.S. intake in 1970 indicated levels well below the "acceptable" level.[9]

REFERENCES

Chlordane and Heptachlor

1. Alvarez, W. C., and Hyman, S.: Lack of toxic manifestations in workers exposed to chlordane, Arch. Ind. Hyg. Occup. Med. 8:480, 1953.
2. Ambrose, A. M., Christensen, H. E., Robbins, D. J., and Rather, L. L.: Toxicological and pharmacological studies on chlordane, Arch. Ind. Hyg. Occup. Med. 7:197, 1953.
3. Curley, A., Copeland, F., and Kimbrough, R. D.: Chlorinated hydrocarbon insecticides in organs of stillborn and blood of newborn babies, Arch. Environ. Health 19:628, 1969.
4. Dadey, J. L., and Kammer, A. G.: Chlordane intoxication, report of a case, JAMA 153:723, 1953.
5. Derbes, V. J., Dent, J. H., Forrest, W. W., and Johnson, M. F.: Fatal chlordane poisoning, JAMA 158:1367, 1955.
6. Infante, P. F., Epstein, S. S., and Newton, W. A.: Blood dyscrasias and childhood tumors and exposure to chlordane and heptachlor, Scand. J. Work Environ. Health 4:137, 1978.
7. International Agency for Research on Cancer: IARC monographs on the evaluation of the carcinogenic risk of chemicals to man: Some organochlorine pesticides (Vol. 5), Lyon, France, pp. 173–184, 1973.
8. Lensky, P., and Evans, H. L.: Human poisoning by chlordane, JAMA 149:1394, 1952.
9. Report on carcinogenesis bioassay of chlordane and heptachlor, Technical Background Information, USDHEW, NIH, NCI, Bethesda, Maryland, September, 1977.
10. Special Pesticides Review Group (Fitzhugh, O. G., and Fairchild, H. E., chairmen): Pesticidal aspects of chlordane in relation to man and the environment. U.S. Environmental Protection Agency, Government Printing Office, Washington, D.C., 6 pp. 1975.

Chlordecone (Kepone)

CHLORDECONE (known under the trade name Kepone) is a chlorinated insecticide used against leaf-eating insects, ants, cockroaches and the larvae of flies. More than 90% of the production has been for export and only 0.8% for domestic use, mainly as bait in ant traps.[5]

In 1975, an epidemiologic investigation of a Kepone manufacturing plant was initiated by NIOSH as a result of a finding by the

Center for Disease Control of a high blood level of Kepone in a worker exhibiting symptoms of marked weight loss, nystagmus and tremors. Of 113 active and former employees studied, more than half had clinical symptoms of Kepone poisoning, including tremors ("Kepone shakes"), visual disturbances, nervousness, vertigo, insomnia, chest and abdominal pain and weight loss. In a few cases, infertility and loss of libido were reported.[6] Manufacturing was discontinued in July, 1975.

Subsequent studies at the Medical College of Virginia of 32 former Kepone-exposed employees indicated that half were unable to work at the beginning of the study because of neurologic disorders, including tremors, stuttered speech and memory lapses, and 11 patients had severely depressed sperm counts.[1]

Cholestyramine, an ion exchange resin that has been used clinically to bind bile salts and cholesterol, has been found to increase significantly the excretion of Kepone. In the Virginia study, all patients were greatly improved after 6 months of cholestyramine therapy and only 3 continue to have abnormally low sperm counts, indicating some reversibility of this effect.

Technical-grade chlordecone has been found to cause a significant increase in the incidence of hepatocellular cancer as compared to controls in high dose level rats and at both dose levels mice after oral feeding for 80 weeks at average dose levels of 8 and 24 ppm for male rats, 18 and 26 ppm for female rats, 20 and 23 ppm for male mice and 20 and 40 ppm for female mice. Clinical signs of toxicity were observed in both species, including generalized tremors and dermatologic changes.[5]

Adverse effects of chlordecone on reproduction in mice have been reported by Good et al.[3] and Huber.[4] Huber found the reproductive capacity of treated mice inhibited or severely reduced, particularly in the female mice. Data collected by means of vaginal smears, hormone bioassays, histologic examinations and results of matings indicated disturbances in the female hormonal system.

The author noted "the occurrence of constant estrus, the development of large follicles, the absence of corpora lutea in their ovaries, and the failure to reproduce are indications that the treated females were under a prolonged stimulation of FSH and estrogen, but insufficient LH stimulation."[4]

In August, 1975, the U.S. Environmental Protection Agency ordered the manufacturers to stop the sale and use of the compound and prohibited further manufacture.

In January, 1976, the NIOSH recommended that Kepone be considered a potential human carcinogen and that the workplace environmental level be limited to 1 $\mu g/m^3$ as a time-weighted average for up to a 10-hour workday and a 40-hour workweek.

REFERENCES

Chlordecone (Kepone)

1. Cohn, W. J., et al.: Treatment of chlordecone (Kepone) toxicity with cholestyramine, N. Engl. J. Med. 298:243, 1978.
2. Cueto, C., Page, N., and Saffiotti, U.: Report of Carcinogenesis Bioassay of Technical Grade Chlordecone (Kepone). National Cancer Institute, Bethesda, Md., 1976.
3. Good, E. E., Ware, G. W., and Miller, D. F.: Effects of insecticides on reproduction in laboratory mouse: I. Kepone, J. Econ. Entomol. 53:754, 1965.
4. Huber, J. J.: Some physiological effects of the insecticide Kepone in the laboratory mouse, Toxicol. Appl. Pharmacol. 7:516, 1965.
5. NIH-HEW Report on Carcinogenesis Bioassay of Kepone. National Cancer Institute, Bethesda, Md., April, 1976.
6. National Institute for Occupational Safety and Health: Recommended standard for occupational exposure to kepone. DHEW, PHS, NIOSH, 1976.

Chloroprene

$$H_2C{=}\underset{\displaystyle Cl}{\underset{|}{C}}{-}CH{=}CH_2$$

CHLOROPRENE, 2-chlorobutadiene, is used to manufacture polychloroprene latex and neoprene rubber. The NIOSH estimates that about 2,500 workers in the United States could be potentially exposed to chloroprene during its production and polymerization. In 1974, about 190 million kg (410 million lb) were produced in the United States.[2]

In 1936, von Oettingen et al.[5] reported findings of altered reproductive function in rats and mice after exposure to chloroprene by skin absorption (skin painting) and by inhalation. Exposure levels for inhalation studies over 8 hours ranged from 12 ppm to 152 ppm in mice and from 121 to 6227 ppm in rats. The animals had delays in reproduction and reduced numbers of young; some were sterile. In the rats, the testes showed pathologic changes, including epithelial degeneration with giant cell formation; the spermatic canals contained cellular debris derived from degenerated spermatozoa, and degenerative changes were described in the spermatogonia. In these initial studies of minimal lethal doses there were no differences in susceptibility between males and females, but males were found to show altered reproductive function and histologic changes at exposure levels that produced no such changes in females. Culik et al.[3] reported that there were no effects on male reproductive function in rats at exposures of 25 ppm (90 mg/m^3) and also no histologic changes in the testes of rats.

Evidence of reproductive toxicity of chloroprene in male workers exposed to it has been reported by Sanotskii,[4] who described functional disturbances in spermatogenesis after exposure to chloroprene for 6–10 years and morphologic disturbances after exposure of 11 or more years. In addition, the author found, through a questionnaire survey, a threefold incidence of spontaneous abortion in the wives of 143 chloroprene workers as compared with a control group of 100 male factory and office workers in an electrical engineering plant. Environmental data, particularly in regard to air concentrations of chloroprene, work, and health and safety practices (skin absorption) and presence of other air contaminants, were lacking. However, the author includes the findings of an inspection of a factory in the U.S.S.R., where a chloroprene-based latex was used, and indicated levels of 1–7 mg/m^3 in air and low levels of ammonia (2–4 mg/m^3) as the most frequent other volatile substance in the latex.

Mutagenicity studies of chloroprene in microorganisms have shown variable results. Bartsch et al.[1] have reported positive mutagenicity findings from chloroprene (origin acetylene) in *Salmonella typhimurium* TA 1530 and TA 100; in the latter there was a linear increasing mutagenic response from 0.5% up to 8% of 2-chlorobutadiene in air. Litton Bionetics[2] reported negative mutagenicity findings of chloroprene (origin butadiene) with *Saccharomyces cerevisiae* and some Salmonella tester strains but positive findings in TA 1535. No clear data on mutagenic effects of chloroprene on mammalian cells are available.

There is no conclusion to date that chloroprene is carcinogenic, although there is evidence associating chloroprene with skin and liver cancers.[2]

Reports indicating chloroprene as a teratogenic substance are limited and somewhat conflicting. Sanotskii[4] reported that chloroprene exposure in a concentration of 4 mg/m^3(1.1 ppm) during the entire pregnancy of rats resulted in an increase in over-all embryonic mortality, a decrease in fetal weight and a disturbance in vascular permeability noted in histologic sections. However, the same dose given days 5–6, 9–10, 11–12 or 13–14 of pregnancy produced teratogenic effects of cerebral hernia (mostly days 5–6) and hydrocephalus (mostly days 11–12, none days 13–14). On the other hand, Culik et al.[3] reported that inhalation during the full pregnancy of chloroprene of 1.0, 1.1, 10 or 25 ppm led to no clearly teratogenic effects, although the highest concentration used may have increased the incidence of abnormal vertebral centra in pups of the exposed pregnant rats.

The present OSHA standard for chloroprene is an 8-hour time-weighted average of 25 ppm (90 mg/m^3). The NIOSH recommended standard is a ceiling limit of 1 ppm (3.6 mg/m^3). "The adverse risk of genetic abnormalities being transmitted to subsequent generations by an agent with the mutagenic properties of chloroprene is the main reason for the NIOSH's recommendation for its current value."[2] The level of 1 ppm has been selected because it can be measured readily under field conditions by the analytic methods currently available. Studies of reproductive performance and effects on both male and female workers exposed to chloroprene are needed to elucidate the safety of 1 ppm as a standard for chloroprene.

REFERENCES

Chloroprene

1. Bartsch, H., Malaveille, C., Montesano, R., and Tomatio, L.: Tissue-mediated mutagenicity of vinylidene chloride and 2-chlorobutadiene in *Salmonella typhimurium*, Nature 255:641, 1975.
2. National Institute for Occupational Safety and Health: Criteria for a recommended standard . . . occupational exposure to chloroprene, DHEW, PHS, NIOSH 77–210, 1977.
3. Culik, R., Kelly, D. P., and Clary, J. J.: Beta-chloroprene (2-Chlorobutadiene-1,3)—Embryotoxic and Teratogenic Studies in Rats. Wilmington, Del., E. I. du Pont de Nemours and Co., Haskell Laboratory for Toxicology and Industrial Medicine, 1976, 18 pp. (cited in NIOSH Criteria Document[2]).
4. Sanotskii, I. V.: Aspects of the toxicology of chloroprene—immediate and long-term effects, Environ. Health Perspect. 17:85, 1976.
5. von Oettingen, W. F., Hueper, W. C., Deichman-Gruebler, W., and Wiley, F. H.: 2-Chloro-butadiene (chloroprene)—its toxicity and pathology and the mechanism of its action, J. Ind. Toxicol. 18:240, 1936.

Dibromochloropropane

DIBROMOCHLOROPROPANE (1,2-dibromo-3-chloropropane, $CH_2Br\text{-}CH_2Cl$) (DBCP) has been used as a fumigant and nematocide in agriculture since 1955, with about 12 million kg (25 million lb) manufactured and used in the United States each year. In 1961, Torkelson et al.[8] investigated the effects of DBCP on experimental animals. In rats, they found a dose-level response to inhalations of DBCP, which included a decrease in the mean weight of the testes, degenerative changes in the seminiferous tubules, a reduction in the number of sperm cells and an increase in the proportion of abnormal sperm cells. Guinea pigs and rabbits exposed to vaporized DBCP showed significant decreases in the mean weight of the testes. The studies indicated that in subacute exposures there was an antispermatogenic effect in the male rat and a nephrotic effect in both sexes, but especially in the female rat. The effect of DBCP on the testes was not altered beneficially by adrenocorticotropic hormone (ACTH), cortisone or testosterone.

Rakhmatulayev[5] also found dose-related

results of reductions in the weight of testes and in the duration of motility of spermatozoa in rats administered DBCP by mouth in subacute (17.5–70 mg/kg for 2½ months) and chronic (0.0005–5 mg/kg for 8 months) exposures. In the chronic exposure study, effects were manifest at the 0.05 mg/kg but not at the 0.005 mg/kg dose level.

Faydysh and co-workers[2,3] found necrosis of the testes in rats given oral doses of 70 mg/kg DBCP. The dose level was such that 5 rats died between days 20 and 25 of the experiment and another 5 lived through the 45 days of the experiment. Daily doses of 0.5 mg/kg given over an extended period produced the same testicular damage, suggesting that the action of the DBCP may be cumulative on this target organ.

Reznik and Sprinchan[6] studied the gonadotropic actions of DBCP in both male and female rats exposed to single oral doses of 100 mg/kg or daily oral doses of 10 mg/kg administered over a 4–5-month period. In the males, the single large dose produced a decreased sperm count in the semen and decreased duration of motility of the spermatozoa. The repeated lower doses had the same effect after 4 months. In the female rats, the single large dose resulted in a prolonged estrus and diestrus. The repeated lower dose produced a typical estrus by the first month in 24% of the rats and by the fifth month in 70%. By the fifth month, 57% of the female rats also became acyclic. These findings would indicate the necessity for considering the reproductive physiology of both male and female employees with occupational exposure to DBCP.

The mutagenic activity of DBCP was investigated by Rosenkranz[7] utilizing two strains of *E. coli* and two of *Salmonella typhimurium*. DBCP was mutagenic for the first tester strain but not for the second. The principal effect was on the DNA. It was found that base-substitution types of mutations are induced by DBCP.

Concern for the hazardous nature of occupational exposure to DBCP was raised in August, 1977, when the Oil, Chemical and Atomic Workers Union asked the National Institute for Occupational Safety and Health to conduct a health hazard evaluation of a California plant based on reports that a number of workers there had abnormally low sperm counts. Tests were conducted on 86 male workers in a plant manufacturing DBCP. It was found that 47 had no or low sperm counts, the break point being 20 million sperm/ml of semen. Sixty-one men were chosen for follow-up and 35 of these agreed to a second test in November. Seven of the 35 showed sperm counts increasing from less than 20 million to more than that count. Five men who had no sperm in August showed a "significant number" in the November test. The findings presented by Whorton[9] at the NIOSH-sponsored Workshop of Methodology for Assessing Reproductive Hazards in the Workplace indicated recovery where there had been exposure for only a short period. Other toxic factors and control measures for DBCP may be found in the NIOSH Criteria Document.[1]

Kapp[4] reported certain studies of human sperm utilizing fluorescent darkfield microscopy to monitor for Y chromosomal dysfunction, which may result from certain toxic substances. He noted that in 30-year-old healthy men without exposures, the over-all background rate is 1.3% Yff sperm. With DBCP exposure in a group of 30 men (average age 33), 12 were azoospermic and the Yff was 3.8%. He suggested the feasibility of monitoring for Y chromosomal dysfunction in sperm in exposed workers, pointing out that the disorder of spermatogenesis (gametogenesis) takes about 4 weeks to be revealed after the toxic exposure.

Major producers of DBCP in the United States stopped production in late August, 1977, and began a recall campaign. The Environmental Protection Agency suspended sale and use of the nematocide in late October, 1977.*

*DBCP manufacturing resumed in April, 1979, in a plant in California.

OSHA established a new standard, effective April 17, 1978, that limits exposure to DBCP to 1 ppm of air averaged over an 8-hour workday and prohibits eye and skin contact. Based on current findings, these limits should afford an ample margin of safety for all workers and for the fetus.

REFERENCES

Dibromochloropropane

1. National Institute for Occupational Safety and Health: Criteria for a recommended standard . . . occupational exposure to dibromochloropropane. DHEW, PHS, NIOSH, 78–115, 1978.
2. Faydysh, E. V., and Avkhimenko, M. G.: Effect of the nematocide nemagon on the reproductive function of an organism, Trans. Uzb. Nauchno-Issld. Inst. Sanit. Gig. Profzabol 8:42, 1974 (Russian) (cited in NIOSH Criteria Document[1]).
3. Faydysh, E. V., Rakhmatulayev, N. N., and Varshavskii, V. A.: The cytotoxic action of nemagon in a subacute experiment, Med. Zh. Uzb. 1:64, 1970 (Russian) (cited in NIOSH Criteria Document[1]).
4. Kapp, R. W.: A New Screening Technique for Assessing Adverse Effects in Human Sperm. Annual Meeting of the Society for Occupational & Environmental Health, Washington, D.C., Dec. 10–13, 1978.
5. Rakhmatullaev, N. N.: Hygienic characteristics of the nematocide nemagon related to the sanitary protection of bodies of water, Gig. Sanit. 36:19, 1971 (Russian) (cited in NIOSH Criteria Document[1]).
6. Reznik, Y. B., and Sprinchan, G. K.: Experimental data on the gonadotoxic effect of nemagon, Gig. Sanit. 76:101, 1975 (Russian) (cited in NIOSH Criteria Document[1]).
7. Rosenkranz, H. S.: Genetic activity of 1,2-dibromo-3-chloropropane, a widely-used fumigant, Bull. Environ. Contam. Toxicol. 14:8, 1975.
8. Torkelson, T. R., Sadek, S. E., Rowe, V. K., Kodama, J. K., Anderson, H. H., Loquvan, G. S., and Hine, C. H.: Toxicologic investigations of 1,2-dibromo-3-chloropropane, Toxicol. Appl. Pharmacol. 3:545, 1961.
9. Whorton, D.: Dibromochloropropane. Workshop of Methodology for Assessing Reproductive Hazards in the Workplace, April 19, 1978, SOEH/NIOSH, Bethesda, Md.

Diethylstilbestrol

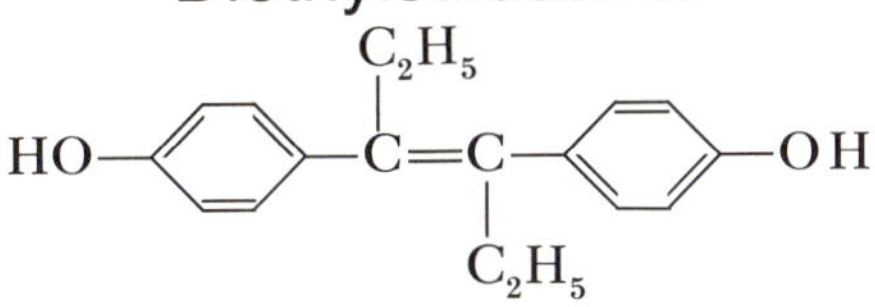

DIETHYLSTILBESTROL (DES), a potent estrogenic compound, was synthesized initially by Dodds in 1938 in England. Because of a potency similar to natural estrogens and because it was inexpensive to prepare and could be administered orally, it was used extensively in women with threatened pregnancies in the late 1940s and 1950s, up to the beginning of the 1970s. Welch[9] estimated that approximately 500,000 –2,000,000 women probably received DES during pregnancy in that interval. As a result of that experience, a sufficient number of cases of carcinoma of the genital tract in offspring of women treated with DES have been reported to suggest that DES is the first apparent transplacental carcinogen in humans.

Between 1966 and 1969, Herbst et al.[5] encountered 7 young females with clear cell adenocarcinoma of the vagina (a relatively rare tumor) and noted that all of these patients were products of pregnancies during which the mothers received DES. Subsequently, a registry for such cases was established at Massachusetts General Hospital, and Welch[9] reported the findings of 150 cases in the registry as of June, 1976. In every instance where adequate maternal histories were obtained, DES had been administered prior to the 18th week of gestation. The ages at time of diagnosis ranged from 7 to 28 years, with an average in the late teens and the majority past puberty. Vaginal bleeding and discharge were the manifestations for which medical attention was sought; however, one-sixth of the patients were asymptomatic and the tumor was detected on routine gynecologic examination, including Papanicolaou smears. (Cytologic examination alone may not detect the tumor and such examination needs to be combined with adequate pelvic examination and appropriate biopsies.) Subsequently, Greenwald et al.[3] reported 5 additional cases of clear cell vaginal adenocarcinoma in young women, all of whose mothers received synthetic estrogens (4 DES, 1 dienestrol) early in pregnancy. These findings can be compared with those of Lanier et al.[6] in a follow-up study of 1719 persons (818 females, 901 males) exposed to estrogens in utero and born between 1943 and 1959. The follow-up interval ranged between 11 and 30 years and the median age was 22 years. No cases of adenocarcinoma of the vagina or cervix were found in any of the young women. On the basis of their study, the authors estimate an incidence of vaginal or cervical adenocarcinoma associated with in utero exposure to estrogens to be no greater than 4 per 1000 cases, and for those exposed in the 1st trimester, no greater than 9 per 1000. The authors indicated that the estrogenic dosage in their series may have been a little less than 100 mg/day, the prevailing recommended dose level at the time.

In addition to the malignancies, nonmalignant anomalies have been found in the in utero exposed populations, including vaginal adenosis and vaginal and cervical ridges.[9] In one study, Herbst et al.[5] noted that adenosis was present in 73% of offspring where the drug was administered prior to the 8th week of gestation, but in no one exposed after the 18th week. Although it has been suggested that adenosis is a premalignant condition, malignant transformation of adenosis has not as yet been observed. Welch[9] noted that some investigators have predicted that glycogen-poor (metaplastic) squamous epithelium that is associated with adenosis will result in increased rates of squamous cell malignancy.

Studies by McLachlan and his associates using radioactive tagged DES in pregnant mice have indicated that DES crosses the placenta, initially very slowly, but after an appropriate time reaches the fetus in a considerable amount and accumulates in the fetal reproductive tract. In one study, analysis of selected fetal tissues for ^{3}H-DES content, ½ hour after treatment, showed an approximately fourfold accumulation of parent compound relative to the fetal plasma in the genital tract.[7]

Prenatal toxicity of DES was studied in pregnant mice, using subcutaneous treatment with DES in corn oil on the 9th through 16th day of gestation, and the offspring evaluated for altered genital tract function. Altered function was reported in both female and male offspring.[7] In the females there were found dose-related decreases in reproductive capacity, ranging from minimal subfertility at the lowest dose to essential sterility at the two highest doses. Notably, the highest dose used was 100 μg/kg, which is 1/20 the maximal average daily dose based on body weight given to pregnant women therapeutically (100 mg/day). Lesions of the genital tract found in female mice included cystic hyperplasia of the endometrium, uterine adenocarcinoma and histologic changes in epithelium resembling adenosis and/or adenocarcinoma.

Male mice exposed to DES in utero also showed impaired genital tract function,[7] but the effect occurred only at the highest dose of 100 μg/kg and not at the lower doses studied. The findings included sterility in 60%, undescended testes in 25%, epididymal cysts in 33% and in 25% nodular enlargement of the seminal vesicles and/or coagulating glands, which were associated with squamous metaplasia.

Abnormal findings in human male offspring of DES-treated mothers have been reported by Gill et al.[2] from a follow-up study of male offspring of DES-exposed mothers compared to placebo-exposed mothers, all of whom were participants in a prospective study at the Chicago Lying-In Hospital during the early 1950s. The more common genital lesions found were epididymal cysts, hypotrophic testes, capsular induration of the testes and microphallus (flaccid penis less than 4 cm in length) in more than 25% of the 163 DES-exposed males, as compared to a 6.5% incidence in the 168 control males. Severe pathologic changes in spermatogenesis and abnormal spermatozoa were found in 28% and 46%, respectively, of 39 DES-exposed males compared with 0% and 12% in 25 controls. No cases of genitourinary malignancies were found in the follow-up study of 901 males by Lanier et al.,[6] mentioned previously.

In the late 1960s, estrogens had been used in the prevention of ischemic heart disease, but the practice was discontinued because of adverse side effects. Among the less severe side effects noted within a few months of treatment with doses of 5–10 mg/day of equine estrogens or 5–25 mg/day DES were breast enlargement (100%), reduced testicular size (82%), increased areolar pigmentation (77%) and decreased or absent libido (74%).[1]

Occupational exposure to DES is largely in the pharmaceutical industry, where DES is produced and packaged and used in the production of hormonal products.[8] Hyperestrogenism has been reported in female pharmaceutical workers, manifested mostly as intermenstrual bleeding and breast enlargement and tenderness and in male workers as clinical gynecomastia with or without increased areolar pigmentation and decreased libido and impotence.[4] To date there have been no studies in the United States on the reproductive capacity and/or function in such workers or on the effects of such exposure in their offspring.

No threshold for occupational DES exposure has been established. It is recognized that DES can be absorbed through the skin as well as by inhalation. The correlative findings in both animal and human studies of the effects of DES on the genital system in both males and females and the transplacental effects reported in the offspring of exposed animals and humans indicated some dose relationship. Occupational exposure to DES should be kept to a minimum.

REFERENCES

Diethylstilbestrol

1. Coronary Drug Project: JAMA 214:1303, 1970.
2. Gill, W. B., Schumacher, G. F. B., and Bibbo, M.: Structural and functional abnormalities in the sex organs of male offspring of mothers treated with diethylstilbestrol (DES), J. Reprod. Med. 16:147, 1976.
3. Greenwald, P., Barlon, J. J., Nasca, P. C., et al.: Vaginal cancer after maternal treatment with synthetic estrogens, N. Engl. J. Med. 285:390, 1971.
4. Harrington, J. M., Rivera, R. O., and Lowry, L. K.: Occupational exposure to synthetic estrogens—the need to establish safety standards, Am. Ind. Hyg. Assoc. J. 39:139, 1978.
5. Herbst, A. L., Ulfeder, H., and Poskanzer, D. C.: Adenocarcinoma of the vagina: Association of maternal stilbestrol therapy with tumor appearance in young women, N. Engl. J. Med. 284:878, 1971.
6. Lanier, A. P., Noller, K. L., Decher, D. G., Elvebach, L. R., and Kurland, L. T.: Cancer and stilbestrol; a follow-up of 1719 persons exposed to estrogens in utero and born 1943–1959, Mayo Clin. Proc. 48:793, 1973.
7. McLachlan, J. A.: Male as Well as Female In Utero Exposure to Diethylstilbestrol. Proc. Conf. on Women and the Workplace, Soc. of Occup. and Environ. Health, Washington, D.C., June 17–19, 1976.
8. Morbidity and Mortality Weekly Report: Epidemiologic Notes and Reports: Occupational

Exposure to Synthetic Estrogens, Puerto Rico, April 1, 1977, Vol. 26, No. 13.
9. Welch, W. R.: Transplacental Carcinogenesis; Prenatal Diethylstilbestrol (DES) Exposure; Clear Cell Carcinoma and Related Anomalies of the Genital Tract in Young Females. Proc. Conf. on Women and the Workplace, Soc. of Occup. and Environ. Health, Washington, D.C., June 17–19, 1976.

Epichlorohydrin

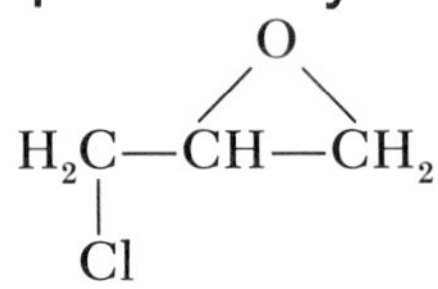

PRODUCTION of epichlorohydrin in the United States in 1978 was estimated at more than 320 million kg (715,000,000 lb); 58% is used in the manufacture of synthetic glycerin and the remainder, in its refined form, to manufacture epoxy resins, surface-active agents, pharmaceuticals, insecticides, agricultural chemicals, textile chemicals, coatings, adhesives, ion exchange resins, solvents and plasticizers. The NIOSH estimates that 50,000 employees may be exposed to epichlorohydrin in the United States.[2]

Epichlorohydrin has been reported to cause sterility in animals.[1,4] Hahn[4] gave male rats of demonstrated fertility a dose of 15 mg/kg body weight orally for 12 days (total dose 180 mg/kg body weight) and evaluated the fertility of the animals after 7 days by the number of uterine implantations in pre-estrus females placed in the cages of the treated males. Within 1 week, the males became infertile, but the effect was reversible within the succeeding week. Histologic examination of the testes, epididymis, prostate and seminal vesicles on the twelfth day of treatment showed no differences between test and control animals, and sexual libido and ability to ejaculate were unaffected.

Epstein and co-workers[3] gave a single intraperitoneal dose of 150 mg/kg of epichlorohydrin to male Swiss mice and recorded the number of total live implants and early and late fetal deaths. Late fetal deaths were very rare, and the authors reported no effects of epichlorohydrin on early fetal deaths or other reproductive characteristics, including male fertility.

Cooper et al.[1] administered epichlorohydrin orally to 3 groups of 5 adult male rats; one group received doses of 20 mg/kg for 5 days (total 100 mg/kg), another group was given 50 mg/kg for 5 days (total 250 mg/kg) and a third group 100 mg/kg as a single dose. The 5 doses of 20 mg/kg resulted in lost fertility during the first 2 weeks, but this was reversed in the third week. Five doses of 50 mg/kg resulted in sterility throughout the 2-week period observed. A single dose of 100 mg/kg resulted in reduced litter size during the 10 weeks and, by 12 weeks, large retention cysts were present in the ductuli efferentes and proximal caputs in 4 of the 5 test animals that were sterile.

In rats, but not mice, therefore, it appears that epichlorohydrin causes sterility that is both dose and time dependent.

Epichlorohydrin has been reported to produce tumors in mice at subcutaneous injection sites but not by skin painting.[5] The NIOSH Criteria Document[2] references several reports indicating that epichlorohydrin has induced a high frequency of positive results in point mutation tests in fungi, other microbial organisms and the fruit fly. Also noted is the report that the urine of workers exposed to 25 ppm of epichlorohydrin influenced the genetic mechanisms of *Salmo-*

nella typhimurium. The Criteria Document further states that there have been experimental attempts to cause teratogenesis by exposing pregnant animals to epichlorohydrin, but these efforts have been negative.

The present OSHA standard for epichlorohydrin is 20 mg/m^3 (5 ppm). The NIOSH recommends that this be reduced to 2 mg/m^3 (0.5 ppm), with a ceiling of 19 mg/m^3. This recommendation follows consideration of the limited available data on reproductive and carcinogenic effects, plus effects on the kidneys, liver, respiratory tract and skin. Additional studies are needed on the reproductive effects, including effects on the male.

REFERENCES

Epichlorohydrin

1. Cooper, E. R. A., Jones, A. R., and Jackson, H.: Effect of alpha-chlorohydrin and related compounds on the reproductive organs and fertility of the male rat, J. Reprod. Fertil. 38:379, 1974.
2. National Institute for Occupational Safety and Health: Criteria for a recommended standard . . . occupational exposure to epichlorohydrin, DHEW, PHS, NIOSH 76–206, 1976.
3. Epstein, S. S., Arnold, E., Andrea, J., Bass, W., and Bishop, Y.: Detection of chemical mutagens by the dominant lethal assay in the mouse, Toxicol. Appl. Pharmacol. 23:288, 1972 (cited in NIOSH Criteria Document[2]).
4. Hahn, J. D.: Post-testicular antifertility effects of epichlorohydrin and 2,3-epoxypropanol, Nature 226:87, 1970.
5. Van Duuren, B. L., Goldschmidt, B. M., Katz, C., Seidman, I., and Paul, J. S.: Carcinogenic activity of alkylating agents, J. Natl. Cancer Inst. 53:695, 1974.

Ethylene Dibromide

$BrCH_2—CH_2Br$

APPROXIMATELY 135,000,000 kg (300 million lb) of ethylene dibromide are produced annually in the United States. Ethylene dibromide, a volatile liquid, is used primarily as a lead scavenger in leaded fuels (to reduce lead deposition in engines, a decreasing use as the consumption of leaded gasoline decreases), as a soil, grain and fruit fumigant, as an intermediate in the synthesis of dyes and pharmaceuticals and as a solvent for resins, gums and waxes. The NIOSH estimates that approximately 9000 employees (U.S.) are potentially exposed during the course of these uses. In addition, gasoline station attendants are potentially exposed to very low levels of ethylene dibromide.[5]

Skin contact with ethylene dibromide may cause chemical burns as well as systemic effects due to absorption of ethylene dibromide through the skin. Ethylene dibromide may also cause adverse effects to the liver, kidneys, heart and other internal organs and systems. Reported adverse health effects of employees chronically exposed to ethylene dibromide may include the induction of cancer and sterility, as well as malformations and heritable changes in offspring.[5]

Studies on the effect of ethylene dibromide on reproduction have been very few. However, of those reported, there have been none that have indicated a no-effect dose level. Experimental data from animal studies indicate that ethylene dibromide can induce sterility and altered spermatogenesis. Daily doses of 2 mg/kg during various periods of development in newborn and adult bulls resulted in abnormalities, including abnormally shaped sperm, decreased sperm motility and decreased sperm counts after 2 weeks of treatments.[1–3] In one report, the spermatogenic abnormalities were reversible after discontinuation of ethylene dibromide administration, but renewed dosing produced recurring effects that persisted longer.[1] Reduced litter size has been reported from female rats mated with males given intraperitoneal injections of ethylene dibromide at a dose of 10 mg/kg body weight for 5 days. The latter effect occurred during the third and fourth weeks following administration of ethylene dibromide, corresponding with the maturation cycle of the spermatids in the genital tract of rats.[4] Studies on the effect of ethylene dibromide on reproduction in females are limited to avians (chickens), where reductions in weight, number of eggs laid and fertilization have been reported. Of note is that the male chickens have not been found to be affected.[5] No mammalian studies of ethylene dibromide on reproductive toxicity in females have been reported.

Studies on the mutagenic potential of ethylene dibromide are referenced in the NIOSH Criteria Document,[5] noting that such potential has been established in vertebrate cell cultures, insects, bacteria, plants and fungi. The NIOSH notes that the ability of ethylene dibromide to produce mutations in a wide variety of test systems is suggestive of its potential for mutagenesis in humans, although quantitation of such risk is not possible at this time.[5]

Only one study on the teratogenic effect of ethylene dibromide has been noted in the Criteria Document, indicating significant fetal abnormalities in mice and rats exposed to ethylene dibromide (31.6 ppm X 23 hours/day) during gestation (days 6–15) as compared to an unexposed control group. The abnormalities produced were different and more frequent than those produced in a control group of feed-restricted animals to simulate malnutrition.[7]

Carcinogenicity of ethylene dibromide has been noted in one report of studies in mice and rats given daily doses (half the maximal tolerated dose) into the stomach for up to 62 weeks; this produced a large percentage of squamous cell carcinomas of the stomach.[6]

The present OSHA standard for ethylene dibromide is 153.6 mg/m^3 (20 ppm). The NIOSH recommends a reduction in the standard to 1 mg/m^3 (0.13 ppm). In view of the lack of animal data indicating a no-effect level of exposure to ethylene dibromide and the reports of altered spermatogenesis in bulls fed only 2 mg/kg per day, there is a concern for such effect in humans even at low levels of exposure. Further studies in this regard are indicated.

REFERENCES

Ethylene Dibromide

1. Amir, D.: The sites of the spermicidal action of ethylene dibromide in bulls, J. Reprod. Fertil. 35:519, 1973.
2. Amir, D.: Individual and age differences in the spermicidal effect of ethylene dibromide in bulls, J. Reprod. Fertil. 44:561, 1975.
3. Amir, D., and Volcani, R.: Effect of dietary ethylene dibromide on bull semen, Nature 209:99, 1965.
4. Edwards, K., Jackson, H., and Jones, A. R.: Studies with alkylating esters. II. A chemical interpretation through metabolic studies of the anti-fertility effects of ethylene dimethanesulphonate and ethylene dibromide, Biochem. Pharmacol. 19:1783, 1970.
5. National Institute for Occupational Safety and Health: Criteria for a recommended standard . . . occupational exposure to ethylene dibromide, DHEW, PHS, NIOSH 77-221, 1977.
6. Olson, W. A., et al.: Induction of stomach cancer in rats and mice by halogenated aliphatic fumigants, J. Natl. Cancer Inst. 51:1993, 1973.
7. Short, R. D., Jr., Minor, J. L., Ferguson, B., Unger, T., and Lee, C.: Toxicity Studies of Selected Chemicals. 1—The Developmental Toxicity of Ethylene Dibromide Inhaled by Rats and Mice during Organogenesis. Report No. EPA 5601, 6-76-018. USEPA, Off. of Tox. Subst., 1976 (cited in NIOSH Criteria Document[5]).

Ethylene Oxide

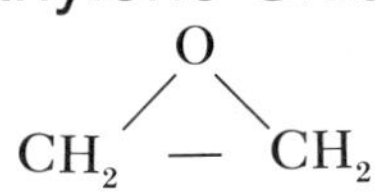

ETHYLENE OXIDE (ETO) is a colorless gas used as an intermediate in the production of ethylene glycol (antifreeze), polyester fiber and film, as an agricultural fungicide, a fumigant for foodstuffs and textiles and for sterilization of surgical instruments, equipment and heat-sensitive materials in medical facilities. It is one of the top 25 chemicals (by volume) produced in the United States,[13] annually about 2 million kg, and about 865 million kg in Europe. Between 5500 and 6000 hospitals in the United States have ETO sterilizers, and an unknown number of industries, which are scattered throughout the country, have such sterilizers; consequently, the NIOSH estimates that up to 100,000 employees may be directly or casually exposed.[13]

Acute effects include conjunctival irritation, headaches, respiratory tract irritation and primary irritation and sensitization of the skin.[9] Gross et al.[8] noted neurologic effects varying from incoordination to recent memory loss and delayed nerve conduction.

Hollingsworth et al.[10] and Jacobson et al.[11] studied the effects of repeated doses of ETO vapors on various animal species. There was no evidence of damage to the gonads of rats, mice, guinea pigs, rabbits, dogs and monkeys when ETO was inhaled at dose levels of 49 ppm, 100 ppm and 113 ppm in air for 6 or 7 hours per day, usually on a 5-day-per-week basis, with the total number of exposures per animal ranging from 122 to 157. At 204 ppm, ETO in air administered 7 hours per day with 122–157 exposures over 176–226 days produced slight testicular tubal degeneration in the rat. At this dose level, 22 of 40 exposed rats died. The primary cause of death was secondary respiratory infection. At 357 ppm for 7 hours per day with 123 exposures over 176 days there was degeneration of testicular tubules in male guinea pigs. All 16 exposed guinea pigs survived. Dose levels of 841 ppm given for 7 hours per day with 1–8 exposures over 10 days were lethal to all rats, guinea pigs, rabbits, mice and monkeys exposed.

The mutagenic potential of ETO has been studied in at least 14 different species, and in 13 of these there was an increased frequency of mutation. The exception was a bacteriophage of *Escherichia coli*.[12] Evidence of chromosomal damage has been reported in rats. Strekalova[14] found statistically significant increases in aberrations in femur bone marrow cells after the administration of a single oral dose of 9 mg ETO/kg. Embree and Hene[5] exposed rats to 250 ppm ETO in air for 7 hours per day for 3 days. Twenty-four hours after the last exposure, they observed isochromatid and chromatid gaps and breaks in bone marrow cells. They also investigated the mutagenic potential of ETO, using the dominant-lethal assay in rats. They exposed male rats to 1000 ppm ETO for a 4-hour inhalation period. There was a significant increase in implantations that died in female rats mated to treated males at 1, 2, 3 and 5 weeks after exposure.

Ethylene oxide is a highly strained three-membered ring epoxide that is broadly reactive to cellular nucleophils. Reactions with protein[6] and nucleic acid[4,7] have been measured. Covalent chemical bonding between ETO and DNA probably can occur spontaneously to form altered biomolecules, which may account for the mutagenic properties of ETO. Furthermore, ETO exposure may saturate the detoxicating mechanisms in vivo.[1,4] This action could be a factor contributing to the mutagenesis.

The studies on mutagenesis suggest the possibility that continual occupational exposure at significant levels of ETO may induce an increased frequency of mutations in humans. There is, at present, little information on exposed worker populations. Ehrenberg and Hallstrom[3] studied a group of workers in a factory manufacturing and using ETO. Seven workers who had been exposed to high levels of gaseous ETO for 2 hours during an industrial accident showed a significantly higher number of chromosomal abnormalities than did a comparable control group.

There are no data concerning the teratogenic effects of ETO. However, ethylene chlorohydrin, a reaction product of ETO, was found to be teratogenic when administered to the developing chick embryo.[13]

In 1978, Hogstedt and co-workers[9] from the Department of Occupational Medicine at the Regional Hospital in Örebro, Sweden, reported their investigation and findings on a group of ethylene oxide-exposed workers from a small factory with a warehouse (storage hall) (68 women and 2 men were employed). They described 1 case of chronic myeloid leukemia, 1 case of acute myelogenetic leukemia and 1 case of primary macroglobulinemia (Waldenström), which occurred between 1972 and 1977. Levels of ETO in the warehouse were 2–70 ppm with an 8-hour, time-weighted average concentration (in the breathing zone) calculated as 20 ± 10 ppm.*

The expected cumulative incidence of leukemia during that period was calculated by multiplying the person-years of observation and the sex- and age-specific national leukemia incidence for 1972.[2] Without considering any latency time or minimal exposure, a 0.2 case incidence of leukemia would have been expected.

At present, the OSHA standard for occupational exposure to ethylene oxide is 50 ppm parts of air (90 mg/m^3) as an 8-hour, time-weighted average concentration (TWA). The NIOSH recommends that the short-term exposure limit should be no higher than 75 ppm (135 mg/m^3) for a period of up to 15 minutes.

Based on the conclusions of the Hogstedt report, the Swedish threshold limit value for ethylene oxide has been lowered to 10 ppm as an 8-hour, time-weighted average concentration limit. Reduction of worker exposure through improved industrial hygiene practices is vital. Epidemiologic studies of workers potentially exposed to ETO, including reproductive data, are urgently needed in order to assess the adequacy of the current and proposed standards.

REFERENCES

Ethylene Oxide

1. Arias, I. M., and Jakoby, W. B. (eds.): *Glutathione: Metabolism and Function,* (New York: Raven Press, 1976).
2. Cancer Incidence in Sweden 1972. Stockholm, National Board of Health and Welfare, p. 44, 1977.
3. Ehrenberg, L., and Hallstrom, T.: Haematologic studies on persons occupationally exposed to ethylene oxide, in International Energy Agency Report; SM 92/26, pp. 327–334, 1967 (cited in NIOSH Criteria Document[13]).
4. Ehrenberg, L., et al.: Evaluation of genetic risks of alkylating agents: Tissue doses in the mouse from air contaminated with ethylene oxide, Mutat. Res. 24:83, 1974.
5. Embree, J. W., and Hene, C. H.: Mutagenicity of ethylene oxide, Toxicol. Appl. Pharmacol. 33:172, 1975.
6. Frankel-Conrat, H.: The action of 1,2 epoxides of proteins, J. Biol. Chem. 154:227, 1944.
7. Frankel-Conrat, H.: Chemical modification of viral ribonucleic acid. Part I. Alkylating agents, Biochem. Biophys. Acta 49:165, 1961.
8. Gross, J. A., Haas, M. L., and Swift, T. R.: Ethylene oxide neuropathy, Neurology 28:355, 1978.
9. Hogstedt, C., Malmqvist, N., and Wadman, B.: Leukemia in workers exposed to ethylene oxide, JAMA 241:1132, 1979.

*The authors noted that in sterilizing hospital equipment, 50% ethylene oxide and 50% methyl formate had been used since 1968 (methyl formate has much less volatility than ETO, and is permitted as a food additive).

10. Hollingsworth, R. L., et al.: Toxicity of ethylene oxide determined on experimental animals, A.M.A. Arch. Ind. Health 13:217, 1956.
11. Jacobson, K. H., Hackley, E. B., and Feinsilver, L.: The toxicity of inhaled ethylene oxide and propylene oxide vapors, A.M.A. Arch. Ind. Health 13:237, 1956.
12. Loveless, A.: Influence of radiomimetic substances on desoxyribonucleic acid synthesis and function studied in *Escherichia coli* phage systems. Part 3: Mutation of T2 bacteriophage as a consequence of alkylation in vitro, Proc. R. Soc. Lond. (Biol.) 150:497, 1959.
13. National Institute for Occupational Safety and Health: Special occupational hazard review with control recommendations: Use of ethylene oxide as a sterilant in medical facilities, DHEW, PHS, NIOSH 77-200, 1977.
14. Strekalova, E. E.: Mutagenic action of ethylene oxide on mammals. [CA75-1077251]. Toksikil. Nov. Prom. Khim Veshchesto 12:72, 1971 (Russian) (cited in NIOSH Criteria Document[13]).

Ethylene Thiourea

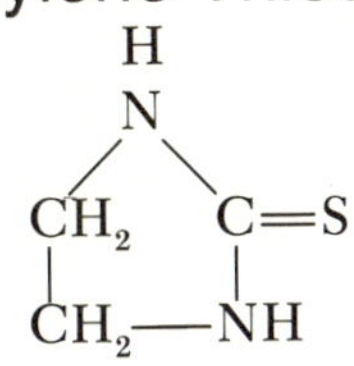

ETHYLENE THIOUREA (ETU) is a white crystalline solid that is used extensively as an accelerator in the curing of polychloroprene (the synthetic rubber trademarked Neoprene) and other elastomers. The NIOSH estimates that approximately 3500 workers in the rubber industry have potential occupational exposure to ethylene thiourea.[4] Not to be overlooked is that exposure to ETU can result from the very widely used ethylene bisdithiocarbamate fungicides, as ETU may be present as a contaminant in these fungicides and can also be formed when food containing the fungicides is cooked.

Ethylene thiourea is a thyroid depressant in laboratory animals, producing myxedema, goiter and other manifestations related to decreased thyroid hormone.[4] In rats, ETU has also been found to produce thyroid carcinoma.[1,2,6]

In addition, ETU has been found to be a significant teratogen in laboratory animals.[3,5] Stula and Krauss[5] reported fetal malformations in all of 73 fetuses taken on the 20th day of gestation from pregnant rats in which ETU (50 mg/kg body weight) had been applied to the skin on the 12th and the 13th day of gestation whereas no abnormalities were found in the fetuses of the controls. Their studies further demonstrated that the teratogenic effects were related to the dose and exposure time in the pregnancy. Utilizing the same dose of 50 mg ETU/kg body weight on gestation days 10 and 11 did not result in any fetal abnormalities.

At present, there is no OSHA standard for ETU exposure or a proposed limit by the NIOSH. It would be prudent, however, to minimize any exposure to this substance, including skin exposure.

REFERENCES

Ethylene Thiourea

1. IARC Monographs on the Evaluation of Carcinogenic Risk of Chemicals to Man, 7:45, 1974.
2. Innes, J. R. M., et al.: Bioassay of pesticides and industrial chemicals for tumorigenicity in mice: A preliminary note, J. Natl. Cancer Inst. 42:1101, 1969.
3. Khera, K. S., and Tryphonas, L.: Ethylene thiourea-induced hydrocephalus: Pre- and postnatal pathogenesis in offspring from rats given a single oral dose during pregnancy, Toxicol. Appl. Pharmacol. 42:85, 1977.
4. National Institute for Occupational Safety and Health: Current intelligence bulletin #22:

Ethylene thiourea, DHEW, PHS, NIOSH 79-109, 1978.

5. Stula, E. F., and Krauss, W. C.: Embryotoxicity in rats and rabbits from cutaneous application of amide-type solvents and substituted ureas, Toxicol. Appl. Pharmacol. 41:35, 1977.
6. Ulland, B. M., et al.: Thyroid cancer in rats from ethylene thiourea intake, J. Natl. Cancer Inst. 49:583, 1972.

Glycidyl Ethers

Carl Zenz, M.D.

THE MAJOR USE of the glycidyl ethers is as reactive diluents in epoxy resins applications. Most of the glycidyl ethers are liquids, but a few are solid and are characterized by the presence of the 2,3-epoxypropyl group and an ether linkage to another organic group. They have a generalized formula:

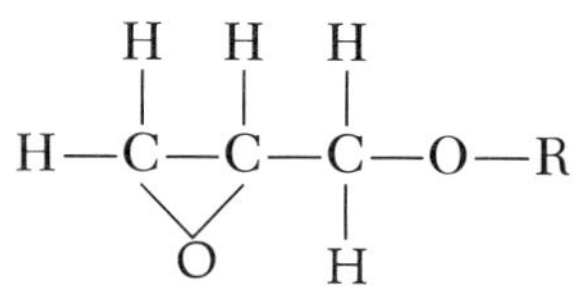

These compounds have relatively low vapor pressures, and dermocontact is the major route of exposure, with inhalation a possible secondary route. Exposure to the epoxide moiety in certain glycidyl ethers and epoxy resins may occur until the resin is completely cured. Therefore, workers must be considered to be at some risk of exposure from the time the glycidyl ethers are synthesized until the curing process of the epoxy resin is complete.

Occupations with potential exposure to glycidyl ethers: adhesive makers and users, automobile workers, cable makers, casting and molding workers, custom-blended epoxy resin system production workers, dental laboratory technicians, dentists, electrical appliance production workers, electronic equipment production workers, flooring makers, glycidyl ether production workers, laminators, nurses, paint makers, physicians, soft drink canners, telephone production workers and telephone installers. The NIOSH estimates that 118,000 workers in the United States are exposed to glycidyl ethers and that an additional 1,000,000 workers are exposed to epoxy resins. There are no specific diagnostic tests to determine the extent of absorption into the worker's body, and environmental controls by sampling the worker's breathing zone are necessary.

The most commonly used glycidyls, along with their acronyms and the presently allowable concentrations (1978), are:

Allyl glycidyl ether (AGE)	45 mg/m^3 (9.6 ppm)
Isopropyl glycidyl ether (IGE)	240 mg/m^3 (50 ppm)
Phenyl glycidyl ether (PGE)	5 mg/m^3 (1 ppm)
n-Butyl glycidyl ether (BGE)	30 mg/m^3 (4.4 ppm)
Di(2,3-epoxypropyl)ether (DGE)	1 mg/m^3 (0.2 ppm)

Because epoxy resins have such a wide range of applications, workers often must handle glycidyl ethers and the uncured resins containing them in processes such as tooling and molding, manufacturing and using adhesives, roof and floor construction and applying protective coatings. Uncured resins used in protective coatings often are applied by spraying, so the applicators could be exposed to large quantities of vapors and mists containing glycidyl ethers. Work practices appropriate for handling glycidyl ethers should be adhered to in processes involving an uncured epoxy resin system.

Glycidyl ethers such as PGE and BGE

are synthesized by adding the appropriate alcohol to epichlorohydrin in the presence of a catalyst. The intermediate chlorohydrin is not isolated and undergoes dehydrochlorination to yield a glycidyl ether. Commercial manufacture of glycidyl ethers takes place within an enclosed system, but workers may be exposed to glycidyl ethers during drumming operations at the end of the process. Very small quantities of glycidyl ethers are used for other purposes, most of which are proprietary in nature; in these instances, identification of exposed workers and estimation of their extent of exposure become difficult.

Human toxicologic data concerning these compounds are scarce, but information available reveals that glycidyl ethers are primary skin and eye irritants and that they are potential skin-sensitizing agents. There are data suggesting that di(2,3-epoxypropyl) ether should be regarded as a potential occupational carcinogen and that *n*-butyl glycidyl ether is a mammalian mutagen. Some glycidyl ethers have also produced cytotoxic effects in animals. Although there are no reports of carcinogenic, mutagenic, teratogenic or reproductive effects of the glycidyl ethers in humans, there have been reports of animal studies demonstrating testicular degeneration in several animal species after exposure to AGE, DGE, PGE and triethylene glycol diglycidyl ether.[3,5,7,11] Necrosis of the testes was reported in rats that received 6 dermal applications of DGE at 250 or 500 mg/kg[5] or 4 injections of AGE at 400 mg/kg.[7] Testicular atrophy with decreased spermatogenic activity was seen in mice receiving high intraperitoneal doses of triethylene glycol diglycidyl ether.[11] Atrophied testes were found in 2 rabbits that died after a single 24-hour exposure to DGE at 24 ppm (128 mg/m^3) and possibly in a dog that received 6 12.5 mg/kg intravenous doses of this compound.[5] In chronic inhalation experiments, 1 of 15 rats exposed to DGE at 3 ppm (16 mg/m^3) had necrosis of testicular tubules after 19 exposures; 5 of 10 rats exposed at 0.3 (1.6 mg/m^3) had "poorly defined" focal degeneration in the testes after 60 exposures.[5] In rats exposed to PGE at 1.75–11.2 ppm (10–71 mg/m^3) for 19 days, focal degeneration of the seminiferous tubules was observed in 5 of 24, but the investigator considered that this damage was of questionable significance and probably was not treatment related.[3] Only in the PGE study was any attempt made to correlate testicular damage with effects on reproduction, and this study showed no significant mutagenic or reproductive effects.[3]

Lack of data on most of the glycidyl ethers makes it difficult to correlate variations in the results of tests of their mutagenicity and carcinogenicity with differences in the structure of particular compounds within the class. Thus, only tentative conclusions can be drawn about the potential of glycidyl ethers to cause cancer or mutations.[1]

Following occupational exposures to certain substances such as styrene, for example, metabolic breakdown epoxides are formed that are very reactive and are considered to be potentially of significance in possible tumorigenesis. Since glycidyl ethers contain the epoxide group, they would be expected to undergo the types of reactions that have been demonstrated for this moiety, with potential reactions that have significance for biologic systems.[2,9]

Experimental evidence also indicates that glycidyl ethers are very reactive biologically. They have been used for tumor inhibition because of their alkylating properties.[11] They have produced chromosomal aberrations in plants,[6,8,9] and Hine[5] and Kodama et al.[7] have demonstrated their radiomimetic effects on blood cells. BGE has been shown to be mutagenic in mammals,[10] and all glycidyl ethers tested have shown some mutagenic activity in bacterial systems.[3,10,12] However, very high doses generally were required to produce these effects, and attempts to find consistent structure-activity relationships among var-

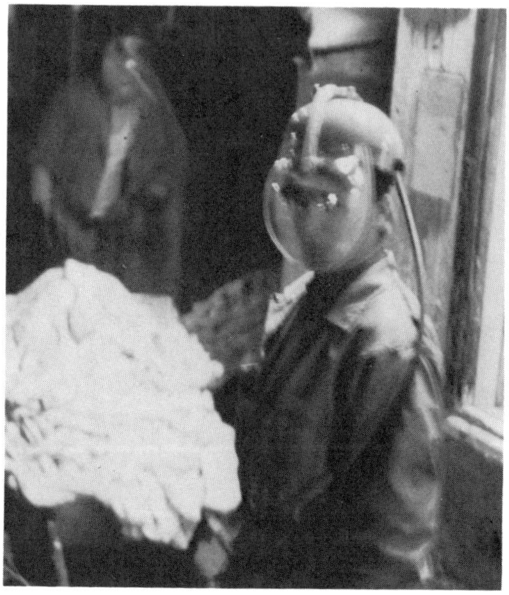

Fig 3-1.—A worker in a synthetic-fiber plant where carbon disulfide is used. Note the special air-supplied helmets and face pieces provided.

ious glycidyl ethers have met with little success.[4,7]

The National Institute for Occupational Safety and Health[1] states that gross skin contact with glycidyl ethers may represent an important hazard to worker health, and, because of demonstrated mutagenicity, the

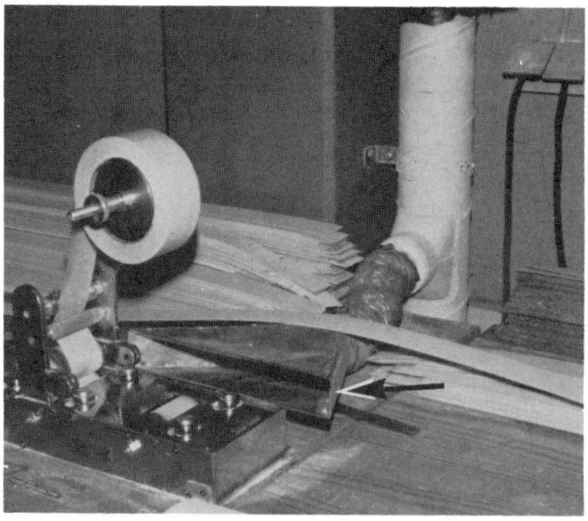

Fig 3-2.—Epoxy-fiberglass material used for manufacturing laminated skis. Arrow indicates the exhaust system located at this cutting stage.

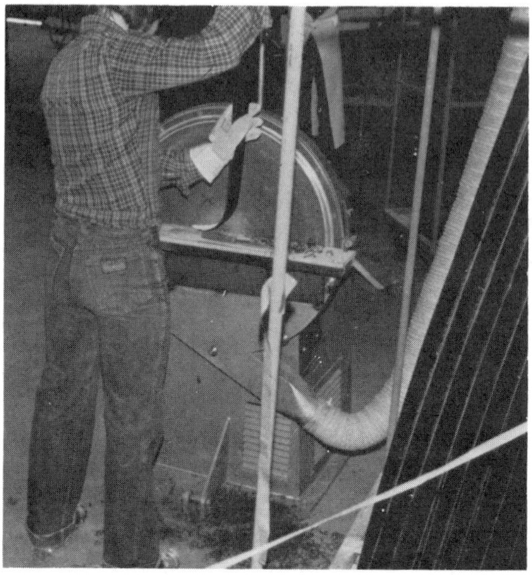

Fig 3-3.—Exhaust system at the grinding stations for manufacturing skis of epoxy fiberglass.

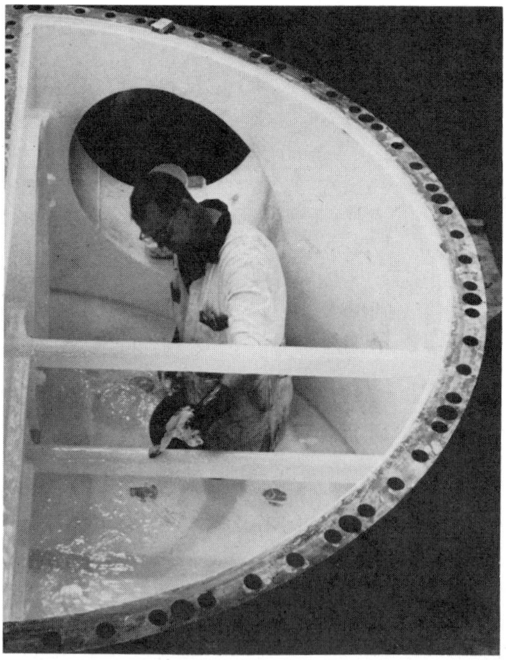

Fig 3-4.—A workman hand brushing epoxy resin on a large steel object for corrosion resistance. Note protective clothing. With downdraft exhaust ventilation, no respiratory protective equipment is needed.

glycidyl ethers should, in the absence of adequate carcinogenicity test data on individual compounds, be regarded as potentially serious hazards.

Several glycidyl ethers are combustible or flammable liquids presenting fire hazards. Since many of them may polymerize violently after heating, stringent precautions must be taken to prevent fire. In addition, inhalation of the chemicals can be minimized by enclosing processes and providing suitable and adequate ventilation systems with specifically placed exhaust hoods (Figs 3–1, 3–2, 3–3 and 3–4), and all epoxy-based adhesives containing these substances should be used only with adequate ventilation. As with most potentially toxic substances, eating and drinking must not be permitted in the work areas nor must food or beverages be allowed to be stored in workplaces, and employees must be advised to wash their hands before eating or using toilet facilities. Workers should also be cautioned not to touch or rub their eyes with fingers or hands, which may be contaminated.

REFERENCES

Glycidyl Ethers

1. National Institute for Occupational Safety and Health: Criteria for a recommended standard . . . occupational exposure to glycidyl ethers, DHEW, PHS, NIOSH 78-166, 1978.
2. Fournier, P. E., and Gervais, P.: Toxicological study of epoxy resins, Occup. Health Rev. 17:19, 1964.
3. Haskell Laboratory Reports on Glycidyl Ethers, No. 164-75, 225-74, 133-76, 163-75. Unpublished report submitted to NIOSH by E. I. du Pont de Nemours & Co., Employee Relations Dept., Medical Division, February, 1978, 14 pp.
4. Hendry, J. A., Homer, R. F., Rose, F. L., and Walpole, A. L.: Cytotoxic agents. II. Bis-epoxides and related compounds, Br. J. Pharmacol. 6:235, 1951.
5. Hine, C. H., et al.: Effects of diglycidyl ether on blood of animals, Arch. Environ. Health 2:37, 1961.
6. Kihlman, B. A.: Factors affecting the production of chromosome aberrations by chemicals, J. Biophys. Biochem. Cytol. 2:543, 1956.
7. Kodama, J. K., et al.: Some effects of epoxy compounds on the blood, Arch. Environ. Health 2:56, 1961.
8. Lane, G. R.: Chromosome Breakage by Diepoxide and by X-rays, in Bacq, Z. M., and Alexander, P. (eds.), *Proceedings of the Radiobiology Symposium* (New York: Academic Press, 1955), pp. 265–274, 277–281.
9. Loveless, A.: Qualitative aspects of the chemistry and biology of radiomimetic (mutagenic) substances, Nature 167:338, 1951.
10. Pullin, T., and Legator, M. S.: Integrated Mutagenicity Testing Program. Unpublished report submitted to NIOSH by Dow Chemical Co., Dow Chemical USA, Health and Environmental Research, Midland, Michigan, December, 1977, 71 pp.
11. Shimkin, M. B., et al.: Bioassay of 29 alkylating chemicals by the pulmonary-tumor response in strain A mice, J. Natl. Cancer Inst. 36:915, 1966.
12. Wade, M. J., Moyer, J. W., and Hine, C. H.: Mutagenic Action of a Series of Epoxides, publication No. 78-2. San Francisco, University of California, School of Medicine, Dept. of Pharmacology (Toxicology Activity), 1978, 12 pp.

Hypoxia

ERIC P. KINDWALL, M.D., and CARL ZENZ, M.D.

CABIN attendants and stewardesses in commercial aircraft constitute a large body of the work force in the air transport industry, and there is the potential danger of hypoxia to the fetus of a stewardess at a normal cabin pressure. Commercial jet aircraft are pressurized to maintain a cabin altitude of about 1500–2100 m (5000–7000 ft). Hypoxic symptoms in passengers and/ or crew begin above this level and are most noted above the altitude of 3000 m (10,000 ft).[3] Fetal anomalies have been demonstrated in experimental animals exposed to very high degrees of hypoxia.[5, 12, 13, 17] Pregnant mice, when exposed to reduced pressure equivalent to 7600 m (25,000 ft) for 8 hours have delivered anomalous infants. Although the effects of high altitude on reproduction in the Bolivian Andes have been studied, there is little evidence in the literature of occupational exposure under hypoxic conditions. In addition, such conditions are encountered seldom except under unusual circumstances. There are isolated reports of defects in children born of mothers who were subjected to an acute episode of hypoxia early in pregnancy arising from exposure to an anesthesia or to carbon monoxide in suicide attempts.

Kamat[14] reported that for the first time in the 1960s, defense forces of any country were located at an altitude of 4000 m for a prolonged period (India). In 1964, defense force personnel carried 40 male and female ducks from the plains to this altitude. The ducks were supervised with the aid of expert advice and protected from cold weather. The animals gained weight but were noticed to mate infrequently, and no eggs were laid during the first 8 months. Only one egg was laid during the succeeding 10 months. At the plains during this period, a comparable group laid several hundred eggs. After sacrifice, all ducks were inspected for any unlaid eggs or ova, of which none were found (unpublished observation). A 2-year attempt to breed a colony of pigs at 4000 m was also unsuccessful. The piglets were weak, small and lethargic.

Raina[20] has reported that cows in the Himalayas experienced a vague, weak and short period of heat. Rat species are plentiful, but diminutive, in the Ladakh area. Fertility has been shown to be impaired at altitudes above 3200 m.[6] Weihe[23] has reported poor lactogenesis in various animals living at altitudes above 3000 m. Several army personnel stationed at high altitudes have complained of impaired fertility, and, on investigation, scanty specimens of semen were collected, exhibiting low-count spermatozoa.

Scholten[21] summarized the oxygen requirements of the developing embryo and fetus, reviewing the work of Cameron[4] and others. The fetus normally grows at oxygen tensions that would be considered severely hypoxic for the normal child or adult.[1] The important figures to consider are the percent arterial oxygen saturation and the partial pressure of oxygen in the blood measured in millimeters of mercury. Of equal importance is the phenomenon called "oxygen cascade," a term used to describe the progressively falling partial pressure of oxygen (Po_2) from the inspired air, through the circulation to the capillaries of the tissue being oxygenated at the end of the cascade.[2, 11]

At sea level, the Po_2 in the inspired air is about 150 mm Hg, which drops to a little over 100 mm Hg in the alveoli in the arterial blood. By the time the capillary bed is reached, the Po_2 is a mean of 60 mm Hg and, on return through the circulation, is 37 mm Hg in the mixed venous blood. These are the normal values at sea level.

At 2438 m (8000 ft), the upper limits of normal cabin pressurization, the inspired air has a Po_2 of about 110 mm Hg, down from the sea level of 150. The alveolar air and the arterial blood have a Po_2 of about 64, a considerable drop from the normal 100. Capillary levels decline from the 60 at sea level to a mean of 46 at 2438 m (8000 ft); on the venous side, the drop is only from 37 to 32. Thus, there is a relatively large drop in the inspired oxygen partial pressure, which results in a very much smaller decrease in the mean capillary Po_2. At the same time, the oxygen saturation curve shows considerably less decline as altitude increases, because of the protective buffering features of the oxygen dissociation mechanisms in human blood.[8, 11] As the atmospheric pressure goes down, oxygen dissociates from the hemoglobin cycle at an increased rate and maintains the oxygen saturation of the blood. Oxygen saturation falls as low as 90% at an alveolar partial pressure of 50–72 mm Hg, a pressure that corresponds to about 3048 m (10,000 ft). Most authorities would agree that hypoxia begins to be noticed only at or above this altitude.[18,19]

The fetus normally lives in a hypoxic atmosphere.[1] At sea level it exists with a Po_2 of 32 in its cord arterial blood and 10.6 in the venous blood returning through the umbilical cord.[22,24] This is in contrast to the maternal figures of 100 and 37, respectively; thus, partial pressures of oxygen in the fetal circulation are about one-third those of the mother.[7]

When the mother is breathing 15% oxygen, equivalent to 2438 m (8000 ft), her arterial partial pressure drops to 64, but the effect on fetal oxygenation is much less. While the mother's Po_2 drops from 100 to 64, the fetal Po_2 drops from 32 to 25.6 and the oxygen saturation drops even less. This is due to several factors. First, the fetal hemoglobin dissociation curve operates at a much lower partial pressure of oxygen than the maternal and, under the same conditions, the O_2 saturation of fetal blood is greater than that of maternal blood. Second, in relatively hypoxic states there is a protective shift in pH of fetal blood to the alkaline side, which enhances the fetal dissociation curve so that more oxygen is taken up at a given partial pressure.[19]

Thus, it would appear that the fetus is able to withstand hypoxia much better than does an adult. The level of hypoxia reached by passengers and crew under normal circumstances on modern commercial jet transport aircraft has no adverse effect on the fetus. However, these studies were carried out on pregnant women who were the equivalent of sedentary passengers. There are no similar data on pregnant women doing moderate to heavy work at equivalent altitudes, as stewardesses would be. In Denver, at 1615 m (5300 ft), there are no greater numbers of spontaneous abortions or rates of anomalies than in seacoast cities, although the average birth weights in Denver are slightly less than in areas of lower altitudes.[9,15,16]

Billings[3] stated that "The question of whether hypoxia at normal cabin altitudes has a detrimental effect on the young fetus is unanswered; it is thought that it does not. I believe that pregnant women, especially early in pregnancy, should receive supplemental oxygen during flights above 3000 m in unpressurized aircraft."

REFERENCES

Hypoxia

1. Barcroft, J.: *Researches on Pre-Natal Life* (Springfield, Ill.: Charles C Thomas, Publisher, 1947), p. 259.
2. Bartels, H., Moll, W., and Metcalfe, J.: Physiology of gas exchange in the human placenta, Am. J. Obstet. Gynecol. 84:1714, 1962.
3. Billings, C. E.: Aerospace Medicine—Occupational Health Aspects, in Zenz, C. (ed.), *Occupational Medicine: Principles and Practical Applications* (Chicago: Year Book Medical Publishers, 1975), pp. 157–190.
4. Cameron, R. G.: Should air hostesses continue flight duty during the first trimester of pregnancy?, Aerospace Med. 44:552, 1973.
5. Carter, C. O.: Incidence and Aetiology, in Blackwell, A. P. N. (ed.), *Congenital Abnormalities in Infancy* (Oxford: Oxford University Press, 1963).
6. Cook, S. F., and Krum, A. A.: Determination of mouse strains exposed for long periods to low atmospheric pressure, J. Exp. Zool. 128:561, 1955.
7. Dawes, G. S.: Oxygen Supply and Consumption in Late Fetal Life and the Onset of Breathing at Birth, in *Handbook of Physiology*, Section 3, Vol. II, *Respiration* (Washington, D.C.: American Physiological Society, 1965).
8. Dawes, G. S.: The umbilical circulation, Am. J. Obstet. Gynecol. 84:1634, 1962.

9. Grahn, D., and Kratchman, J.: Variation in neonatal death rate and birth weight in the United States and possible relations to environmental radiation, geology and altitude, Am. J. Hum. Genet. 15:329, 1963.
10. Hellman, L. M., and Pritchard, J. A.: *Williams Obstetrics* (14th ed.; New York: Appleton-Century-Crofts, 1971).
11. Hurtado, A.: Animals in High Altitudes, Resident Man, in Dill, D. B., (ed.), *Handbook of Physiology*, Section 4, Adaptation to the Environment (Washington, D.C.: American Physiological Society, 1964).
12. Ingalls, T. H.: Environmental Factors in Causation of Congenital Anomalies, in Wolstenholme, G. E. W. (ed.), *Ciba Foundation Symposium on Congenital Malformations* (London: Livingston-Churchill, 1960).
13. Ingals, T. H.: Experimental production of congenital anomalies, N. Engl. J. Med. 247:758, 1952.
14. Kamat, S. R.: Fetal growth retardation and increased infant mortality at high altitude, Arch. Environ. Health 33:150, 1978.
15. Lichty, J. A.: Studies of babies born at high altitude, A.M.A. J. Dis. Child. 93:666, 1957.
16. Lubchenco, L. O.: Sequelae of premature birth, Am. J. Dis. Child. 106:101, 1963.
17. Mazess, R. B.: Neonatal mortality and altitude in Peru, Am. J. Phys. Anthropol. 23:209, 1965.
18. Metcalfe, J., Bartels, J. H., and Moll, W.: Gas exchange in the pregnant uterus, Physiol. Rev. 47:782, 1967.
19. Metcalfe, J., Novy, M. J., and Peterson, E. N.: Reproduction at High Altitudes, in Benirschke, K. (ed.), *Comparative Aspects of Reproductive Failure* (New York: Springer-Verlag, 1966).
20. Raina, S. S.: Diagnosis of early pregnancy in cows, Indian Vet. J. 39:507, 1962.
21. Scholten, P.: Pregnant stewardess—should she fly?, Aviat. Space Environ. Med. 47:77, 1976.
22. Tominaga, T., and Page, E. W.: Accommodation of the human placenta to hypoxia, Am. J. Obstet. Gynecol. 94:679, 1966.
23. Weihe, W. H.: Influence of altitude and cold on pregnancy and lactation of rats on two different diets, Int. J. Biometeorol. 9:43, 1965.
24. Wulf, H.: Gas exchange in the mature placenta in man, I., Z. Geburtsh. Gynaek. 158:117, 1962.

Mercury*

PLACENTAL TRANSFER of mercury has been found to vary with the chemical nature of mercury compounds.[5,6,17,25] Suzuki et al.[25] noted that the placenta acts as a barrier to inorganic and phenyl mercury to a similar extent but not to methyl mercury. Clarkson et al.[7] studied the transplacental passage of elemental mercury in rats and found that after injection of elemental mercury, the fetal content was more than 10 times greater than maternal blood and, after inhaling mercury, approximately 40 times greater than after an equivalent dose of inorganic mercury. Utilizing data from both of these studies, Koos and Longo[15] summarized the relative placental permeability for the various forms of mercury as phenyl: 1, inorganic: 2, elemental: 10–20 and methyl: 20.

After acute exposure to inorganic mercurials, the greatest concentrations are in the kidneys, liver, spleen, muscle and blood.[5] Metallic mercury, which is more lipid soluble, can penetrate into the brain and achieve much higher levels (10×) there than ionic mercury compounds. Phenyl mercury is rapidly degraded to inorganic mercury and follows the distribution of mercuric ions.[15, 26] Methyl mercury is much more stable, is lipid soluble, readily diffuses through cell membranes and can attain appreciable quantities in the brain.[10] Yang et al.[28] found by oral feeding of methyl mercuric chloride in rats that the percentage of the mercury dose in all parts of the brain of

*The reader is referred to the section on mercury by Knight[14] in *Occupational Medicine, Principles and Practical Applications* for a general discussion of mercury, its industrial uses, occupational exposures, biologic and toxicologic effects, diagnosis, treatment and hygienic control measures.

the mother remained essentially the same over the 5-day postfeeding period studied. On the other hand, in the fetus there was a threefold increase in uptake of mercury in brain parts from day 1 to day 5, and the fetal brain accumulated a higher concentration of mercury than did the maternal brain.

Mercury has been found in breast milk of women exposed to methyl mercury through the ingestion of contaminated food. In an Iraqi experience,[4] milk levels of the total mercury correlated closely with whole blood levels and averaged 5% of simultaneous concentrations in maternal blood, consisting of 40% in the inorganic form and 60% as methyl mercury. Similar findings have been reported by Skerfving[21] in 15 lactating women exposed to methyl mercury found in fish, except that the methyl mercury component was only 20%. Even with the relatively low concentrations of mercury in milk, suckling infants have been noted to accumulate significant amounts of mercury in the blood if their mothers had been heavily exposed.[1]

The reproductive effects of exposure to mercury (methyl mercury in particular) were brought into focus largely by the epidemic of mercury poisonings in Minamata, Japan, beginning in 1953. This epidemic resulted from the ingestion of fish and shellfish from Minamata Bay that had been contaminated with effluent containing methyl mercury from a nearby factory. During the epidemic, 23 cases (more since) of prenatally exposed infants with severe psychomotor signs of brain damage (including cerebral palsy and mental retardation) were recorded. It is possible that these infants may also have had postnatal intake of mercury from breast milk. In contrast to the infants, the mothers were found to be asymptomatic or to have mild paresthesias.[12] Most of these patients were examined some time after the onset of poisoning, and no documentation on dose or maternal and fetal blood or brain levels of methyl mercury was possible.

Since the 1953 epidemic, additional epidemics involving pregnancy and methyl mercury poisoning from ingestion of contaminated food have been reported in Iraq[2,4] and in the USSR,[3] and isolated cases have also been noted elsewhere.[19,22]

In Iraq, the source of the poisoning was traced to ingestion of homemade bread prepared from wheat treated with a methyl mercury fungicide. From February, 1972 to August, 1972 there were 6530 patients with poisoning admitted to hospitals and 459 hospital deaths in Iraq. Bakir et al.[4] observed that the admission of pregnant women with diagnosable poisoning was low (31 observed compared to 150 expected) and that the frequency of pregnant females was also low when computed on the basis of the rural population, possibly indicative of an effect on fertility by the mercury. From this exposed population, Amin-Zaki et al.[2] reported the clinical and laboratory findings of 15 infant-mother pairs exposed to methyl mercury during pregnancy. They found that in all but 1 case, the infants' blood mercury levels were higher than their mothers' during the first 4 months after birth, indicating the transplacental passage of methyl mercury from the mother to the fetus and the maintenance of neonatal blood mercury levels from ingestion of mercury in mothers' milk.

Clinically, 6 of the 15 mothers and at least 6 of the infants had positive manifestations of mercury poisoning. In 5 severely affected infants there was gross impairment of motor and mental development. In contrast to the reported findings in Minamata, there was only 1 infant-mother pair in which the infant was affected and the mother free from clinical manifestations. All of the pregnancies were full term, but in 5 cases there was a history of unduly prolonged labor as opposed to easy deliveries in prior pregnancies. No congenital anomalies were described. Among the clinical manifestations noted in the infants were reduced head circumference, fretfulness, irritability, excessive crying, blindness, hearing impairment, altered reflexes and mental retardation. (The investigators estimated a level of 400 ppb of mercury in blood as the level above which all mothers exhibited signs and symptoms of poisoning. The lowest infant blood mercury level associated with signs of poisoning was 564 ppb.) An attempt was made to relate the degree of effect to the period of pregnancy in which the major exposure took place. Three severely affected infants were exposed only in the 3d trimester and the others throughout pregnancy, particularly in the 1st trimester. The number of cases, however, in each trimester, namely, 4, 4 and 8, was too small on which to base any conclusions.[1,2]

Of particular interest in the isolated instances of reported mercury poisonings is the experience of a family in New Mexico affected by the ingestion of meat from hogs fed seed grain treated with a methyl mercury fungicide. The mother of the family was pregnant and ingested the contaminated meat from the 3d to the 6th month of pregnancy. Other than having elevated urinary mercury levels during the 7th and 8th months of gestation, her examination did not reveal any abnormalities, and she was without symptoms except for slight slurring of speech during a 2-week period during the pregnancy. The male infant delivered at term weighed 3062 gm, displayed intermittent, gross tremulous movements of the extremities and had elevated urinary mercury levels. The infant had progressive neurologic abnormalities and after 3 months his originally normal electroencephalogram became progressively abnormal, with an epileptiform pattern. At 1 year of age, the child had normal physical growth, but he could not sit up or see. It is noteworthy that no detectable mercury was found in the urine of this infant at 6 weeks and that he was not breast fed, so the mercury exposure was solely intrauterine.[19,22]

Genetic mutations and chromosomal aberrations have been produced by organic compounds of mercury experimentally in certain plants and Drosophila.[20] Although all of the organic mercury compounds tested produced c-mitosis, methyl and phenyl mercury are among the most active agents found to produce this effect.[9,20] Fahmy[9] indicated that inorganic mercury is about 200 times less effective than are organic mercury compounds in producing c-mitosis. Studies on inbred CBA mice have failed to demonstrate dominant lethal mutations from organic mercury compounds,[20] but single doses given parenterally on day 10 of gestation resulted in a high frequency of resorbed litters and an increased percentage of dead fetuses.

Skerfving[21] reported a statistical increase in chromosomal breaks in blood cells of 23 human consumers of large amounts of fish containing methyl mercury (0.5–7 mg/kg) as compared with 16 people with low to moderate intake of oceanic fish. The mercury levels in blood were 1.4–11.6 μg/100 ml in the exposed group and 0.3–1.8 μg/100 ml in the nonexposed. There was a statistical relationship between blood mercury and frequency of chromosomal breaks. On the other hand, Firman, in an unpublished report to the WHO task force,[27] reported that a study in progress did not disclose a statistical difference in chromosomal breaks between mercury-exposed persons and a control population. Similarly, Harada et al.[11] reported normal chromosome patterns in 7 adult victims of Minamata disease and 1 infant victim with severe noncongenital Minamata disease. In summary, genetic effects of mercury compounds are meager and somewhat contradictory.

There are no existing data on human exposure in utero to implicate mercury as a teratogen. However, teratogenic effects have been reported in animals. Administration of single high-level doses of methyl mercury phosphate to pregnant rats on day 10 of gestation resulted in reduced birth weight of offspring and an incidence of 31.6% of cleft palates.[18] Spyker and Smithberg[23] found that single doses of methyl mercury that did not affect the pregnant females of two strains of mice produced retarded growth and development, death and congenital malformations in fetuses. Differential effects of methyl mercury were dependent on strain of mice, dose and stage of embryonic development. For both strains, only treatment on day 9 and later had significant embryocidal or teratogenic effects (cleft palates and micrognathia).

There is no information on the effects of mercury on germ cells or fertility in humans, although Bakir et al.[4] suggest that the number of pregnancies in the Iraq epidemic seemed to be low. Suter[24] has reported small but significant decreases in fertility in mice reproduction capacity studies. Male mice injected intraperitoneally with 10 mg/kg methyl mercury hydroxide showed significant small reductions in numbers of implants after about 7.5 days post-treatment. Similarly treated females showed a significant small decrease in number of offspring and living embryos when mated within 4.5 days after treatment. Lee and Dixon[16] also noted reduced male fertility in mice with 1 mg/kg methyl mercury hydroxide intraperitoneal doses and their studies suggested a spermatogenic effect. Studies on the reproductive capacity of men as well as women workers exposed to mercury are needed.

The present OSHA inorganic mercury standard for occupational exposure is a ceiling of 0.1 mg/m^3. In a 1973 criteria document, the NIOSH recommended 0.05 mg/m^3 for a TWA over a 10-hour day.[8] The WHO task force recommends this same level for elemental and inorganic mercury compounds, but notes that this level does not consider the sensitive groups in the general population. In view of the apparent greater susceptibility of the fetus and newborn to these exposures as compared with adults, one must question whether this limit is sufficiently safe for occupational exposure of pregnant women and indirectly for the fetus in utero. For organic mercurials, the WHO task force recommends continued adherence to the advice of the 1969 MAC Committee of WHO that women of childbearing capacity not be exposed to methyl mercury compounds.[27] As a result of a comprehensive review of the subject of mercury toxicity, the pregnant woman, fetus and newborn infant, Koos and Longo[15] recommend the following as exposure limits for women of childbearing capacity: mercury vapor, < 0.01 mg/m^3; inorganic mercury salts (aerosols) and phenyl mercury compounds, < 0.02 mg/m^3; and methyl mercury, none.

REFERENCES

Mercury

1. Amin-Zaki, L., Elhassani, S., Majeed, M. A., et al.: Studies of infants postnatally exposed to methyl mercury, J. Pediatr. 85:81, 1974.
2. Amin-Zaki, L., Elhassani, S., Majeed, M. A., et al.: Intra-uterine methyl mercury poisoning in Iraq, Pediatrics 54:587, 1974.
3. Bahulina, A. V.: The effect of a subacute ethyl mercury coated grain poisoning on the progeny, Sov. Med. 31:60, 1975 (cited in Koos, B. J., and Longo, L. D.[15]).
4. Bakir, F., Damaluji, S. F., Amin-Zaki, L., et al.: Methyl mercury poisoning in Iraq, Science 181:230, 1973.
5. Berlin, M., and Ullberg, S.: Accumulation and retention of mercury in the mouse, Parts I, II and III, Arch. Environ. Health 6:589, 1963.
6. Clarkson, T. W.: The pharmacology of mercury compounds, Annu. Rev. Pharmacol. 12:375, 1972.
7. Clarkson, T., Magos, L., and Greenwood, M. R.: The transport of elemental mercury into fetal tissues, Biol. Neonate 21:239, 1972.
8. National Institute for Occupational Safety and Health: Criteria document for a recommended standard . . . occupational exposure to inorganic mercury, DHEW, PHS, NIOSH (HSM 73-11024), 1973.
9. Fahmy, F. Y.: Cytogenetic Analysis of the Action of Some Fungicide Mercurials, Ph.D. Thesis, 1951, Institute of Genetics, University of Lund, Sweden (cited in Environ. Res. 4:64, 1971).
10. Friberg, L. T. (Chairman): Expert Committee: Maximum Allowable Concentrations of Mercury Compounds. Report of an Interna-

tional Committee, Arch. Environ. Health 19:891, 1969.
11. Harada, Y., et al.: Clinical study (Rinshoto Kenkyu) 48:1431, 1971 (cited in WHO Env. Health Criteria I: Mercury[27]).
12. Harada, Y.: Congenital (Fetal) Minamata Disease, in Katsuna, M. (ed.), *Minamata Disease* (Kuonamoto University, 1968), p. 93.
13. Hazards of Mercury, Special Report to HEW Sec's. Pesticide Advisory Committee, Environ. Res. 4:1, 1971.
14. Knight, A. L.: Mercury and Its Compounds, in Zenz, C. (ed.), *Occupational Medicine: Principles and Practical Applications* (Chicago: Year Book Medical Publishers, 1975), pp. 668–677.
15. Koos, B. J., and Longo, L. D.: Mercury toxicity in the pregnant woman, fetus and newborn infant, Am. J. Obstet. Gynecol. 126:390, 1976.
16. Lee, I. P., and Dixon, R. L.: Effects of mercury on spermatogenesis studied by velocity sedimentation cell separation and serial mating, J. Pharmacol. Exp. Ther. 194: 171, 1975.
17. Mansour, M. M., Dyer, N. C., Hossman, L. H., et al.: Maternal-fetal transfer of organic and inorganic mercury via placenta and milk, Environ. Res. 6:479, 1973.
18. Oharazawa, H.: Effects of ethyl mercuric phosphate in the pregnant mouse on chromosome abnormalities and fetal malformation, J. Jpn. Obstet. Gynecol. Soc. 29:14, 1968 (cited in Environ. Res. 4:67, 1971).
19. Pierce, P. E., Thompson, J. F., Likosky, W. H., et al.: Alkyl mercury poisoning in humans, JAMA 220:1439, 1972.
20. Ramel, C.: Genetic effects of organic mercury compound, Hereditas 57:445, 1967.
21. Skerfving, S.: Conference of Environmental Effects of Mercury, Brussels, November, 1973, in Publicaties om bet Institut voor Wiltenschappen om bet haefmilieu, p. 103, Brussels, Vrije University (cited in Environ. Health Criteria I: Mercury[27]).
22. Snyder, R. D.: Congenital mercury poisoning, N. Engl. J. Med. 284:1014, 1971.
23. Spyker, J. M., and Smithberg, M.: Effects of methyl mercury on prenatal development in mice, Teratology 5:181, 1971.
24. Suter, K. E.: Studies on the dominant-lethal and fertility effects of the heavy metal compounds methyl mercuric hydroxide, mercuric chloride and cadmium chloride in male and female mice, Mutat. Res. 30:365, 1975.
25. Suzuki, T., Matsumoto, N., Miyania, T., and Katsunuma, H.: Placental transfer of mercuric chloride, phenyl mercury acetate and methyl mercury acetate in mice, Ind. Health 5:149, 1967.
26. Takeda, Y., Kunugi, T., Hoshino, O., and Uketa, T.: Distribution of inorganic aryl and alkyl mercury compounds in rats, Toxicol. Appl. Pharmacol. 13:156, 1968.
27. World Health Organization Environ. Health Criteria I; Mercury, Geneva, 1976.
28. Yang, M. G., et al.: Deposition of mercury in fetal and maternal brain, Proc. Soc. Exp. Biol. Med. 141:1004, 1972.

Polychlorinated Biphenyls (PCBs)

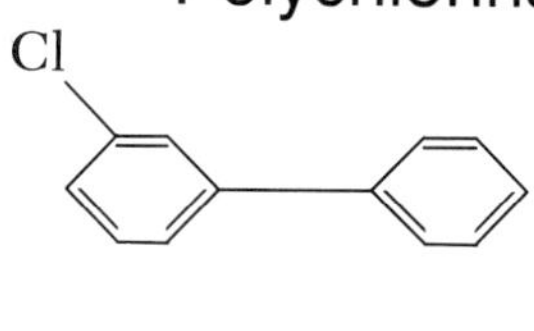

3-chlorobiphenyl

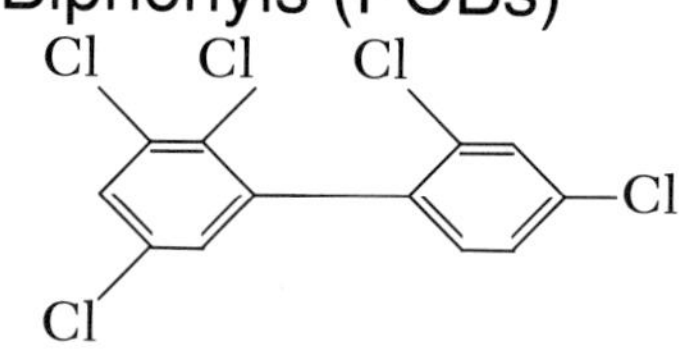

2,2′,3,4′,5-pentachlorobiphenyl

POLYCHLORINATED BIPHENYLS (PCBs) are groups of compounds manufactured commercially by the progressive chlorination of biphenyls in the presence of a suitable catalyst. Among the major uses are for the insulation of electric capacitors and transformers, as plasticizers, investment casting waxes and molds and heat exchange units. PCBs have been used in "carbonless carbon paper." The NIOSH estimates that 12,000 U.S. workers currently have potential occupational exposure to these compounds, the majority in capacitor production and in investment casting processes.[4]

PCBs are very resistant to degradation and persist in the environment. Workers, in addition to their occupational exposure, may be further exposed to PCBs carried into their homes from the workplace and from general contamination of the air, water and food supply. Within workplaces, PCBs have been shown to remain in the air and on surfaces long after their use is discontinued.[7] The role of the impurities known to be present in commercial PCBs, namely, chlorinated dibenzofurans and chlorinated naphthalenes, in the etiology of the adverse effect of PCBs requires further clarification.

PCBs are well absorbed via the gastrointestinal tract, skin and lungs but are poorly metabolized and can accumulate in human and animal tissues.[6] The accumulation, particularly in high-lipid tissues, seems to be greater for the penta and more highly chlorinated compounds. Surveys of human adipose tissue of nonexposed subjects in several countries have shown most samples to contain PCBs around 1 mg/kg or less in contrast to occupationally exposed men, who have shown levels up to 700 mg/kg.[17] National surveys indicate levels in blood around 0.3 μg/100 ml for nonoccupationally exposed populations and levels approaching 200 mg/100 ml in men occupationally exposed, with or without skin lesions.[17]

Placental transfer of PCBs has been found in "Yusho" patients in Japan[14] as well as in various species of animals.[4,17] PCBs have been quantitatively measured in animal and human milk, in the latter in concentrations averaging 0.02 mg/l but reaching levels as high as 0.1mg/l.[19]

In 1968 in Japan, numerous cases of poisoning from PCBs occurred from the ingestion of rice bran oil contaminated with Kanechlor 400, a 48% chlorinated biphenyl, which leaked through small holes in heat transfer pipes immersed in the oil during an oil purification process. The rice oil was also contaminated with chlorinated dibenzofurans, and the role of these impurities needs to be clarified.

By 1975, almost 1300 cases of the disease called "Yusho" were registered. The major manifestations included acneiform eruptions (chloracne), enlargement and hypersecretion of the meibomian glands of the eyes, with swelling of the eyelids and hyperpigmentation of the nails and mucous membranes.[4] In addition, there were alterations in liver enzymes, an increase in serum triglycerides (up to 4 times normal level)[15] and changes in the microanatomy of liver cells, indicative of microsomal enzyme stimulation.[10] Offspring of "Yusho" mothers were smaller than normal and exhibited dark brown skin pigmentation, which persisted for several months after their birth. In 4 babies studied at birth, retarded intrauterine growth was noted in 3, edematous face and exophthalmic eyes in 3, retarded dentition in 2, calcification of the skull and wide-open sagittal suture of the skull in 3.[8] These findings were not persistent, and postnatal mental and physical development appeared normal in these and other "Yusho" children. Only 1 case of "Yusho" from PCB exposure during nursing was observed.[19] In 80 female patients with "Yusho" disease, 60% had changes in their menstrual cycles after the exposure.[12] PCB levels were found for many years in the blood adipose tissue and milk of mothers and in the blood of offspring.[4,17] This occurrence in Japan clearly indicated that PCBs can be transmitted transplacentally to the fetus and also from mothers' milk during lactation.

Data pertinent to reproductive effects from PCBs in humans other than the "Yusho" cases are very limited. In 1936, Schwartz[13] reported that impotence in men was one of the health problems associated with occupational exposure to chlorobiphenyls. Inoue et al.[11] reported on exposure to PCBs among workers in family-owned silk thread glossing factories in Japan. Among those exposed was a woman in her 10th month of pregnancy with a PCB level of 24 ppb in her blood serum. Subsequent to the birth of the child, it was found that the mother's breast milk contained 0.25 ppm PCB, and breast feeding was discontinued. At the time of the report, mother and child exhibited no abnormalities.

Animal studies have indicated such reproductive effects as increased fetal resorptions, lower fertility, decreased survival and teratogenesis, the effects occurring primarily at higher doses. Studies of rhesus monkeys are of particular interest because this animal has been found to respond to PCBs in a fashion similar to humans with "Yusho" disease.[4]

Allen et al.[2] fed female rhesus monkeys a diet containing 25 ppm Arochlor 1248 for 2 months. There was lower fertility in females, which persisted for at least 8 months after the dose was discontinued. Barsotti et al.[3] and Allen and Barsotti[1] fed male and female rhesus monkeys 2.5 ppm and 5.0 ppm Arochlor 1248 in a commercial diet for 6 months. Menstrual cycles became irregular and there was prolonged and excessive menstrual bleeding. There was lower fertility and increased resorptions and abortions compared with the controls, and the offspring had lower body weights. The infants developed signs of PCB poisoning after nursing for less than 2 months and there was a 50% rate of infant mortality during the nursing period. (Milk levels were 0.154–0.397 ppm PCB.)

A report of the findings of a study conducted at the Karolinska Institute by Westöö and Norén[16] reiterates the persistence of PCBs in the environment. They measured levels of organochlorine pesticides and polychlorinated biphenyls (PCBs) in pooled samples of human milk from Stockholm for different periods from April, 1967 to March, 1977. These pooled milk samples were obtained from the Mothers' Milk Center in Stockholm and analyzed for the pesticide levels. Reported average PCB level was 10–20 mg/kg of milk during a period from April to July, 1967, and an average level of 24–30 mg/kg of milk was found from the samples taken between April, 1976 and March, 1977. Despite the fact that PCBs have been severely restricted since June, 1972, special licenses having been required for the importation, production, sale and use of PCBs in Sweden, the authors speculate that PCB discharges from other Baltic countries and global fallout may make a major contribution to the PCB levels in Swedish fish, which are thought to be the main source of PCBs for the mothers.

Studies in animals and microorganisms have shown PCBs to have very weak mutagenic potential. Green et al.[9] found no statistically significant chromosomal aberrations in spermatogonal or bone marrow cells or evidence of dominant lethal mutations in rats fed varying doses of Arochlor 1242 or 1254. In the Ames test, higher chlorinated PCBs showed very little activity, although 4-chlorobiphenyl showed some activity.

The carcinogenic potential of PCBs has been suggested in view of the formation of arene oxides as an intermediate in the metabolism of PCBs and the demonstration of binding of PCB metabolites to nuclear components of liver cells in monkeys, rats and in vitro studies. Dose-related increased incidences of liver tumors, including neoplastic nodules, hepatomas and hepatocellular carcinomas, in rats and mice were noted.[4,17] Confirmation of carcinogenicity of the PCBs has not been obtained in humans. Follow-up of deceased "Yusho" patients indicated a possible increase in cancer incidence, but no consistency as to types of cancer found has been reported.[4]

There is no existing OSHA standard for occupational exposure to PCBs. The NIOSH proposes as the standard a time-weighted average for up to a 10-hour workday, 40-hour workweek, 1 $\mu g/m^3$, which is the minimal detectable level with present methodology. NIOSH has considered the effects on reproduction in establishing this standard and considers that this recommended level will protect unborn babies. The WHO task force has noted that the most sensitive species to PCBs is man and that at intake rates of 0.1 mg/kg body weight per day it seems unlikely that effects on reproduction would be apparent. Based on conversion data suggested by Ferguson[5] for air concentrations and potential dose of a 1 $\mu g/m^3$ for an 8-hour day, if totally absorbed, would be equivalent to 0.14 $\mu g/kg$ for adult males and 0.12 $\mu g/kg$ for adult females.

REFERENCES

Polychlorinated Biphenyls (PCBs)

1. Allen, J. R., and Barsotti, D. A.: The effects of transplacental and mammary movement of PCBs on infant rhesus monkeys, Toxicology 6:331, 1976.
2. Allen, J. R., Carstens, L. A., and Barsotti, D. A.: Residual effects of short-term, low-level exposure of non-human primates to polychlorinated biphenyls, Toxicol. Appl. Pharmacol. 30:440, 1974.
3. Barsotti, D. A., et al.: Reproductive dysfunction in rhesus monkeys exposed to low levels of polychlorinated biphenyls (Arochlor 1248), Food Cosmet. Toxicol. 14:99, 1976.
4. National Institute for Occupational Safety and Health: Criteria for a recommended standard . . . occupational exposure to polychlorinated biphenyls (PCBs), DHEW, PHS, NIOSH 77-225, 1977.
5. Ferguson, D. M.: Toxicological problems related to the employment of women: Health of Women at Work, Society of Occupational Medicine, London, England, April, 1976.
6. Finklea, J., et al.: Polychlorinated biphenyl residues in human plasma expose a major urban pollution problem, Am. J. Public Health 62:645, 1972.
7. Fujiwara, K., et al.: Discovery of PCB pollution at a textile factory. II. Follow-up study on causes of environmental pollution, Jpn. J. Public Health 22:461, 1975 (Japanese) (cited in NIOSH Criteria Document[4]).
8. Funatsu, I., et al.: Polychlorinated biphenyls (PCBs) induced fetopathy. I. Clinical observation, Kurume Med. J. 19:43, 1972 (cited in NIOSH Criteria Document[4]).
9. Green, S. G., et al.: Lack of cytogenetic effects in bone marrow and spermatogonal cells in rats treated with polychlorinated biphenyls (Arochlor 1242 and 1254), Bull. Environ. Contam. Toxicol. 13:14, 1975 (cited in NIOSH Criteria Document[4]).
10. Hirayama, C., et al.: Fine structural changes of the liver in a patient with chlorobiphenyls intoxication, Fukuoka Acta Med. 60:455, 1969 (Japanese) (cited in NIOSH Criteria Document[4]).
11. Inoue, Y., et al.: Discovery of PCB pollution in a textile factory. 1. PCB level in blood serum of laborers and results of physical examination, Jpn. J. Public Health 22:461, 1975 (cited in NIOSH Criteria Document[4]).
12. Kusuda, M.: Study on the female sexual function suffering from the chlorobiphenyls poisoning, Sankato Fujinka 4:1063, 1971 (Japanese) (reviewed in WHO Environmental Health Criteria 2[17]).
13. Schwartz, L.: Dermatitis from synthetic resins and waxes, Am. J. Public Health 26:586, 1936.
14. Tsukamoto, H., et al.: The chemical studies on detection of toxic compounds in the rice bran oils used by the patients of Yusho, Fukuoka Acta Med. 60:496, 1975 (Japanese) (cited in WHO Environmental Health Criteria 2[17]).
15. Uzawa, H., et al.: Clinical and experimental studies on the hyperglyceridemia induced by oral ingestion of chlorinated biphenyls, Acta Med. 62:66, 1971 (Japanese) (cited in NIOSH Criteria Document[4]).
16. Westöö, G., and Norén, K.: Organochlorine contaminants in human milk, Stockholm 1967–1977, Ambio 7:2:62, 1978.
17. WHO Environmental Health Criteria 2: Polychlorinated Biphenyls and Terphenyls. Geneva, 1976.
18. Wyndham, C., et al.: The in vitro metabolism macromolecular binding and bacterial mutagenicity of 4-chlorobiphenyl, a model PCB substrate, Res. Commun. Chem. Pathol. Pharmacol. 15:563, 1976 (cited in NIOSH Criteria Document[4]).
19. Yoshimura, T.: Epidemiological study on Yusho babies born to mothers who had consumed oil contaminated by PCB, Acta Med. 65:74, 1974 (Japanese) (cited in NIOSH Criteria Document[4]).

Tetrachloroethylene (Perchloroethylene)

$Cl_2C{=}CCl_2$

TETRACHLOROETHYLENE is a chlorinated organic solvent widely used as a dry cleaning agent, a degreaser, a fumigant and as a chemical intermediate in the manufacture of other chemicals. The NIOSH estimates that approximately 500,000 workers currently are at risk of exposure to trichloroethylene in the United States.[3]

There have been two animal studies concerning exposure to tetrachloroethylene with reproductive effects. Schwetz et al.[4] exposed 17 rats and 17 mice for 7 hours daily to 300 ppm tetrachloroethylene on days 6–15 of gestation. The controls consisted of 30 unexposed rats and 30 unexposed mice. The exposure was associated with a decrease in maternal weight gain in the rats and an increase in the maternal relative weight gain in the mice. There was a higher percentage of fetal resorptions in exposed rats but no difference in the skeletal anomalies among the exposed litters relative to the controls. Fetal mice, on the other hand, showed decreased body weights and an increased incidence of subcutaneous edema, delayed ossification of skull bones and split sternebrae, as compared with the controls.

In another study, Carpenter[1] evaluated the effects of exposures to 70 ppm, 230 ppm and 470 ppm of tetrachloroethylene on the fertility of female rats between the ages of 70 and 250 days. There were 10 control and 12 test rats in each of the exposure groups. He found a slight drop in fertility at 70 ppm and a slight increase at the higher levels and concluded that it was unlikely that these findings were due to the tetrachloroethylene exposure.

The usefulness of the information furnished by these two animal studies in the consideration of occupational exposure of pregnant women is indeterminate at this time. The teratogenic effect of tetrachloroethylene suggested by Schwetz et al.'s study needs further evaluation, particularly in regard to the difference reported between the effects on the mice and rats. The exposure level used in the study, namely, 300 ppm, is higher than the present OSHA air standard of a time-weighted average exposure of 100 ppm and ceiling of 200 ppm and the proposed NIOSH recommendation in 1976 of 50 ppm time-weighted average and ceiling of 100 ppm (15 minutes).

Of further note is information published by the NIOSH in its 1978 Current Intelligence Bulletin #20, Tetrachloroethylene,[3] from a study by the National Cancer Institute (NCI) with findings of excess hepatocellular carcinomas in male and female mice exposed by forced feeding to tetrachloroethylene as compared with controls. The exposure dosages over 78 weeks were 536 or 1072 mg/kg per day for male mice and 386 or 772 mg/kg per day for female mice. The NIOSH notes that a 70-kg man breathing a typical 10 m^3 per day (over an 8-hour shift) would have an inhalation exposure equivalent to 100 mg/kg per day. Although the dosages used in the NCI studies and those in the previously mentioned animal studies referable to reproductive effects were considerably in excess of the exposure a worker might receive in work areas controlled at recommended levels, further studies are needed to determine what margin of safety, if any, exists at these levels for both the possible neoplastic and reproductive effects of tetrachloroethylene.

REFERENCES

Tetrachloroethylene (Perchloroethylene)

1. Carpenter, C. P.: The chronic toxicity of tetrachloroethylene, J. Ind. Hyg. Toxicol. 19:323, 1937.
2. National Institute for Occupational Safety and Health: Criteria for a recommended standard . . . occupational exposure to tetrachloroethylene (perchloroethylene), DHEW, PHS, NIOSH 76-185, 1976.
3. Current Intelligence Bulletin #20, Tetrachloroethylene (Perchloroethylene). NIOSH-DHEW, January 20, 1978.
4. Schwetz, B. A., Leong, B. K. J., and Gehring, P. J.: The effect of maternally inhaled trichloroethylene, perchloroethylene, methyl chloroform and methylene chloride on embryonal and fetal development in mice and rats, Toxicol. Appl. Pharmacol. 32:84, 1975.

Vinyl Chloride

$H_2C{=}CHCl$

VINYL CHLORIDE, also known as vinyl chloride monomer (VCM), chloroethylene and chloroethene, is a gas at normal temperature and atmospheric pressure. It is the parent compound of a series of thermoplastic resin polymers and copolymers that are widely used for containers, wrapping tissues, electrical insulation, pipe, conduit and a variety of other products. Annual world production of vinyl chloride exceeds 10 billion kg, 25% of this in the United States, where it has been produced commercially since 1939. For a detailed discussion of vinyl plastics and occupational exposures, control measures and related hygienic aspects, the reader is referred to *Occupational Medicine, Principles and Practical Applications*.[2]

Observations over the years have indicated toxic effects of vinyl chloride on the lung, liver, selected bones of the fingers (acro-osteolysis) and central nervous system. However, VCM has been recognized as a human carcinogen since a report made to the NIOSH in 1974 of angiosarcoma of the liver in a small number of employees at the B. F. Goodrich Chemical Company and subsequent epidemiologic studies in the United States, as well as abroad, of workers exposed to VCM, the findings of which confirmed similar data from animal studies since 1971. Both animal and human studies indicate that VCM produces excess tumors not only in the liver but also in the lung and lymphatic and central nervous systems.

Effects of VCM relative to its reproductive toxicity have also been reported. Vinyl chloride has been found to be mutagenic in microbial test systems,[1] in Drosophila[9] and in hamster cells.[6]

Excess chromosomal aberrations in lymphocyte cultures have been reported in male vinyl chloride workers.[3,5] In a study of vinyl chloride monomer workers that compared them with an age-matched control of rubber workers with no known toxic chemical exposure, Infante et al.[7] reported a significant excess of fetal mortality in the wives of the VCM workers as compared with wives of the controls (15.8% and 6.1%, respectively). Fetal mortality (any product of conception not born alive) was not significantly different between the two groups prior to the VCM exposure (8.8% and 6.9%, respectively).

A report by Infante[8] of excess birth defects (particularly anencephaly and spina bifida) in residents of an Ohio community where a polyvinyl chloride manufacturing plant was located was followed by a subsequent case-controlled study of these birth defect cases. Comparison of subject and control data failed to indicate any relationship between occupational and geographic exposure to VCM with the birth defects noted.[4]

In view of the mutagenic responses to VCM in microbial test systems, increased chromosome aberrations in VCM male workers and increased fetal mortality in the wives of such workers, vinyl chloride can be considered a possible reproductive toxin in human males. The effect in females has not as yet been evaluated.

OSHA and the NIOSH have recognized VCM as a carcinogen, and requirements of environmental and medical surveillance pertinent to known carcinogens are mandated. The present OSHA environmental limit is 1 ppm averaged over 8 hours with a maximum of 5 ppm for any 15-minute period.[10]

REFERENCES

Vinyl Chloride

1. Bartsch, H., Malaveille, C., and Montesano, R.: Human rat and mouse liver-mediated mutagenicity of vinyl chloride in *S. typhimurium* strains, Int. J. Cancer 15:429, 1975.
2. Beliczky, L. S., and Zenz, C.: Occupational Health Aspects of Plastics and Rubber Manufacturing, in Zenz, C. (ed.), *Occupational Medicine: Principles and Practical Applications* (Chicago: Year Book Medical Publishers, 1975), pp. 786–815.
3. Ducatman, A., Herschborn, K., and Selekoff, I.: Vinyl chloride exposure and human chromosome aberrations, Mutat. Res. 31:163, 1975.
4. Edmonds, L.: Birth defects and vinyl chloride, in Proceedings of Conference on Woman and the Workplace. Society of Occupational & Environmental Health, Washington, D.C., pp. 114–119, June 17–19, 1976.
5. Funes-Cravioto, F., et al.: Chromosome aberrations in workers exposed to vinyl chloride, Lancet 1:459, 1975.
6. Huberman, E., Bartsch, H., and Sachs, L.: Mutation induction in Chinese hamster V79 cells by two vinyl chloride metabolites, chloroethylene oxide and 2-chloroacetaldehyde, Int. J. Cancer 16:639, 1975.
7. Infante, P. F., et al.: Genetic risks of vinyl chloride, Lancet 1:734, 1976.
8. Infante, P. F.: Oncogenic and mutagenic risks in communities with polyvinyl chloride production facilities, Ann. N.Y. Acad. Sci. 271:49, 1976.
9. Magnussen, J., and Ramel, C.: Mutagenic effects of vinyl chloride in Drosophila melanogaster, Mutat. Res. 38:114, 1976.
10. OSHA, U.S. Dept. of Labor: Emergency Temporary Standard for Exposure to Vinyl Chloride; Fed. Register 39:12343, 1974.

Waste Anesthetic Gases and Vapors

OCCUPATIONAL EXPOSURE to waste inhalation anesthetic gases can occur in medical, dental and veterinarian facilities where gaseous and volatile liquid agents are administered for anesthetic purposes. Halothane and nitrous oxide currently are the two most widely used agents in the United States. Other agents are chloroform, cyclopropane, trichloroethylene, fluroxene, methoxyflurane and isoflurane. The NIOSH estimates that there are approximately 50,000 hospital operating room personnel (excluding surgeons) exposed daily to waste anesthetic gases in the United States. Others who are potentially exposed include about 100,000 dentists and dental assistants and 50,000 veterinarians and their employees.[10]

Current scientific evidence suggests that chronic exposure to anesthetic gases increases the risk of spontaneous abortions and congenital abnormalities among offspring of both male and female workers. In 1967, Vaisman[16] conducted a survey by questionnaire of 303 Russian anesthesiologists (193 men and 110 women) who were exposed to diethyl ether, nitrous oxide, halothane and other anesthetic agents. In 31 pregnancies there were 18 spontaneous abortions and 2 premature births, and 2 women discontinued work because of threatened abortions. There was 1 congenital malformation. There was no scavenging of waste anesthetic gases. Concentration levels were not reported and there were no controls for comparison. The anesthesiologists with abnormal pregnancies were exposed 25 hours per week or more whereas those with normal pregnancies did not exceed 15 hours per week.

A questionnaire survey of Danish nurses and male and female anesthetists conducted by Askrog and Harvald[2] showed a 10% abortion rate in pregnancies with onsets before exposure and a 20% spontaneous abortion rate in pregnancies started after exposure. Wives of exposed male anesthetists also had an increased abortion rate. There were 570 usable questionnaires and information was included on 212 pregnancies started before exposure and 392 started during exposure.

There was no significant difference in frequency of congenital malformations.

Cohen et al.[6,7] interviewed 67 female operating room nurses and 92 general duty nurses and did a questionnaire survey of 50 female anesthesiologists and 82 female physicians in other specialties. In both studies, they found increased spontaneous abortions in the exposed group as compared with the control group, and the abortions in the exposed group tended to occur earlier in the pregnancy.

From Sweden, Götell and Ståhl[12] reported teratogenic effects, liver damage and addiction to halothane and indicated that fatigue, headache, tiredness and irritability are common symptoms in hospital operating room personnel. Based on their studies of operating room personnel at the Regional Hospital in Örebro, they stated that an anesthetist may be exposed to about 2 "patient doses" of halothane per year (25,000–30,000 ppm hours).

Knill-Jones et al.[13] conducted a questionnaire survey among physicians in Great Britain. The exposed-to-anesthetics group and the control group were matched for maternal smoking habits, birth order, maternal age at the time of birth and paternal age at the time of response. They found that female exposure was associated with an increased frequency of spontaneous abortion and a possible increase of minor congenital abnormalities. There also was an increased frequency of congenital abnormalities in live-born children of exposed men.

Corbett and co-workers[9] did a questionnaire survey of female nurse anesthetists and found a higher incidence of birth defects in children whose mothers worked during pregnancy (16.4%) compared with those who did not (5.7%).

The American Society of Anesthesiologists[1] reported increased risk of spontaneous abortion and congenital abnormalities among offspring of exposed personnel. Children of exposed female nurse anesthetists compared with children of unexposed nurses had an increase in congenital abnormalities of 60%; a 25% increase in congenital anomalies was found in offspring of exposed male physicians. A comparison was made of dentists in general practice and oral surgeons exposed for at least 3 hours per week during the calendar year preceding their spouses' pregnancies and those with no exposure to anesthetics. Spontaneous abortion was increased by 78% and fetal abnormalities by 15% in the former.

The German Anesthesia and Reanimation Association report by Garstka et al.[11] found increased abortion frequency, premature births and complications of pregnancy among exposed female anesthesiologists but not among wives of exposed male anesthesiologists. The exposed female anesthesiologists also reported a higher incidence of premature births and complications during pregnancy. Those who reported malformed offspring had been exposed to halothane for an average of 20 months before pregnancy and for 6–7 months during the pregnancy. Exposure levels were not given.

In the epidemiologic studies discussed, except where indicated, there was no information on the types of anesthetic agents or on the concentration levels of exposure.

The effects of inhalation anesthetics on reproduction in experimental animals have been reported by many investigators and are cited in the NIOSH Criteria Document, to which the reader is referred for more details.[10] In Sprague-Dawley rats, Chang et al.[3-5] reported that teratogenic effects may follow exposure to halothane at levels likely to occur in occupational environments, i.e., 10 ppm. Schwetz et al.[14] reported that exposure of rats to chloroform at levels of 30, 100 or 300 ppm produced dose-related fetal abnormalities.

Animal studies have demonstrated increased resorptions and fetal anomalies on exposure. Epidemiologic studies of persons with chronic exposure to waste anesthetic gases suggest an increased incidence of spontaneous abortions and congenital malformations among the children of exposed females and wives of exposed males. Spence et al.[15] conducted a comparative analysis of data from 3 large retrospective surveys in the United States and the United Kingdom, reaffirming an increased incidence of spontaneous abortion among female physicians working in the operating room. The liveborn children of female physicians exposed in the operating room also had substantially more congenital abnormalities. Male anesthetists, compared with nonanesthetist physicians, had an increased incidence of hepatic disease; there was also an increased frequency of congenital abnormalities in their children. The incidence of spontaneous abortion in wives of male anesthetists and the rate of cancer among exposed male anesthetists was similar to controls. Despite differences in survey methods and analysis (which were explained), there was remarkable agreement in conclusions drawn from the independent studies.

There are no occupational exposure standards at present in the United States for gaseous and volatile chemicals when used as anesthetics. Specific occupational standards promulgated by OSHA are chloroform—50 ppm, 8-hour TWA; trichloroethylene—100 ppm, 8-hour TWA with a ceiling limit of 200 ppm and a 300 ppm maximal peak above the acceptable ceiling for 5 minutes in any 2 hours; and diethyl ether—400 ppm, 8-hour TWA.

The NIOSH recommends that exposure to all anesthetic gases be controlled so that it is limited to the lowest detectable level, using established sampling and analytic techniques such as charcoal absorption collection and gas chromatographic analysis. This would limit exposure to 2 ppm of halogenated anesthetic agents, based on the weight of the agent collected from a 45-liter air sample by charcoal absorption over a period not to exceed 1 hour. For nitrous oxide alone, a limit of 25 ppm TWA concentration during anesthetic administration is recommended.

It is important that there be continued studies on the effects of anesthetic gases on reproduction. Further animal studies are indicated at levels that simulate occupational exposure, and data on the outcome of pregnancies in exposed women and wives of exposed men should be compiled.

REFERENCES

Waste Anesthetic Gases and Vapors

1. American Society of Anesthesiologists: Anesthesiologists express concern over long-term effects of gases, JAMA 226:609, 1973.
2. Askrog, V., and Harvald, B.: Teratogenic effect of inhalation anesthetics, Nord. Med. 83:498, 1970 (Danish) (cited in NIOSH Criteria Document[10]).
3. Chang, L. W., Dudley, A. W., Jr., Katz, J., and Martin, A. H.: Nervous system development following in utero exposure to trace amounts of halothane, Teratology 9:A-15, 1974.
4. Chang, L. W., Dudley, A. W., Jr., Lee, Y. K., and Katz, J.: Ultrastructural studies on the pathological changes in the neonatal kidney following in-utero exposure to halothane, Environ, Res. 10:174, 1975.
5. Chang, L. W., Lee, Y. K., Dudley, A. W., Jr., and Katz, J.: Ultrastructural evidence of the hepatotoxic effect of halothane in rats following in-utero exposure, Can. Anaesth. Soc. J. 22:330, 1975.
6. Cohen, E. N., Belvill, J. W., and Brown, B. W., Jr.: Anesthesia, pregnancy, and miscarriage. A study of operating room nurses and anesthetists, Anesthesiology 35:343, 1971.
7. Cohen, E. N., Brown, B. W., Bruce, D. L., Cascorbi, H. F., Corbett, T. H., Jones, T. W., and Whitcher, C. E.: Occupational disease among operating room personnel—a national study, Anesthesiology 41:321, 1974.
8. Cohen, E. N., et al.: A survey of anesthetic health hazards among dentists, J. Am. Dent. Assoc. 90:1291, 1975.
9. Corbett, T. H., Cornell, R. G., Endres, J. L., and Lieding, K.: Birth defects among children of nurse-anesthetists, Anesthesiology 41:341, 1974.

10. National Institute for Occupational Safety and Health: Criteria for a recommended standard . . . occupational exposure to waste anesthetic gases and vapors, DHEW, PHS, NIOSH 77–140, 1977.
11. Garstka, K., Wagner, K. L., and Hamacher, M.: Pregnancy complications in anesthesiologists. Presented at 159th Meeting, Lower Rhine-Westphalia Gynecology and Obstetrics Assoc., Bonn, West Germany, June 23, 1974. Bonn, The Women's Clinic, Bonn University (German) (cited in NIOSH Criteria Document[10]).
12. Götell, P., and Ståhl, R.: Exposure of nurse anesthetists to halothane, Läkartidningen 69:179, 1972.
13. Knill-Jones, R. P., Newman, B. J., and Spence, A. A.: Anaesthetic practice and pregnancy. Controlled survey of male anaesthetists in the United Kingdom, Lancet 2:807, 1975.
14. Schwetz, B. A., Leong, B. K. J., and Gehring, P. J.: Embryo- and fetotoxicity of inhaled chloroform in rats, Toxicol. Appl. Pharmacol. 28:442, 1974.
15. Spence, A. A., Cohen, E. N., Brown, B. W., Knill-Jones, R. P., and Himmelberger, D. U.: Occupational hazards for operating room-based physicians. Analysis of data from the United States and the United Kingdom, JAMA 238:955, 1977.
16. Vaisman, A. I.: Working conditions in surgery and their effect on the health of anesthesiologist, Eksp. Khir, Anesteziol. 3:44, 1967 (Russian) (cited in NIOSH Criteria Document[10]).

RF/Microwave Radiation

THE MOST COMMONLY OBSERVED biologic effect of radiofrequency (RF) microwave radiation is thermal. The reported health effects data are difficult to interpret, since effects at 27 megahertz often are compared with effects at 30 gigahertz. These radiation frequencies differ by a factor of 1000, and the effect at the molecular level may be entirely different. Little information is provided in the literature on depth dose distribution in irradiated tissue even in those cases where information is given on the power density and frequency.

Continuing inferences in the popular literature[1] and occasional reports in the technical literature keep one aware that electromagnetic radiation arising in the frequency range from 10 megahertz to 10 gigahertz may have an effect on the fetus and sperm cells. Because of these considerations, the question remains: Is the present standard of 10 milliwatts/cm^2 for continual exposure safe for fetal and sperm cell exposure in the frequency range from 10 MHz to 100 GHz? Background exposure for the U. S. population is less than 1 microwatt/cm^2.[6] What follows is a summary of what has been reported on human exposures and its adverse effects on the reproductive cycle.

Two organs of the human body have poor temperature regulation due to lack of blood flow in and around the organs. One is the lens of the eye and the other is the testicle. Consequently, any stress, such as RF/ microwave radiation, that will increase the temperature in these organs may cause damage.

In an investigation of 3 male technicians, average age 33 years, with an average of 8 years' exposure to electromagnetic radiation in the frequency range 3.6–10 GHz, a significant decrease was noted in normal motile sperm compared to an unexposed control group.[3] The exposed group also had a greater incidence of complaints regarding decreased sex drive. No differences were noted in hormone production (17-ketosteroids and total gonadotropins). Another study involving 841 Polish workers noted no differences in sex drive between high and low microwave-exposed groups.[10] Accurate quantitative exposure data were not available.

The evidence that microwave exposure causes sterility in men is of questionable reliability. Two reports of an anecdotal nature have been reported in the literature.[7,8] In both cases, the exposure reported was in the region where heat effects would be produced. The reports involved a microwave radar repairman and a repairman for microwave ovens in which the safety mechanism was bypassed for the convenience of the worker. The levels of microwave radiation reported were lower than what might be assumed is necessary to cause sterility, and the microwave oven repairman's medical history indicated that he might have accompanying medical problems that could have caused sterility.

The medical literature associating microwave exposure and miscarriages is equally difficult to evaluate. Single case reports from the United States[9] and from Italy[2] suggest the possibility of RF-induced miscarriages.

The Polish literature[5] reports impaired embryo development in both humans and animals following RF radiation, especially during the initial stages of embryogenesis. All of these cases reported in Western and Eastern literature concerning human female exposures leading to miscarriages apparently involved diathermy treatment and, therefore, the dose received by the fetus was considerable, but no exposure measurements were given. A report from Czechoslovakia[4] suggests a much broader range of effects, such as changes in menstrual patterns, retarded fetal development, congenital defects in newborns, decreased lactation in nursing mothers and an increased incidence of miscarriages for women working with microwaves. As a result of such occupational exposure reports, women of reproductive capacity are prohibited from working with RF radiation sources in Czechoslovakia. Intimations exist in the Western technical literature about the potential genetic effects of RF/microwave exposures. In 1965, a report[11] suggested a possible correlation between paternal radar exposure and mongoloidism in their offspring.

OSHA (29 CFR 1910.97) has adopted ANSI C95.1, 1974 as a guide for occupational exposure limits and the permissible exposure is 10mW/cm^2 (between 0.3 MHz and GHz) averaged over a 6-minute period. This is based on thermal effects and the subject of safety for the fetus is not addressed. ANSI has a draft of a revised standard for RF/microwave (C95.4, November 2, 1979) which bases permissible limits on exposure time, frequency and intensity, the latter measured either in power density (far field) or in units of electric and/or magnetic field (near field). Of note is the fact that reproductive effects have not been addressed in this draft either.

REFERENCES

Microwave

1. Brodeur, P.: *The Zapping of America* (New York: W. W. Norton & Company, Inc., 1977).
2. Cocozza, G., Blasio, A., and Nunziata, B.: Remarks on short wave embryopathy, Pediatria revista d'igiene med. e chor dell' infanzia 68:7, 1960 (Italian).
3. Lancranjan, P., et al.: Gonadic function in workman with long-term exposure to microwaves, Health Phys. 29:381, 1975.
4. Marha, K., Musil, J., and Tuba, H.: *Electromagnetic Fields and the Living Environment,* State Health Publishing House, Prague, Czechoslovakia, 1968. Trans. SBN 911 302-13-7, San Francisco Press, Inc., San Francisco, 1971.
5. Minecke, L.: Effect of an RF electromagnetic field on embryonal development, Med. Pracy 15:307, 1964 (in Polish).
6. Radiological Quality of the Environment in the United States. EPA 520/1-77–009, U.S. EPA, Office of Rad. Programs, Washington, D.C., 1977.
7. Rose, V., Gellin, G., Powell, C., and Bourne, H.: Evaluation and control of exposures in repairing microwave ovens, Am. Ind. Hyg. Assoc. J. 30:137, 1969.
8. Rosenthal, D., and Berrung, S.: Hypergonadism after microwave radiation, JAMA 205:105, 1968.
9. Rubin, A., and Erdman, W. I., II: Microwave exposure of the human female pelvis during early pregnancy and prior to conception, Am. J. Phys. Med. 38:219, 1959.

10. Siekierzynski, M., et al.: Health surveillance of personnel occupationally exposed to microwaves. III. Lenses translucency, Aerosp. Med. 45:1146, 1974.
11. Sigler, A. T., Lilienfeld, A. M., Cohen, B. H., and Westlake, J. E.: Radiation exposure in parents of children with mongolism, Bull. Johns Hopkins Hosp. 117:374, 1965.

Ionizing Radiation

IONIZING RADIATION is capable of causing dose-related damage to all biologic tissues. Despite this serious potential, the radiation industry has proved to be one of the safest places to work.

The National Council on Radiation Protection and Measurements (NCRP) has for many years been considered the responsible source of recommendations about occupational exposure to ionizing radiation. The NCRP has published recommendations on exposures to fertile and pregnant women over the years, most recently in their Report No. 53.[1] Report No. 53 recommends the same exposure limits as their Report No. 39, which is reviewed by Voelz in *Occupational Medicine*.[2]

In brief, the NCRP recommends that the dose equivalent to the embryo or fetus from occupational exposure of the mother be limited to 0.5 rem. In the usual occupational setting, actual exposure measurements to an embryo or fetus within the worker's uterus are not made. Rather, the worker is monitored and the relationship of the reading of a pregnant employee's exposure badge and the dose to an embryo or fetus can vary depending on the location of the monitoring device, the geometry, type and energy of the radiation, as well as the thickness of the overlying maternal tissues.

The occupational dose limit in effect is 5 rem per year whole body, or 1.5 rem per quarter. A pregnancy may go undiagnosed for several weeks, but if radiation exposure is within the acceptable limits and relatively stable as to dose rate, considering the attenuating effects of maternal tissues, an embryo or fetus would not be likely to receive more than 0.5 rem prior to the time of the diagnosis of pregnancy. When this occurs, the recent exposure records can be reviewed and a decision made about any further exposure as long as the estimated or calculated dose to the fetus is kept below 0.5 rem through the term of the pregnancy. The NCRP recommendations in Report No. 53 are stated to be based on limits that would not unreasonably restrict the employment of fertile women in the radiation industry, yet provide safety to the products of conception.

Ionizing radiation is considered a teratogen and a carcinogen, and the effects are dose related. For a detailed discussion of the calculated risks, in part extrapolated from animal data, see the entire Report No. 53.[1]

REFERENCES

Ionizing Radiation

1. National Council on Radiation Protection and Measurements, Radiation Dose Limits for Embryo and Fetus in Occupationally Exposed Women. NCRP Report No. 53, 1977.
2. Voelz, G. L.: Radiologic Health in Occupational Medicine Practice, Zenz, C. (ed.), *Occupational Medicine, Principles and Practical Applications* (Chicago: Year Book Medical Publishers, 1975), pp. 499–551.

4 / Preplacement Medical Evaluation and Recommendations

MARCUS B. BOND, M.D., and JACQUELINE MESSITE, M.D.

THE PRECEDING two chapters have provided considerable assurance that men and nonpregnant women do not differ sufficiently in their responses to hazardous substances or conditions in the workplace for the difference to be of major importance in recommendations about job placement. In physical strength, aerobic capacity and tolerance to hot environments there is a wide range of capabilities in men and women, and there is much overlap. Thus, the "between individual" variations are more important than the "between sex" differences. Except for pregnancy, we believe that there are no medical reasons to make job placement recommendations solely on the basis of the sex of the worker.

NONPREGNANT WOMEN

Medical examinations prior to placement of workers in jobs that can be described as strenuous and/or potentially hazardous are required by most large and some small employers. Physicians and employers usually believe that these examinations are effective in determining those candidates whose health or safety might be adversely affected by such jobs. This is a reasonable premise insofar as it pertains to persons with gross abnormalities of structure or functions. The scope of preplacement examinations generally has been adequate to detect significant abnormalities in the special senses (especially vision and hearing), gross abnormalities in the musculoskeletal and nervous systems, such as balance and coordination, symmetry, motor power and joint motion, the presence of significant organ or systemic disease and gross abnormalities in mental status.

Preplacement examination experiences were reported by M. B. Bond at the October, 1977 joint meeting of the American Academy of Occupational Medicine and the American Academy of Industrial Hygiene. In the telephone industry, medical examinations such as those mentioned above were given to men and the results correlated with job performance in outside craft jobs. Attrition was about 1.5% in 6 months. Recently, women have similarly been evaluated and placed in these same jobs, but the attrition has been much greater. The reasons for the difference in performance by the women has not been poor health but rather inadequate muscle strength, small stature, fear of heights (from ladders and poles) and awkwardness with tools and machinery. These abilities have not traditionally been evaluated adequately in a preplacement medical evaluation. The total exertion in these jobs over a working day is not high as compared with other construction and service jobs, but heavy exertion is required for short periods for several of the tasks, such as using extension ladders, removing manhole covers and climbing telephone poles. In addition to a high rate of attrition, women have initially shown a rate of accidental injuries 2–3 times that of men doing the same work.

A review of these experiences indicated the need to improve in the selection and/or training process and to provide modifications of the job and equipment. Some success has been gained from efforts in all these areas. Over a period of several months, specialists in psychometrics, headed by Mary L. Tenopyr, Ph.D., of the AT&T Company, developed a series of physical tests that are simple to administer and correlate well with success in performance and in reducing on-the-job accidents.

These tests are conducted so that interpretation of results is straightforward and objectively scored. Thus, the tests are validated statistically and are used in the same way as aptitude tests. They can be conducted by nurses or by nonprofessional personnel trained to administer them. Preliminary results with a battery of three tests (static arm strength, balance and skinfold measurements) are assisting in selecting those men and women who are expected to have an improved rate of job success as well as fewer on-duty injuries. Preplacement medical examinations continue to be used as before. Individuals who fail to pass the Physical Abilities Test may retake the test after a few months following a training program to improve fitness.

Lessons from this experience can be applied in other jobs and other industries. In particular where the job tasks are strenuous, thus requiring persons with above-average physical strength and agility, simple tests can be designed to measure these abilities in job candidates. Initially, the chosen tests must be validated for the particular jobs by testing successful incumbents and by testing a suitable number of persons selected for placement by the new methods. Those in the latter group should be observed over a period of weeks or months and their safety and performance correlated with test results. From these results, a pass/fail set of scores can be determined to assist in selecting those men and women with strength and agility characteristics that lead to safe and satisfactory job performance[3] (Fig. 4–1).

Regulations of the U.S. Department of Labor implementing Section 503 of the Rehabilitation Act of 1973 require that any medical examinations or test that might discriminate against persons who are handicapped, as handicapped is defined under the law, must be job related. Thus, jobs that involve lifting of objects would be suitable for the development of lifting tests as a preplacement screening technique. Chaffin et al.,[2,3] after research in this area for several years, working with a number of large employers, reported that the incidence and severity of low back and other musculoskeletal on-the-job injuries vary directly with maximal weight lifted and with the frequency of lifts. Furthermore, workers with varying lifting requirements have been given static lift strength tests and the results compared with the actual lifts required on the job. Those whose lift strength test results indicated high lifting capacity strength as compared with lift required on the job had fewer low back incidents than those lifting nearer their maximum. Efficiency of job performance and attrition rate were not included as study variables, but it is reasonable to think that those persons lifting at or near their maximal capacity would have less efficient production and higher attrition rates.

The two techniques discussed represent a realistic approach to improving the value of preplacement screening to predict job success and safety. The testing methods apply to individuals rather than to gender and should be related to tasks required in certain jobs. A considerable degree of job analysis is required to obtain measures of lifting and carrying strength, balance, coordination or other requirements. It is likely that simple tests and measurements will suffice and, likewise, the "person-tests" may also

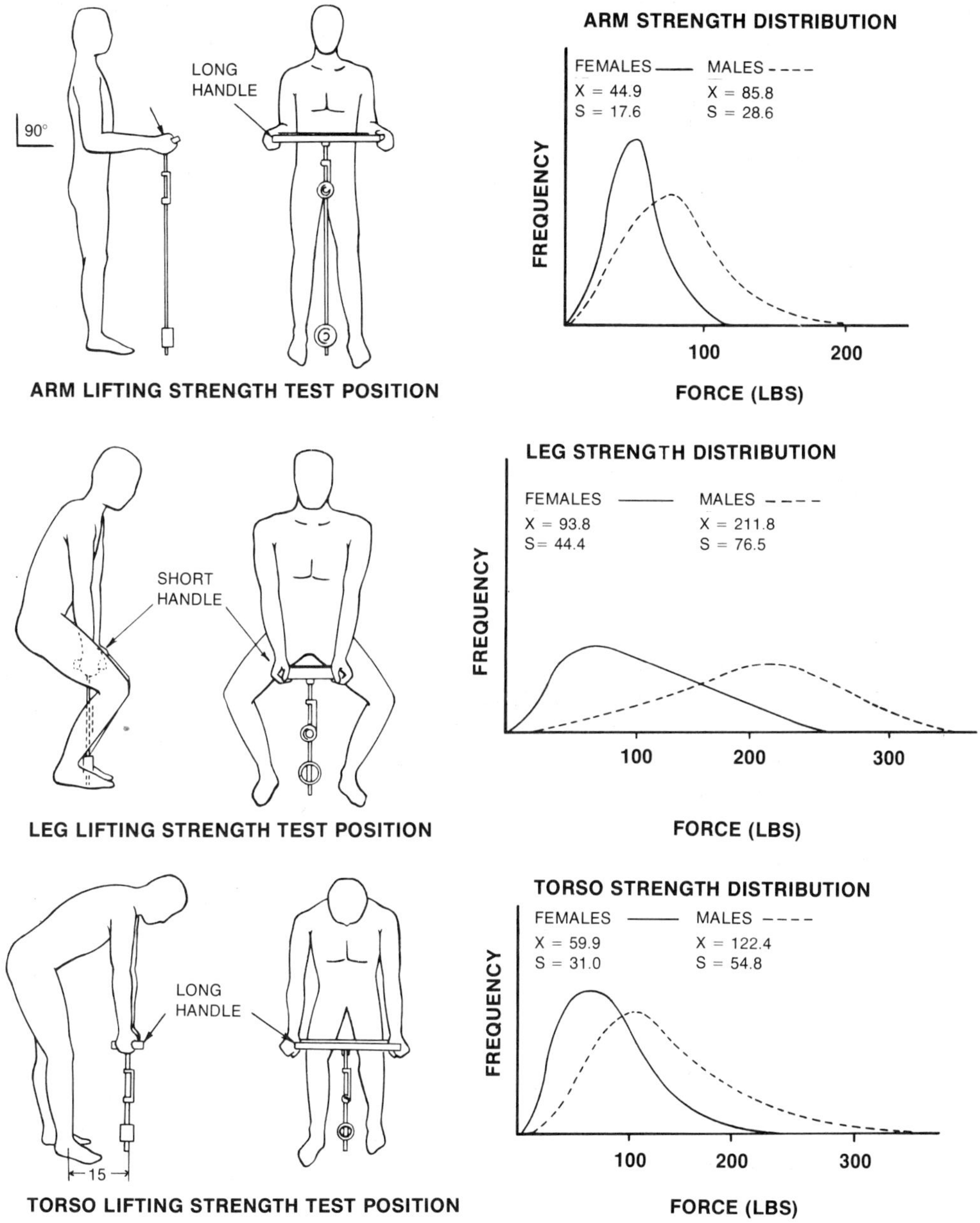

Fig 4–1.—(Adapted and modified from Chaffin et al.[2])

be simple rather than sophisticated measures such as the maximal aerobic capacity discussed earlier. Safe and efficient job performance depends heavily on factors other than strength and agility of the worker.

Job and equipment modification are additional areas that should be explored further to improve the person-machine interface. Too often work areas and equipment have been designed for persons of average size and, in the past, primarily for males, who traditionally have predominated in the jobs.

This offers barriers to persons who vary from these averages and produces artificial and adverse reasons for lack of job success.

In summary, men and nonpregnant women do not differ enough in their response to hazardous substances identified to date to justify medical recommendations for such work exposures based on gender.

PREGNANCY AND JOB PLACEMENT PHYSICAL STRESSES

As in the nonpregnant state, women who are pregnant vary greatly in ability to do physically stressful work. Therefore, it is not possible nor even legally correct to make medical recommendations about the amount of lifting, for example, that is acceptable for pregnant women as a group. The Guidelines on Pregnancy and Work published in 1977 by the American College of Obstetricians and Gynecologists[1] under a NIOSH contract indicate:

> The normal woman with an uncomplicated pregnancy and a normal fetus in a job that presents no greater potential hazards than those encountered in normal daily life in the community may continue to work without interruption until the onset of labor and may resume working several weeks after an uncomplicated delivery.

There was unanimous agreement among obstetric and occupational medicine representatives who prepared these Guidelines on all points in the above statement except in specifying return to work after delivery, and the term "several weeks" (more than 2) was chosen as a term that would recognize variations in persons. Many women may not wish to work until the onset of labor, and, furthermore, some women may have minor symptoms of backache, fatigue and/or a feeling of awkwardness, but which are not a threat to safety or health of the woman or her pregnancy and, therefore, would not require a medical recommendation to cease work. Physicians should resist requests of either employers or employees to make recommendations for nonmedical reasons.

Communication is necessary between the occupational physician and the obstetrician, particularly when the pregnancy is abnormal and/or the woman suffers from an abnormality or disease. Each case must be evaluated on the basis of the clinical status and nature of the job.

Medical recommendations about pregnant women in jobs that are strenuous require careful individualization. Strength and fitness of the individual must be considered, particularly as they relate to the proportion of maximal capacity required by the job. Pregnancy does use a portion of the reserve capacity in the cardiovascular and respiratory systems, and this must enter into clinical judgment.

Special consideration must be given to physical hazards inherent in the job. This includes working at heights (ladders, platforms, poles) and the operation of certain types of heavy equipment and machines in which an accident likely would cause serious damage to the woman and to the fetus, particularly after the uterus has enlarged out of the pelvis. Beginning about midpregnancy, posture becomes slightly distorted and this increases to term due to the increased spinal curvatures to accommodate the protruding abdomen. This may cause a potential hazard in jobs requiring frequent rapid movements of both upper and lower extremities and well-coordinated agility. The problem is compounded if the surface for footing is unsteady or slippery. Such jobs as airline flight attendants, some waitress jobs, certain factory work and certain construction jobs have these characteristics. Many pregnant women may be uncomfortable in such jobs beyond about midterm, but each pregnant woman must be individually evaluated as to her condition and the particular job. Frequent re-evaluation by the occupational physician or nurse and the obstetrician will assist women wanting to work as long as is safely possible during their pregnancy. In some jobs that are particularly strenuous or hazardous, both obstetricians and occupational physicians may agree that some women may not be able to work beyond the 1st trimester in their regular jobs. Nonmedical factors also may intervene and require a change in jobs or cessation of work during pregnancy if work efficiency declines below that considered acceptable due to a combination of minor symptoms that are not truly harmful or dangerous to the woman. Transportation to and from the job, home responsibilities and social activities are factors to be considered also.

HAZARDOUS SUBSTANCES OR CONDITIONS IN THE WORKPLACE

Toxicology of the reproductive process is discussed in detail in Chapter 3. Discussion here will include only medical preplacement recommendations with respect to the embryo or fetus for women who are pregnant or who are fertile.

A dilemma exists with both medical and societal aspects in regard to undiagnosed pregnancy. Since neither the woman nor anyone else can know of the existence of pregnancy until at least several days and usually a few weeks postconception, harm to the fertilized ovum or embryo could occur from work exposures that are considered safe for the nonpregnant worker. The question that logically follows is: Are there work exposures considered acceptable for the nonpregnant woman but from which the risks of harm to the embryo are so great as to make it wise to forbid the woman of childbearing capacity to experience them? Certainly this is more than just a medical question. But it is a medical responsibility to define the risks and make recommendations based on the best scientific knowledge available. If the latter is inadequate, dependence on the informed opinion of a knowledgeable physician would be required. The "opinion" becomes increasingly important when it is realized that we do not have adequate information on the teratogenicity or fetotoxicity in humans of many substances that may be in the work environment. To a certain extent, this situation perhaps always will be with us because of new substances being introduced daily plus the difficult problem of determining whether a particular agent actually causes fetal damage. Even under existing laws and regulations (Toxic Substances Control Act, Occupational Safety and Health Act and others), we do not have assurance that required testing and surveillance will reveal information on potential harm to the embryo or fetus. Rather than conceding defeat by these discouraging words, it is suggested that the only responsible way to proceed is by more and better epidemiologic studies on humans and by cautious extrapolation from animal research. In 1974, Hernberg,[9] the scientific director of the Institute of Occupational Health in Helsinki, Finland, was one of the first investigators to address in a positive fashion the problems of women of reproductive age employed in lead industries. Gordon[4] has discussed this subject on the basis of long experience in a large chemical firm and Lerner[5] has discussed the specific problems with lead.

For the woman who is pregnant or planning pregnancy, exposures to substances or conditions known or highly suspected to cause fetal malformations, abortions, fetal toxicity or transplacental carcinogenesis should not be recommended unless the exposure level is known to be or can be assumed to be below the recommended standards and that such standards take into consideration the reproductive effects. Dose-response data are not always known or, more frequently, the data are inconclusive, particularly as to what the threshold dose for fetal harm is. For example, the NRCP Report No. 53[6] recently reviewed the data on ionizing radiation and potential harm to the embryo or fetus and reaffirmed the recommended permissible total dose to the fetus of 0.5 rem, as had been provided in Report No. 39 in 1971. Since photon energy and dose rate are important in ionizing radiation, the Council pointed out in

1971 that if a woman were exposed to a rather steady amount of radiation within the permitted nonpregnant adult exposures of 1.25 rem per quarter, considering the intrauterine exposure to be attenuated by maternal tissues, a fetus would not receive more than 0.5 rem by the time pregnancy is diagnosed. At this time, a detailed assessment can be made of the probable dose to the fetus and exposure should be kept within 0.5 rem. Medical x-ray should be included, if known, in the calculation.

There are many data on ionizing radiation, but much less on many chemical substances known or suspected to be teratogens, abortifacients, fetotoxins or transplacental carcinogens. Therefore, it is essential that the occupational physician keep abreast of all the pertinent toxicologic information on the exposure as it relates to pregnancy and obtain detailed information about the nature and degree of exposure associated with the particular operation(s) in question. At times, particularly where sporadic high and unanticipated exposures may occur even with good general control, it may be prudent to recommend that women who are pregnant or planning a pregnancy not be subjected to such risks to their embryos and fetuses.

For women who are not pregnant and not planning a pregnancy, but are of childbearing capacity, there is no real consensus about work exposures among those interested or even among well-informed physicians. There appear to be at least two alternatives that could be followed. One is to consider the woman capable of childbearing in the same group just discussed, viz., the pregnant or likely to be soon, and exclude them from exposure to teratogens or fetotoxins. Certainly this would be considered the safest practice to many of those concerned, including employer or legal representatives. At least a few employers have had this practice in effect with lead exposures, for example, and fertile women are forbidden in lead areas. Similar practices are in effect by many employers with substances known or suspected to be harmful to the fetus. On the other hand, in the health care and research areas, such practices are not routine even though most laboratory and x-ray technicians and operating room personnel are women and there are potential hazards to the fetus from biologic agents, chemicals and radiation.

Such exclusionary practices are not considered reasonable by many persons for one or more of the following reasons:

1. A large number of productive employees would be excluded from jobs.
2. This practice probably is a violation of EEOC Regulations.
3. No similar consideration is made for male workers whose reproductive function may be impaired and who may be subject to mutagenic damage to sperm from certain exposures.
4. Such exclusions are not considered in traditionally female jobs in the health industry, such as operating room personnel, nurses and x-ray and laboratory technicians.

Therefore, an alternative is needed, and one such alternative is to make *individual* medical evaluations of the risks present, using medical judgment when precise information is not available.

Employee education is essential for all women who are or may be exposed to substances or conditions that may harm the fetus. It applies equally to women who are pregnant or who are capable of being pregnant. Information must be provided to such women in order that they may participate in decisions about when and where they work. To the extent possible, information should be quantified by describing the relative toxicity of the substances or conditions concerned and to what extent they are present in the workplace, i.e., regularly, irregularly or only potentially, and at what levels relative to known effects. For example, a hazardous chemical might be present only at intervals of a week or a month and for only a few minutes or hours each time as associated with maintenance or cleanup operations. Also, a process might be completely enclosed but, with certain accidental conditions, the material could be released into the workplace, causing unavoidable exposure. Of course, the levels of potentially hazardous substances or conditions present must be known by adequate surveys and measurements and related to existing standards. With the quantitative information and a consideration of the relative toxicity of the materials, employees can be advised with reasonable confidence of the exposures and risks associated with a particular job.

The other variable of importance is the likelihood of pregnancy in a woman capable of becoming but not planning to be pregnant soon. The employee must be fully informed as described and then must be completely straightforward with the occupational physician or nurse. These conditions are necessary for frank discussion between the employee, who should be satisfied that she is not subjecting her fetus to an unusual risk, and a physician who has enough information about the employee as well as the exposures in order to make a recommendation about placement. Ultimately it is the employer who must make a decision about placement, but the physician's recommendations generally will be followed. However, in the alternative just described, the employer's legal advice may not agree with a medical recommendation to permit a fertile woman to work in an environment that is potentially hazardous to the fetus. However, provisions of EEOC Regulations and of Title VII of the Civil Rights Act may forbid such work restrictions. Reconciling such conflicting pressures is beyond the scope of this discussion. The fetus is in the workplace involuntarily and may have legal rights to sue an employer or even the mother for alleged damages during gestation.

To summarize, there may be times when women who are or expect to become pregnant soon should not be recommended for work where there are significant exposures to substances known to be or seriously considered to be abortifacients, teratogens, fetotoxins or transplacental carcinogens. The decision to label a substance or condition as having these deleterious qualities is more difficult than deciding what to recommend once a label has been chosen.

For women not pregnant nor expecting to be soon but capable of pregnancy, the safest recommendation would be to prohibit such exposures. This is not acceptable to many in our society. A suggested alternative is to do individual medical evaluations on women subject to such exposures. An informed woman can make a judgment of the risks and decide whether or not she wishes to work at that job. But if she decides to work at that job, the physician must advise both the employee and the employer of the risks based on a medical evaluation of that individual, her pregnancy and the particular job.

Whether a woman should be able to choose a high risk to the fetus is not really a medical question. Although it is the employer who finally must decide when a person will be placed at a particular job, it is the job of the occupational physician to adequately and properly inform both the employer and the employee of the risks involved.

REFERENCES

1. American College of Obstetricians and Gynecologists: Guidelines on Pregnancy and Work, NIOSH Contract 210–76–0159, 1977.
2. Chaffin, D. B., et al.: Pre-employment Strength Testing in Selecting Workers for Material Handling Jobs. University of Michigan, NIOSH publication CDC 99–74–62, 1976.
3. Chaffin, D. B., Herrin, G. D., and Keyserling, W. M.: Pre-employment strength testing, J. Occup. Med. 20:403, 1978.
4. Gordon, H. L.: Placement of workers in high risk areas. Proceedings of Conference on

Women and the Workplace. Society for Occupational and Environmental Health, 1976.

5. Lerner, S.: Job placement of workers in the lead trades. Proceedings of Conference on Women and the Workplace. Society for Occupational and Environmental Health, 1976.
6. National Council on Radiation Protection and Measurements: Radiation Dose Limits for Embryo and Fetus in Occupationally Exposed Women, NCRP Report No. 53, 1977.
7. Rose, L. M.: Low back pain in industry, J. Occup. Med. II:161, 1969.
8. Tenopyr, M. L.: American Telephone & Telegraph Co., Basking Ridge, N. J., unpublished data, 1977.
9. Hernberg, S.: Lead, in Zenz, C. (ed.), *Occupational Medicine: Principles and Practical Applications* (Chicago: Year Book Medical Publishers, 1975), p. 749.

5 / Women in Manufacturing Industries—Ergonomic Factors and Deficiencies

MARSHA KAPLAN, M.S., and SHERI KNUTSON, M.S.

DURING THE 1940s, occupational safety and health of women workers was an area of limited concern. The United States Department of Labor's Women Bureau compiled statistics on industrial accidents to females and published pamphlets regarding safe work conditions for women. In the early 1940s, others investigated and identified safety and design problems for women workers.[1, 19, 28] However, the results of our studies have shown that these problem areas still exist.[18] Since the Occupational Safety and Health Act (OSHA) of 1970, women in the workplace are receiving a resurgence of interest, primarily concerned with exposures of women to toxic materials and their potential effects on pregnant workers.[14, 20, 23]

A review of the literature for the past several years has shown an apparent void of research in the area of human factors and safety related to female workers. Library computer searches were conducted at the engineering and medical libraries at the University of Wisconsin along with a computer search of more than 300,000 international articles by the National Institute for Occupational Safety and Health (NIOSH). These searches yielded few papers that referred to women in regard to safety and ergonomic factors, and relevant articles that were listed focused mainly on health problems for women in industry, along with a few military studies using anthropometric data with sex as a variable.[29] Hand searches of trade journals and safety publications revealed little in the way of pertinent information.

During a symposium on Women and the Workplace, March, 1977, in Oakland, California, highlighting health hazards and pregnant workers, only one presentation concerning ergonomics and women workers was given. Bond described changes made by the American Telephone & Telegraph Company as women moved into nontraditional jobs such as telephone installers and maintenance work (see Chap. 4).

A systems study of women in the workplace was proposed, with emphasis on human factors design because: (1) No widescope investigation on the topic had been undertaken for more than 30 years, (2) there was preliminary evidence of design problems that affected women primarily, such as improper fit of personal protective equipment and inadequate tool design,[3, 4, 7, 8] and (3) with the increase of women in nontraditional jobs, design problems resulting from inadequacies of tools or equipment for one group when designed for another group

EDITOR'S NOTE: Although some aspects of this chapter are anecdotal, these authors bravely entered workplaces, bringing into the open the longstanding deficiencies involving varied health and safety factors of women on the job. Their efforts are pioneering, at least in the United States, and ought to serve as worthy examples to those concerned with improvement in working conditions for the growing numbers of women in the workplace.

(to be discussed) might restrict women from reaching their full potential in the job, thus hampering their success or achievement and, at the same time, may unduly expose them to certain hazards.[9, 10, 15, 21, 24–26]

Based on the increasing number of accidents of women workers, the need for a survey, or overview, of women in selected Wisconsin industries, with an emphasis on human factors, design and safety, was apparent. In order to yield a wide perspective on the topic, statistical and data analyses as well as field studies were performed.

The study of women working in Wisconsin revealed an increasing number of women working in manufacturing industries and in specific "nontraditional" occupations such as carpenters, electricians, mechanics, grinders and fork-lift truck drivers, etc. The increase in accidents that involve female workers is paralleling the employment increases. However, in certain industry groups, women have a greater chance of injury than does a man, regardless of employment. The following industry groups are among those experiencing high numbers of female accidents: miscellaneous, manufacturing plastics, household appliances, miscellaneous electrical equipment and supplies, engines and turbines, miscellaneous plastics and electrical and industrial apparatus.

Analysis of all industrial accidents that occurred in Wisconsin in 1975 and 1976 showed that women experienced differential patterns of accidents. For example, women received high percentages of wrist and arm injuries, including "tendinitis" and "ganglions" and high percentages of "rubbed and abraded" types of injuries.

WOMEN IN THE WISCONSIN LABOR FORCE

The state of Wisconsin, with slightly more than 4,600,000 inhabitants, is highly industrialized and may serve as a "macrocosm" for occupational health and safety problems encountered throughout the United States and elsewhere as well.[2]

On the national level, women now constitute nearly half of the labor force, with a growing number entering jobs traditionally held by males. This phenomenon is not new, since women took over many of the so-called men's jobs during World War II. During this wartime period, women worked as foundry workers, welders, crane operators, etc., there being few occupations that were not held by women.

In 1970, women made up 37% of Wisconsin's work force (Table 5–1). The percentage of women workers in the labor force has been steadily rising. The number of women working in Wisconsin has increased by 183,878 from 1960 to 1970. In the United States, more than 58% of women with school-age children are working (1978); this trend is noted in Britain and France, where more than 40% of the labor force is composed of women, and more than 50% in Japan and some Scandinavian countries.[30]

In 1970, Wisconsin made up 25% of all employees working in manufacturing industries (Table 5–2).

Wisconsin manufacturing industries employing the largest number of women in 1970 were electrical machinery, equipment and supplies (18,930 women), which includes 13,076 workers in the electrical machinery, equipment and supplies (not elsewhere classified) industries, machinery except electrical (17,462 women), which includes engines and turbines (5214 women), and machinery except electrical (not else-

TABLE 5–1.—WISCONSIN EMPLOYMENT

YEAR	NO. MEN	NO. WOMEN	TOTAL	WOMEN % OF TOTAL
1940	829,322	231,086	1,060,408	22
1950	995,125	359,429	1,354,554	26
1960	1,011,324	457,307	1,468,631	31
1970	1,085,629	641,185	1,726,814	37

Source: U.S. Census data.

TABLE 5–2.—WISCONSIN MANUFACTURING EMPLOYMENT

YEAR	NO. MEN	NO. WOMEN	TOTAL	WOMEN % OF TOTAL
1940	270,021	45,063	315,084	17
1950	414,601	86,218	500,819	21
1960	483,783	102,034	585,817	21
1970	528,407	130,602	659,009	25

Source: Authors' analysis of U.S. Census data and Wisconsin Department of Industry, Labor and Human Relations, Research and Statistics.

where classified) industries (5249 women).*

In the nondurable manufacturing industries, 10,973 females worked in food and kindred products (meat, 2184 women; dairy, 3129 women), paper and allied (7002 women), printing, publishing and allied (8936 women), and leather products (7223 women), of whom 5286 were in footwear industries.*

Occupational data in 1970 showed that clerical and kindred workers accounted for 30% of employed females, operatives, except transport (13%), service workers except households (19%), etc.* (Table 5–3).

OCCUPATION CHANGES

There were 40% more women working in 1970 than in 1960 in Wisconsin. However, the rate of increase of women in specific occupations is much higher than the overall increase of 40% (Table 5–4). From these tables it can be seen that women are entering certain jobs that traditionally were held by males and, in some cases, these increases are high, which may serve to indicate occupational groups of women where design problems with machinery, tools, personal protective equipment, workplace or training may exist.

TABLE 5–3.—TEN INDUSTRY GROUPS EMPLOYING THE LARGEST NUMBER OF WOMEN WORKERS IN 1970—WISCONSIN

INDUSTRY	NO. WOMEN
1. Electrical machinery, equipment and supplies	13,076
2. Machinery except electrical	5,249
3. Engines and turbines	5,214
4. Printing, publishing, allied	5,632
5. Footwear, except rubber	5,286
6. Apparel	5,302
7. Pulp, paper and paperboard mills	3,333
8. Dairy	3,129
9. Motor vehicles and equipment	3,436
10. Metal stamping	3,454

Source: 1970 U.S. Census data.

*U.S. 1970 Census data.

ACCIDENTS IN WISCONSIN BY INDUSTRY

A computer listing of all female workers' compensation accidents in Wisconsin during 1975 and 1976 divided into industry groups (using the Standard Industrial Codes, SIC) was requested from the data processing department of the Wisconsin Department of Industry, Labor and Human Relations (DILHR). The purpose of these data requests was to point out industries that were experiencing large numbers or percentages of female accidents and to aid in selecting companies to visit for possible study. Nonmanufacturing industry groups such as retail and hotels were requested by 2-digit SIC classifications. Our study focused primarily on manufacturing operations, requiring 3-digit SIC codes for manufacturing industries. Three-digit codes are more specific than 2-digit codes (3-digit codes are contained within a 2-digit classification, i.e., 20 is food and kindred products and 201 is meat products). Table 5–5 reveals that the period 1975–1976 was sufficient to reflect an accurate picture of the current accident situation for females in Wisconsin industries.

The preceding sections provided a general picture of the employment and accident situation of women workers in Wisconsin, and the data served as a background in order to initiate investigations on possible ergonomic factors that might contribute to hazardous situations for women in the workplace.

TABLE 5–4.—OCCUPATION CHANGES

	NO. IN 1960	NO. IN 1970	% INCREASE
Nontraditional Occupations			
Carpenters	69	232	236
Electricians	19	126	563
Auto mechanics	46	246	434
Grinding operatives	49	344	602
Fork-lift and towmotor operatives	10	128	1,180
Craftsmen and kindred	176	471	139
Welders, flame-cutters	465	913	96
Machinists	247	463	87
Freight and materials handlers	564	1,023	81
Traditional Occupations			
Assemblers	10,672	14,728	40
Checkers, examiner inspectors; manufacturing	4,602	6,677	45
Clerical, kindred	127,988	193,175	51
Laundry, dry cleaning operatives	2,025	3,103	53
Service workers (except private)	75,230	120,888	61
Salesworkers	39,601	46,476	17
Bottling, canning	399	301	−14 (decrease)
Ironers, pressers	2,667	2,000	−25 "
Sewers, stitchers	8,398	7,948	− 5 "
Shoemaking operatives	2,757	1,367	−50 "
Textile operatives	1,885	1,554	−18 "

Source: U.S. Census data, authors' analysis.

TABLE 5–5.—INDUSTRIES WITH THE HIGHEST NUMBER OF WOMEN'S ACCIDENTS (1975–1976)

SIC	NAME OF INDUSTRY GROUP	NO. OF WOMEN'S ACCIDENTS	% WOMEN'S ACCIDENTS TO TOTAL ACCIDENTS
201	Meat	582	19
351	Engines and turbines	492	28
307	Miscellaneous plastics	403	40
362	Electrical industrial apparatus	342	35
346	Metal forging and stamping	332	13
203	Canning	259	29
202	Dairy	225	13
363	Household appliances	222	51
314	Footwear except rubber	203	59
243	Millwork	201	23
251	Household furniture	201	34

Source: Authors' analysis of Wisconsin workers' compensation data.

WISCONSIN ACCIDENT STATISTICS AND ACCIDENT PATTERNS

The number of women experiencing industrial accidents and illnesses appeared to be rising steadily, as was the percentage of female accidents to total accidents and the percentage of females to total employment (Table 5–6).

Scope of Investigations

AVAILABLE DATA.—Data from the Wisconsin Workers' Compensation Case History File was utilized in the following phases of our study, as Wisconsin is among several states that have thorough accident data-keeping systems with all work-related accidents resulting in 4 or more lost workdays recorded. Accidents and illnesses are summarized, coded and computerized by type of accident ("fall," "caught in," etc.), source of accident ("grinder," "saw," "dust," etc.), part of body affected ("finger," etc.), nature ("silicosis," "fracture," "tendinitis," etc.), occupation of injured ("assembler," "electrician," etc.), kind of injury ("fatal," "permanent partial disability," etc.) as well as sex, date reported, benefits paid, employer, etc. This information can be requested and analyzed through a "Report Generator," a program developed for accident analysis. Combinations and interactions of the above-mentioned factors can be examined.[5,11]

TABLE 5–6.—PERCENTAGE OF WOMEN'S ACCIDENTS TO TOTAL ACCIDENTS AS COMPARED TO THE PERCENTAGE OF WOMEN TO TOTAL EMPLOYMENT

YEAR	NO. WOMEN ACCIDENTS	% WOMEN TO TOTAL ACCIDENTS	% WOMEN TO TOTAL EMPLOYMENT
1940	1,663	7.1	22
1960	3,642	12.9	31
1970	7,116	17.9	37
1975	9,852	20.4	39

Source: U.S. Department of Labor; Monthly Labor Review, 1945; U.S. Census data, U.S. Department of Labor; Geographical Profile of Employment and Unemployment, 1975 (Bureau of Labor Statistics, 1977, Report 481); Wisconsin Department of Industry, Labor and Human Relations Research and Statistics, workers' compensation accident statistics.

Another source of accident information available is reports of accident investigations of workers' compensation accidents performed by the Wisconsin State Safety Inspectors. These reports contain detailed information related to the accident as well as interviews with the injured party and witnesses. A case is investigated if, on reading the Employer's First Report of Injury, an inspector or administrator determines that a violation of a state or OSHA safety standard appears to have been an important factor in the accident. Therefore, these reports represent a rather biased sample of accidents, since they are investigated if a violation seems to be likely. Nonviolations, as well as violations, were examined in our study.

Information from the sources described above was utilized in the following analyses for the isolation of patterns or factors related to ergonomic problems for women.

Analysis of Workers' Compensation Accidents

All Wisconsin workers' compensation accidents that occurred in 1975–1976 were analyzed as to the following factors: source of accident, type of accident, nature of accident, part of body injured and occupation of the injured. The number of female accidents associated with each of these codes was printed in the output, computing the percentage of total accidents that involved women for each of the above factors. In this way, the incidence of female accidents that were related to a certain source, occupation, etc., relative to men, depicting patterns or problem areas was studied.

Keeping in mind that women made up 39% of the Wisconsin work force in 1975, they have more than 53% of all injuries to "arms-multiple" and 77% of all Colles' fractures. Women experience about half of arm-hand tendinitis, tenosynovitis and ganglion

TABLE 5–7.—ANALYSIS OF WORKERS' COMPENSATION ACCIDENTS IN WISCONSIN (1975–1976*)

PART OF BODY	TOTAL NO. OF ACCIDENTS	NO. OF WOMEN'S ACCIDENTS	% TOTAL ACCIDENTS INVOLVING WOMEN
TOTAL	96,217	20,504	21
Eyes	2,418	330	14
Upper extremities	14,768	3,850	26
Back	20,534	4,583	22
Legs	14,024	2,706	19
Fingers	14,795	3,081	21
Feet	7,246	1,072	15
Head-neck	4,748	1,047	22
Trunk	9,817	1,771	18
Specific Examples			
Arms, multiple	36	19	53
Colles' fracture	9	7	77
Coccyx	209	99	47
Tibia, fibula	24	10	42
Bronchial tubes	48	19	40

*Women made up 39% of the work force in Wisconsin in 1975.
Source: Authors' analysis of Wisconsin workers' compensation data.

TABLE 5–8.—ANALYSIS OF WORKERS' COMPENSATION ACCIDENTS IN WISCONSIN (1975–1976)

NATURE OF INJURY	TOTAL NO. OF ACCIDENTS	NO. OF WOMEN'S ACCIDENTS	% OF TOTAL ACCIDENTS INVOLVING WOMEN
TOTAL	96,217	20,504	21
Sprain-strain	37,583	8,336	22
Dermatitis, poisoning	1,357	419	31
Cut, laceration	16,434	2,876	18
Contusion	13,304	2,989	22
Fracture	9,861	1,727	18
Burn	3,112	677	22
Specific Examples			
Tendinitis	379	180	47
Tenosynovitis	85	43	50
Ganglion	98	48	49

Source: Authors' analysis of Wisconsin workers' compensation data.

cases, about half of all "rubbed and abraded" types of injuries and "injuries resulting from violence." Eight-nine per cent of all meat wrappers injured are women, 87% of all sewers and stitchers, 43% of all upholsterers and 40% of all assemblers (Tables 5–7–5–11).

OCCUPATIONAL DISEASES

A short analysis was done for 1 year (1975) on occupational diseases relating to women from a computer run categorized by the standard industrial classification. Not surprisingly, "skin diseases" and "repetitive trauma" turned up as the most frequent types of occupational diseases. Included in the category of skin diseases was "dermatitis" or "allergies." Repetitive trauma included "tendinitis," "tenosynovitis," "ganglion" or "other inflammation" or "irritation of joints, tendons and muscles"; hearing loss is in this category also. Tables 5–12 and 5–13 show lists of those industries reporting

TABLE 5–9.—ANALYSIS OF WORKERS' COMPENSATION ACCIDENTS IN WISCONSIN (1975–1976)

TYPE OF INJURY	TOTAL NO. OF ACCIDENTS	NO. OF WOMEN'S ACCIDENTS	% OF TOTAL ACCIDENTS INVOLVING WOMEN
TOTAL	96,217	20,504	21
Fall from elevation	6,102	939	15
Fall same level	9,050	3,256	36
Struck self	10,704	1,620	15
Struck by someone, something else	627	157	16
Struck onto, against	6,902	1,463	21
Buried	168	11	7
Struck	10,733	1,516	14
Caught in machinery	7,586	1,643	22
Highway wrecks	2,230	201	9
Pedestrian struck on highway	153	20	13
In-plant traffic accident	2,079	190	9
Electrical mishaps	229	30	13
Explosion	352	54	15
Extreme temperature	2,615	593	23
Rubbed, abraded	1,421	691	49
Toxic contact	2,052	628	31
Extreme noise	379	6	2
Specific Examples			
Rubbed, abraded by repeated motion	1,028	560	54
Rubbed, abraded by repeated pressure	258	112	43
Violence	1,325	634	48

Source: Authors' analysis of Wisconsin workers' compensation data.

TABLE 5–10—ANALYSIS OF WORKERS' COMPENSATION ACCIDENTS IN WISCONSIN (1975–1976)

OCCUPATIONS	TOTAL NO. OF ACCIDENTS	NO. OF WOMEN'S ACCIDENTS	% OF TOTAL ACCIDENTS INVOLVING WOMEN
TOTAL	96,217	20,504	21
Assemblers	2,543	1,025	40
Meat wrappers	75	67	89
Upholsterers	44	19	43
Sewers, stitchers	234	205	87

Source: Authors' analysis of Wisconsin workers' compensation data.

TABLE 5–11.—ANALYSIS OF WORKERS' COMPENSATION ACCIDENTS IN WISCONSIN (1975–1976)

SOURCE OF ACCIDENT	TOTAL NO. OF ACCIDENTS	NO. OF WOMEN'S ACCIDENTS	% OF TOTAL ACCIDENTS INVOLVING WOMEN
TOTAL	96,217	20,504	21
Assembling press	80	38	47
Metal stamper	14	11	78
Eyeglasses	56	29	52
Fiberglass	40	21	52
Glove	9	5	55
Carbon tetrachloride	16	11	69
Nitric acid	4	3	75
Acetone	4	3	73
Belt conveyor	149	43	29

Source: Authors' analysis of Wisconsin workers' compensation data.

TABLE 5–12.—OCCUPATIONAL DISEASES (1975)

SIC	TOTAL CASES	WOMEN'S CASES	WOMEN'S % OF TOTAL
Skin Diseases			
201 Meat packing	37	14	38
351 Engines and turbines	24	15	62.5
361 Electric transmission and dist. equip.	7	5	71
373 Ship and boat building/repair	9	5	55.5
581 Eating and drinking places	12	8	66.6
805 Nursing and personal care industries	15	15	100
806 Hospitals	25	23	92
Repeated Trauma			
201 Meat packing	46	15	32.6
202 Dairy	4	3	75
251 Household furniture	5	4	80
262 Paper mills	12	5	41.6
265 Paperboard containers	6	3	50
273 Books	6	5	83.3
302 Rubber, plastic footwear	13	13	100
307 Misc. plastic	8	8	100
314 Footwear except rubber	7	5	71.4
342 Metal forgings	61	12	19.6
351 Engines/turbines	23	19	82.6
362 Electrical ind. apparatus	13	8	61.5
363 Household appliances	20	16	80
806 Hospitals	7	5	71

TABLE 5–13.—TOTAL OCCUPATIONAL DISEASES ACROSS INDUSTRIES (1975)

	TOTAL CASES	WOMEN'S CASES	WOMEN'S % OF TOTAL
Skin diseases	552	203	37
Dust diseases of lungs	52	2	.04
Respiratory conditions due to toxic agents	109	23	21
Poisoning	81	18	22
Disorders due to physical agents	133	21	16
Repeated trauma	729	269	37

NOTE: Dust diseases, respiratory conditions, poisoning and disorders due to physical agents did not show up significantly by specific industrial classifications for women.

the highest proportion of occupational disease affecting women workers.

INSPECTORS' INVESTIGATIONS

Inspectors' investigations of accident reports for the years 1970–1976 were obtained and all accident reports of female injuries were analyzed to discern possible human factors design problems that may have contributed to the accident under investigation. For this period, almost 10,000 inspectors' investigations were examined, but a comparison between men and women accident investigations was not feasible. (It is possible that many of the problems isolated for women would also cause problems for men in industry; see Chaps. 4, 6 and 10.) The basic aim of this pilot study was to determine the factors rather than trying to prove that women have more accidents because of ergonomic considerations.

The analysis centered around the following areas: *problems with safety glasses, protective gloves, personal protective clothing, hair getting caught, training, physical size, machine and work environment*.

A general summary of possible human factors design problems was isolated from the inspectors' investigations (Table 5–14). Frequency counts were not recorded because an exact count of the number of inspectors' investigations was not available. Specific questions relating to human factors are not asked by the inspectors; they are included only incidentally in the report. Pertinent information was listed rather than providing artificial counts or percentages based on a biased sample (inspectors generally investigate all fatalities and those accidents where an employer possibly was negligent). In certain instances, the inspection reports indicate multiple human factors design problems combined at the time of the accident.

TABLE 5–14.—SUMMARY OF INSPECTORS' INVESTIGATIONS (1970–1976)

No respirator—bad ventilation
No safety shoes
Poor design of work environment
Inadequate training, instruction, work procedures, lack of training in operating equipment
New employee not familiar with work operation
Nervous about operation
Glove, mitten caught in gears, rollers, etc.
Gloves too big
Gloves not provided
Arms not long enough to reach controls
Too short to reach shutoff switch
Small hand
Equipment not adjusted for women
No eye protection provided
Safety glasses gave employee a headache
No side shields provided on safety glasses
Improper fitting of safety glasses and side shields
Hair caught in gears of machinery
Shirt caught in moving gears
Tripped operating lever with sleeve of shirt
No protective clothes provided
Protective clothing provided too big, resulted in getting caught in machinery

PROCESS OF SELECTING COMPANIES FOR VISITS

Factors taken into account when choosing companies to visit included: (1) companies that belong to an SIC group that is experiencing high numbers of accidents to female workers (data obtained from analysis described earlier), (2) companies and SIC groups that employ large numbers of women (data obtained from 1970 Census data and 1973 Wisconsin Manufacturers Association Guide, listing the number of women employed in each company), (3) companies that may have women working in nontraditional female jobs (industries where the number of women has increased in the past few years; previous analysis of Census data provided insight into this factor), (4) companies that may be more likely to utilize personal protective equipment, tools, etc. (may be implied from the operations or finished product that a plant produces), (5) budgetary constraints, plants within 120 km radius preferably and, of importance, (6) companies that voluntarily agreed to let us in.

Procedures

Based on the literature search, statistical research, inspectors' investigations, interviews with safety suppliers, manufacturers, union officials and workers, major human-factor problem areas were determined. These factors include personnel protective equipment, machinery, equipment, operations, workspace and training.[22–25] A questionnaire was developed focusing on these areas (Fig 5–1).

Interviewing Procedure

Permission to visit plants was obtained by telephone communication with plant management, followed by a letter describing the proposed study. Once at the plant, plant

Male __________ Female __________ How long on job. __________

Size __________ Work activity __________

____

__________ Pace __________

Training

Did you receive specific training for your job? __________

What type of training? __________

____

____

Do you feel comfortable (understand, familiar) with machine, tools operations?

____

____

Do you feel the need for increased training? If so, in what areas? __________

____

Machinery—Work space

Do you feel that any of these machinery or tools should be changed or designed differently to meet your needs (make working more comfortable)? How?

____

____

Does your work area allow you space to work safely? __________

____

Do you have difficulty reaching? Do operations require uncomfortable positions?

____

____

Personal Protective Equipment

What personal protective equipment is necessary for your job? __________

What personal protective equipment do you use? __________

Was this equipment provided or did you purchase it yourself? __________

Were there problems in obtaining proper fit? __________

____

Do you feel the need for other safety equipment? If so, what? __________

____

Do you feel the need for improved design or fit of equipment? How? __________

Fig 5–1.—A questionnaire to determine major human factors problem areas.

management (personnel, safety, plant manager, nurse or supervisors) were interviewed, with ideas relating to the area of human factors and women workers discussed. Although the questionnaire was used as a guideline in interviewing employees, the interviews were kept as informal and open-ended as possible, taking place while the employee was working. It seemed that workers may feel more comfortable talking about their job while they were actually performing it, rather than in an isolated office or lunchroom; also, ideas and details may be less likely to be overlooked when the interview takes place in the normal work environment. Workers' names were not taken and interviews were on a one-to-one basis with the worker and one of the authors, and brief, unobtrusive notes were taken during the 10–15-minute interview to avoid disrupting the flow of conversation. The authors tried to remain as objective as possible when conducting the interview to avoid leading or biasing the responses, and workers were told at the outset that the purpose of the interview was to gain their perspective on any hazards or problems that they might experience in the workplace.

Approximately 20 workers were interviewed in each plant, representing different operations in the plant. Although most of those interviewed were women, males were interviewed if they were performing the same job. (The authors took pictures of possible ergonomic problems, when permitted.)

Results of Interviews in Factories

Frozen foods manufacturer (SIC 203)—420 workers; one-half women, 3 shifts, young work force (25 and under); 24 interviewed (19 women); (women did not work in stockrooms or shipping; most worked on conveyor lines). Worker comments regarding human factors inadequacies: Cloth gloves provided by company were too big for women, so clumsy and uncomfortable that workers often would not wear them (even when handling frozen foods), flour dust, heat and poor ventilation were mentioned as irritating, heights of some conveyor belts were too low, resulting in backaches from bending and twisting, speed stress from working on the lines, continual changing of jobs made some workers feel uncomfortable with their operations and machines and some believed that more training was necessary. (See Figs 5–2–5–8.)

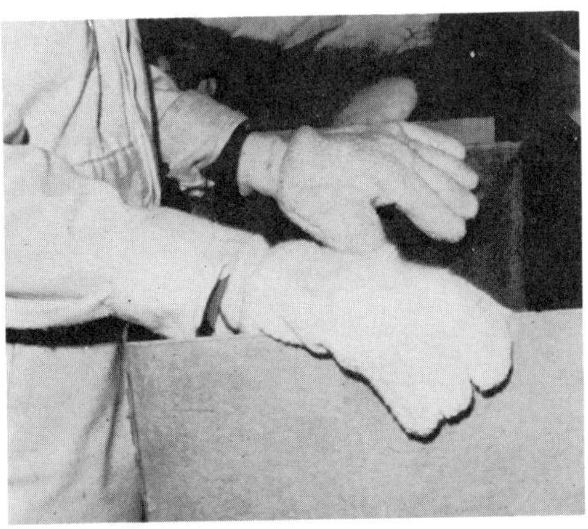

Fig 5–2.—Gloves are too big, uncomfortable, clumsy, often not worn even when handling frozen goods.

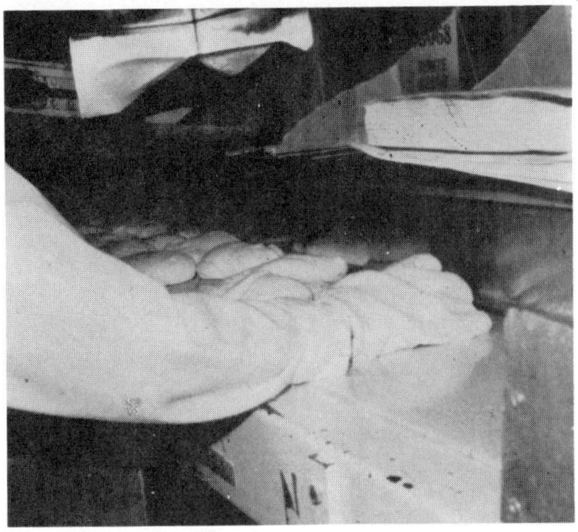

Fig 5–3.—Large gloves can get caught in conveyor parts, causing hand injury.

Battery manufacturer (SIC 369)—rural area, 180 workers; two-thirds women, 2 shifts; 19 females interviewed, representing all departments and machinery where women were employed. Women were employed as machine operators, on packaging lines, in graphite areas but not in mixing room or as shippers. Men were not observed to be working on lines. Workers moved to different jobs, based on production needs and to relieve tedium. Worker comments regarding human factors inadequacies: Some felt nervous or uncomfortable around their machines and thought that more training may have been helpful in getting used to the machine. One woman es-

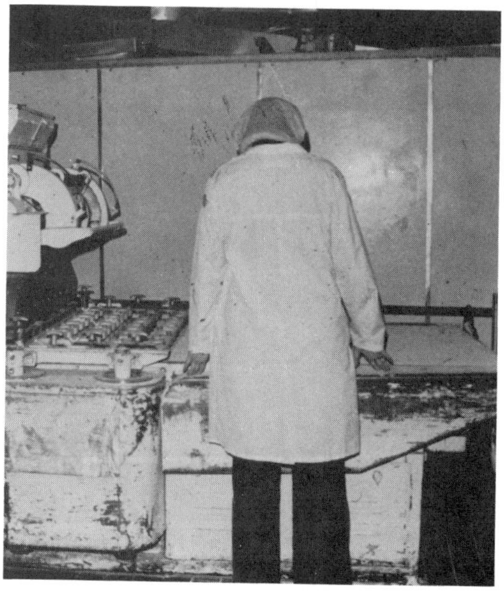

Fig 5–4.—Low height of workplace causes back problems.

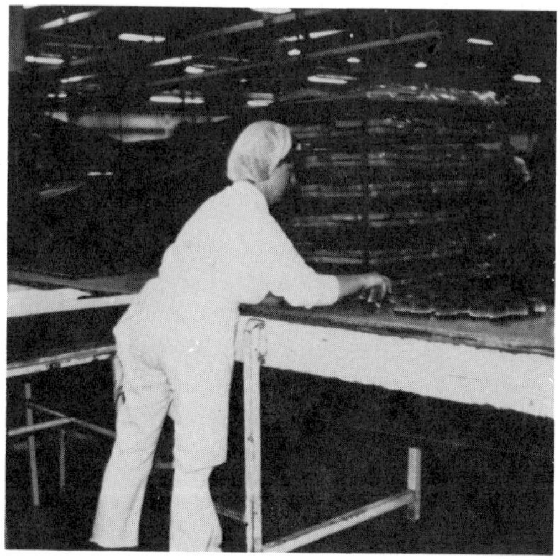

Fig 5–6.—Operating under speed stress. Height of workplace requires constant reaching. Job requires repetitive twisting and turning.

pecially related that the "dust mask" did not fit tightly and thought that she "still breathed a lot of black dust" (graphite); lack of ventilation, heat caused discomfort and made gloves and dust masks hot to wear, fatiguing, painful body positions, back strain from lifting boxes, "sore arms" from packing and lifting boxes, "tired shoulders and back" from sitting, "tired fingers" from packaging. Most jobs were rotated hourly. The machinery was custom made for the company, and the designers seemed to have considered the probability of it being operated by women. Each worker was fitted by the plant nurse for personal protective equipment (gloves and glasses). The nurse

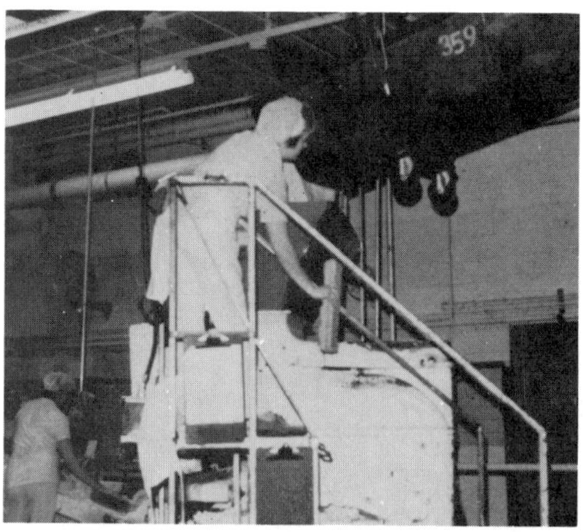

Fig 5–5.—Operating crane controls requiring awkward position on precarious platform.

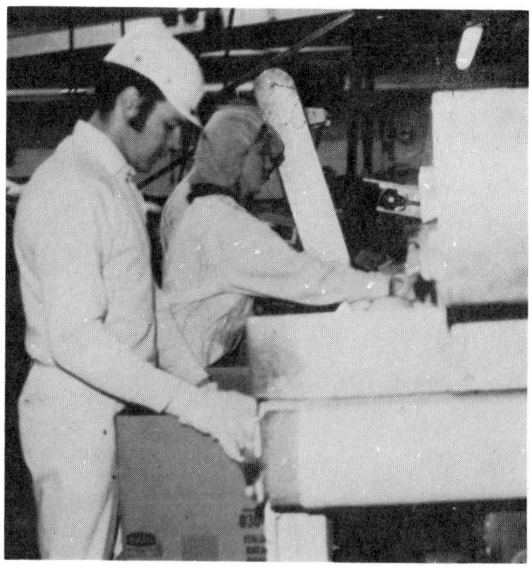

Fig 5–7.—Operating requires different work position for men and women workers—woman has to bend and reach farther.

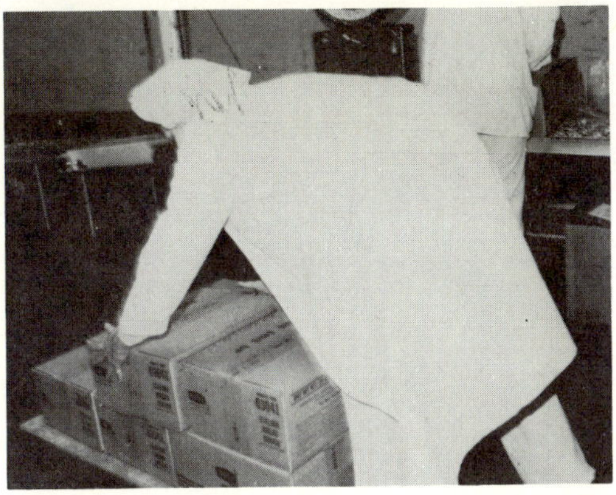

Fig 5–8.—Repeatedly bending and lifting 18-kg boxes.

monitored workers for mercury, with special surveillance of pregnant workers. She prepared lists of toxic substances and posted these in each department. These listed chemicals contained in substances found in each department and outlined their physiologic effects. (N.B., this plant had a low accident rate.)

Household appliance manufacturer (SIC 363) having foundry, metal stamping and metal fabrication operations. During 1976, women's incidence of accidents was twice as great as men's in this plant, 500 workers; 73 women, of whom 43 worked in manufacturing plant, 2 shifts with the work force generally over 25 years of age. Men and women worked in assembly areas, packaging, press operations and grinding operations, but no women were employed in the foundry or paint area. Thirteen women were interviewed, representing all operations where women were employed. Worker comments regarding human factors inadequacies: Face shield for grinders permits space where dust and wire could hit face and eyes, face shields "push against eyeglasses," earmuff pressure causes eyeglasses to "dig in behind ears," coveralls for grinding were mentioned as being inappropriate, as pieces of metal brush from hand grinder "fly through the garment"; one worker said that she "couldn't hear at the end of a day" in the grinding area although earmuffs were worn, banding tools and crimpers "too large to handle," requiring "a lot of arm strength" and "difficult for a woman to handle," a small hand grinder "causes stiff, swollen fingers" for the grinder, "never really comfortable with the press," sitting or standing all day presented discomfort, lifting up to 23 kilos presented a problem to some, ventilation was claimed to be poor around grinding area, "breathing paint dust from grinding causing burning eyes." (See Figs 5-9–5-11.)

Plastics manufacturer (SIC 307)—a complete plastic-making process from designing molds to packaging and shipping finished products; 3 shifts, 367 workers, 197 women primarily employed as operators of injection molding machines and on assembly lines. There were no women in maintenance jobs or operating machines in the blow molding

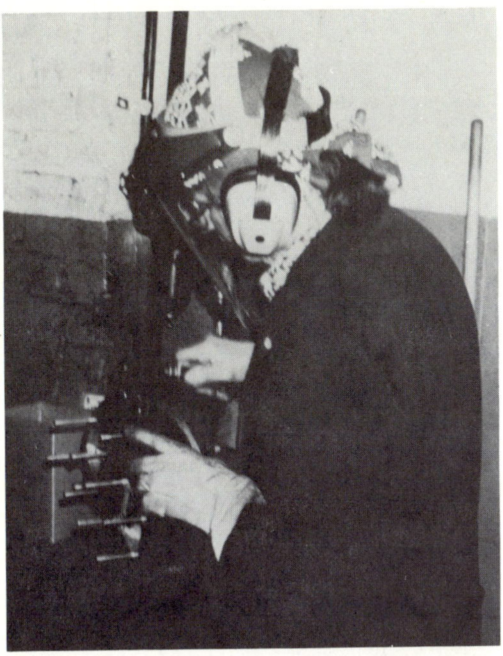

Fig 5–9.—Despite using hand grinder, wearing gloves, hearing protection, face shield and glasses, worker still is affected by noise, flying particles and vibration. Pieces of metal fly through coveralls; face shield leaves gaps where dust and wire can reach eyes; vibration causes stiff, swollen fingers.

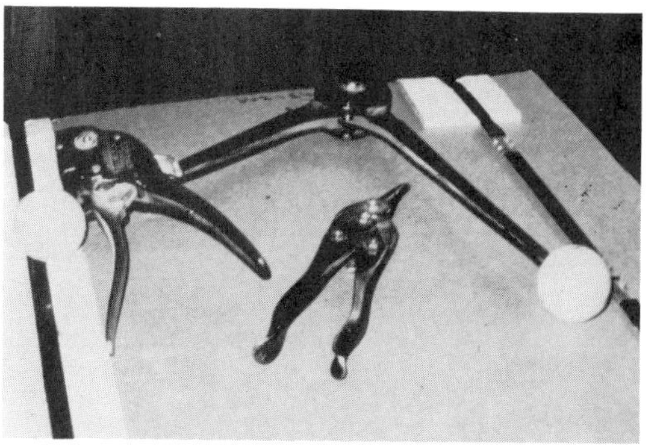

Fig 5–10.—Grips on tools are too large, require considerable arm strength.

unit, as these larger machines apparently "required more strength and reach" than injection molding machines. A few women were employed as inspectors and in the warehouse area (primarily in paperwork jobs). Eleven women were interviewed, representing various operations in the plant. Worker comments regarding human factors inadequacies: Paint and solvent fumes, standing all day, fast pace of work, crowded work area at lines, height of work area inadequate when sitting or standing, "strain from lifting," "hammering all day," "possibility of burns from flaming operation (rotating a plastic item by hand in a flame)," "continual use of nippers to trim off excess plastic causes hand fatigue," "some lines are very crowded, working side by side to one another—there's no elbow room, creating extra strain on arm and shoulders when pounding." (See Fig 5-12.)

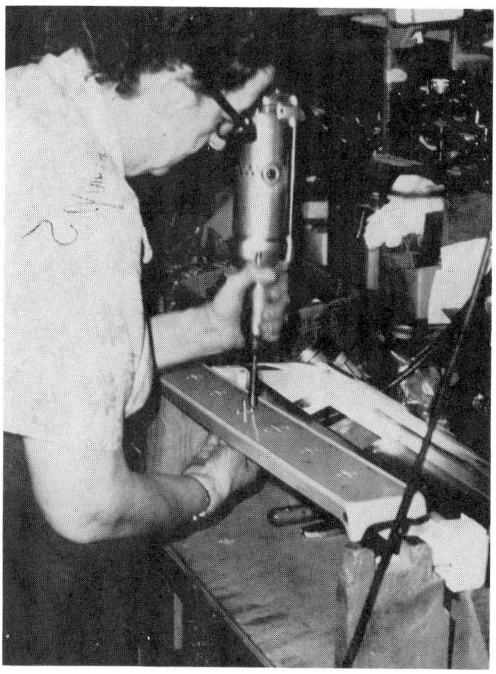

Fig 5–11.—Use of powered hand tools. Suspended tool reduces muscle fatigue but height of work surface requires constant bending.

Paper company (SIC 265)—manufactures corrugated paper boxes; 180 workers, 2 shifts, one-fifth women. Women were employed mainly in the finishing department, operating smaller machines, lifting and stacking finished boxes. Men ran fork-lift trucks and larger machines and presses, which apparently require a great deal of strength to operate. The plant manager said that women were considered equally for the same positions as men, so he believed that the difference between the jobs held by men and women "was a natural occurrence." Women had tried operating

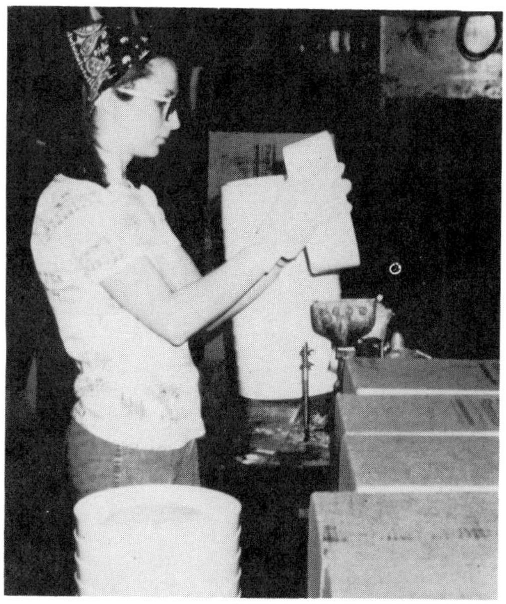

Fig 5–12.—Burns to hand can result from flame; potential carbon monoxide exposure.

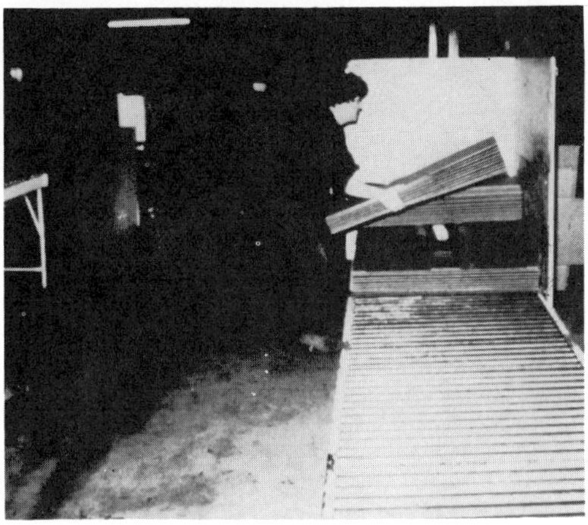

Fig 5–13.—This workplace and job design require bending and lifting, with insufficient room at work station.

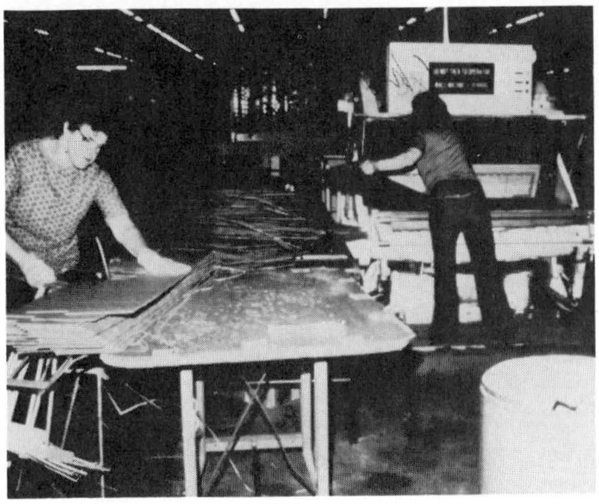

Fig 5–15.—Workplace and job design require repeated twisting and turning and, at the same time, constant attention operating machine. Worker at left uses hand tool repetitively (note left elbow bandage).

one of the heavy presses, but were forced to leave "because the work was too strenuous." Worker comments regarding human factors inadequacies: Safety shoes were required for all workers and hearing protection was required in certain areas. Several women stated that the "safety shoes had to be ordered by mail, so they couldn't be fitted before purchasing the shoes," some stating that "their shoes were very uncomfortable and too big."

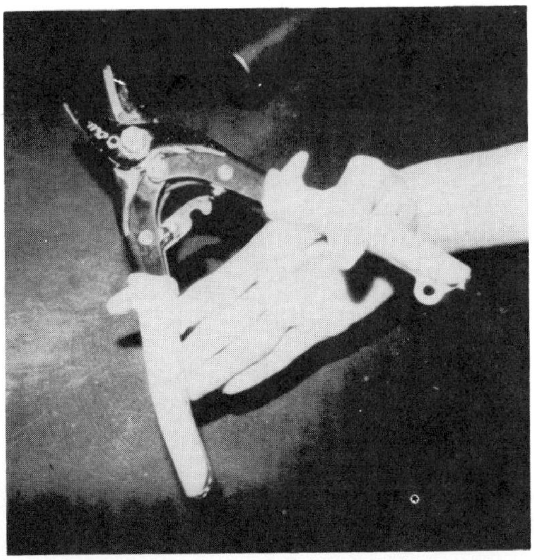

Fig 5–14.—Hand tool designed for large hands. Requires two hands to operate by average woman.

This company had initiated their own lifting standard based on the size and weight of the box being handled, and workers were told to get help whenever anything was too heavy to lift alone, but it failed to eliminate complaints of backaches from lifting boxes that were awkward to handle or from pushing boxes on conveyor lines. (See Figs 5–13–5–15.)

SUMMARY OF WISCONSIN STUDIES

The results of the data analyses indicate that the differences in male and female accidents and illness patterns appear to be related more to differential job placement and inherent job tasks rather than simply biologic differences; the most outstanding finding occurring in the plants surveyed involved inadequate availability or fit of personal protective equipment for women. (There are no OSHA standards for women's shoes.)[6, 22] Gaps may exist between safety glasses and side shields or face shields; gloves often are too large and clumsy; most work clothing is manufactured only in men's sizes. The plants studied utilized machines or tools that do not accommodate individual's needs; lack easy access to machine levers and controls; tools have large grips or require excess strength; inadequate training for new employees or new operations is prevalent. Inadequate job design producing monotony or stress, restricted social interaction and workplace design, such as inadequate height of work surface, or operations requiring repetitive standing, reaching, etc., are commonplace.

DIRECTIONS FOR FUTURE ACTIONS

In-depth studies are needed to analyze accidents or illnesses (such as "tendinitis," "ganglion," "dermatitis") and accident sources (air tools, etc.) that have a high proportion of female occurrences. Design problems related to machines, equipment, tools and training specific to nontraditional female jobs need further, intensive examination.

Engineers, planners, management, workers and unions should take into consideration the complicated interaction between people, machines, work environment and social factors in their workplaces, especially in the light of the enlarging role of women in industry.[30,31] Improvements, however minimal, undoubtedly would serve to improve the capabilities of women to work more effectively and efficiently in these predominant industry groups, thus enhancing management's goals in the long run.[12 31]

ACKNOWLEDGMENTS

We thank Professors Howard Harrison, Robert Miller and Gordon Robinson of the University of Wisconsin, Dr. Patrick Coleman and our colleagues of the State of Wisconsin's Occupational Safety and Health Research Unit and the staff of the University of Wisconsin's School for Workers for their support and assistance. We also wish to thank the Wisconsin companies, their workers and management and other individuals and groups too numerous to mention, who cooperated so willingly in providing information and direction for this study. Finally, we would like to express a special thanks to Dr. Karl Smith, Professor Emeritus, University of Wisconsin, who provided ideas and encouragement for our endeavor.

REFERENCES

1. Baetjer, A. M.: *Women in Industry—Their Health and Efficiency* (Philadelphia: W. B. Saunders Company, 1946).
2. Bartholomew, A. B.: Women in industry, Occup. Health Nurs. (N. Y.) 27:18, 1975.
3. Chaffin, D. B.: Human strength capability and low-back pain, J. Occup. Med. 16:248, 1974.
4. Chaffin, D. B., et al.: Pre-Employment Strength Testing in Selecting Workers for Materials Handling Jobs, University of Michigan (Ann Arbor, Mich.), sponsored by NIOSH, USDHEW, CDC-99-74-62, October, 1976.
5. Coleman, P.: Hazard management. Wis. DILHR, Research and Statistics Bureau, Risk Management Section, Madison, Wi., 1976.
6. Cook, W. I.: A Report of the Performance of Women's Safety-Toe Footwear. USDHEW, NIOSH, HEW Publication No. (NIOSH) 76-199, July, 1976.
7. Davis, L. E., and Taylor, J. C. (eds.): *Design of Jobs* (London: Cox and Wyman, Ltd., 1972).
8. Ducharme, R. E.: Problem tools for women, Industrial Engineer, pp. 46–50, September, 1975.
9. Ducharme, R. E.: Women workers rate "male" tools inadequate, Hum. Factors Soc. Bull., Vol. 20, No. 4, April, 1977.
10. Ginnold, R.: Females—a Job Safety Priority. School for Workers, University of Wisconsin Extension, unpublished, 1976.
11. Gottlieb, M., and Coleman, P.: Workers' awareness of industrial hazards. Wis. DILHR, Research and Statistics Bureau, Risk Management Section, Madison, Wi., 1976.
12. Greenburn, L., and Chaffin, D.: *Workers and Their Tools: A Guide to the Ergonomic Design of Hand Tools and Small Presses* (Midland, Mich.: Pendell Publishing Co., 1977).

13. Hricko, A. M.: Two fifths of the nation's workforce, J. Curr. Social Issues, pp. 18–22, Spring, 1975.
14. Hricko, A. M., and Brunt, M.: Working for your life: A woman's guide to job health hazards. Labor Occup. Health Program/Health Research Group, June, 1976.
15. Hricko, A. M., and Marrett, C. B.: Women's occupational health: The rise and fall of a research issue. Presented at the Am. Assoc. for Advance of Science Mtgs., New York, N.Y., January 28, 1975.
16. Hunt, V. R.: Occupational health problems of pregnant women. A report and recommendations for the Office of the Secretary, HEW, April, 1975.
17. Jaworski, A.: An analysis of the favorable and unfavorable features of 13 types of guards or devices used to guard or protect the "point of operation" or "danger zone" of power press dies. Wis. Ind. Comm., Industrial Safety and Buildings, September, 1964.
18. Kaplan, M., and Knutson, S.: A systems approach to the study of women in the workplace: A hazard analysis focusing on human factors. Wis. Dept. of Ind., Labor & Human Relations, Research & Statistics Bureau, Risk Management Section, Madison, Wi., 1977.
19. Knoenberg, M. H.: Working conditions for female employees, JAMA 124:677, 1944, (cited in Baetjer[1]).
20. Kuntz, W. D.: The pregnant woman in industry, Am. Ind. Hyg. Assoc. J. 37:423, 1976.
21. McConville, J., and Churchill, E., Webb Assoc., Yellow Springs, Ohio: Human Variability and Respirator Sizing. Contract No. HSM 99-73-15, NIOSH, USDHEW, March, 1976.
22. National Safety News: Toe, foot and leg protection, 115:45, 1977.
23. Prieve, C.: Lead and women, a unique problem? Symposium on Women and the Workplace, sponsored by the Society for Occup. & Environ. Health, Washington, D.C., June, 1976.
24. Reinhart, V.: Ergonomic studies improving life on the job, Job Safety and Health 3:12, 1975.
25. The Respiratory Protective Devices Manual. Am. Ind. Hyg. Assoc. & Am. Conf. of Gov. Ind. Hyg., Braun and Brumfield, Ann Arbor, Mi., 1963.
26. Snook, S. H., and Ciriello, V. M.: Maximum weights and work loads acceptable to female workers, J. Occup. Med. 16:527, 1974.
27. Stellman, J. M.: *Women's Work, Women's Health, Myths and Realities* (New York: Pantheon Books, Inc., 1978).
28. U.S.D. of Labor, Women's Bureau, Special Bulletin No. 19. Mohr, J.: The Industrial Nurse and the Woman Worker, pp. 24–25, 1944.
29. Van Cott, H. P., and Kinkade, R. G., (eds.): Human engineering guide to equipment design. Sponsored by Joint Army-Navy-Air Force Steering Committee, Washington, D.C., Bumed., USN, 1972.
30. Wall Street Journal: Women at work: As their ranks swell, women holding jobs reshape U.S. society, Vol. LVIII, No. 221, August 28, 1978.
31. Watkeys, J. D.: Women in the work environment, J. Occup. Med. 17:308, 1975.

PART THREE

The Physical Working Environment

6 / Practical Ergonomics

O. BRUCE DICKERSON, M.D., M.P.H.

ERGONOMICS crosses boundaries between many scientific and professional disciplines and utilizes data, findings and principles from all of them. Zenz[17] depicts scientific disciplines involved in ergonomics under the three general headings: (1) Engineering and Physical Sciences, (2) Biologic Sciences and (3) Behavioral Sciences. Van Wely[16] best brings the field into focus by stating that the goal of ergonomics is to develop "a kind of eternal triangle among efficiency, comfort, and health."

Often the terms ergonomics and human factors engineering are used interchangeably; however, some authors believe that ergonomics is more physiology oriented and human factors engineering more engineering and physical sciences oriented. A few authors point to geographic differences, stating that the American professional societies in this field are more interested in the engineering approach and the European societies in the physiology approach. Chapanis[1] writes that "a greater faction of our ergonomic effort in America has been concerned with military systems, large computer systems, and automated systems in general. On the other hand, I think I see in Europe somewhat more emphasis on mining, forestry, agriculture, railroading, and industry in which human operators are still important sources of mechanical power."

Practical ergonomics implies that we link various disciplines and resources together in such a way as to be able to favorably influence task-individual interfaces in our everyday practices and actions. For instance, Figure 6–1 presents some important ergonomic components of an agriculture worker's activities in using the "short-handle hoe." In a study performed for the state of California it was concluded that use of the short-handle hoe could result in permanent low back disability. Subsequently, the California Supreme Court reached a decision eliminating its use by agriculture workers. Although evidence had existed for some time pointing to permanent low back impairment with this type of work, union and management attitudes were the ergonomic factors that precipitated the change in work design.

The worker in Figure 6–2 is an individual performing microscope work in the modern semiconductor industry. She is viewing through a high-power (X650) lens the pattern shown at the bottom right part of the picture. Factors influencing the successful task-individual interface of a microscope worker are depicted. First, job analyses of various types of microscopes are performed. Applicants for microscope work then are vision tested, with vision profile results evaluated against visual criteria consistent with job analyses. In a study reported by me,[2] only 73% of employees were capable of full-time work with low- and high-power microscopes. Another 13% were capable of microscope work on a part-time basis of not more than 4 hours a day, preferably with low-power microscopes, and the remaining 14% were not recommended for microscope work. Of equal importance to job analyses and vision testing for proper placement of workers are proper microscope maintenance

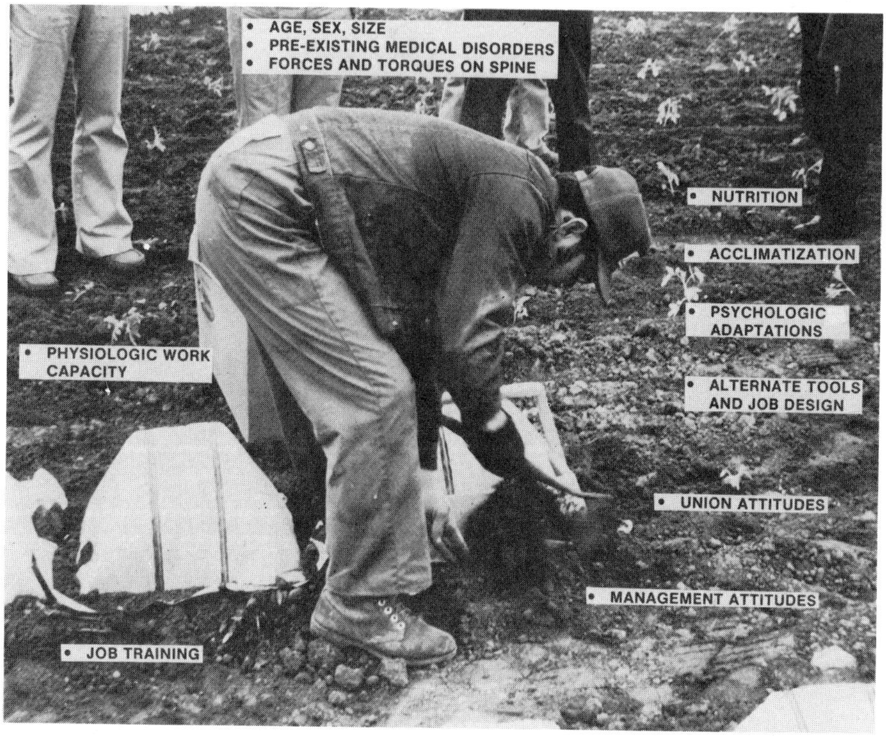
• AGE, SEX, SIZE
• PRE-EXISTING MEDICAL DISORDERS
• FORCES AND TORQUES ON SPINE
• NUTRITION
• ACCLIMATIZATION
• PSYCHOLOGIC ADAPTATIONS
• PHYSIOLOGIC WORK CAPACITY
• ALTERNATE TOOLS AND JOB DESIGN
• UNION ATTITUDES
• MANAGEMENT ATTITUDES
• JOB TRAINING

Fig 6–1.—Human factors in farm worker using the short handle hoe.

and job training. Microscopes often need recalibration and cleaning, especially if the job requires working with high-power magnification. Several factors are important in training individuals to use microscopes correctly. Methods of focusing microscopes are taught to individuals in the semiconductor industry with the realization that they may bring a field into focus hundreds of times a day. Training an individual to periodically relax his/her eye muscles by looking up from the microscope into the distance is an extremely important part of the orientation. Continual near-point accommodation can cause spasms of the ciliary muscles and temporarily change the vision of the microscope worker. During accommodation, the ciliary muscle contracts and, by contracting, relaxes the suspensory ligament. This permits the inherent elasticity of the lens to make the lens assume a more spherical shape, thereby increasing its refractive power and allowing it to focus on near objects. When viewing distant objects, the ciliary muscle relaxes and the lens flattens. MacLeod and Bannon[9] have contributed valuable suggestions to combat eyestrain while using the microscope.

Söderberg et al.[14] studied 75 microscope operators in two different electronic factories in the Stockholm area with special reference to eye function and visual strain. Three investigations (independent of one another) were performed: (1) standardized interviews focused on symptoms of visual strain, (2) examinations of the refractive state as well as possible diseases of the eye and (3) examinations of the binocular vision. They showed that 80% of the operators who worked exclusively with microscopy reported various symptoms of visual strain, and statistical analysis showed a significant connection with visual strain and astigmatic refractive errors, quality of the binocular vi-

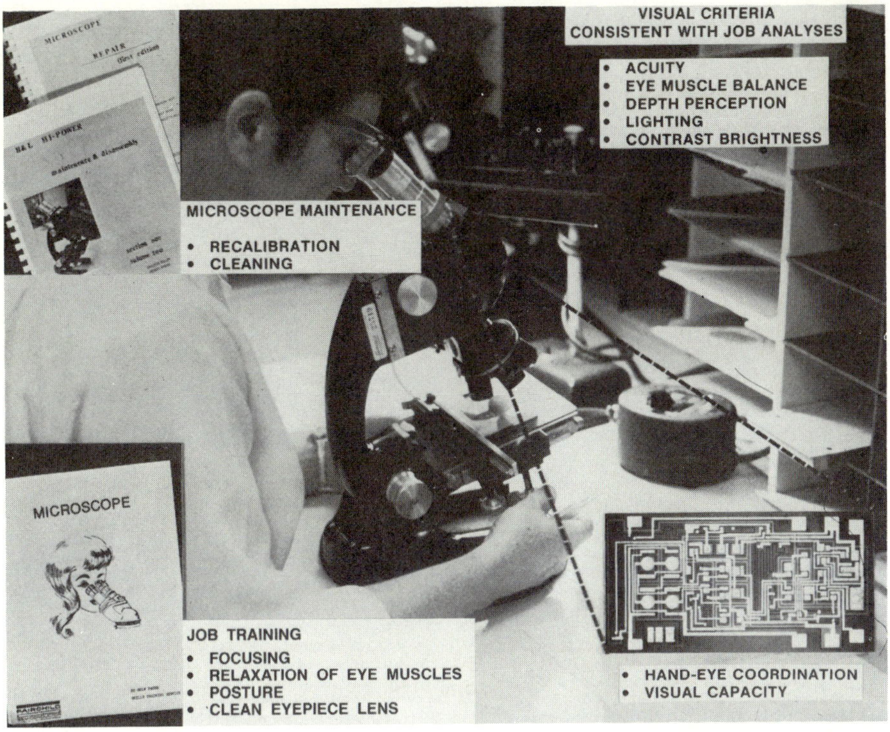

Fig 6–2.—Ergonomics involved in microscope work in the semiconductor industry. For details, see text.

sion and the duration of work (microscopy) during a shift.

In addition to the visual requirements described, worker position demands attention to lessen discomfort and fatigue during prolonged microscope work, especially that encountered in many clinical, research and hospital laboratories for cell and chromosome counting (Figs 6–3 and 6–4). Orthopedist Gunnar Andersson of Göteborg and co-worker Sven Lundberg, Chief of the Cytology Laboratory at the Jönköping Hospital, developed an innovative arrangement as seen in Figure 6–5. The seat was obtained from the Volvo automobile factory and adapted to the table and base for the technician and microscope and first used in the general hospital in Malmö.[13] (These photographs were provided by Mr. Per Thermaenius, Editor of *Arbetarskydd,* the monthly journal of Sweden's ARBETARSKYDDSSTYRELESEN, equivalent to the U. S. OSHA. The "sitting machine" is manufactured by Elecktromekano i Bredaryd AB, S-330, 10, Bredaryd, Sweden.)

The use of hand tools is an area that is receiving considerable attention recently. Tichauer and Gage[15] have developed an excellent article on ergonomic principles basic to hand tool design. These authors state that the primary ergonomic consideration in designing hand tools is optimization of forces, that a tool should be designed to extend and reinforce range, strength and effectiveness of a limb, or limbs, performing a given task. They believe that in the past to accomplish this function designers frequently followed only the rule to maximize the ratio of tool force output to hand force input. This obviously leaves much to be desired, as it does not take into consideration effective sensory feedback during the task or precise

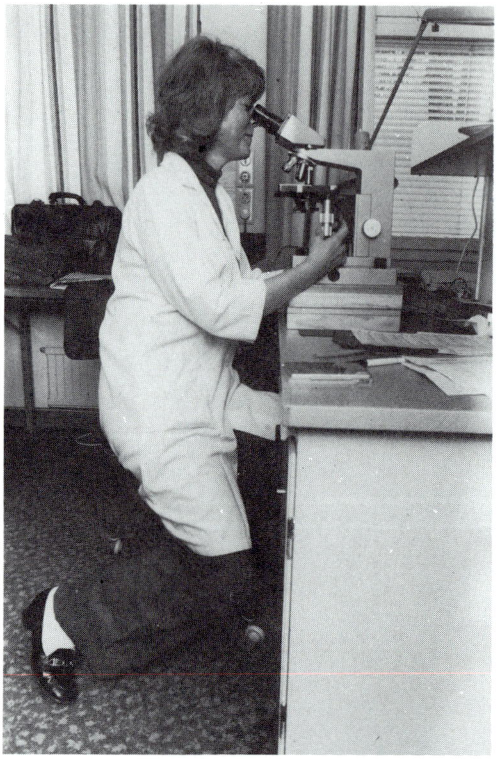

Fig 6–3.—Hospital laboratory worker with a poor sitting position. (Figs 6–3—6–5 courtesy of Mr. Per Thermaenius, Editor of *Arbetarskydd,* Stockholm.)

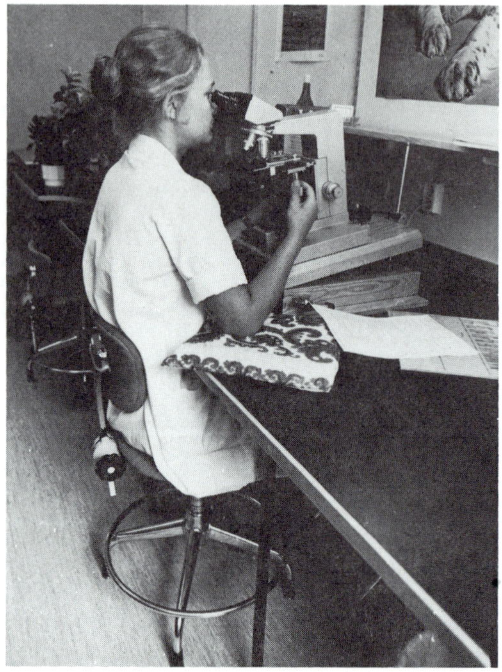

Fig 6–4.—Better than Figure 6–3, but still not good—a hospital cytology laboratory.

concentration of applied forces toward the desired location of the workpiece. For instance, the authors point out that without sensory feedback in a thread-tapping job, if the ratio is too large the applied force may be excessive and result in stripped threads.

Distribution of contact pressures on surfaces of the hands and anthropometric characteristics are of extreme importance in designing hand tools. Garrett[6] has written of anthropometric and biomechanical variations in hands, and his data point to the need to design hand tools that are not restricted to the fit of the average hand but rather designed so as to fit the dimensions of the wide range of hands found throughout the working population. In many cases, hand tools to be used by women should have dimensions different from those to be used by men.

In practice in the electronics industry, I have encountered cases of tenosynovitis with prolonged use of a simple tool such as tweezers. Figure 6–6 shows the old type of tweezers used by a technician to handle hundreds of silicon wafers per day. Many employees using this type of tweezers complained of finger and forearm pains and a significant number experienced tenosynovitis. Numerous redesigns were attempted until the tweezers shown in Figure 6–7 were developed. Much less pressure was required to lift silicon wafers with the new tweezers, and symptoms disappeared with introduction of the newly designed tool into the work force.

The electronic data processing industry is growing rapidly in the United States and ergonomic problems are emerging almost in pace with the industry growth. Figure 6–8

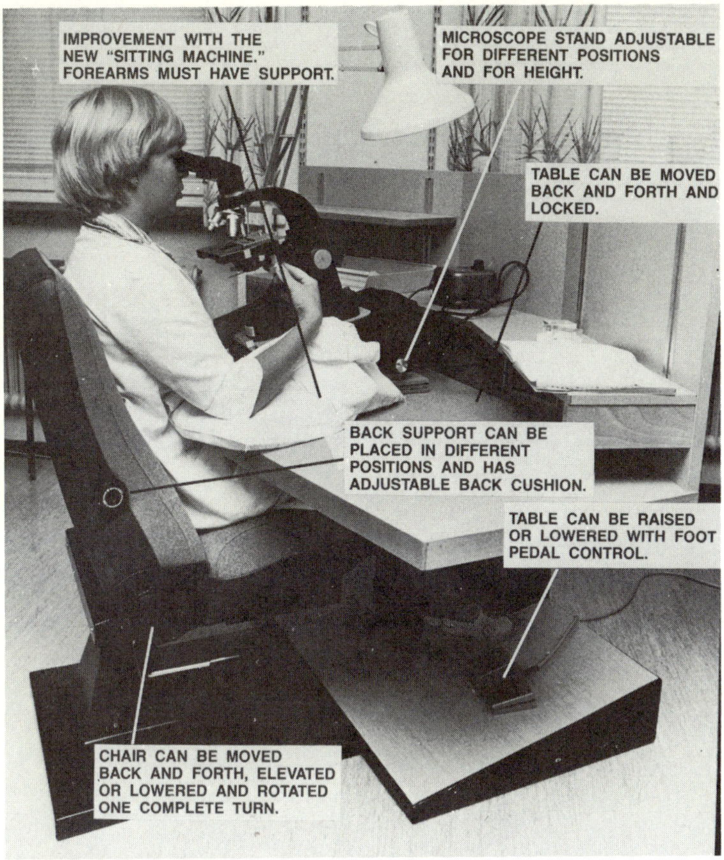

Fig 6–5.—The new seating equipment for microscope work in hospital laboratories. (Manufactured by Elecktromekano i Bredaryd AB, S-330, 10, Bredaryd, Sweden.)

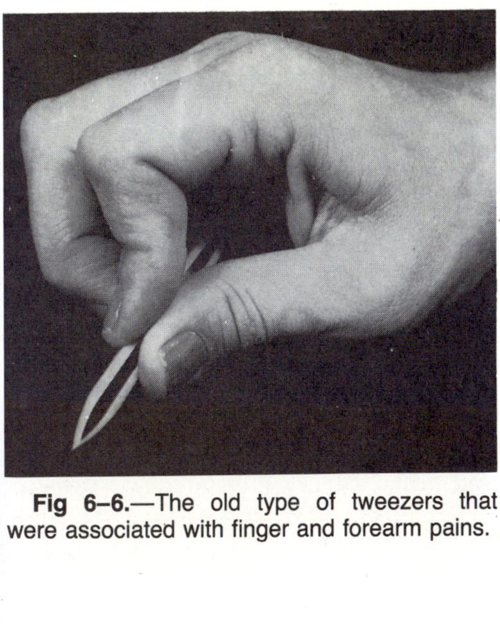

Fig 6–6.—The old type of tweezers that were associated with finger and forearm pains.

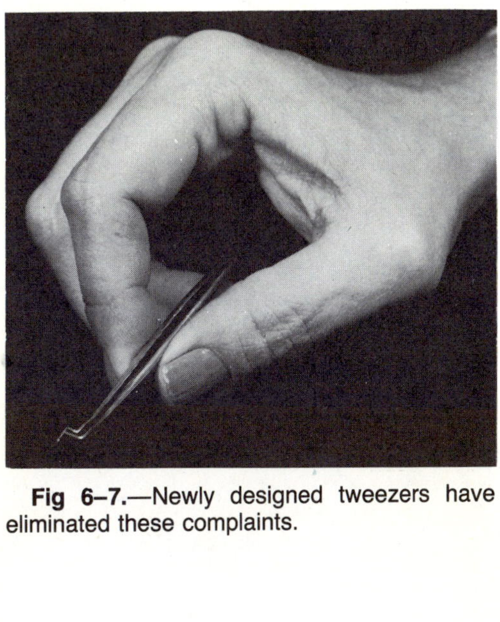

Fig 6–7.—Newly designed tweezers have eliminated these complaints.

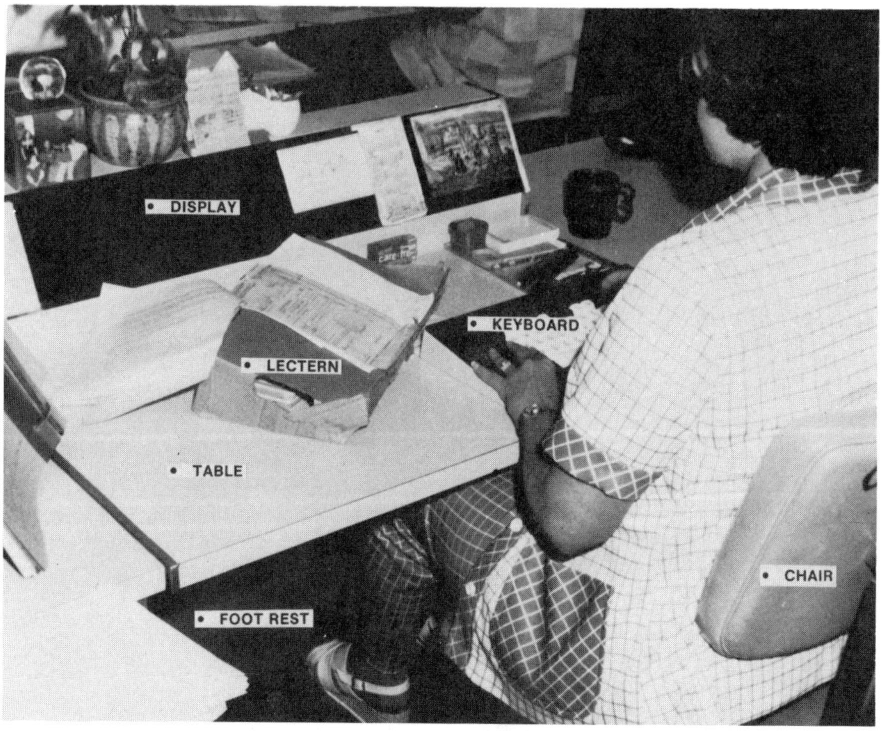

Fig 6–8.—Human factors—keypunch operator. For details, see text.

shows the workplace layout of a typical keypunch equipment operator in a data entry department. I have seen significant numbers of cases of upper-extremity tenosynovitis from this operation. Literature review confirms this experience, as numerous articles[3-5, 8] have been written detailing conditions that can result from keypunch operations. Ferguson[4] describes "telegraphists' cramps and myalgia"; Duncan and Ferguson[3] and Kroemer[8] further expand on this subject with experimentally obtained results from individuals working with keyboards. Kroemer[8] states that the keyboard in use today causes unnecessary tension on the hands, wrists and forearms. He notes that the hand performing the stroking movements is close to the anatomic limit and kept there while repetitively moving the fingers for long periods. Trying to relieve some of the tensions, keypunch operators tend to lift the elbow laterally and forward. Then part or the whole of the arm can become involved, especially if the person is susceptible to strains and holds his/her arm in an unusual position for extended periods. To relieve these stresses, Kroemer suggests lateral tilting of keyboards. In his findings,[8] work with the laterally tilted keyboard showed no stroke frequency advantage over the standard keyboard, but "aches and pains" given as reasons for quitting were much less frequent, and only half as many errors were committed. Duncan and Ferguson[3] obtained medical results from faulty body positions versus keyboard operations and concluded that body positions of extended periods of shoulder abduction (elbow away from body), ulnar deviation of the wrist (palm down, hand turned outward) and wrist extension (palm down, back of hand turned upward) were important predictors of keyboard operators' medical symptoms.

Suggested keyboard designs that could change these positions and reduce medical symptoms are as follows: (1) To correct the shoulder abduction, the keyboard should be positioned near the front edge of the table and be movable so that it can be turned in a horizontal plane. (2) To correct the ulnar deviation, again, having the keyboard in a movable horizontal plane is of prime importance. (3) To correct the pronation and extension of the wrists, the keyboard should have a lateral tilt. If both hands are used regularly by the keypunch operator, the keyboard should be divided in the middle so that each half is tilted toward the hand in use.

Another important factor in properly designing a workplace for keypunch operators is to have a lectern that can hold the document from which the operator reads. Continually looking up and down from documents on a flat surface to a vertical display screen can aggravate existing cervical disorders. A movable and adjustable lectern would correct this problem. In Figure 6–8, the operator has constructed her own lectern of cardboard.

Visual problems are the largest source of operator discomfort in keypunch operations. Visual fatigue from reading print on documents is the most common complaint. Often, source documents are handwritten and hard to read, and not infrequently, the paper and ink are of poor quality. Other operator complaints relate to reflection from displays and glare from the table and keyboard surfaces.

Since the vision demands of a keyboard operator are considerable, even the most minor defects in the operator's visual functions might be important. Professor Olov Östberg,[11] a leading expert in workplace design considerations, has written me regarding visual problems with individuals using CRT (cathode ray tube) display terminals. He believes that display terminal manufacturers have designed their products poorly in this regard. For instance, the visual distance of display screens is 60 cm (see Fig 6–8) whereas 33 cm is the normal reading distance used in judging the need for spectacles. Professor Östberg further notes that wearing bifocals that are designed according to visual ophthalmologic practice (e.g., 33 and 200 cm) can result in considerable problems unless the ophthalmologist is made aware of the particular work an individual is performing. A gratifying trend, however, is that a few data entry equipment manufacturers now are developing displays that are adjustable in distance from the eyes.

Of particular importance as we enter this new era of electronic marvels is how the visually handicapped and older workers can perform with their eyes. If the average young adult is defined as having normal vision, all differences from this condition would be called abnormal. As in other areas in ergonomics, we must be careful not to design electronic equipment that favors one part of our population over another in the job market. From the point of view of the young adult having "normal vision," increasing age is accompanied by abnormalities in the physiology of the eye and visual system that reduce visual ability. Age markedly affects the accommodative ability of the eyes. The lens loses elasticity. The pupil also changes in size (becomes smaller) with age. This decreases the amount of light reaching the retina, which is one of the causes of loss of visual sensitivity with age, particularly at low luminance levels. Another important loss is the reduction in visual acuity, even with the best possible refractive correction. There is also an increase in sensitivity to disabling glare as a function of age. Last, there is a loss of contrast sensitivity. Job designs in this electronics revolution must allow for these changes, and individuals encouraged to have their vision checked at regular intervals.

The Swedish government issued directives for work regularly involving reading display screens that became effective January 1, 1979.[12] These are as follows:

1. General lighting must be suitably adapted. Special importance must be attached to lighting conditions at workplaces where reading of display screens occurs regularly. Generally, the lighting required is weaker than that often used in ordinary office work. In workplaces where work is continually conducted at display screens, a lighting power of between 200 and 300 lux* may be suitable.

NOTE: Lower lighting power levels may be appropriate in certain working environments of a special nature (e.g., monitoring and traffic control).

2. When general lighting is subdued as per point 1, additional lighting must be provided for other working areas near the display screen. Additional lighting must be adjustable and fitted with antidazzle arrangements.
3. Excessive differences of luminance in the field of vision produce what is termed contrast dazzle. The workplace, therefore, should be organized in such a way that the background to the display screen is of a suitable luminance and the employee's field of vision does not include a window or any other powerful light source. Bright reflections in the display screen are to be avoided.
4. The visual distance to the display screen and the angle of inclination of the display screen should be individually adjustable with due regard for other ergonomic requirements. In the case of employees who wear glasses, it is important that the optical correction is well adapted to the visual distance and vice versa.

NOTE: Ordinary glasses for private use often are unadapted to the visual distances occurring in display screen work. Traditional bifocal spectacles are unsuitable in many cases, because they often entail a strenuous work posture when used for display screen reading.

5. If an employee has a refractive error and incurs visual discomfort in connection with display screen work when using glasses intended for normal purposes, the display screen must be moved to a position where the discomfort is eliminated. If this is not possible, the employer is to provide the employee with special glasses that have been tested for display screen work.
6. If eye fatigue or visual discomfort tends to develop, the work must be organized in such a way that the employee can intermittently be given periods of rest from work involving more conventional visual requirements.

Other items of interest in keypunch operations are chairs and footrests. Regarding chairs, a slight give in a back rest is important. However, a play of more than 1 inch is undesirable.[8] Recent literature stresses the importance of designing a work chair with a forward-tilting seat.[10] A seat tilt of 15° forward instead of the usual present practice of 5° backward pushes the individual forward to a more comfortable and relaxed position for bent-forward work such as keypunching. Also, normal curves in the spine are maintained with the forward-tilting seat and, therefore, less strain of back musculature occurs. With the tilted seat, sufficient seat cover friction is needed to keep from sliding forward. Easily adjustable footrests are important, and the surface of the footrest may be inclined up to 30 degrees.[7]

Last, regarding data entry equipment, Professor Östberg et al. have furnished me examples of "purpose-designed terminal desks" now on the market in Sweden (Fig 6–9).

Another interesting visual ergonomics problem that I was asked to investigate related to complaints from workers required to read computer printouts that recently had been changed (see Fig 6–10 for new printout at the left side of the picture versus the old printout at the right side). The number of lines had been changed from 60 lines per page to 80 lines per page, leaving almost no spacing between lines. The cost savings would have been considerable if the new

*A measure of light intensity; for light falling on a surface, the unit of measurement is the lux. 1 lux (lx) = 1 lumen (lm) per square meter. (The industrial hygienist can make these measurements.)

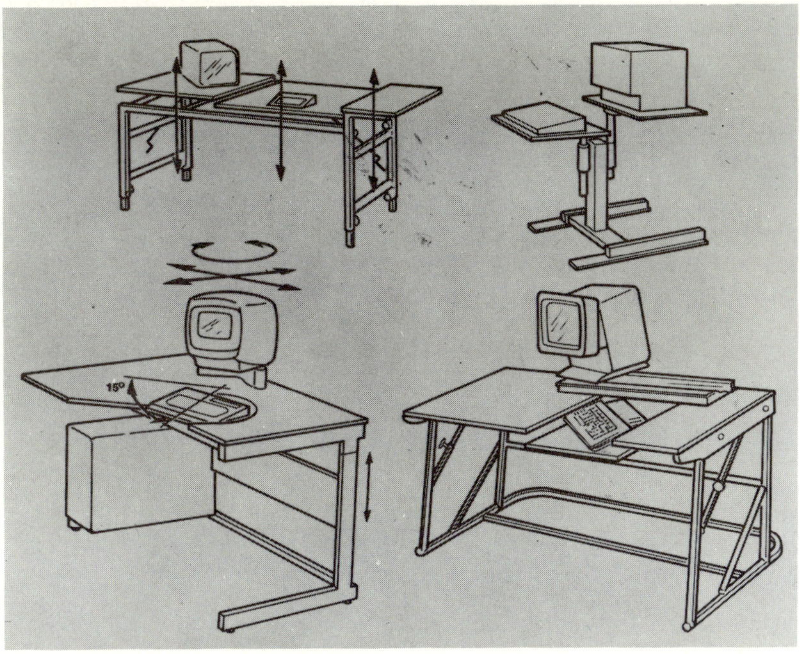

Fig 6–9.—Human factors in designing data entry equipment. (Modified from Östberg.[11])

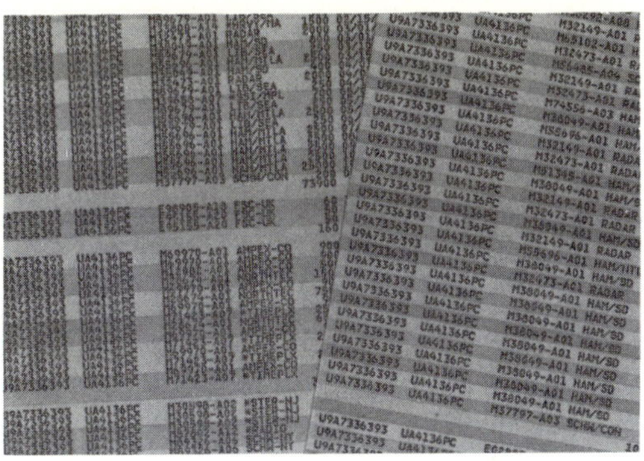

Fig 6–10.—New computer printout at left side of picture caused eye fatigue and headaches.

format could be used. A survey of workers using the new printout revealed numerous instances of eye fatigue and headaches, worse in individuals required to use the printout as a "working document" and less among individuals required to use it as a "reference document." As soon as the new printout was discontinued, eye fatigue and headache complaints disappeared.

ACKNOWLEDGMENTS

Appreciation is given to Glen Reid, Bill Steffan, Art Carter and Robert E. Swencicki, M.D. for their helpful suggestions.

REFERENCES

1. Chapanis, A.: Relevance of physiological and psychological criteria to man-machine systems: The present state of the art, Ergonomics 13:337, 1970.
2. Dickerson, O. B.: Visual criteria aid in job placement, Int. J. Occup. Health Safety 45:39, 1976.
3. Duncan, J., and Ferguson, D.: Keyboard operating posture and symptoms in operating, Ergonomics 17:651, 1974.
4. Ferguson, D.: An Australian study of telegraphist's cramp, Br. J. Ind. Med. 28:280, 1971.
5. Ferguson, D., and Duncan, J.: Keyboard design and operating posture, Ergonomics 17:731, 1974.
6. Garrett, J. W.: The adult human hand: Some anthropometric and biomechanical considerations, Hum. Factors 13:117, 1971.
7. Kroemer, K. H.: Seating in plant and office,

Am. Ind. Hyg. Assoc. J. 32:633, 1971.
8. Kroemer, K. H.: Human engineering the keyboard, Hum. Factors 14:51, 1972.
9. MacLeod, D., and Bannon, R. E.: Microscopes and eye fatigue, Ind. Med. 42:7, 1973.
10. Mandal, A. C.: Work-chair with tilting seat, Ergonomics 19:157, 1976.
11. Personal correspondence from Professor Olov Östberg, Institute Work Sciences, University of Luleå, Sweden, February, 1977.
12. Reading of display screens, Directions No. 136, ARBETARSKYDDSSTYRELSEN, Fack, S-100 26, Stockholm, August 2, 1978.
13. Sittmaskin i labortoriet, Arbetarskydd No. 7, p. 8, September, 1976.
14. Söderberg, I., Calissendorff, B., Elofson, S., Knave, B., and Nyman, K. G.: Mikroskoparbete I. Utredning av ögonbesvär hos mikroskop-operatörer på en elektronisk industri, Arb. och Hälsa 16, Stockholm, 1978.
15. Tichauer, E. R., and Gage, H.: Ergonomic principles basic to hand tool design, Am. Ind. Hyg. Assoc. J. 38:622, 1977.
16. van Wely, P. A.: Ergonomics in a major European industry, Am. Ind. Hyg. Assoc. J. 32:131, 1971.
17. Zenz, C.: Ergonomics: Work Effort, Determination of Energy Expenditure and Fatigue, in Zenz, C. (ed.), *Occupational Medicine: Principles and Practical Applications* (Chicago: Year Book Medical Publishers, 1975), p. 424.

7 / Health and Safety Hazards of Truck Drivers

JOSEPH LaDOU, M.D.

THERE ARE APPROXIMATELY 2.1 million truck drivers in the United States, including both line-haul (or intercity) and local pickup and delivery drivers.[68] These drivers accounted for 244.5 billion miles of driving in 1972, the latest year for which data are available.[74] In 1975, motor carriers are estimated to have accounted for 761 billion ton-miles and registered 24.6 million trucks.[3]

Motor carriers fall in two broad categories: private and for hire. Private carriers are shippers that use their own or leased vehicles to transport their own products. For-hire carriers provide transportation of freight for others and may operate interstate, intrastate or locally. Intrastate and local operators usually are regulated by state or local agencies. Interstate operations are regulated at the federal level by the Interstate Commerce Commission (ICC).

For-hire carriers fall in three distinct types—common carriers, contract carriers and exempt carriers. Common carriers are certified by the ICC to serve the general public; contract carriers serve specific shippers on a regular basis; and exempt carriers include carriers of livestock and agricultural commodities, newspapers, and the like, and vehicles used incidental to air transport and certain other limited uses. Interstate common and contract carriers are regulated by the ICC and consequently often are referred to as regulated carriers. They are also responsible for observing Department of Transportation (DOT) regulations. The ICC approves rates, routes, types of service and types of commodities transported. DOT establishes safety and equipment standards and regulations concerning hours of service of drivers. Interstate exempt carriers and private carriers are not subject to economic regulation by the ICC but are subject to DOT regulations.

In trucking, two types of vehicles are used primarily—straight trucks and tractor-trailer trucks.

Straight trucks typically are vehicles with 3 axles and 10 wheels. They are equipped with van, flatbed, tank, dump or similar bodies. These vehicles are used mainly for local pickup and delivery. Their drivers constitute about 70% of the nation's truckers. They frequently work a 10-hour day, with sporadic rest periods and mealtimes. Drivers who haul commodities and construction materials also follow a rigorous schedule and are required to load and unload their cargoes as well.

Tractor-trailer combinations consist of a front unit, or tractor, and one, two or occasionally three rear units, or semitrailers. Vehicles with two semitrailers are known as "double rigs" and may exceed 70 feet in length and 40 tons in gross weight. These rigs are used for line-haul transport of goods. Their drivers are subject to any of the following work schedules, depending on the type of rig that they drive.

TURNAROUND OR SHORT RELAY.—With this type of haul, a driver leaves his home terminal at a specified time and drives for

4–5 hours. At a predetermined point, he meets another driver, they exchange vehicles and he returns to his home base driving the second vehicle.

LONG RELAY.—Long-relay hauls are similar to short relays except that the trucker drives for up to 10 hours before reaching the exchange point and by law is required to take an 8-hour rest period before driving the exchange vehicle back to his home terminal. Truckers who have driven several long-relay hauls consecutively usually are given time off to compensate for the long work time.

STRAIGHT-THROUGH HAULS ("ROLL AND REST").—In this type of run, a driver may travel across several states or span the entire continent. He alternately drives for 10 hours and rests in a motel for 8 hours. At his destination, he is given a new load to be hauled to a point that may or may not be his home terminal. With succeeding cargo changes, several weeks may elapse before his cargo destination permits him to return to his home base.

SLEEPER HAULS.—Sleeper hauls are a variation of straight-through hauls except that there are two drivers who alternate driving and sleeping in a sleeper berth built into the rear of the truck cab. Typically, each driver drives for 4 hours and rests for 4 hours, but they may change at longer intervals. Sleeper drivers stop regularly for rest breaks and to eat or shower. At their destination, they may be required to uncouple the trailer, hitch up to a loaded trailer that is waiting and depart immediately for another destination. Drivers on this type of haul may be on the road for several weeks before returning to their home terminals. Owner-operators frequently follow this type of schedule.

The physical demands of trucking, together with a stressful work environment, may impose particular mental and physical stresses as well as psychosocial problems. Moreover, drivers have a higher rate of job-related injuries and illnesses than do workers in other fields. For example, in Maryland in 1974, 16% of the state's death claim awards were for truckers; in California in 1973, truckers accounted for 3% of disabling work injuries and 7% of work fatalities even though they represented only slightly more than 1% of the employees covered by workers' compensation.[4]

The job factors in this occupation that create mental stress include schedule shifting, irregular work/rest cycles, irregular mealtimes and poor nutrition, unsatisfactory sleeping accommodations, delays in departure and en route traffic problems, prolonged periods of driving, anxiety over meeting delivery schedules and economic pressures.

Physically stressful factors are related to handling the big rigs. They require constant visual and auditory monitoring and extreme mental alertness during driving. Stresses are compounded when driving at dusk or night, in adverse weather, in heavy traffic or on poorly surfaced or mountainous roads. The driving position creates another problem, because this position, when maintained for many hours, results in blood pooling in the lower extremities, postural fatigue and stiffening of the joints and muscles. Research studies using chair rest to evaluate the physiologic effects of immobilization have shown that physical fitness deteriorates with prolonged seated immobility.[42]

To the above factors must be added the stresses of vibration, noise, heat and the monotony of driving.

Many truckers must also perform a number of physically stressful tasks that are not related to driving, including putting on chains during heavy snow, changing tires, loading and unloading heavy cargo, coupling and uncoupling trailers and cargo inspection and adjustment.

Finally, the schedules observed by most truckers are not conducive to a positive family or social life. Drivers may be on the road for weeks before seeing their wives and children or sweethearts again. Wife-husband driving teams avoid the problem of separation, but other problems may occur because both are subjected to stresses. The importance of psychosocial factors cannot be ignored. In some cases, they may have tragic effects because trucking accidents have been found to occur after drivers have experienced domestic conflicts, separation, divorce or the serious illness or death of close friends or relatives.[24]

These tight schedules and the economic pressures associated with them are also responsible for the problem of drug and alcohol abuse among drivers,[81] because some drivers attempt to drive for as long and as far as possible with insufficient sleep. The prevalent use of caffeine and nicotine among drivers also results from stressful schedules and lack of sleep.

The following discussion examines the various factors that dominate the trucker's work environment.

ACCIDENTS AND INJURIES

There are few accurate statistics on accident and injury rates among truckers, largely because of differences in reporting methods of various agencies. The U.S. Bureau of Labor Statistics provides injury and illness data for employees in trucking and warehousing but makes no breakdown between the two occupations, nor do these statistics identify fatality cases. The U.S. National Center for Health Statistics provides information on deaths from motor vehicle accidents but does not indicate whether the figures pertain to trucks, buses or automobiles. Reports from other agencies, both federal and state, are no more definitive. Consequently, figures on deaths and injuries among truckers, both on the highway and during loading, are at best imprecise.

Taking these reporting limitations into account, the following figures are given for the 1973–1975 period. The U.S. National Center for Health Statistics reported deaths for all motor vehicle accidents at 54,600 in 1970, 46,400 in 1974 and 45,900 in 1975. The decline noted between 1970 and 1975 probably is due largely to the reduction in the highway speed to 55 miles per hour. The agency also provides the following data on deaths and death rates involving motor vehicles (again not identified as to trucks, buses or passenger cars):

Deaths 1965	1970	1973	1974	1975	
48,050	53,493	54,347	45,314	44,820	Traffic
1,113	1,140	1,164	1,088	1,033	Nontraffic
Rate per 100,000 Resident Population					
24.8	26.3	25.9	21.4	21.0	Traffic
0.6	0.6	0.5	0.5	0.5	Nontraffic

The U.S. Bureau of Labor Statistics has published the following information on trucking and warehousing:

Occupational Injury and Illness Rates (per 100 full-time employees)

Total Cases			*Lost Workday Cases*			*Nonfatal Cases—No Lost Workdays*		
1973	1974	1975	1973	1974	1975	1973	1974	1975
17.2	18.0	14.8	7.9	8.4	7.5	9.2	9.5	7.3

Lost Workdays		
1973	1974	1975
139.8	152.2	144.7

The data, as indicated, are not broken down by trucking operations or warehousing or according to death, injuries and illnesses.

A highly controversial *New York Times* article published in late 1977 stated that the percentage of fatal highway accidents involving trucks rose from 7.8% of all accidents in 1975 to 8.9% in 1976.[66] The author also claimed that although all fatal accidents had increased by only 1–2% over the 1975–1976 period, those involving heavy trucks had risen by 16.8%. (The source of these figures was identified only as federal government.)

The foregoing figures on mortality on the job in the trucking industry indicate that currently available data are neither definitive nor dependable. If useful data are to be obtained, standards will have to be established for reporting by all government agencies and industry organizations.

The National Safety Council reports that passenger cars have an accident frequency rate significantly higher than that of trucks[51] (Table 7–1). However, fatalities and injuries of greater severity are more likely to occur in accidents where trucks are involved. The Keystone-AAA Auto Club has cited statistics comparing the number of fatalities when each of three different kinds of trucks collides with a passenger vehicle.[17] When a pickup truck collides with a passenger car, there are 3 fatalities per 1000 persons involved; when a trailer truck collides with a passenger car, 71 persons are killed per 1000 involved; when a tandem trailer combination collides with a passenger car, 133 persons are killed for every 1000 persons involved. Thus, the fatality rate with the tandem trailer would be double that of a single trailer and 50 times that of a pickup truck.

TABLE 7–1.—VEHICLE FATALITIES AND INJURIES—1973 VS 1975

Number of Fatalities

All vehicles
- 1973—55,113
- 1975—45,500
  - Reduction: 14.4%

BMCS trucks
- 1973—3,058
- 1975—2,232
  - Reduction: 27%

Number of Injuries

All vehicles
- 1973–2,835,664
- 1975–2,808,323
  - Reduction: 1%

BMCS trucks
- 1973—35,245
- 1975—26,374
  - Reduction: 25.2%

The State of California Division of Labor Statistics and Research has presented a comprehensive report of the experience in California.[82] The survey underlying the report indicated that lost-time, work-connected injuries in trucking increased by 30% between 1964 and 1973 whereas employment increased by only 24% over the same period. Fatalities were also high, with more than 280 trucking employees losing their lives over the past 7 years (Table 7–2).

Between 1969 and 1973, 230 fatalities were reported by the trucking industry under the California Workers' Compensation Act. Line-haul and short-haul drivers accounted for 200 of these fatalities, or 87%. More than 4 of 5 occurred during motor vehicle accidents, either collisions or single-vehicle accidents (Table 7–3). The remainder consisted primarily of workers run over by vehicles or struck by shifting loads.

Nearly 50% of the disabling injuries reported were sustained by line-haul drivers, either working for common carriers or under special contracts. Employees of local trucking companies accounted for 36% of

TABLE 7–2.—FATAL AND DISABLING WORK INJURIES, CALIFORNIA TRUCKING INDUSTRY, 1964–1973

YEAR	TOTAL	FATAL
1964	6567	33
1965	6846	36
1966	7227	38
1967	7127	41
1968	7572	43
1969	7886	45
1970	7623	45
1971	7282	44
1972	7732	42
1973	8562	54

TABLE 7–3.—TYPE OF ACCIDENT INVOLVING HIGHWAY MOTOR VEHICLES

ACCIDENT TYPE	NUMBER	%
TOTAL	188	100.0
Overturning, running off road	72	38.3
Collision with other moving vehicle	65	34.6
Collision with fixed or other object	31	16.5
Run over or struck by	11	5.8
Caught between moving vehicle and other object	4	2.1
Struck by shifting load or object falling from vehicle	3	1.6
Others	2	1.1

the injuries and the remainder consisted of injuries to employees of moving and storage companies.

More than half of driver accidents occurred during loading and unloading, and 8% were sustained while climbing on or off a vehicle or loading dock. Thirty percent were injured in strain or overexertion accidents, usually when lifting or carrying containers or household goods. Twenty-five percent of the injuries were caused by being struck by or striking against an object. Vehicles were responsible for the great proportion of accidents in which workers were struck. Injuries from falls or slipping constituted the third highest cause, with most occurring while the injured worker was stepping off a vehicle, dock or stairs. Falling or flying objects, such as containers and hand tools, also were responsible for a large number of accidents. Vehicles were responsible for 1 of 4 accidents, with trucks accounting for 50%. Other vehicles responsible were fork-lifts and manually operated equipment, such as handtrucks and dollies.

Strains, sprains, dislocations and hernias were the most frequent nondriving injuries, amounting to 1014 injuries, or 46% of the total. Other injuries included contusions, abrasions, lacerations and puncture wounds.

The survey concluded that the recordable injury and illness rates for California truckers were 25% higher than figures for the U.S. trucking industry as a whole and 30% higher than the rate for all U.S. industries. Thus, rates for California would appear to be substantially higher than those for the nation as a whole. It should be noted, however, that California is widely recognized as having the most reliable reporting system for worker injuries. Thus, the higher rates recorded in California very probably indicate that the experience in other states has been severely underreported.

As indicated earlier, the primary physical stressors in trucking are vibration, noise, heat engine emissions and postural requirements during driving.

Vibration

Many studies have been conducted on the physiologic effects of vibration, but few conclusive studies have been undertaken on the effects of vibration in over-the-road trucks. Vibration is the motion (oscillating, reciprocating or otherwise) that forces a body or medium out of a position or state of equilibrium. It generally is measured in terms of frequency, amplitude, velocity and acceleration. Frequency is expressed in cycles per second (Hz), amplitude in displacement units, velocity in displacement units per second and acceleration in displacement units per second squared or in the nondimensional unit of "g."[12] Vibration can occur from either direction in any one of three axes—front to back chest, which is designated as the "x" axis; front chest to lower back, designated "y"; and head to foot, "z," which appears to be the most significant axis.

Most research has been concerned with laboratory effects of vibration along the z axis, including biodynamics, subjective evaluation, behavior and performance and physiology.[2, 10, 23, 25, 26, 67] Biodynamic studies have revealed that man exhibits a major response to vibration in the z or vertical direction at about 5 Hz. The most critical frequency band is 4–8 Hz in the vertical direction, with whole-body vibration occurring at approximately 5 Hz. Sinusoidal vibration generally is uncomfortable at acceleration amplitudes above 0.1 g, distressing or painful at 1 g and injurious above 2 g if maintained for longer than a few cycles.[12]

Vibration in the 3–7 Hz frequency range produces major physiologic effects. At about 5 Hz, chest pain may occur, balance and the ability to sit erect be impaired and physical fatigue result. Even very-low-frequency vibration can be a problem; vibration at 1 Hz results in motion sickness and at 2 Hz can cause sleepiness. At frequencies above 10 Hz, visual acuity and coordination can be impaired.[26]

Truck cabs vibrate at a frequency of up to 20 Hz, with major structural resonances occurring anywhere within this range. In comparison, smooth-riding city buses have a mean acceleration level of 50 cm/sec or 0.05 g, whereas typical over-the-road trucks have an acceleration level 3–5 times higher.

Although the physiologic effects of whole-body vibration on truck drivers have not been studied extensively, research to date indicates that the primary effects are related to the circulatory, gastrointestinal, genitourinary and musculoskeletal systems.[23] In a comprehensive comparison of the medical histories of truck drivers, bus drivers and air traffic controllers—all of whom work in the seated position with and without vibration—truck drivers (highest degree of vibration) had a significantly higher incidence of the following problems: bone deformities and vertebrogenic pain syndrome, hemorrhoids, kidney disease and peptic ulcer.[25]

The bone deformities observed in truck drivers are primarily spine deformities, which these drivers exhibit to a significantly greater degree than do bus drivers (less vibration) or air controllers (little if any vibration). There is more than twice the incidence of premature, degenerative deformities of the spinal column among line-haul truck drivers than there is among bus drivers.[5]

Whole-body vibration and the faulty posture assumed by drivers to compensate for vibration discomfort, as well as the heavy manual work required of truck drivers, may contribute to the significantly higher incidence of vertebrogenic pain exhibited by these drivers as compared with bus drivers. This situation probably occurs because line-haul truck design is concerned with aspects other than riding comfort. The problems experienced are vertebrogenic pain syndrome with displacement of intervertebral disks, sacroiliac problems and, to a lesser degree, joint ankylosis. Vibration is traumatic to the spine. The intervertebral disks serve as "shock absorbers" during vibration. If the individual is exposed to vibration over a prolonged period, the intervertebral disks appear to become susceptible to premature, degenerative deformities.

Truckers often compensate for discomfort from vibration by changing their positions. If the assumed posture is incorrect, the stress is applied along other axes, with similar effects. The problem may stem not only from the exposure to vibration but also from the manual labor in trucking, as well as the cab-over-engine configuration of much truck construction, which permits greater vibration to be felt by the driver.

Truck drivers have a significantly higher incidence of hemorrhoids than do bus drivers. This complaint may result from whole-body vibration, since large intraluminal pressures can build up in the 4–7 Hz vibration range and be transmitted to the hemorrhoidal veins, with the possibility of damage to those veins.[79] However, the poor dietary habits of truck drivers, with emphasis on low-residue foods, may also be a contributing factor.

Kidney disease may be more prevalent among line-haul truck drivers, and some investigators believe that vibration is the cause.[14] Pain in the region of the kidneys and frequent urination with some burning have been complaints of many operators of vehicles that have a high range of vibration. Heavy seat vibrations may serve as a stimulus to diuresis, and the impact of the bladder against the pelvis and abdomen during vibration may stimulate urination.[14] Further research will be required, however, before genitourinary disease can be unequivocally attributed to truck vibration.

A higher incidence of peptic ulcer has been found among truck drivers than among either air traffic controllers or bus drivers.[25] Although whole-body vibration may be a factor in the development of peptic ulcer, there is little conclusive evidence to that end. Both air traffic controllers and bus drivers usually eat meals at regular intervals and have time to eat hot, well-prepared and nutritious meals. Truck drivers, on the other hand, tend to eat meals hurriedly and irregularly—meals that often are high in "junk" foods and low in nutrition. The further factor of a high use of alcohol, caffeine and nicotine among truck drivers would suggest that whole-body vibration, although it may be a factor, is not the entire cause.

Truck drivers have been found to have a high frequency of appendicitis. Although their poorer eating habits may contribute to this complaint, whole-body vibration cannot be entirely ruled out as a contributor. Increased intraluminal pressures resulting from vibration may impede the flow of blood to and from the colon and into the appendiceal mucosa, thereby contributing to appendicitis. In this regard, research has indicated that sustained intraluminal pressures in the area of the appendix can cause changes in the wall of this organ.[78]

Laboratory studies also have indicated that vibration can affect performance adversely.[34] In a series of experiments, investigators exposed 12 subjects to vibration of 6 Hz at 0.1 g_z while requiring them to perform tracking tasks. The ability of the subject to perform these tasks deteriorated during vibration in both the vertical and horizontal tracking directions.

The effects of various stressors are closely interrelated, so the effects of one stressor cannot always be isolated from those of another. Thus, no one stressor can be judged to be entirely responsible for the physiologic problems related to truck driving. Consequently, vibration should be further studied as a contributor to musculoskeletal, gastrointestinal and circulatory problems in truckers.[25]

Noise

Noise is defined as any essentially random oscillation of sound pressure within the audible frequency range of 20–20,000 Hz that does not impart information to the human ear. The measure most commonly used to assess noise intensity is related to the response curve of the human ear. It is the frequency-weighted sound level across the range of 20–10,000 Hz, with weighting values assigned according to the "A-Scaling" procedure. It is measured in decibels as a quantity 20 times $\log_{10}$ of the ratio of noise sound pressure to a specified reference pressure (0.002 dynes/cm).

The most effective short-term index of noise response is the temporary threshold shift (TTS), which indicates the immediate reaction of the human ear to excessive noise exposure. When the TTS occurs, the individual temporarily loses the ability to hear at the level where he normally would be able to hear. If TTSs occur repeatedly over prolonged periods, permanent hearing losses may occur. When an individual is exposed to destructive noise levels over a prolonged period, noise-induced permanent threshold shifts (NIPTS) occur. NIPTSs indicate that a permanent, irreversible hearing loss has occurred.

The National Institute for Occupational Safety and Health (NIOSH) has established 90 decibels (dB) as the noise level at which hearing damage is likely to occur.[53] Exposure at this level, however, is damaging to hearing only after a long period. Exposure to high-pitched noise is also more damaging than exposure to low-pitched noise. Some persons in the hearing field have suggested that NIOSH should reduce its noise standard to 85 dB, indicating that they believe that hearing impairments may occur at a lesser noise level.

Cabs of older interstate trucks often reach noise levels that exceed 90 dB. Moreover, because of highway noises, drivers may be exposed briefly to noise at intensities greater than 110 dB. Exposure to this level of noise even for brief periods may cause temporary hearing loss that requires several days to alleviate. There are problems also at lesser levels of noise. Noise in excess of 70 dB can result in communication problems stemming from a loss of understanding of signals. Even low-to-moderate levels can create difficulties for noise-sensitive individuals, including profound emotional responses, distraction and abnormal behavior.

In addition to hearing loss, a number of nonspecific responses have been observed following exposure to high-level noise. They include elevated heart rate, elevated blood pressure and increased urinary excretion of adrenalin and noradrenalin.[1] These responses are indicative of a physiologic reaction to stress.

In the tracking studies referred to above, noise alone or in combination with vibration was found to have little consistent effect on performance. It has been noted in other research, however, that noise in truck driving virtually eliminates audition in the transmission of information, with even horns and sirens having only minimal effect.[30]

There appear to be three primary concerns with regard to the effect of environmental noise on truck drivers: (1) that prolonged exposure will lead over time to permanent hearing loss, (2) that it may deprive drivers of information that is vital to driving safety and (3) that it will result in fatigue leading to decrements in performance.

The National Board of Occupational Safety and Health of Sweden demonstrated its concern regarding reports that infrasound and ultrasound may be damaging to health by establishing new threshold limit values that came into effect October 1, 1978. Infrasound and ultrasound at high levels can give rise to complaints of nausea, tiredness and discomfort. Compressors, large diesel engines and discharges of steam are among potential sources of infrasound on work sites. Infrasound also occurs inside vehicle cabs, especially when traveling with a window open. The TLV stipulated by the Board for infrasound is an acoustic pressure level of 110 dB within the 2–20 Hz frequency range for 8 hours exposure per day. A level of 130 dB can be accepted for up to 1 hour per day. The TLVs for ultrasound are 105 dB at 20,000 Hz, 110 dB at 25,000 Hz and 115 dB for 31,500 Hz and upward. These figures can be increased by 3 dB for up to 4 hours total daily exposure and by 9 dB for up to 1 hour total daily exposure. It is unlikely that ultrasound far above the hearing range causes hearing damage, but undertones within the audible range can cause hearing impairment, added to which they often are extremely irritating. The National Board of Occupational Safety and Health of Sweden already has instituted a TLV of 80 dB for noise of frequency range 20 through 20,000 Hz.[36]

In an extensive study of the ergonomic and work conditions for truck drivers, Hansson et al. reported measurements and assessments on 17 different trucks manufactured in 1974–1975.* The trucks carried out distribution, sanitation, route traffic, long-distance traffic, oil transport, forestry haulage and gravel haulage assignments. A questionnaire study comprising 122 drivers was

*Hansson, J-E., Klussel, L., Svensson, G., and Wikström, B-O.: Arbetsmiljön i lastbilshytter, 104 pp., Arb. och Hälsa, Stockholm, 1976.

conducted and included drivers of both old and new vehicles.

The questionnaire study disclosed that all the drivers were most irritated by the noise, dust and climate in the cab and with provisions for getting in and out of cabs. In view of the importance of these matters to them, measures are required to improve the climate (too warm in summer and too drafty in winter) and noise level in cabs, followed by measures to make getting in and out of cabs safer and more convenient. The drivers expressed concern about the driver's seat, seating position, visibility and eliminating exhaust fumes in the cab, but these conditions were believed to be less of a problem than the four factors mentioned earlier. However, 43% of the drivers were dissatisfied with the standard lighting on their trucks, especially with dipped beams. In a number of cases, the problems perceived varied with the driving assignment. The ergonomic and hygienic measurements and assessments revealed major differences between different truck types and driving assignments. The authors noted that certain measures should be adopted in order to improve trucks and recommendations are suggested and explained. The main results are summarized as follows:

> Facilities for getting in and out of cabs were regarded as being unsatisfactory in most cases and radical changes should be made in the design of trucks used for distribution and sanitation.
>
> Headroom in cabs was regarded as being too low to allow a tall driver to sit at a comfortable height and headroom should be increased to a minimum of 150 cm (59 inches).
>
> The driver's seat is too close to the door and the rear cab wall (cab too short) in certain trucks so that the driver is exposed to drafts in winter; certain minimum measures are proposed.
>
> Trucks should be fitted with seats that can be raised and lowered easily and simply (45 ± 5 cm, i.e., 17¾ inches ± 2 inches).
>
> With respect to design, location and operation, controls were regarded as being satisfactory. High control resistance was found in a number of older vehicles. Adjustable steering wheels were believed desirable to enable both tall and short drivers to find comfortable positions.
>
> Visibility to the front was judged to be good. Visibility to the right of the truck was found to be poor and should be improved. The windshield wipers on certain trucks impaired visibility (further studies are proposed).
>
> The strength and spread of dipped headlamps were found to be poor in most cases, which could have an adverse effect on safety at high speeds (further studies are proposed).
>
> Heat in many cabs in summer is a major stress factor, as are drafts in winter.
>
> In most cases, the noise level in the vehicles studied was under the level producing damage to hearing, but still should be reduced for the sake of greater driver comfort. Improved maintenance of the trucks in this respect and continued improvements in design were believed to be urgent.
>
> Vibration stress to drivers was greatest in semitrailer tractors and tank trucks. On the basis of the ISO 2631 standard, the exposure, in most cases, was not regarded as being deleterious to health but was creating "fatigue—decreased proficiency." Drivers' seats that reduce vibration should be used.
>
> Dust measurements in trucks hauling gravel to and from a quarrying plant disclosed high levels in cabs. Drivers working under such conditions for many years run the risk of contracting pneumoconiosis (further studies are recommended).

Detailed drawings of the truck cabs studied, showing all views, are included, as well as dimensions, forward visual fields, with wiper areas diagramed, and areas seen through the rear-view mirrors. Forward lighting areas with intensities are shown and interior cab noise levels in city driving with and without loads are graphically displayed, including highway driving at 70 km/hr with and without loads.

Heat

The NIOSH has specified that a hot environment is one in which temperature, humidity, radiation and wind speed combine to create a wet-bulb temperature (WBGT) that exceeds 79° F.[52] For drivers exposed to heat for 8–10 hours, 80° F WBGT is considered to be the conservative upper limit if they take suitable rest breaks every 2–3 hours.

Heat stress is evidenced in a number of

ways. Perspiration is the most immediate effect as the body attempts to maintain thermal equilibrium. Blood pressure declines as the blood flow shifts from the interior of the body to the skin, with systolic pressure exhibiting a greater decline than diastolic. Finally, heart rate increases, urinary excretion of 17-hydroxycorticosteroids decreases and production of adrenalin and noradrenalin declines. All of these responses are accompanied by a rise in rectal body temperature. The decline in catecholamine production has also been observed when individuals are required to perform monotonous tasks for a long period[56] and is associated with failure to respond to important events during the extended performance of routine tasks.[54]

Fortunately, the body has a strong mechanism for adapting to heat. The primary response in this adaptive process is a shift of the blood from the interior of the body to the skin to create a heat loss through radiation and convection. This shift is accomplished by cutaneous vasodilation. Under normal conditions, 5% of the blood flow is directed to the skin. During heat adaptation, however, up to 20% of the flow will be directed to the skin. The immediate drop in blood pressure when this happens occurs because of the increased vascular space. When the blood flow is directed to the skin, it is pulled away from other organs. To compensate for this loss, cardiac output must be increased and, consequently, heart rate increases. This compensation is not sufficient in some individuals, however, and cerebral ischemia results because of inadequate blood flow to the brain. Heat exhaustion then occurs, the first indications being extreme fatigue, nausea and dizziness. Syncope follows if the cerebral flow declines further. Although heat exhaustion generally is not a major medical problem, any reduction in cerebral blood flow is serious in motor vehicle operators because it can create serious performance problems.

The body not only begins to react immediately to a hot environment but it also acclimatizes over a period of 4–7 days, depending on the individual. Acclimatization is more effective in persons who work from 1 to 4 hours intermittently in a hot environment than in those who rest during heat exposure. It also occurs more rapidly in physically fit individuals and apparently is unaffected by age. When an individual has been acclimatized, heat discomfort disappears, body temperature and heart rate decrease and perspiration becomes more profuse and dilute. Total blood volume and venomotor tone also increase, enhancing the refilling rate of the heart so that it need do less work to maintain normal blood pressure. Following acclimatization in hot, dry environments, total blood volume gradually returns to normal. The same is not true, however, in hot, wet environments.

Physical symptoms of heat stress appear in most individuals at WBGTs of around 79° F. At WBGTs higher than about 88° F, neither adaptation nor acclimatization is possible. Not only temperature but also sex has a bearing on response to heat stress. Thus, women are more susceptible to heat stress than are men because of the higher skin temperature at which women perspire.[31]

It has been well established that body temperature and performance are interrelated and that peak performance generally occurs at the time of peak body temperature in the circadian temperature rhythm.[11,12] These findings, however, refer to normal body temperature rhythms, which rarely change by more than 1.2° over a 24-hour period. In contrast, during exposure to heat, body temperature rises more rapidly and to a greater degree. Current knowledge suggests that mental working capacity deteriorates progressively as body temperature exceeds 100.4°.[11,60] It is not known, however, how long drivers would be able to function under such conditions.

Heat stress throughout much of the United States during the summer could be sufficient to impair the driving ability of truck drivers. Moreover, heat stress can exacerbate existing physiologic conditions, such as heart disease and emphysema, and many line-haul truck drivers are between 40 and 60 years of age—an age group that has a relatively high incidence of cardiopulmonary diseases.[76] Consequently, prolonged exposure to heat must be considered a hazard to the safety and health of truck drivers.

Engine Emissions

Although considerable research has been conducted on the effects of gasoline engine emissions, little has been done with regard to emissions from diesel engines. The Environmental Protection Agency has begun to request studies in this area, but several years could elapse before the results are available.[61] The findings of such studies may have a significant impact on the trucking industry, whose drivers may be exposed to diesel exhaust fumes for long periods because of leaks in exhaust and ventilation systems. Exposure to fumes in truck cabs may cause dizziness, drowsiness, headache, nausea, degraded mental performance and decrements in visual acuity. Any of these conditions could be hazardous to highway safety. Carbon monoxide exposure will be studied together with diesel fumes in the near future.[61]

Postural Requirements

Line-haul truck drivers spend many hours each day in the seated position. They must cope with a multi-ton vehicle and, to control the large steering wheel, they are forced to assume a rigid, upright position. This position, when held for any length of time, causes stiffening in the neck, back and extremity muscles. Discomfort soon results, followed by postural fatigue.

Prolonged seated immobility may also lead to the deterioration of physical fitness. Blood pooling occurs in the lower extremities, draining the blood from the upper body and heart. Orthostatic intolerance as well as metabolic and cardiovascular changes commonly occur. Studies on the physiologic effects of immobilization, using chair rest as the means of immobilization, showed that physical deconditioning occurred within a few days.[42] Total blood volume and red blood cell mass decreased and orthostatic and exercise tolerance diminished progressively the longer the chair rest was in effect. Other research has indicated that pulse frequency is reduced, blood pressure declines and stroke volume is lowered.[76] The immediate implications for truck drivers are obvious. But the effects on the cardiovascular system of prolonged sitting posture over months or years are not known.

Considerably more is known about the effects of prolonged sitting on the musculoskeletal system. In one very comprehensive study, the medical histories of 440 subjects with back problems and 494 matched and unmatched controls without back problems were reviewed.[39,40] The subjects ranged in age from 20 to 64 years. The study was conducted to determine whether a correlation existed between occupation and the occurrence of acute herniated lumbar intervertebral disks (HIVD). It demonstrated that truck drivers exhibited a higher incidence of HIVD than did nondrivers. Moreover, those who drove but did not drive commercially had a higher incidence of HIVD than did individuals who did not drive at all.

Twenty-two of the subjects had jobs in which they spent 50% or more of their work time seated in a motor vehicle whereas their matched controls did not. There were also 8 pairs in which the controls spent more than half of their work time in a motor vehicle whereas the subjects did not. The difference between those who drove motor vehicles for a livelihood and those who did not was statistically significant ($p > 0.02$), leading the investigators to estimate that drivers of motor vehicles have a relative risk factor of 2.75. Thus, truck drivers apparently are 3 times as likely to experience herniated intervertebral disks as are individuals whose occupation does not require long hours of driving. The study also indicated that persons of either sex who drive are more likely to develop acute herniated lumbar disks than those who do not drive at all. The investigators could not attribute these associations to any of the other variables considered during the study—that is, age, sex or body weight.

PSYCHOSOCIAL STRESSORS AND EMOTIONAL STRAIN

In addition to the physical stresses of commercial driving, line-haul drivers are faced with a number of psychosocial stresses, many of which can be conducive to job-related injuries and illnesses. These stresses include irregular work/rest cycles and sleep deprivation; disorganization of circadian rhythms; prolonged driving; job monotony and frustration; overburden; delays and schedule shifting; poor work, family and social relationships; and economic pressures. The effects of many of these stressors are interrelated.

Hans Selye, a leading authority on stress, has said that "The secret of health and happiness lies in successful adjustment to the ever-changing conditions on this globe; the penalties for failure in this great process of adaptation are disease and unhappiness."[65] The initial response to psychosocial stress usually is emotional strain, which results as the individual tries to cope with or combat a negative life situation. With all types of stress it becomes more difficult for the individual to cope with the stressor if it occurs repeatedly or too frequently. When that happens with psychosocial stressors, the individual can suffer mental fatigue and exhaustion, decrements in performance, accidents or illness. Particularly high accident risk factors and clusters of illnesses seem to be prevalent when motor vehicle drivers are having difficulty adapting to negative life situations.[24]

Sleep Deprivation, Fatigue and Driving Performance

Many studies have been conducted on the effects of various psychosocial stressors on driving performance. Methods used have included driving simulators, driving vehicles on closed-circuit driving tracks, open-road driving and driver performance tests administered both before and after prolonged driving. Much of the research has been concerned with the effects on driving performance of sleep deprivation, fatigue and prolonged periods of driving. Each of the methods used has inherent uncontrollable variables; consequently, research findings with each method may be open to question.

Study results on sleep deprivation are among the more consistent regardless of the method used. Sleep deprivation is common among many line-haul drivers, particularly owner-operators who must drive long hours to meet economic pressures. There appears to be little disagreement among investigators that sleep deprivation results in degraded performance.

One team of investigators measured the driving performance of 10 subjects under two conditions of sleep deprivation—cumulative sleep deprivation (5 subjects with 4 hours of sleep per night for 3 nights) and extreme sleep deprivation (5 subjects with no sleep for 24–36 hours).[18] The subjects drove test vehicles for 5 hours, covering 200 miles over a 4-lane highway during that period. The vehicle was equipped with dual braking and steering controls. All subjects served as their own controls, since they previously had driven the highway when they were not sleep deprived. The performance of those subjected to cumulative sleep deprivation did not differ significantly from that during their "normal" (no sleep deprivation) runs. For those exposed to extreme sleep deprivation, however, the differences between the normal and test conditions were significant in terms of lane drifting, unnecessary speed changes, eye blinking and instrument checking. The findings of other studies agree with the premise that fatigue results in decrements in driver performance.

Prolonged driving time—even without sleep deprivation—also appears to have a significant deteriorative effect on driver performance. Various performance variables have been noted to change following prolonged driving. Studies using simulators have shown that the ability of drivers to maintain the proper lane position declines as a function of driving time.[29, 47, 69] The findings of these studies have been reinforced by the results of studies conducted on the open road.[15, 43, 70] Increased variability in vehicle velocity control has also been observed during prolonged driving.[49, 55, 70] Some investigators have also found that steering wheel reversal rates and judgment decrease over time on the open road,[22, 48, 63] on a closed-circuit track[55] and in a simulator.[29] Judgmental errors, including risky maneuvers and discourteous actions, have been observed to increase as a function of driver time at the wheel.[8, 55, 59]

Physiologic changes have also been observed during prolonged driving. EEG recordings have shown an increase in slow-frequency, 8–13 Hz, alpha waves.[7, 29, 57] Average heart rate has been found to decrease with prolonged driving over a closed-circuit track[8, 55] and on the open road.[44, 57] One investigator also reported that heart rate variability increased in correlation with decrements in driver performance.[43] Respiration rate has been observed to decrease,[45, 55] and changes have occurred in eye movement[38] and eosinophil counts in the blood.[47]

Circadian Desynchronization

All physiologic systems within the human body function according to certain rhythms. Most of these rhythms approximate a 24-hour pattern and, as a result, have been termed "circadian rhythms" (meaning "about a day"). When these rhythms are disrupted—as occurs when a truck driver's schedule is shifted from driving in daylight to driving at night—a state of stress is produced that can result in impairment of physical health, emotional and behavioral problems, sleep difficulties, altered responses to medication and decrements in work performance and safety awareness. It may also increase the individual's susceptibility to the effects of other stressors.[9, 12, 50, 80] (See Chapter 10 for a more detailed discussion.)

Changes in circadian rhythms in motor vehicle drivers need to be studied to assess whether a measurable correlation exists between circadian desynchronization and the rate of injury and illnesses among drivers. In view of the consistent findings that circadian desynchronization creates both physiologic and emotional changes,[72, 80] it would seem reasonable for employers to consider carefully the advisability of shifting drivers repeatedly from day to night schedules and back. The more frequently the schedule is shifted the more serious the desynchronization, because the body has insufficient time to adapt before it must adapt again. In fact, schedules should not be shifted any more frequently than every 3 weeks or once a month.[72]

Job Monotony and Frustration

Long-haul truck driving is a monotonous experience. The nation's carefully engineered system of highways stretches monotonously straight. Usually, all that the driver sees is mile after mile of highway stretching to infinity; most drivers call it a "long, dreary ride." Individuals have difficulty remaining alert in a monotonous situation. Even in physically fit and healthy individuals, monotony results in drowsiness, which is followed by lethargic fatigue. Repetitive driver tasks that require intense eye fixation and scanning are also difficult to perform under monotonous conditions. The implications for highway safety, of course, are considerable. When one driver signals another in passing, he is not only observing a courtesy of the road but also "casting a lifeline" by breaking the monotony.

Frustration is another inherent part of truck driving. Frustration results from poor road conditions, heavy traffic, inconsiderate drivers, delays en route and at terminals and shifts in schedules. It occurs when an individual is blocked from achieving his immediate goal or goals by physical obstacles, conflicts or his own deficiencies. When frustrations occur, the individual either will react immediately or will not react at all. In the latter case, he will develop attitudes that will have more enduring consequences. Frustration usually is met either by aggression or by apathy. In aggression, the anger that is aroused when the individual is blocked tends to be expressed in some form of direct action—that is, the individual strikes back immediately at the source of the frustration. In the trucker's case, he might "tailgate" an inconsiderate driver or unleash a string of invectives at a terminal employee who caused a delay.

If the source of the frustration is impersonal, inaccessible or too powerful to attack, displaced aggression occurs. In this case, the aggression is focused on an innocent person or an object rather than on the true source of the frustration. The implications of aggression for highway safety are serious, since aggressive driving behavior has been the cause of many accidents.

Apathy is the opposite response to frustration. When resistance to the source of frustration is futile, the frustrated individual may become sullen and withdrawn. This situation has been observed when extremely frustrating conditions persist over a long period and the individual has no hope of being free from them.[32] The apathetic person is incapable of remaining alert.

Job Dissatisfaction

The major sources of job dissatisfaction among truck drivers are unsatisfactory human relationships in the work environment, work overload and lack of opportunities for the development or control of one's own destiny.

HUMAN RELATIONSHIPS IN THE WORK ENVIRONMENT.—Unsatisfactory relationships with supervisors, co-workers or business associates can have a deteriorative effect on a trucker's health and well-being. French and Caplan[19] have defined poor work relationships as "those which include low trust, low supportiveness, and low interest in listening to and trying to deal with problems that confront the organizational member." Kahn and associates[37] determined that one source of unsatisfactory human relationships on the job is a feeling of threat from superiors and colleagues.

Lack of consideration by supervisors also creates job tension. In one study using the Fleishman leadership questionnaire to evaluate this aspect of worker relationships, managerial consideration was graded in terms of "friendship," "respect" and "feelings of warmth between employee and supervisor." Workers who believed that their supervisors were inconsiderate complained that they showed favoritism, took advantage of them, criticized them unfairly and not constructively and "pulled rank." The investigators concluded that inconsiderate behavior by supervisors "contributed significantly to feelings of job pressure."[46]

Poor work relationships also occur when there is a conflict over how a job should be done, what the priorities should be and when inadequate information is given.

All deteriorative human work relationships can result in psychologic stress in the worker.

WORK OVERLOAD.—Quantitative work overload—that is, assigning more work than the individual can realistically accomplish in the time required—is a widespread practice in U. S. industry and is not uncommon in the trucking industry. The overload results in job tension, which often leads to the development of personal habits that can be harmful to health, such as smoking.[20]

The length of time worked per day is another aspect of quantitative overload. In this regard, a positive correlation has been found between the number of hours worked per day and the incidence of coronary disease. In a study of mortality rates among men in California, investigators found that workers in light industry who spend more than 48 hours a week on the job faced twice the risk of a fatal heart attack compared with workers of a similar age who worked 40 hours or less per week.[6] In a study of young coronary patients, 25% were found to have been working at two jobs and 45% were working 60 or more hours per week.[62]

LACK OF JOB CONTROL.—The lack of an opportunity to progress or to have a voice in decisions that directly affect a person's job can result in job indifference, frustration, depression and antagonism. Investigators have suggested that a correlation exists between frustrated job aspirations and mental illness.[41,71] In the trucking industry, drivers who work for large companies have little control over their work destinies, which can be a frustrating situation. Although owner-operators, on the other hand, would appear not to face this problem, they must submit to the will of their customers, terminal managers and demanding business associates if they are to survive financially.

Economic Pressures

Drivers for large motor freight lines and other company-owned transport systems can earn as much as $30,000 per year and face few, if any, economic pressures. Owner-operators, however, who constitute a large proportion of the nation's truck drivers, often are faced with severe economic pressures. Most have loan payments to make on their vehicles, and the increasingly higher costs of fuel and maintenance, as well as rampant inflation, add to their financial problems. Consequently, they must work long hours at the greatest possible speed just to keep up financially. They may be known as independent operators, but, as one owner-operator expressed it, "The independent trucker today is about as free as a man in chains."

The financial risk of purchasing or leasing a truck, its costly upkeep and management (state and federal highway use taxes range from $1834 a year for a 3-axle tractor-trailer to $3941 a year for a 5-axle truck and trailer) and the intense competition for loads and the better routes all contribute to the stress of driving for a livelihood. Many owner-operators fail to make the financial grade and return to working as company-employed drivers. Most manage to continue on a marginal basis. Some enjoy relative success but face additional costs and stresses, as well as a greater risk to health and safety than do company-employed drivers.

Those who manage to acquire more than one vehicle employ drivers who share their goal of delivering goods the greatest distance in the shortest possible time. Drivers for small independents are relatively unsupervised and sometimes press dangerously for rapid delivery with the aid of drugs and the falsification of DOT-required driving records. They generally lack the benefits of union representation, prefer a working life that replaces a time clock with a demanding haul and demand a life style free from supervision. Together with their employers, they make distance and load their primary objectives. With the aid of amphetamines and other drugs, they may drive a thousand miles without sleep. To such drivers, the CB radio becomes not only a means of checking the weather ahead but also a vital means of staying awake.

Economic pressures on the owner-operators who do not lease to major motor carriers are compounded by dependence on brokers for loads. Typically, such an owner-operator will be forced to pay 10% of his delivery fee to obtain a load; his profit may be even further diminished by even greater "skimming" on the part of the broker. Additional costs occur if he feels compelled to offer payment to the dispatcher to ensure prompt loading of his cargo. In some cities, particularly on the East Coast, the owner-operator's profits would be even further diminished because he would be required to pay for a lumper's unloading fee.* Moreover, many drivers complain that they are subjects of extortion schemes. They are met at the loading dock by men who demand the right to load or unload their cargoes or demand payment if they are not permitted to do so. If the driver refuses to pay, he may wait days to be scheduled into a dock or warehouse. Law enforcement efforts against extortion, violence and violation of ICC regulations are inconsistent and sometimes nonexistent.

In light of these financial pressures, it is not surprising that many owner-operators are barely surviving and that one-third of them will go out of business in any given year. On a typical run, one owner-operator drove 928 miles in 27 hours with only 4 hours of fitful sleep and earned about $450. Deducted from this amount was $126.80 for fuel and $12.00 for food, leaving him a total profit of $311.20, not taking into account overhead expenses and depreciation on his vehicle.[73]

The foregoing economic pressures place owner-operators and drivers for small for-hire trucking companies at a greater risk of serious occupational safety and health problems than those experienced by drivers employed by regulated carriers. Owner-operators and their drivers will achieve financial rewards, such as they are, at the cost of seriously impairing their physical and mental well-being.

Mental and Emotional Illnesses

A possible correlation between mental illness, including alcoholism and drug dependence, and stressful conditions in the work environment has received increasing attention since World War II. Mental problems in the work environment take the form of job dissatisfaction, low self-esteem, job tension, impaired personal relationships and psychosomatic illnesses. These problems stem from various stressors in the work environment, including role conflict and ambiguity, quantitative and qualitative overload, personal conflicts with supervisors and co-workers and lack of worker autonomy.

Mental illnesses among vehicle operators have been the concern of a number of studies, with the primary objective being to determine the role played by mental disorders in traffic accidents.[13,58,77] A series of accident investigations conducted by Southwest Research Institute for the National Highway Traffic Safety Administration revealed that of 198 automobile drivers involved in accidents 24% had severe impairment of their mental functions at the time of the accident and that 72% suffered from some degree of mental disturbance ranging from mild to severe[13] (Table 7–4). In nearly 50% of those who were severely functionally impaired, the problem resulted from alcohol and drug abuse. In a similar study conducted in the District of Columbia, investigators found that drivers suffering from schizophrenia, anxiety neuroses and depressive neuroses had 50% more accidents than did members of an appropriate control group.[58] They also had the highest accident rate of all of the impaired drivers studied. A California study showed that drivers with a mental illness, other than alcoholism or drug dependence, had about twice as many accidents as did their mentally healthy counterparts.[77]

The use of alcohol is thought to be widespread among truck drivers despite the fact that Federal Motor Carrier Safety Regulations prohibit commercial drivers from consuming alcoholic beverages (regardless of the percentage of alcohol content) either while on duty or for 4 hours prior to going on duty. During a comprehensive study of problems in the work environment conducted for the Department of Health, Education, and Welfare,[81] interviews were

*A lumper is defined as a person who controls access to loading areas and who purports to be an official loader and unloader. The Federal Bureau of Investigation has begun to investigate cases of physical abuse of truck drivers who refuse to be intimidated by this extortion scheme.

TABLE 7–4.—DIAGNOSED MENTAL DISORDERS OF A GROUP OF DRIVERS INVOLVED IN TRAFFIC ACCIDENTS

CLASSIFICATION	NO. OF CASES	DIAGNOSIS	NO. OF CASES
Psychotic disorders	4	Paranoid schizophrenia	1
		Acute schizophrenia	1
		Schizophrenia	1
		Reactive depressive psychosis	1
Neurotic and personality disorders	19	Anxiety neurosis	1
		Depressive neurosis	1
		Hypochondriacal neurosis	2
		Cyclothymic personality	3
		Schizoid personality	1
		Explosive personality	4
		Obsessive compulsive personality	2
		Antisocial personality	2
		Immature personality	3
Emotional or adjustment disorders	20	Habitual excessive drinking	10
		Alcohol addiction	1
		Drug dependency	3
		Transient disturbances	3
		Epilepsy	1
		Senile brain disease	2
Mental retardation	4	Borderline mental retardation	3
		Unspecified mental retardation	1

conducted to determine the extent of alcohol use among workers in heavy industry. Responses indicated that many workers drank heavily during the lunch break to face the sheer monotony of their jobs. The same study also revealed that there is substantial on-the-job use of drugs by younger workers, particularly assembly-line workers and long-haul truck drivers.[81]

Federal Motor Carrier Safety Regulations specify that "No person shall operate a commercial vehicle if under the influence of, or frequently using, any of the following substances: (1) a depressant drug, (2) a stimulant drug or (3) any other substance to a degree adversely affecting arousal, mood, personality or behavior."[24] Thus, habit-forming narcotic, barbiturate, tranquilizing, stimulating or hallucinogenic drugs are unacceptable for use by commercial drivers.

Despite the above restrictions, it is recognized that the use of drugs, particularly stimulant drugs such as amphetamines, is widespread among truck drivers because of the need to stay awake for prolonged periods. Most drivers, of course, would not admit to using drugs, so the chances of learning how widespread the practice is are limited. One research group seeking answers to this question devised a different approach to the problem.[28] Instead of asking drivers whether they used drugs "occasionally" or "regularly," they asked, "Among *other* drivers that you know, what percent would *occasionally* use some sort of pill, like Benzedrine, to pep them up when they get tired on long hauls?" Later, the same question was asked, but with the word "frequently" substituted for the word "occasionally." Although the percentages obtained do not represent the absolute incidence of use, they do give some indication of usage. About 45% of those interviewed stated that they knew drivers who use pep pills occasionally, and 30% indicated that they knew drivers who use them regularly (Table 7–5). Those who drove more than 2000 miles a week and those under 30 years of age were more likely to "know" drivers who use pep pills to combat fatigue.

When similar questions were asked regarding the use of alcohol, the resulting fre-

TABLE 7–5.—KNOWLEDGE OF DRIVERS WHO USE PEP PILLS (BY TYPE OF CARRIER)

AMOUNT OF USE	OWNER-OPERATORS (N = 202)	COMMON CARRIERS (N = 100)	PRIVATE CARRIERS (N = 98)	ALL DRIVERS (N = 400)
Yes, know drivers who use pills occasionally	45	42	47	37
No, do not know drivers who use pills occasionally	32	38	38	46
Do not know whether they do or not	23	20	15	18
Yes, know drivers who use pills regularly	31	24	34	23
No, do not know drivers who use pills regularly	46	54	50	59
Do not know whether they do or not	23	22	16	18

NOTE: Numbers reflect percentage of all respondents.

quencies were very similar to the drug-use responses. The investigators believed that "The similar patterns of response may . . . lend some credence to the assertion that there is significant use of both drugs and alcohol by some truck drivers engaged in long-haul operations."[28]

In a recent survey, Dr. Daryl Wyckoff disseminated 65,000 four-page questionnaires related to problems in trucking. Approximately 10,500 were returned, half from company drivers and half from owner-operators.[35, 83] The findings indicated that 34% of drivers 25 years of age used amphetamines and 27% of those aged 25–50 and 9% of the over 50s used "uppers."

The use of alcohol, stimulants and barbiturates by drivers has serious implications for highway safety. Moreover, not only are these drugs dangerous when a person is driving but their physiologic impact also differs when they are taken at different times of the day. Alcohol, for example, has a much greater effect when taken early in the day. In studies of mice injected with a large amount of alcohol at various times during the day, the injections proved to be lethal when administered at the end of the animals' rest span.[27] Whereas 60% died when injected at their usual time of awakening, only 12% died when injected late in the day.

With other drugs also, there is a period during the day when the organism is highly resistant to the drug and another period when it is highly vulnerable. Amphetamines, for example, have the greatest effect at the peak of an individual's activity period. In studies of rats injected with lethal amounts of amphetamine at 2-hour intervals, only 6% died when injected at 0600 hours whereas 77.6% died when injected at midnight (their activity peak).[64] Furthermore, when taken at certain times of the day, amphetamines can cause mania and psychosis, particularly when the drug has been used for prolonged periods.

Drugs not only are affected by human rhythms but also may change those rhythms. Investigators have found, for example, that sodium pentobarbital will suppress the adrenal hormone rhythms in animals.[64] When animals were given a fast-acting barbiturate in the evening, the drug blocked the morning rise in hormone levels. This did not occur when the drug was given at other times during the day. In humans, this reaction may explain why the drug sometimes causes a hangover effect after total excretion or metabolism.

OUTLOOK FOR HIGHWAY SAFETY

Truck transportation has become a major factor in American business and industry. Federally regulated ton-miles of truck traffic have doubled since 1960; the Highway Users Federation predicts that the figure will double again over the next 15–20 years.

Of the 4 million trucks operating in the

United States, 1 million weigh up to 80,000 pounds and some, by special permit, weigh up to 130,000 pounds. The weight limit was raised to 80,000 pounds in 1974 at the height of the energy crisis, when the 55-mile-an-hour speed limit was put into effect. The increased weight has been accepted by most states. On the East Coast, Maryland is one of the last barriers to the unobstructed movement of 80,000-pound trucks between Florida and New England. Another barrier exists in the Middle West, where several states that have not approved the 80,000-pound truck have created a chain from north to south, frustrating east-west truck travel. How long these barriers will continue, however, is questionable.

The introduction of more trucks, heavier trucks and longer trucks will have a direct impact on highway safety and on the structural integrity of the nation's highways. With regard to highway safety, collisions between trucks and passenger cars result in a mortality rate that is significantly higher than that resulting from the collision of two or more automobiles. A combination of economic factors and energy issue pressures is creating larger and heavier trucks and smaller and lighter automobiles. This situation creates an extremely unequal contest when trucks collide with cars.

With regard to the safety aspects of truck drivers, Wyckoff's survey has indicated that regulated truckers have better safety records than exempt carriers and owner-operators.[83] Nearly half the drivers employed by exempt carriers reported that they "regularly" drive longer than the 10-hour limit, and about one-third of them reported using multiple log books to circumvent the hours of service rules. In contrast, only about 3.5% of company drivers working for common carriers regularly violate hours of service regulations and less than 2% use multiple logs. Cruising speeds are also higher among drivers for nonregulated carriers, averaging 63 mph in contrast to the 58.85 average of drivers for regulated carriers. Similarly, moving violations, when reduced to incidents per 100,000 miles, showed exempt owner-operators to be high, with a rate of 1.33, and drivers for common carriers to be low, with 0.41.

Doctor Wyckoff's findings conflict with data published by the Bureau of Motor Carrier Safety, which show that regulated carriers have a higher accident rate than nonregulated carriers. In the Wyckoff survey, exempt owner-operators were high, with an accident rate of 0.70 per 100,000 miles, whereas drivers for common carriers were low with 0.19 per 100,000 miles.

"My interpretation of the conflict between BMCS data and what the drivers told us is quite simple," said Doctor Wyckoff. "The only people playing by the rules or reporting accidents when they are supposed to (when there is property damage of $200 or more, or personal injury) are the regulated and private companies. The owner-operator, by his own admission, has a higher accident rate. The only time he reports an accident is when he has a major disaster." The Department of Defense, recognizing the disparity in safety records of owner-operators, prohibits those on a trip-lease from transporting hazardous materials and ammunition/explosives.

The integrity of the highway system must also be considered a critical factor in highway safety because structural breakdowns of U.S. highways would contribute to highway accidents. Highway engineers have predicted that, under the continual stress of 80,000-pound trucks, pavement life could be decreased by 25–40% and bridges on interstate highways (which are stronger than noninterstate bridges) would be overstressed by up to 36%.

Smaller cars driving at lower speeds are producing less fuel tax revenues for the building and maintenance of highways. This declining source of highway funds, coupled with increased use of highways by all vehicles, results in a less than optimistic outlook for highway safety.

Government agencies, particularly at the federal level, have established few realistic standards for health and safety of truck drivers.[4] Although the Occupational Safety and Health Administration (OSHA) has established continually expanding health and safety standards for other industries, little has been done at either the federal or state level to protect the millions of individuals whose jobs require long hours of driving. Senator Charles Percy of Illinois has sponsored legislation to provide this protection—the Truck Safety Act of 1978.

The Department of Transportation (DOT) has established some safety standards, but they cover only drivers in interstate commerce and do not apply to drivers in intrastate transportation or local drivers. DOT standards often are delayed, weakened or not applied to vans, trucks, tractor-trailers and buses. For example, DOT standards for door latches and seat belts became effective for trucks many years after they were established for passenger vehicles. Similarly, some standards for safety features are established for passenger vehicles but not for trucks[4] (Table 7-6). DOT, however, does continually sponsor research aimed at improving conditions for truckers as well as for the rest of the driving public. State agencies, on the other hand, often exhibit a permissive attitude toward safety and health infractions in the trucking industry.

Government agencies, for the most part, consider their obligation to safety and health in the trucking industry to be fulfilled by writing regulations and conducting spot checks of truckers' daily logs and load weights. In some cases, the regulations are so unrealistic that they obviate compliance. In the case of owner-operators and jobshoppers in particular, the minimal profit margins in this area of trucking make restrictive regulations on permitted driving hours almost impossible to obey. Consequently, the percentage of violations in this group is extremely high.

The most recent proposed DOT regula-

TABLE 7–6.—EXAMPLES OF FEDERAL MOTOR VEHICLE SAFETY STANDARDS DELAYED OR NOT APPLIED TO TRUCKS

FMVSS NO.	DESCRIPTION	EFFECTIVE DATES PASSENGER CARS	TRUCKS 10,000 LB
105	Hydraulic Service Brake, Emergency Brake, Parking Brake Systems	1-1-68	---
109, 119	New Pneumatic Tires (109—passenger cars; 119—other vehicles)	1-1-68	3-1-75
110	Tire Selection and Rims	4-1-68	---
111	Rear-view Mirrors	1-1-68	2-12-76
117	Retreaded Pneumatic Tires	1-1-72	---
201	Occupant Protection in Interior Impact	1-1-68	---
202	Head Restraints	1-1-69	---
203	Impact Protection for the Driver from the Steering Control System	1-1-68	---
204	Steering Control Rearward Displacement	1-1-68	---
206	Door Locks and Door Retention Components	1-1-68	1-1-72
207	Seating Systems	1-1-68	1-1-72
208	Occupant Crash Protection (Seat Belts)	1-1-68	7-1-72
210	Seat Belt Assembly Anchorage	1-1-68	7-1-71
212	Windshield Mounting	1-1-70	---
214	Side Door Strength	1-1-73	---
216	Roof Crush Strength	8-15-73	---
301	Fuel System Integrity	1-1-68	---

tions (issued May 15, 1978) are even more restrictive than previous rules with regard to permitted length of driving time, off-duty time and length and timing of relief periods.[16] Under these regulations, no driver can be on duty more than 60 hours in any 7-day period, and during this period he must have at least 36 consecutive hours off duty. During any duty period, a driver is not permitted to remain on duty for more than 12 hours; moreover, he is permitted to drive for no more than 10 hours in that 12-hour period or a distance of 450 miles, whichever occurs first. Drivers must also take a relief period every 2½ hours, which must be no shorter than 30 minutes; a meal period of 1 hour must be taken every 4 hours. During the 36-hour off-duty period, employers and their agents or representatives are not permitted to contact the drivers in any way; if they do so, the off-duty period is increased by an additional 4 hours. The duty period must start as close to the beginning of the calendar week as possible. Finally, schedule time for a run cannot slip any more than 3 hours in any 1 day or a total of 6 hours during 1 calendar week. The outlook for violations of these restrictions is monumental, particularly in view of the limited funding and personnel allotted to the policing agencies.

Jurisdiction over safety in interstate trucking is governed by the Bureau of Motor Carrier Safety (BMCS). BMCS operations are limited by a severe lack of funds and insufficient personnel. For example, the agency has only 128 people to handle all enforcement activities against 4 million drivers. Consequently, action is taken against only the most flagrant violations. Agency management admits that their enforcement agents are able to give audio-visual inspection to only about 80,000 vehicles a year, or only 2% of the 4 million trucks on the road.

Overloading is believed to be a common practice in the nonregulated trucking industry, with drivers frequently leaving the highway to bypass weigh stations. The policing of truck load weight is left to the states, few of which enforce the weight restrictions stringently.

The situation in the trucking industry concerning safety and health is serious and is of considerable concern both to the industry itself and to the federal government. It may be expected to become more serious as the number of trucks and passenger vehicles increases and truck weights rise. Solutions will not be easy, and some undoubtedly will be costly. The latter factor presents a particularly difficult hurdle because profit margins are narrow for much of the trucking industry, and for many owner-operators they are almost nil.

Four primary areas must be addressed if highway safety and health of motor vehicle drivers is to be improved—the vehicle, the driver, the highways and the legislative standards that govern them.

In any industry, well-designed, well-maintained equipment is essential to the well-being of the worker. In the trucking industry, it can be a matter of life and death. Design improvements that are needed in trucks include control of vibration, noise, heat and engine emissions and better seating and cab conditions. All such improvements will contribute to the greater comfort of the driver and to his safety and health. It has been argued that providing a comfortable environment for the driver, combined with the monotony of the present highway system, will lull drivers into a soporific state that will result in fatal single-vehicle accidents. But that has not been the experience of one operator of a 1500-truck fleet who installed air conditioning, insulation, improved seats and engine emission controls while achieving an excellent safety record.

The relation of a truck's loaded weight to its power source is reflected in its ability to maintain speed on a grade. Results of one study have indicated that in 7 of 8 collisions occurring on an upgrade that involved a truck, the truck was struck from the rear.

Inadequate braking ability, which is also related to loaded weight, was found to be a primary factor in collisions on a down grade or level when the truck was the striking vehicle.[4] If such collisions involve a passenger vehicle, the occupants of the car are more likely to be killed than is the truck driver. Truck improvements in this area consequently would benefit all highway users.

In most industries, fail-safe mechanisms are incorporated into equipment to protect workers from human and other failures. For example, some machines are equipped with automatic off-switches to avoid hand or finger mutilation; others are controlled by electric sensing devices that stop the machine before an injury occurs. Today's microelectronic technology soon may offer passive devices that will enhance truck safety. Padded dashboard and air bag restraints should be provided on all trucks. One of the primary goals of vehicle design should be protection of the drivers and the occupants of passenger cars involved in collisions with trucks.

The design of heavy motor vehicles should also include doors that can be readily opened after collisions and alternative escape routes, because extrication of the occupants following collisions has been a serious problem with tractor-trailers. In one study, it was found that at least 8 of 41 truckers who died after collisions were trapped in the cab (no fire involved) for periods of up to 3½ hours.[4] Rescuers were unable to free them because of jammed doors, smashed cabs, shifted loads or turnover of the tractor-trailer.

Drivers also need education, particularly those who have been on the road for many years or are very new to the occupation. The Teamsters Union has objected to the requests of some commercial operators to send their drivers to training classes, arguing that the drivers were professionals and did not require further training. In any field, however, additional training always is desirable. With such training, drivers will learn newer operating methods, be conditioned to use seat belts and other safety devices and be taught to eat properly and exercise sufficiently. Truckers should also be taught basic lifesaving techniques so that they will be able to help other truckers and passenger car occupants who are in need. This is particularly important because most accidents occur far from sources of medical help and the longer the accident victim remains without medical help the less the opportunity for recovery.

Highway standards must also be improved. Highway signs are not always understandable or clear, and instructions that apply to passenger vehicles may not always be applicable to trucks. The design of some highways also is not conducive to highway safety. Divided highways that are not limited-access highways present a particular problem. Collisions occur when vehicles pull onto the highway from a side road or turn left into the path of an oncoming tractor-trailer. Road designs that permit vehicles to intersect the paths of fast-moving trucks are an invitation to fatal accidents. One study revealed that 40% of the fatal accidents surveyed were caused by vehicles entering a highway from a side road or turning left across oncoming traffic. A possible solution could lie in eliminating or modifying such intersections or restricting heavy truck traffic to limited-access highways.[4]

Finally, legislation is needed to provide truckers with a working environment in keeping with the intent of OSHA, which states its objectives "to assure so far as possible every working man and woman in the Nation safe and healthful working conditions and to preserve our human resources."[75] At present, large numbers of workers in the trucking industry have not been provided with this assurance.

As an example of what can be done to improve the situation, let us consider the innovative approach taken by a private carrier that operates a highly specialized fleet of nearly 1500 rubber-tired vehicles.[21] The company's program stresses both safety and health. All drivers are required to take driver education courses and all are instructed in the benefits of following proper eating and exercise habits. They are provided with lists of nutritional foods to be eaten on the road and alerted that proper and regular meals will ease nervousness during the stress of operating the vehicle and help them to reduce the tendency to smoke and drink. They are also requested to perform a set of simple exercises during travel to improve their physical fitness.

Since the company also wants its drivers to stop and assist motorists and other truckers who are in trouble, all drivers are required to take courses in firefighting and first aid.

Finally, all drivers are monitored periodically by a team of company physicians who specialize in occupational medicine.

The company has also used an innovative approach in the design of its trucks. Primary among design changes is a "pulsating" seat to relieve drivers from restricted blood circulation in the lower extremities resulting from the postural requirements of driving. The seat consists of a series of 6 tubes that vibrate to stimulate the driver's circulation. Its developer believes that the pulsating seat will add to a driver's health and safety by overcoming blood pooling in the lower extremities.

The company's heavy-duty trucks also contain built-in air conditioning equipment and insulation for noise control. Furthermore, they are equipped with considerably more instrumentation than most trucks have. The main instruments are tachographs that monitor truck speed so that the 55-mile-per-hour speed limit can be maintained, which the company insists on. A pyrometer is also included and rigged to an alarm that is triggered when exhaust temperature reaches 900 degrees; it is coupled to a fuel bypass system that forces the driver to ease up on the throttle and shift into another gear. As an added environmental benefit, this equipment has reduced truck emissions by 52%.

The program's safety record has been outstanding; in the 11 years that it has been in existence, no company truck has been involved in a highway fatality and no driver has been hospitalized because of a highway accident. Moreover, unit operating costs per mile have been reduced significantly.

This illustration indicates the steps that can be taken by employers to improve the safety and health potential of their long-haul truck drivers. Such a program not only benefits the drivers but also benefits the employer by extending the productive life of his workers.

REFERENCES

1. *A Study of Heat, Noise, and Vibration in Relation to Driver Performance and Physiological Status*. Human Factors Research, Incorporated. Prepared for the National Highway Traffic Safety Administration. PB-238-829. December, 1974.
2. Allen, G.: Human reaction to vibration, J. Environ. Sci., Sept./Oct., 1971, pp. 10–15.
3. *American Trucking Trends, 1976, Statistical Supplement*. Department of Economics and Public Relations Department, American Trucking Association, Inc., Washington, D.C.
4. Baker, S. P., Jackson Wong, M. P. H., and Baron, R. D.: Professional drivers: Protection needed for a high-risk occupation, Am. J. Public Health 66:649, 654, 1976.
5. Barbaso, E.: Incidence of spine changes in drivers of one bus company, Med. Lav. 49:10, 1958.
6. Breslow, L., and Buell, P.: Mortality from coronary heart disease and physical activity of work in California, J. Chronic Dis. 11:615, 1960.
7. Brown, I. D.: Decrement in skill observed after seven hours of car driving, Psychonom. Sci. 7:131, 1967.
8. Brown, I. D., Simmonds, D. C. V., and

Tickner, A. H.: Measurement of control skills, vigilance, and performance on a subsidiary task during twelve hours of car driving, Ergonomics 10:665, 1967.

9. Browne, R. C.: The day and night performance in industry. 5th Conf. Soc. Biol. Rhythm. Stockholm: Aco Print, 1961, pp. 61–64.
10. Collins, A. M.: Decrements in tracking and visual performance during vibration, Hum. Factors 15:379, 1973.
11. Colquhoun, W. P.: Temperament, inspection efficiency and time of day, Ergonomics 3:377, 1960.
12. Conroy, R. T. W. L., and Mills, J. N.: *Human Circadian Rhythms* (London: J. & A. Churchill, 1970).
13. Cromack, R. J., et al.: Multidisciplinary Accident Investigation, Interim Report on Contract No. DOT-HS-024-1-115, January, 1973.
14. Dawson, D.: *Over the Road to Preventable Disease* (Pontiac, Mich.: Pontiac Medical Science Laboratories, Inc., 1972).
15. Ellingstad, V. S., and Heimstra, N. W.: Performance changes during the sustained operation of a complex psychomotor task, Ergonomics 13:693, 1970.
16. Federal Register, Vol. 43, No. 90, May 22, 1978.
17. Fellmeth, R.: *The Interstate Commerce Omission* (New York: Grossman Publishers, 1970).
18. Forbes, T. W., Katz, M. S., Cullen, J. W., and Deterline, W. A.: Sleep deprivation effects on components of driver behavior, Highway Res. Abstr. 28:21, 1953.
19. French, J. R. P., and Caplan, R. D.: Organization Stress and Individual Strain, in Marrow, A. J. (ed.), *The Failure of Success* (New York: AMACOM, 1973).
20. French, J. R. P., and Caplan, R. D.: Psychosocial factors in coronary heart disease, Ind. Med. 39:383, 1970.
21. Glines, C.: Robert Allen, guru of the trucking industry, Commercial Car Journal for Fleet Management 134:3, 1977.
22. Greenshields, B. D.: Changes in driver performance with time in driving, Highway Res. Rec. 122:75, 1966.
23. Grether, W. F.: Vibration and human performance, Hum. Factors 13:203, 1971.
24. Gruber, G. J.: *Establishment of Guidelines to Aid Examining Physicians*. Southwest Research Institute, San Antonio, Texas. Prepared for the Bureau of Motor Carrier Safety, Department of Transportation, under Contract No. DOT-FH-11-8274, November, 1976.
25. Gruber, G. J.: *Relationships between Wholebody Vibration and Morbidity Patterns among Interstate Truck Drivers*. Southwest Research Institute, San Antonio, Texas. Prepared for the National Institute for Occupational Safety and Health, under Contract No. CDC-99-74-22, November, 1976.
26. Guignard, J. C., and King, P. F.: Aeromedical aspects of vibration and noise. AGARDograph No. 151. NATO Advisory Group for Aerospace Research and Development, Neuilly sur Seine, France, 1972.
27. Halberg, F., Bittner, J. J., and Gully, R. J.: Twenty-four hour periodic susceptibility to audiogenic convulsions in several stocks of mice, Fed. Proc. 14:67, 1955.
28. Harris, W., and Mackie, R. R.: *A Study of the Relationships Among Fatigue, Hours of Service, and Safety of Operations of Truck and Bus Drivers*. Human Factors Research Incorporated, Goleta, California. Prepared for Bureau of Motor Carrier Safety. Report No. PB-213 963, November, 1972.
29. Heimstra, N. W.: The effects of "stress fatigue" on performance in a simulated driving situation, Ergonomics 13:209, 1966.
30. Henderson, R. L., and Berg, A.: *Vision and Audition in Driving*. Systems Development Corp. Report No. TM(L)-5297/000/00, 1974.
31. Henschel, A.: The Environment and Performance, in *Physiology of Work Capacity and Fatigue* (Springfield, Ill.: Charles C Thomas, Publisher, 1971).
32. Hilgard, E. R., Atkinson, R. C., and Atkinson, R. L.: *Introduction to Psychology* (New York: Harcourt Brace Jovanovich, Inc., 1971).
33. Hornick, R.. J.: Vibration, in *Bioastronautics Data Book* (Falls Church, Va.: Bio Technology, Inc., 1972).
34. Hornick, R. J., and Lefritz, N. M.: A study and review of human response to prolonged random vibration, Hum. Factors 8:481, 1966.
35. "How Truck Rules Affect Driver Safety," *San Francisco Chronicle*, June 26, 1978.
36. Infra and ultra sound, Directions No. 110:1. Arbetarskyddsstyrelsen, Stockholm, Sweden, May, 1978.
37. Kahn, R. L., et al.: *Organizational Stress* (New York: John Wiley & Sons, Inc., 1964).
38. Kaluger, N. A., and Smith, G. L., Jr.: Driver eye-movement patterns under conditions of prolonged driving and sleep depri-

vation, Highway Res. Rec. 336:92, 1970.

39. Kelsey, J.: An epidemiological study of the relationship between occupations and acute herniated intervertebral discs, Int. J. Epidemiol. 4:197, 1975.
40. Kelsey, J., and Hardy, R. J.: Driving of motor vehicles as a risk factor for acute herniated lumbar intervertebral disc, Am. J. Epidemiol. 102:63, 1975.
41. Kleiner, R. J., and Parker, S.: Goal striving, social status, and mental disorder, Am. Soc. Rev. 28:189, 1963.
42. Lamb, L. E., Stevens, P. M., and Johnson, R. L.: Hypokinesia secondary to chair rest from 4 to 10 days, Aerosp. Med. 36:775, 1965.
43. Lauer, A. R., and Suhr, V. W.: The effect of a rest pause on driving efficiency, Percept. Mot. Skills 9:363, 1959.
44. Lecret, F., Pin, M. C., Cura, J. B., and Pottier, M.: Les variations de la vigilance au cours de conduite sur autoroute. Presented to the Sixth SELF Congress, 1968.
45. Lisper, H-O, Laurell, H., and Stening, G.: Effects of prolonged driving and the experience of the driver on heart-rate, respiration-rate, and a subsidiary auditory reaction time. University of Uppsala, Sweden. Report No. 111, 1971 (b).
46. Margolis, B. L., Kroes, W. H., and Quinn, R. P.: Job stress: An unlisted occupational hazard, J. Occup. Med. 16:654, 1974.
47. Mast, T. M., Jones, H. V., and Heimstra, N. W.: Effects of fatigue on performance in a driving device, Highway Res. Rec. 122:93, 1966.
48. McFarland, R. A., and Moseley, A. L.: "Human Factors in Highway Transport Safety." Harvard School of Public Health, Boston, Mass., 1954.
49. Michaut, G., and Pottier, M.: Conduite en situation monotone. Organisme National de Securite Routiere. Bulletin No. 8, 1964.
50. Morgan, B. B., Brown, B. R., and Alluisi, E. A.: Effects on sustained performance of 48 hours of continuous work and sleep loss, Hum. Factors 16:406, 1974.
51. Motor Carrier Safety—The Issue in Perspective. Background. American Trucking Association, Inc. Washington, D.C., March 17, 1978.
52. *Occupational Exposure to Hot Environments*. Criteria for a Recommended Standard. U. S. Department of Health, Education, and Welfare, NIOSH. U.S. Government Printing Office, 1972.
53. *Occupational Exposure to Noise*. Criteria for a Recommended Standard. U.S. Department of Health, Education, and Welfare, NIOSH. U.S. Government Printing Office, 1972.
54. O'Hanlon, J. F.: Adrenaline's effect on human vigilance: Continuous vs. pulsatile infusions, Proc. 79th Annual Convention, APA, 1971, pp. 767–768.
55. O'Hanlon, J. F.: *Fatigue as Estimated from Concurrent Performance and Psychophysiological Measures in Prolonged Driving*. Human Factors Research, Inc. Technical Report No. 1712-1, 1971.
56. O'Hanlon, J. F.: *Vigilance, the Plasma Catecholamines and Related Bio-Chemical and Physiological Variables*. Human Factors Research, Inc. Technical Report No. 787-2, 1970.
57. Pin, M. C., Lecret, F., and Pottier, M.: Les niveaux d'activation lors de differentes situations de conduite. Organisme National de Securite Routiere. Bulletin No. 19, 1969.
58. Pinckney, T. R., and Rogers, A.: Handicapped Drivers Rated. District of Columbia Traffic Safety Reporter 16:1, 1973.
59. Platt, F. N.: A new method of evaluating the effects of fatigue on driver performance, Hum. Factors 6:351, 1964.
60. Poulton, E. C.: *Environment and Human Efficiency* (Springfield, Ill.: Charles C Thomas, Publisher, 1970).
61. Request for Proposal, U.S. Environmental Protection Agency, CI 78-0010, September, 1977.
62. Russek, H. I., and Zohlman, B. L.: Relative significance of hereditary diet and occupational stress in CHD of young adults, Am. J. Med. Sci. 235:266, 1958.
63. Safford, R. R., and Rockwell, T. H.: Performance decrement in twenty-four hour driving, Highway Res. Rec. 16:30, 1967.
64. Scheving, L. E., Vedral, D. F., and Pauly, J. E.: A circadian susceptibility rhythm in rats to pentobarbital sodium, Anat. Rec. 160:741, 1968.
65. Selye, H.: *The Stress of Life* (New York: McGraw-Hill, 1956).
66. Sherrill, R.: "Raising Hell on the Highways," *New York Times,* November 27, 1977.
67. Shoenberger, R. W.: Human response to whole-body vibration, Percept. Mot. Skills 34:127, monograph supplement 1-V34, 1972.
68. *Statistical Abstract of the United States, 1977*. U. S. Department of Commerce, Social and Economics Statistics Administra-

tion, Bureau of the Census, Washington, D.C.

69. Suhr, V. W.: Driving efficiency over a six-hour period by simulated driving performance. Unpublished doctoral dissertation, Iowa State College, 1956, in Lauer, A. R., and Suhr, V. W., The effects of a rest pause on driving efficiency, Percept. Mot. Skills 9:363, 1959.
70. Sussman, E. D., and Morris, D. F.: *An Investigation of Factors Affecting Driver Alertness*. Cornell Aeronautical Laboratory, Technical Report No. VJ-2849-B-1, 1970.
71. Taylor, G. C.: Executive stress, Int. Clin. Psychiatry 6:307, 1969.
72. Teleky, L.: Problems of nightwork: Influences on health and efficiency, Ind. Med. Surg. 12:758, 1943.
73. "The Joy of Truckin'," *Newsweek*, February 20, 1978.
74. U.S. Bureau of the Census: *Census of Transportation*, 1972, Vol. II.
75. U.S. Congress: Occupational Safety and Health Act of 1970. Public Law 91-596, 91st Congress, S 2193. Washington, D.C., December 29, 1975.
76. Vyazitskiy, P. O., and Kumanichkin, S. D.: The effect of hypodynamia on external respiration under various microclimatic conditions, Voen. Med. Zh. 7:38, 1970.
77. Waller, J. A.: Chronic medical conditions and traffic safety—review of the California experience, N. Engl. J. Med. 273:1413, 1965.
78. Wangensteen, O. H., and Bowers, W. F.: The etiology of appendicitis, Arch. Surg. 34:496, 1937.
79. White, G. H., Lange, K. O., and Coermann, R. R.: The effects of simulated buffeting on the internal pressure of man, Hum. Factors 275, 1962.
80. Winget, C., LaDou, J., and Hughes, L.: Physiological effects of rotational work shifting: A review, J. Occup. Med. 20:3, 204, 1978.
81. *Work in America,* Report of a Special Task Force to the Secretary of Health, Education, and Welfare. MIT Press, Cambridge, Mass., 1973.
82. *Work Injuries in Trucking*. State of California: Agriculture and Services Agency, Department of Industrial Relations, and Division of Labor Statistics and Research, June, 1975.
83. Wyckoff Driver Survey Shows Linkage of Regulation, Safety, Transport Topics, June 19, 1978.

PART FOUR

Psychosocial Considerations

8 / Occupational Stress

JOSEPH LaDOU, M.D.

OCCUPATIONAL STRESS is the sum of the factors in the work environment that affect the psychological and physiologic homeostasis of the worker. The stressful factor is termed a "stressor" and the worker's response to that factor is termed "stress." Hans Selye, a leading authority on stress, has described its illusory nature:

> Anyone who feels that whatever he is doing—or whatever is being done to him—is strenuous and wearing, knows vaguely what we mean by *stress*. The feelings of just being tired, jittery, or ill are subjective sensations of stress. But stress does not necessarily imply a morbid change: normal life also causes some wear and tear in the machinery of the body.[54]

and

> Life is largely a process of adaptation to the circumstances in which we exist. A perennial give-and-take has been going on between living matter and its inanimate surroundings, between one living being and another, ever since the dawn of life in the prehistoric oceans. The secret of health and happiness lies in successful adjustment to the ever-changing conditions on this globe; the penalties for failure in this great process of adaptation are disease and unhappiness.[54]

Stress factors are common in the work environment. Some stress factors are inherent in the characteristics of the job itself whereas others result from the policies of the business firm and its operations. Factors that are intrinsic to the job include physical working conditions, territorial limitations, quantitative overload and qualitative overload. Those resulting from company policies and operations are responsibility for other workers, human interrelationships, the role of the individual in the organization and the opportunities available for career development. Many of these factors cannot be strictly categorized but are interrelated and overlapping in their effects. Any one or a combination over time may cause or aggravate medical problems, such as essential hypertension, hypercholesterolemia, coronary heart disease, diabetes mellitus, peptic ulcer, obesity, heavy smoking, neuropsychiatric disease, alcoholism, drug abuse and suicide.

PHYSICAL WORKING CONDITIONS AND TERRITORIAL LIMITS

Unpleasant working conditions can produce debilitating effects in the worker. Unpleasant working conditions include assembly-line operations, insufficient or improper lighting, excessive noise, inadequate work space, depressing surroundings and unsanitary conditions. Kornhauser,[32] in a study of mental health of industrial workers, found a direct correlation between poor mental health and unpleasant working conditions. Repetitive and dehumanizing operations have been demonstrated to create physical and mental health problems for the worker.[34,55] For example, men working on assembly lines have exhibited a higher incidence of angina pectoris than those working in other job settings.[33] At present, however, not enough is known to determine the full impact of working conditions on the health of the worker.

Similarly, occupational stress may be related to what Robert Ardrey[2] has termed the "territorial imperative." Modern business and industrial organizations are highly complex, with numerous functional divisions, departments and sections, and operations frequently require that an individual leave his own area to conduct business in another area or outside the organization. Leaving his own area may create stress in the worker—for example, feelings of insecurity or nervousness.

French and Caplan[21] have studied two aspects of this problem: making work contacts across organizational boundaries and working in a territory where the dominant occupation differs from the individual's. They have found that having to make contacts across organizational boundaries is stressful and that the greater the spatial distance of the contact the more stressful is the response. At NASA's Goddard Space Flight Center, the investigators determined that workers experience less stress when making contacts within their own territories ($r = 0.31$) and that stress increased with increasing time spent in contacts with other bases and centers ($r = 0.39$).* The frequency of outside contacts was positively correlated with job-related tension and feelings of underutilization of skills. When individuals spent more time in contacts within their own territories, on the other hand, they felt less job tension and believed that their skills were utilized to maximal advantage.

Similarly, individuals working in an alien vocational environment were found to experience greater stress than those working within a group following their own vocation. Administrators working in an engineering area experienced greater quantitative and qualitative overload, greater work pressure, higher systolic and diastolic blood pressure and more rapid pulse rate. The stresses on engineers assigned to an administrative unit were related to their not being able to do the type of work they preferred, decreased opportunity for advancement and lowered utilization of skills.

As with many stressful elements in the work environment, the "territorial imperative" is interrelated with other stressors, including role ambiguity and role conflict, which are discussed below.

To date, studies on the effects on workers of physical working conditions and territorial limits are few. Controlled research is needed if we are to be able to assess adequately the problems that occur as a result of these occupational stressors.

QUANTITATIVE AND QUALITATIVE OVERLOAD

A number of studies have been directed toward assessing the effect of work overload on the worker. Overload may be broken down into two types—quantitative and qualitative overload.[21] Quantitative overload occurs when a worker is assigned more work than he can accomplish in the assigned time. Qualitative overload refers to assigning the worker tasks that are beyond his capabilities.

In modern industry, quantitative overload may be the rule rather than the exception. In a national sample survey, 44% of male white-collar workers reported that they were subjected to some degree of quantitative overload. During a study at NASA's Goddard Space Flight Center, the investigators found that 72.6% of the workers experienced this type of overload to varying degrees and that half of their working time was spent under moderate to extreme pressures.

Quantitative overload results in job tension that can lead to personal habits harmful to health. For example, cigarette smoking has been directly correlated with work overload.[22] In a job that entails numerous telephone calls, office visits and meetings per unit of work time, the individual is likely to become a heavier smoker than

*r measures the extent to which two variables are correlated. Correlations can range from $+1.00$ to -1.00, with $+1.00$ indicating that variables are positively and completely correlated and -1.00 indicating that there is a perfect inverse relationship. A 0.00 correlation ($r = 0.00$) would indicate that two variables were completely unrelated.

someone in a less stressful situation. The incidence of coronary heart disease is increased under these conditions, even in young men.[16]

The length of time worked per day is another aspect of quantitative overload. It is well known that performance and proficiency decline steadily after a certain number of hours worked. But less is known about the physical and psychological consequences of long hours. One indication is that a positive correlation has been found between coronary heart disease and the number of hours worked per day. For example, in a study of mortality rates of men in California, investigators discovered that workers in light industry under the age of 45 who were on the job more than 48 hours a week had twice the risk of death from coronary heart disease as workers of similar age and similar employment who worked 40 hours or less a week.[52] Another study of young coronary patients revealed that 25% had been working at two jobs and 45% had been working in jobs that entailed 60 or more hours per week.[9] In 91% of these cases, prolonged emotional strain had preceded the coronary incident; similar stress situations were noted in only 20% of the control subjects.

Quantitative overload has also been found to relate to various stress indicators—escapist drinking ($r = 0.06$), absenteeism ($r = 0.06$), low work motivation ($r = 0.26$), lowered self-esteem ($r = 0.10$) and lack of interest in contributing suggestions to management ($r = 0.17$).[35] The coefficients are small but statistically significant. Additional findings further indicate that quantitative overload is a source of occupational stress.[47, 48]

Qualitative overload—work that is too difficult for the individual—appears to be another source of job-related stress even though research in this area has been neither extensive nor conclusive. The investigators in one study concentrated on both quantitative and qualitative overload in administrators and professors in a large university.[16] By means of medical examinations, questionnaires and interviews, the investigators explored the relationship between work overload—both quantitative and qualitative—and the incidence of coronary heart disease. In studying low self-esteem, one symptom of job-related stress, they found a different pattern among the administrators than among the professors. For the administrators, low self-esteem was associated with quantitative overload whereas for the professors it was linked to qualitative overload. The administrators suffered feelings of low self-esteem when they had too much to do and the professors when their tasks were too difficult. The investigators also found that quantitative and qualitative overload were positively correlated with achievement orientation ($r = 0.42$ and $r = 0.25$, respectively). A later study demonstrated a strong correlation between achievement orientation and the level of serum uric acid ($r = 0.68$).[12] A correlation has also been found between work overload and increased cholesterol level. Friedman and associates[24] determined such a correlation in tax accountants before a tax deadline and Dreyfuss and Czaczkes[17] noted it in medical students who were required to perform medical examinations while being observed.

French and Caplan[21] suggest that quantitative and qualitative overload produce the following physiologic and psychological symptoms: increased cholesterol, accelerated heart rate, job dissatisfaction, job tension, lowered self-esteem, feelings of threat and embarrassment, and increased smoking. The effects of quantitative and qualitative overload cannot be viewed as exclusively job-related stressors, but must be considered in conjunction with the personality of the individual.

HUMAN INTERRELATIONSHIPS

Unsatisfactory relationships with supervisors, colleagues and subordinates can have a debilitating effect not only on the employee but also on the organization for which he works.[3,15] French and Caplan[21] define poor relationships in the work environment as "those which include low trust, low supportiveness, and low interest in listening to and trying to deal with problems that confront the organizational member." Some investigators have concluded that mistrust among workers is closely correlated with strong feelings of role ambiguity, which results in poor communications and psychological strain.[13,30] Kahn and associates[30] found that one source of unsatisfactory human relationship on the job was the feeling of threat from superiors ($r = 0.41$) and colleagues ($r = 0.44$); employees did not have this feeling, however, with regard to their subordinates ($r = 0.12$).

Lack of consideration by managers also creates job tension. Buck[13] used the Fleishman leadership questionnaire in studying this aspect of worker relationships. Managerial consideration was graded in terms of "friendship," "mutual trust," "respect" and "feelings of warmth between employee and supervisor." Workers who believed that their superiors were inconsiderate complained of favoritism, taking advantage of subordinates, criticism that was not constructive and "pulling rank." The investigator concluded that inconsiderate behavior of supervisors "contributed significantly to feelings of job pressure."

Poor work relationships often are found when conflict occurs over the methods to be used and the priorities to be followed in a job or project ($r = 0.24$) or when inadequate information is provided to designate responsibilities, individual job roles and the means of carrying them out. Such conflicts are not easily resolved and frequently the outcome is determined subjectively by the stronger, more aggressive individual involved in the decision. Unsatisfactory human relationships in the work environment—whether caused by such conflicts or by poor communication—produce psychological stress in workers, stress that is reflected in feelings of low job satisfaction and job threat.

JOB RESPONSIBILITY

Responsibility for a job, a project or for other workers is a stress factor that can cause psychological changes in the employee who bears the responsibility. For example, the assembly-line worker who is raised to a supervisory position may develop a peptic ulcer. In a study of military aviators, Miller[40] determined that 17-hydroxycorticosteroid increased in the blood and urine of pilots during maneuvers. In a later study designed to compare the responses of pilots having primary responsibility for performance of the airplane with radiomen who had no such responsibility, Miller also found that the pilots exhibited greater corticosteroid responses than did the radiomen. Heart rate of pilots manning aircraft increased more than the heart rate of copilots; when their roles were reversed, the copilots exhibited an increase in heart rate and the pilots did not.[40]

French and Caplan[21] found a positive correlation between responsibility for other individuals' work and diastolic blood pressure in a group of NASA personnel at Goddard Space Flight Center. Sharp increases in heart rate also resulted when key NASA personnel suddenly were given additional responsibility. The medical director of one NASA program concluded that "something we simply call 'responsibility' often results in extremely high cardiac rates and is probably a much larger factor in rate changes than was formerly thought."[67] The relationship between accelerated heart rate and added responsibility has been observed even among senior executives with a long history of responsibility.[46]

Wardwell and coinvestigators[66] found that individuals who were responsible for people were more subject to heart disease than those responsible for machines. The stress resulting from added responsibility for people can be attributed to a number of factors, including the need to spend more time interacting with people and their problems, having to attend more meetings and being forced to meet more constrictive schedules and deadlines. Responsibility for people has also been related to the following symptoms of stress: heavy smoking (r = 0.31), increased diastolic blood pressure (r = 0.23) and heightened serum cholesterol levels (index of nonlinear association equaling 0.23).[13] The responsibility-for-people stressor particularly affects clerical, managerial and professional workers.

Because individuals with considerable responsibility in the work environment usually are older, the effects of this stressor must be separated from the effects of aging. Pincherle[46] studied 2000 British executives during their medical checkups and found that physical stress symptoms were linked not only to the level of responsibility but also to the age of the individual. Thus, older executives exhibited more symptoms of cardiac disease and more cardiac risk factors. Terhune[63] also established this relationship. Stressors other than responsibility may play a part in the responses of the older executive. These stressors could include awareness that further advancement is unlikely, awareness of approaching retirement and the threat of isolation from the work scene and restriction of interest in the job. Further research is needed to determine the effects of each factor and to isolate the effect of occupational cumulative injury from the normal aging process.

ROLE OF THE INDIVIDUAL IN THE ORGANIZATION

Many workers suffer from uncertainty about their place in the companies that employ them. This uncertainty consists of two stressors: role ambiguity and role conflict. *Role ambiguity* results from a lack of clarity concerning the requirements of the job—that is, the employee does not know the objectives, scope and responsibilities of his job or what is expected of him by his superiors and colleagues; in essence, he does not have adequate information to perform his work properly. *Role conflict*, on the other hand, occurs when conflicting demands are made on the employee by different groups in his organization or when the employee is required to do work that he dislikes or believes to be outside the requirements of his job classification.

The extent of the incidence of this stressor is not known, but studies have indicated that between 34.7% and 60% of workers are affected by role ambiguity.[21,30] Kahn and associates[30] determined that individuals who are affected by role ambiguity exhibit dissatisfaction with their jobs (r = 0.32), feelings of tension on the job (r = 0.41) and lowered self-confidence (r = 0.27). In a study of 205 engineers, scientists and administrators, French and Caplan[21] observed that role ambiguity was closely correlated with job dissatisfaction (r = 0.42) and feelings of threat to physical and mental well-being (r = 0.40); physiologic indicators observed in the subjects included increased blood pressure and heart rate. Other research has established weak relationships between role ambiguity and mental depression (r = 0.12), lowered self-esteem (r = 0.16), dissatisfaction with life (r = 0.08), job dissatisfaction (r = 0.13), lack of motivation to work (r = 0.06) and job switching (r = 0.07).[35]

The degree of role ambiguity that can be tolerated differs from individual to individual. Individuals who are most comfortable in a highly structured environment with a minimum of ambiguity experience the greatest job-related tension when faced with this stressor.[30]

Role conflict is well established as a significant stressor. The most typical conflict situations are caused by the following:

Differing opinions between one organization unit and another concerning what the job should entail.

Conflicting job demands.

Conflicts resulting from the need to get along with people.

Differences of opinion between supervisors and subordinates over what the job should entail.

Problems related to managing subordinates.

Conflicts resulting from having to perform certain duties, such as administrative functions, that are unpleasant or unwelcome.

One national survey has indicated that approximately 48% of U.S. workers are affected by the role conflict stressor.[30] The problem is more pronounced in some organizations than in others. For example, the percentage of individuals affected by it at one NASA center was considerably higher than the national average—67.1% compared with 48% for the nation as a whole.[21] Some jobs also entail more role conflict than others. In the NASA study, the investigators found that administrators experienced problems of role conflict more often than did engineers or scientists.[21] This situation probably occurs because administrators have less time to spend working by themselves (34% as compared with 38% for engineers and 57% for scientists).

Individuals affected by the role conflict stressor exhibit both emotional and physiologic responses. Job dissatisfaction and job-related tension increase and mean heart rate is accelerated.[13] In monitoring the heart rates of 22 men at NASA Headquarters, French and Caplan[22] found that role conflict correlated with increased heart rate (r = 0.61). Heart rate was monitored for 2½ hours during the workday by telemetry; seven measures of role conflict were obtained by a questionnaire.

Shirom and co-workers[56] conducted a comprehensive study concerning role conflict in 762 men, 30 years of age and older, from 13 kibbutzim in Israel. The relationships were studied between occupational stress factors, including role ambiguity and role conflict, and coronary disease (myocardial infarction, angina pectoris and coronary insufficiency), abnormal electrocardiograms and cardiac risk factors (systolic blood pressure, pulse rate, serum cholesterol levels and smoking habits). All data were grouped according to occupation—i.e., white-collar workers, craftsmen, agricultural workers and factory employees. There was a weak but statistically significant relationship (r = 0.19) in white-collar workers between role conflict and abnormal electrocardiogram readings. Occupations entailing the greatest physical exertion, such as agricultural work, had the lowest incidence of role conflict. As physical exertion on the job decreased, coronary heart disease (myocardial infarction, angina pectoris and coronary insufficiency) was found to increase significantly. The investigators also found a strong correlation between role conflict and obesity. Their results suggest that role conflict is most prevalent in clerical, managerial and professional work.

The stress effect of an individual's occupational level, which is another aspect of one's role within the organization, has been the subject of a number of studies. But the findings from these studies have been conflicting. Some have related occupational level to coronary heart disease, with the risk factors increasing with higher occupational level.[9, 36, 53, 61, 66] U.S. and British national statistics support these findings. Conversely, Pell and D'Alonzo,[45] in a study of Du Pont employees, found an inverse relationship between myocardial infarction and salary level. Others have found no correlation between heart disease and occupational level.[5, 6, 44, 57, 58] Conflicting data indicate the need for more carefully controlled research.

CAREER DEVELOPMENT

Occupational stress can also be related to career development, which includes such stressors as overpromotion, underpromotion, status incongruence (lack of a match between an individual's rate of advancement and his experience), lack of security in the job and thwarted ambition.

When an individual is overpromoted and given a position of responsibility beyond his capabilities or underpromoted and not given a position commensurate with his abilities, behavioral disorders and sometimes even mental illness can occur.[11, 31, 43, 62] Brook[11] undertook to prepare 4 case studies on individuals who exhibited behavioral problems as the result of either overpromotion or underpromotion. The problems of these individuals progressed from minor psychological symptoms (palpitations, episodes of panic, etc.) to marked psychosomatic complaints and finally to mental illness. It has been suggested that career development stress results from feelings that work has value solely as a means of "getting on in the world" and "desires for fame and success."[62] Kleiner and Parker[31] proposed that frustrated job aspirations are linked to mental disorders; a later study of urban blacks added support to this hypothesis.[43]

The U.S. Navy undertook a comprehensive research program to assess systematically the problem of status incongruence. The investigators found that promotional lag among naval personnel was significantly related to psychiatric illness.[4] In later work, they observed that job satisfaction increased when the rate of promotion exceeded expectations ($r = 0.085$, <0.01) and decreased when advancement was slow.[19] Individuals who were not promoted commensurate with their expectations suffered the greatest stress. In a later study of more than 9000 Navy ratings, the same investigators found a direct correlation between status incongruence and psychiatric disorders and between status congruence and job performance ($r = 0.64$).[18]

It is understandable that a lack of opportunity for career development in an organization can lead to frustration, depression, job indifference and antagonism. The effects of this job-related stressor, particularly with regard to neuropsychiatric problems, make it a serious problem in the occupational environment and an important point of future research.

DISEASES RELATED TO OCCUPATIONAL STRESS

Humans, like other animals, when faced with stressors that require behavioral adjustment, exhibit an involuntary response—the fight-or-flight response. This response is associated with increased activity of the autonomic nervous system. As a result of this increased activity there are increases in blood pressure, heart rate, respiratory rate, blood flow to the skeletal muscles, metabolism and release of some hormones as the individual prepares for conflict or escape. Because of the continual stresses of modern life, the fight-or-flight response is elicited frequently. But within the mores of our society, fighting or running usually is unacceptable behavior. The result is stress as it currently is envisioned. The combination of excessive stimulation of and a restrictive social attitude toward the fight-or-flight response may cause or aggravate physical and mental disorders, as well as hasten the aging process in general.

Occupational stress has not yet been recognized as a major public health problem, but many investigators are convinced that psychosocial stimuli—including occupational stress—are important contributors to disease or risk of disease, including coronary heart disease, essential hypertension, gastrointestinal problems, neuropsychiatric illnesses, escapist drinking, drug addiction and suicide.

Coronary Heart Disease and Hypertension

Mortality from heart disease has increased drastically since the 1920s. Over the decade of the 1940s, for example, the mortality rate from heart disease among white males between the ages of 35 and 64 increased by 23%.[7] It has become the leading cause of death in the United States. Stressful life events, including job dissatisfaction, economic frustration and excessive work and responsibility, all appear to contribute to the risk of coronary heart disease.[28, 29] In general, most high-risk individuals are exposed to a high degree of responsibility for other people, work overload and role conflicts.

Stress contributes to the development of coronary heart disease through increasing such coronary risk factors as serum cholesterol and essential hypertension, accelerating the rate of development of damage to the intima of the coronary arteries over time and contributing to the aggregation of blood platelets, which combine into arterial plaques, leading to narrowing of the coronary arteries.[26] Stress also contributes to coronary disease by stimulating the discharge of adrenalin and noradrenalin from the adrenal medulla and sympathetic nerve endings. Both adrenalin and noradrenalin can cause arterial damage and myocardial lesions,[49, 50] as well as contribute to platelet production.[8, 60]

The personality of the individual, as indicated earlier, also has a bearing on his response to stress, particularly with regard to coronary heart disease and hypertension, a primary risk factor for this disease. One widely used personality classification identifies all individuals as either Type A or Type B. Type A individuals are overly ambitious and highly competitive, are governed by a strong sense of time urgency and are frequently subject to feelings of hostility and aggression. Type B personalities, on the other hand, are the antithesis of the Type As. Individuals fall in any one of four categories: fully developed As, incompletely developed As, fully developed Bs and incompletely developed Bs. Type A personalities compound their responses to stress because of their character traits whereas Type B personalities exhibit less sharp responses to stressors.

Type A individuals frequently suffer from hypertension and are considered to be coronary prone. In a study of 3400 men known to be free from coronary heart disease, the subjects were classified as to personality type, either Type A or Type B.[1] Two and one-half years later, when the subjects were observed again, the Type A men (aged 39–49) had 6.5 times the incidence of coronary heart disease as did Type B individuals of the same age range. The traits that predispose Type A people to coronary attacks (competitiveness, sense of time urgency, hostility and aggressiveness), when coupled with stressors in the occupational environment, make them prime candidates for coronary heart disease. Their proneness to coronaries may be mediated by their adrenalin/noradrenalin responses. The initial reaction of a Type A individual to an uncontrollable stressor (one that cannot be avoided) is a concerted effort to assert control over the stimulus. With this response, the adrenalin/noradrenalin discharge can be compounded, exerting further injury on the cardiovascular system.

A correlation between work overload and coronary heart disease has also been suggested by a number of studies. Kritsikis and co-workers[33] studied 150 men with angina pectoris among 4000 industrial workers in Berlin and suggested from their findings that this problem was related to the pressures of assembly-line work. Froberg and associates[25] observed that young female invoicing clerks, when subjected to work overload, exhibited increases in excretion of adrenalin and noradrenalin of 40% and 27%, respectively. Others also have concluded that work overload is a probable contributor to coronary disease.[21, 27, 33, 45]

Hypertension has long been considered to be a psychosomatic disease associated with highly stressful situations. Essential hypertension may result from continuing exposure to stressful conditions in the work environment. Mjasnikov[41] found a high incidence of hypertension in telephone operators in a large exchange who were required to complete many transactions per unit of time with few rest periods. Air traffic controllers, who work in a highly stressful occupation, have been found to exhibit an incidence of hypertension 4 times greater than that found in second-class airmen, who are not subjected to the same degree of stress.[14] Moreover, nearly 6 times as many new cases of hypertension occurred annually among air traffic controllers as occurred among the second-class airmen with whom they were compared. Similarly, the incidence of diabetes was 3 times greater in the air traffic controllers.

It has been estimated that cardiovascular diseases account for 12% of time lost from the job annually by U.S. workers, or a loss of $4 billion per year in business and industry.[20] This represents a serious loss to the nation—a loss that is further compounded by the cost in human suffering and human life.

There is a growing awareness that job stress is costly to industry. Decreased quality of work, increased absenteeism, increased turnover and effects on the cost of health insurance for the worker and worker's family are some of the concerns expressed by researchers in the field of occupational stress. In California, awards under workers' compensation for disability held to be work related are causing a rapid increase in the cost of insurance. There is a growing precedent in that state and in many others that diseases as diverse as coronary heart disease, stroke, hypertension, arthritis, alcoholism and obesity are compensable under the workers' compensation system. Unfortunately, the extent and quality of research in the area of occupational stress leaves our legislators and judiciary with no alternative to the conservative position that awards ought not to be given until such time as medical research becomes more definitive about stress-related disease and the impact of the industrial setting.

Stanislav V. Kasl of the Yale University School of Medicine has reviewed the medical literature on occupational stress from the viewpoint of an epidemiologist. His conclusions are both revealing and deservedly critical. He points out that "there is no integrated program of research in which stress at work and cardiovascular health are systematically studied and where new studies build on the results of earlier ones. Instead, the studies are truly a mixed bag, in the sense of variety of methodologies, settings, conceptualizations, and inadequacies. The overall picture is quite suggestive, but there are many gaps and very few individual studies are above methodological criticism or offer an unambiguous interpretation."*

Gastrointestinal Problems

Peptic ulcer, digestive disturbances and related gastrointestinal problems have been found to be related to occupational stress. Duodenal ulcer, which accounts for the bulk of peptic ulcer in males, is known to result from stressful situations in the work environment. It has been observed in first-line supervisors[60] and air traffic controllers.[14] In a study of the latter, medical histories of 4325 male journeyman air traffic controllers were compared with those of 8435 second-class airmen. The incidence of duodenal ulcer was twice as great in the controllers as in the airmen (observed 48; expected 26.3; $p < 0.001$); the disease also appeared at a lower age in the controllers. The study also revealed a statistically significant difference between the incidence of peptic ulcer in individuals working in high-stress versus low-stress environments (observed 29; expected 13.6; $x^2 = 17$, $p < 0.001$). The investigators concluded that, compared with airmen, air traffic controllers have a high risk of developing peptic ulcer, that they develop the disease at a younger age and that the disease is related to job stress.

There also appears to be a relationship between occupational stress and digestive disorders. On the basis of data from a national survey conducted by the Bureau of the Census in 701 counties in the United States, Wan and Wright[65] concluded that digestive disorders were responsible for 13% of occupational limitations in laborers, 4% in foremen and craftsmen and 7% in managers and professionals. Brodsky[10] studied the long-term effects of work stress in prison guards and teachers—both of which

*Kasl, S. V.: Epidemiological Contributions to the Study of Work Stress, in Cooper, C. L., and Payne, R. (eds.), *Stress at Work* (Chichester: John Wiley & Sons, Inc., 1978).

experience the same stresses of responsibility for others, role ambiguity, work overload and fear. It is clear from knowledge of the two occupations that individuals in both are responsible for others and usually are subject to overload. What is less clear is the part that role ambiguity plays. It occurs in both work environments because both are in a status of change and becoming more volatile places, and neither prison administrators nor school administrators have developed firm policies concerning how to cope with the changes. The fear stressor, of course, is easy to understand, since work in a volatile environment where violence may be forthcoming cannot help but result in a fear response in individuals working in that environment. Gastrointestinal disorders were common among the guards and teachers studied. Loss of appetite and digestive and bowel difficulties predominated, with the workers becoming increasingly concerned about their physical conditions.

Neuropsychiatric Illnesses

Poor mental health and psychiatric illness in the work environment have received increasing attention since World War II. Such problems are manifested by low job satisfaction, low self-esteem, job tension, anxiety, impaired interpersonal relationships and psychosomatic illnesses. The stressors creating these problems are role conflict and ambiguity, quantitative and qualitative overload resulting from rapid technologic change, responsibility for managing people, conflicts in human relationships within the work environment and lack of worker autonomy in the organization.[59]

Other established relationships include low economic status with higher rates of psychiatric hospitalization and symptomatology, long periods of unemployment with high suicide rates and psychiatric hospitalization, and a positive correlation between job satisfaction and mental health. Unfortunately, the relationships between occupational stress and neuropsychiatric problems cannot be isolated from biologic, psychological, societal and cultural causes. One relationship that can be established conclusively, however, is that between physically hazardous working conditions and mental illness.[67]

Kornhauser,[32] in a study of 407 automobile assembly-line workers found that about 40% suffered from some symptoms of mental health problems and that the primary explanation is the relationship of job satisfaction and mental health. His study made clear that other variables may play a role, including education, favorable economic conditions and other socioeconomic factors; nonetheless, distinct occupational effects were found when the foregoing factors were held constant. Kornhauser found that:

> Job satisfaction varied consistently with the level of job. Higher-level blue-collar workers exhibited better mental health than nonskilled workers.
>
> Job dissatisfaction depended on the characteristics of the job—dull, repetitive, unchallenging, low-paying jobs were responsible for the greatest job dissatisfaction. Absenteeism correlated closely with job dissatisfaction.
>
> Work was the primary institution in the lives of the workers (above family, leisure and social institutions), yet only 25% responded that they would choose the same type of work if they had another chance.
>
> Many workers suffered from feelings of helplessness, withdrawal, alienation and pessimism. For example, 50% of assembly-line workers believed that they had little influence over the future course of their lives, compared with only 17% of nonfactory workers.
>
> Workers with the lowest scores on mental health and job satisfaction often exhibited escapist or passive reactions in their lives away from work—they watched television and did not vote or participate in community activities.
>
> The challenge of the job and interest in the job were more accurate predictors of mental health than were wages, security and the physical conditions of work.
>
> Self-esteem correlated strongly with job satisfaction and mental health.

The findings of Kornhauser's 20-year study have been generally corroborated by subsequent research.[37, 64, 67] Kornhauser's conclusion concerning the effect of the working environment on mental health presents a realistic picture of the problem:

> Poorer mental health occurs whenever conditions of work and life lead to continuing frustration by failing to offer means for perceived progress toward attainment of strongly desired goals which have become indispensable elements of the individual's self-identity as a worthwhile person. Persistent failure and frustration bring lowered self-esteem and dissatisfaction with life, often accompanied by anxieties, social alienation and withdrawal, a narrowing of goals and curtailing of aspirations—in short . . . poor mental health.

Alcoholism, Drug Addiction and Suicide

Alan McLean, a physician who has studied behavioral problems of white-collar workers in the work environment, has stated that "workers with personality disorders, including alcoholism and drug abuse, may find that their psychiatric disorders stem partially from job insecurity, unpleasant working conditions, or hazardous work."[39]

Research in this area has been limited. Many physicians and sociologists, however, have corroborated this conclusion on the basis of their clinical findings. For example, alcoholism is common among executive personnel who experience occupational stress. Interviews during a comprehensive study conducted in 1973 for the Department of Health, Education, and Welfare on problems in the work environment indicated that many workers in heavy industry drink heavily on the lunch hour to enable them to withstand the pressures and overwhelming monotony of their jobs during the afternoon shift.[67]

The same study also revealed a disturbing amount of drug use on the job among younger workers, particularly assembly-line workers and long-haul truck drivers. The New York Narcotics Addiction Control Commission found that drug use varied significantly by occupation,[67] and a study by a United Auto Workers Local of a plant employing 3400 people revealed 15% of the workers probably were addicted to heroin.[67]

More conservative estimates of the level of drug abuse in New York industry can be found in data from a 1970 survey,[38] which disclosed that:

> Marijuana was smoked by 12.1% of all employed workers, 4% being regular users, one-fourth of whom report smoking marijuana on the job. Sales workers accounted for the highest incidence of regular use and for use while at work.
>
> Heroin was used by 1.3% of all employed workers, 0.5% being regular users, more than one-third of whom reported using heroin while on the job. Sales workers again were the most likely drug users among job categories.
>
> LSD and Methedrine were used by more than 2% of all employed workers.

Although alcoholism and drug abuse most likely do not result from any single cause, occupational stressors do appear to contribute to excessive drinking and drug habituation.[42] Both problems may occur or be aggravated by role ambiguity and its resultant anxiety in the worker. Similarly, quantitative and qualitative overload appear to be important risk factors for both alcoholism and drug addiction.

Although there are no statistics on suicide by occupation, it is known that the suicide rate is higher among white men than among black men and among men than among women. It is probable that suicide is not genetically linked to either race or sex and that the explanation for it is a host of sociopsychological factors. This hypothesis is tentatively supported by the results of a study that found that female doctors and chemists had a higher suicide rate than women in general.[51] Similarly, it has been found that the suicide rates are higher among professional Type A individuals than the national norm. It is also worth noting that suicide rates among blacks are rising even as they are entering occupational fields that formerly employed only whites.

The available data linking job stressors

with alcoholism, drug abuse and suicide are suggestive rather than conclusive. Logically, however, the work environment would appear to play some role (perhaps a more important one than we are aware of). Further knowledge will be needed to determine causal links between these problems and work conditions; such knowledge may be difficult to acquire, however, because of the lack of adequate devices for measurement.

CONCLUSIONS

There are many weaknesses in the methods used in past research, as well as major gaps in our knowledge of occupational stressors and their impact on the physical and mental health of the work force. Nonetheless, present evidence suggests that occupational stress probably is an important contributor to some diseases, along with other factors in the home and social environments. The impact of these various factors must be isolated before the true impact of occupational stress can be known.

Stanislav V. Kasl has pointed out that much of the research on occupational stress has not been adequately planned and too often is focused on conditions in the work environment rather than including the inherent problems of the individual working in that environment. He, and other essayists in *Stress at Work*, are in general agreement that (1) poorly designed cross-sectional studies are to be avoided; (2) research must be longitudinal, preferably designed around natural experiments (significant events and transitions) that will better reveal the way that the work environment affects health and well-being and the manner in which the individual adapts to his environment and changes therein; (3) a frontal attack is needed on the entire issue of defining and measuring environmental stress subjectively and relating it to subjective measures of distress; and (4) more studies are needed on the interrelationships of various life roles—e.g., the work environment with conditions in the home.*

However, even the suggestion that the work environment may have a destructive effect on the worker mandates that changes be made in that environment. French and Caplan[22] have suggested that

> Many of the stresses which are fairly prevalent in national samples and in specific organizational settings appear to be linked in one way or another with strains which produce coronary heart disease. But, the fact that coronary heart disease seems to be as much a part of organizational life as are other traits of organizations (such as size and structure) does not mean that steps cannot be taken to reduce the risk of disease. There are innovative measures available to management. Programs which involve the coordinated effort of management, medical personnel, and organizational psychologists can be developed. Careful evaluation of these programs can be carried out; and through such experimental programs, modern organizations can make potentially important contributions to both management and medical science, with benefits for both the individual's and the organization's well-being and strength.

The development of reasonable controls over problem areas in the work environment and the early diagnosis and treatment of occupational stress are vitally essential, not only from a financial standpoint but, more important, from a humanitarian standpoint.

---

*Kasl, S. V.: Epidemiological Contributions to the Study of Work Stress, in Cooper, C. L., and Payne, R. (eds.), *Stress at Work* (Chichester: John Wiley & Sons, Inc., 1978).

REFERENCES

1. Ardlie, N. G., Glew, G., and Schwartz, C. J.: Influence of catecholamines on nucleotide-induced platelet aggregation, Nature 212:415, 1966.
2. Ardrey, R.: *The Territorial Imperative* (New York: Dell, 1968).
3. Argyris, C.: *Integrating the Individual and the Organization* (New York: John Wiley & Sons, Inc., 1964).
4. Arthur, R. J., and Gunderson, E. K.: Promotion and mental illness in the Navy, J. Occup. Med. 7:452, 1965.

5. Bainton, C. R., and Peterson, D. R.: Deaths from coronary heart disease in persons fifty years of age and younger: A community-wide study, N. Engl. J. Med. 268:569, 1963.
6. Berkson, D.: Socioeconomic correlates of atherosclerotic and hypertensive heart disease, in culture, society and health, Ann. N.Y. Acad. Sci. 84:835, 1960.
7. Borhani, N. O.: Magnitude of the Problem of Cardiovascular-Renal Disease, in Lilienfield, A. M., and Gifford, A. J. (eds.), *Chronic Diseases and Public Health* (Baltimore: Johns Hopkins Press, 1966).
8. Brady, J. V.: Ulcers in the executive monkeys, Sci. Am. 99:75, 1958.
9. Breslow, L., and Buell, P.: Mortality from coronary heart disease and physical activity of work in California, J. Chronic Dis. 11:615, 1960.
10. Brodsky, C. M.: Long-term work stress in teachers and prison guards, J. Occup. Med. 19:133, 1977.
11. Brook, A.: Mental stress at work, Practitioner 210:500, 1973.
12. Brooks, G. W., and Mueller, E. F.: Serum urate concentrations among university professors, JAMA 195:415, 1966.
13. Buck, V.: *Working under Pressure* (London: Staples, 1972).
14. Cobb, S., and Rose, R. M.: Hypertension, peptic ulcer, and diabetes in air traffic controllers, JAMA 224:489, 1973.
15. Cooper, C. L.: *Group Training for Individual and Organizational Development* (Basel: S. Karger, 1973).
16. Cooper, C. L., and Marshall, J.: Occupational sources of stress; a review of the literature relating to coronary heart disease and mental ill health, J. Occup. Psychol. 49:11, 1976.
17. Dreyfuss, F., and Czaczkes, J. W.: Blood cholesterol and uric acid of healthy medical students under stress of examination, Arch. Intern. Med. 103:708, 1959.
18. Erickson, J., Edwards, D., and Gunderson, E. K.: Status congruency and mental health, Psychol. Rep. 33:395, 1973.
19. Erickson, J., Pugh, W. M., and Gunderson, E. K.: Status congruency as a predictor of job satisfaction and life stress, J. Appl. Psychol. 56:523, 1972.
20. Felton, J. S., and Cole, R.: The high cost of heart disease, Circulation 27:957, 1963.
21. French, J. R. P., and Caplan, R. D.: Organizational Stress and Individual Strain, in Marrow, A. J. (ed.), *The Failure of Success* (New York: AMACOM, 1973).
22. French, J. R. P., and Caplan, R. D.: Psychosocial factors in coronary heart disease, Ind. Med. 39:383, 1970.
23. French, J. R. P., Tupper, C. J., and Mueller, E. I.: Workload of university professors. Unpublished research report, Ann Arbor, Mich., University of Michigan, 1965.
24. Friedman, M., Rosenman, R. H., and Carroll, V.: Changes in serum cholesterol and blood clotting time in men subjected to cyclic variations of occupational stress, Circulation 17:852, 1958.
25. Froberg, J., Karlsson, C., Levi, L., and Lidberg, L.: Physiological and Biochemical Stress Reactions Induced by Psychosocial Stimuli, in Levi, L. (ed.), *Society, Stress, and Disease* (London: Oxford University Press, 1971).
26. Glass, D. C.: *Behavior Patterns, Stress, and Coronary Disease* (Hillsdale, N.J.: Lawrence Erlbaum Assoc., 1977).
27. Glass, D. C.: Stress, behavior patterns, and coronary disease, Am. Sci. 65:177, 1977.
28. House, J. S.: Occupational Stress as a Precursor to Coronary Disease, in Gentry, W. D., and Williams, R. B., Jr. (eds.), *Psychological Aspects of Myocardial Infarction and Coronary Care* (St. Louis: The C. V. Mosby Company, 1975).
29. Jenkins, C. D.: Psychologic and social precursors of coronary disease, N. Engl. J. Med. 284:244, 1971.
30. Kahn, R. L., Wolfe, D. M., Quinn, R. P., Snoek, J. D., and Rosenthal, R. A.: *Organizational Stress* (New York: John Wiley & Sons, Inc., 1964).
31. Kleiner, R. J., and Parker, S.: Goal striving, social status, and mental disorder, Am. Sociol. Rev. 28:189, 1963.
32. Kornhauser, A.: *Mental Health of the Industrial Worker* (New York: John Wiley & Sons, Inc., 1965).
33. Kritsikis, S. P., Heinemann, A. L., and Eitner, S.: Die Angina Pectoris im Aspekt ihrer Korrelation mit biologischer Disposition, psychologischen und soziologischen Emflussfaktoren, Dtsch. Gesundheitsw. 23: 1878, 1968.
34. Marcson, S.: *Automation, Alienation and Anomie* (New York: Harper & Row, 1970).
35. Margolis, B. L., Kroes, W. H., and Quinn, R. P.: Job stress: An unlisted occupational hazard, J. Occup. Med. 16:654, 1974.
36. McDonough, J. R., Hames, C. G., Stulb, S. C., and Garrison, G. E.: Coronary heart disease among Negroes and whites in Evans County, Georgia, J. Chronic Dis. 18:443, 1965.
37. McLean, A., and Taylor, G. C.: *Mental*

Health in Industry (New York: McGraw-Hill, 1958).
38. Meiselas, H., and Brill, L.: Drug abuse in industry—issues and comments, Ind. Med. 41:10, 1972.
39. *Mental Health and Work Organizations*, McLean, A. (ed.) (New York: Rand McNally, 1970).
40. Miller, J. G.: Information input overload and psychopathology, Am. J. Psychiatry 8:116, 1960.
41. Mjasnikov, A.: Discussion in Proc. Joint WHO-Czech Cardio. Soc. Symp. Pathogen Essential Hypertension, Prague, 1961.
42. New York Narcotics Addiction Control Commission: Differential drug use within the New York State labor force, July, 1971.
43. Parker, S., and Kleiner, R. J.: *Mental Illness in the Urban Negro Community* (New York: The Free Press, 1966).
44. Paul, O.: A longitudinal study of coronary heart disease, Circulation 28:20, 1963.
45. Pell, S., and D'Alonzo, C. A.: Myocardial infarction in a one year industrial study, JAMA 166:332, 1958.
46. Pincherle, G.: Fitness for work, Proc. R. Soc. Med. 65:321, 1972.
47. Porter, L. W., and Lawler, E. E.: Properties of organization structure in relation to job attitudes and job behavior, Psychol. Bull. 64:23, 1965.
48. Quinn, R. P., Seashore, S., and Mangione, I.: *Survey of Working Conditions* (Washington, D.C.: U.S. Government Printing Office, 1971).
49. Rabb, W., Chaplin, J. B., and Bajusz, E.: Myocardial necroses produced in domesticated rats and in wild rats by sensory and emotional stresses, Proc. Soc. Exp. Biol. Med. 116:665, 1964.
50. Raab, W. E., Stark, E., MacMillan, W. H., and Gigee, W. R.: Sympathetic origin and antiadrenergic prevention of stress-induced myocardial lesions, Am. J. Cardiol. 8:203, 1961.
51. Roman, P. M., and Trice, H. M.: The development of deviant drinking behavior, Arch. Environ. Health 20:424, 1970.
52. Russek, H. I., and Zohlman, B. L.: Relative significance of hereditary diet and occupational stress in CHD of young adults, Am. J. Med. Sci. 235:266, 1958.
53. Ryle, J. A., and Russell, W. T.: The natural history of coronary disease: A clinical and epidemiological study, Br. Heart J. 11:370, 1949.
54. Selye, H.: *The Stress of Life* (New York: McGraw-Hill, 1956).
55. Shepard, J. M.: *Automation and Alienation* (Cambridge, Mass.: MIT Press, 1971).
56. Shirom, A., Eden, D., Silberwasser, S., and Kellerman, J. J.: Job stresses and risk factors in coronary heart disease among occupational categories in kibbutzim, Soc. Sci. Med. 7:875, 1975.
57. Spain, D. M.: Problems in the study of coronary atherosclerosis in population groups, in culture, society and health, Ann. N.Y. Acad. Sci. 84:816, 1960.
58. Stamler, J., Kjelsberg, M., and Hall, Y.: Epidemiologic studies of cardiovascular-renal diseases: I. Analysis of mortality by age—race—sex—occupation, J. Chronic Dis. 12:440, 1960.
59. Survey Research Center, University of Michigan.
60. Susser, M.: Causes of peptic ulcer: A selective epidemiologic review, J. Chronic Dis. 20:123, 1967.
61. Syme, S. L., Hyman, M. M., and Enterline, P. E.: Some social and cultural factors associated with the occurrence of coronary heart disease, J. Chronic Dis. 17:277, 1964.
62. Taylor, G. C.: Executive stress, Int. Clin. Psychiatry 6:307, 1969.
63. Terhune, W. B.: Emotional problems of executives in time, Ind. Med. Surg. 32:1, 1963.
64. *To Work is Human: Mental Health and the Business Community*, McLean, A. (ed.) (New York: Macmillan, 1967).
65. Wan, T. H., and Wright, A.: Occupational differentials in chronic disability, J. Occup. Med. 15:493, 1973.
66. Wardwell, W. I., Hyman, M. M., and Bahnson, C. B.: Stress and coronary heart disease in three field studies, J. Chronic Dis. 17:73, 1964.
67. *Work in America*, ed. O'Toole, J. (Cambridge, Mass.: MIT Press, 1973).

9 / Sickness-Absence in Industry—the Iatrogenic Factor

JOHANN T. METS, M.D.

"SICKNESS-ABSENCE" is used as a convenient short term to denote the phenomenon of being absent when scheduled to work, with such absence accepted as attributable to illness or injury. As long ago as 1957, when the Permanent International Commission on Industrial Medicine met in Leiden, this definition was adopted and since then has been used extensively in the literature. Perusal of that literature shows how complex the phenomenon is.[10] It is determined not only by medical but also by social, economic, cultural, personal, organizational and occupational factors, with psychological factors pervading all these fields. Whether illness or injury leads to absence from work depends to a large extent on the motivation of the worker himself in all those instances where no objective, clearly total incapacity to work exists.

Hogerzeil[5] emphasized that sickness-absence will result only when a person experiences a deviation from his normal status of well-being as markedly impeding his functioning in the work situation. The point where this occurs depends on the person's threshold for reporting sick-absent. This threshold is determined by a host of personal, social, cultural, economic and other variables. De Kock van Leeuwen[1] showed in his doctoral thesis that the tendency of an individual to absent himself from work may be regarded as a semiconstant attribute of a person if conditions external to him do not vary. Gadourek[3] concluded from his study that the nature of the work process and the organizational group of factors are of greater relevance for the study of well-being of workers and absenteeism than personality characteristics. Philipsen,[9] conceding that absenteeism is, in essence, individual behavior, found that the incidence and duration of sickness-absence are semiconstant traits of organizations. Both latter authors indicate, however, that the determining influence on whether to absent oneself from work or not remains the decision of the individual, especially in what they term, with Hogerzeil, the subjective syndromes.

Hogerzeil[5] relates these concepts to the duration of sickness-absence spells, pointing out that the medical diagnoses listed in the International Classification of Diseases are inadequate indicators for sickness-absence. They are designed to diagnose disease and not sickness-absence, which is a social and not a medical phenomenon. Sickness-absence is viewed as a process caused by perceived incapacity to work as a result of disturbance in social functioning and not necessarily by genuine morbidity. An employee seldom is 100% fit one moment and completely incapacitated the next; usually there is gradual development of a disturbance and gradual recovery.

Phases discernible in the process leading to sickness-absence, viewed as explainable by a decision theory (decision being defined as a choice between alternatives made by the individual), are the incipience of a disturbance in well-being, followed by recognition and then by either acceptance of the role of patient and an acting on it or a refusal to heed the disturbance. On return of the feeling of well-being, the reverse takes place or the role of patient is continued.

In terms of duration of absences, short *subjective syndromes* lasting 1–3 days are characterized by a high degree of freedom of decision by the individual.

Objective-subjective syndromes lasting 4–7 days involve a high degree of freedom of decision at the start, less so at the end. Acute respiratory syndromes may fall under both these duration categories.

Objective syndromes, also termed genuine illness, whether physical or psychological, usually last up to 14 days or more. Little freedom of decision by the individual exists at the beginning. The longer such objective syndromes continue to take their course the greater the freedom of decision by the individual to decide when he feels fit to return to work. Hogerzeil regards 3 weeks as a critical duration because a simple disturbance then may become a complex disturbance of functioning of the individual as a totality.

A corollary of this is that the determining influence of the physician on the duration of a sickness-absence of short time (1–3 days) *is very small indeed*. He has little or no influence on the initiation of such absences and hardly any on the termination; the patient usually decides on these. For longer periods, his influence becomes greater, especially for objective syndromes, but only on the termination of such periods. This applies only if the physician makes an active decision on when the patient should return to work and communicates this clearly to his patient.

The shorter the duration of absence the less likely that it is caused by medical factors. Short-term sickness-absence may be regarded as sickness behavior of the individual, especially if he is a repeater[7] or frequently sick,[13] withdrawing himself from his work situation when he feels the need for escape and requires sanctioning of his absence.

Periods of longer duration, with a preponderance of medical factors, are characterized by the occurrence of classic diseases and, therefore, are more likely to be under the control of physicians. Not only therapeutic potential but also the physician's subjective evaluation of the situation of the patient in relation to his work will determine the duration of absence deemed necessary or allowed.

For sickness to be expressed as "sickness-absence," not only the necessity (as in objective syndromes) but also the perceived need to be absent (as in objective and subjective syndromes), as well as the opportunity, are prerequisites.

Among the many factors that influence sickness-absence, the variable—"the physician"—has received comparatively little attention.

THE ROLE OF THE PHYSICIAN

The accepted role of the physician, for which he is trained, is to cure diseases, alleviate symptoms and promote recovery of the patient. Another aspect of his role is his preventive intervention. Only indirectly is he expected to be concerned with the resumption of the patient's social role. A distinction may be made between the occupational physician and his colleagues in family medicine or the specialties.

In the Occupational Health Institute Publication of the then Industrial Medical Association, Felton[2] expressed the role of the occupational physician in illness absenteeism control as follows:

1. One of the functions of the physician in industry is, through his anticipatory health guidance, or preventive, or constructive medical measures, the minimizing of time lost through illness-absence.
2. The significant role of the physician in contributing his aid to absence control is in working thoughtfully with those repeaters whose individ-

ual spells of absence are part of a continuum which comprises their life patterns or life style.

3. The individual, problem beset, poorly motivated worker is the diagnostic, counseling and re-educative task of the practitioner in the plant.

Howe,[6] in a section on illness-absenteeism control, reiterated the formulation as given under 1 and 2 above. He also mentioned that "the attitude of the physician at the work site is not one so much of diagnosing and treating as it is of wanting to understand why certain workers are consistently absent, presumably from illness or injury. In attempting to maintain the worker on his job, the occupational physician and the private practitioner share a common responsibility."

From these quotations, the conclusion seems warranted that the physician, as one of the partners in the triad "patient-employee," "physician" and "employer-society," may not restrict his function to a purely medical one, abrogating his social role.

This social role may be summarized by stating that the physician, whether he is an occupational physician or otherwise engaged in medical practice, must have as his objective guiding his patient to resuming his social role as soon as possible, in his own interest and that of society.

The physician's actions in sickness-absence control will, to a great extent, be determined by the type of sickness-absence he has to deal with, short-duration sickness (absence behavior) or longer-term illness-absence. The degree to which he can influence these two forms of absence depends on the degree of freedom of decision the patient himself has by virtue of the underlying causation, i.e., subjective syndromes, objective syndromes or a mixture of the two.

CERTIFICATION

Many editorials and correspondence columns in medical journals throughout the world, as well as discussions during medical conferences, have been devoted to this subject. Robb[12] stated: "Medical certification may widely be regarded as a chore, but it is much more than this. It is an essential attribute to the practice of medicine and must be carried out with full attention to the moral, ethical and legal implications. To prescribe 'rest from work' or 'work' may be as much part of the treatment a doctor administers as the prescription of drugs or other forms of therapy. Whilst no workman should be returned to work unless he is fit to perform a particular task, it is not in the best interest of the workman himself to delay unnecessarily his return to work."

Society charges the physician with the task of sanctioning the absence of a worker on the grounds of incapacity resulting from illness or injury, thereby relieving the patient of his social duty to work. Also, if sick benefits are payable to the employee certified as sick, the sick certificate represents a check to be drawn on the sick fund, whether the insurance institution is private or state-controlled.[11] The physician is paid the compliment of being regarded as the most reliable and acceptable person capable of attesting accurately to the fact that incapacity to work exists.

The physician must be counsel for the defense, counsel for the prosecution, judge and jury at the same time in reaching a verdict of whether or not an employee should be relieved of his duties. Integrity of the physician and honesty of the patient are conditions to be fulfilled for a fair trial, resulting in a certificate that must satisfy the contractual relationships between patient, physician and society.

Grossmark and Shares[4] found, in a group practice in England catering to 10,500 people, that 18% of their patients requested certificates. Only 48% of these cases had obvious illness, 36% showed no signs of illness and 13% had certificates issued for hospital treatment (3% were not classified).

As an example of the determining influence of physicians on absences of long duration, the 1957 study by Moss et al.[8] may be noted. They found, in a sample of 229 physicians (surgeons, general practitioners and occupational physicians), that recommended times before returning to work ranged from 1 to 10 weeks for light work and 2 weeks to 6 months for heavy work after an uncomplicated inguinal herniorrhaphy.

Tordoir et al.[14] investigated the role of physicians and the procedures of medical treatment in search of factors that had prolonged sickness-absence. They found that physicians tended to be unsure about the point in time that their patients should return to work for long duration periods due to objective and subjective-objective syndromes. Quoting a survey by Querido (1963), they observed that in 260 of 389 investigated cases, prolongation of absence as a result of shortcomings in the organization of medical investigations and treatment had occurred. An important cause for delay was the lack of communication between physicians, patients, specialists and hospitals (45.9% of the waiting days lost). They also quoted an investigation by van Mansvelt (1974–1975), who found that in 15% of cases of long-term duration, "iatrogenic invalidity" had resulted from lack of communication between curative and insurance physicians. Last, they referred to Heasman (1972), who found a great variation in the number of days patients were in the hospital before and after operations for an inguinal hernia in Scotland. They regarded it as very difficult to evaluate the professional element as a factor in sickness-absence spells of long duration.

THE SURVEY

As part of a more comprehensive study of sickness-absence, an attempt was made to evaluate the influence of physicians on short-term absences. From scrutinizing incoming sick certificates and a pilot survey, an impression had been gained that some physicians actually seemed to contribute to sickness-absence by their certification habits. That there is an iatrogenic factor in long-term sickness-absences already has been indicated. The objective of this survey was to establish whether an iatrogenic factor could be shown for short-term sickness-absence as well, even though this type of sickness-absence is characterized by a great degree of freedom of decision by the patient.

MATERIAL AND METHODS

Certificates for hourly rated white, colored and African employees, all blue-collar workers, were investigated. These employees all have to register with a specific physician on a panel. Physicians are paid a fixed fee per patient per annum and are not influenced by economic considerations when they see patients or ask them to return for checkups, nor by a fear of losing patients. It is the physician's attitude toward patient and society and the degree of his knowledge of patient and work situation that mainly determine his certification habit.

A basic assumption was made that there were *"permissive" physicians* from whom it was easy to obtain a sick certificate, whether or not a patient was objectively ill; *"strict" physicians*, who would tend to restrict the sickness-absence they certified to a minimum, compatible with their findings; and an *intermediate* group of physicians. Data for "permissive" physicians were, where possible, compared with data for all other physicians combined as controls. There were 12 physicians serving the working population under study. Two group practices (one "permissive" and one "intermediate") were selected as well as 5 single doctors (2 "permissive," 1 "intermediate" and 2 "strict"). Sick pay regulations and other occupational and organizational factors of possible influence were very nearly the same for the groups of employees investigated. All employees incorporated in the survey had had at least 6 months' service with the company. The average service duration was 17 months and the median service duration was 13 months. Age could not be taken into account. Over-all sickness-absence rates and absence frequency rates did not vary materially during the periods investigated. Where short periods of a few months only were compared, care was taken to avoid high-frequency seasonal variations due, for example, to influenza. Absences of more than 14 days' duration were held to be caused by objective syndromes. Attendance certificates for patients not being marked off for longer than the time they spent for the consultation were also counted.

Striking features are the absence of attendance certificates, the lower proportion of 1–3-day absences and the higher median duration of spells for the certificates issued by the "permissive" physician as well as the higher number of days marked off by "permissive" physicians per 100 certificates, mainly attributable to the higher proportion of 7–14-day periods.

As it was known that sickness-absence levels varied among the ethnic groups, a survey was done of certificates issued to colored and African employees.

On a slightly different scale than that reflected in Table 9–1, the "permissive" physicians represented in Table 9–2 issued certificates showing similar features, i.e., very few attendance certificates, a lower proportion of 1–3-day spells and a higher number of days booked off per 100 certificates than all other physicians combined. The total number of days certified "off sick" by all physicians combined during the period of 4 months was 4044 calendar days. Whereas the 2 permissive physicians had issued 761 certificates (51%), the other 10 physicians had issued only 732 certificates (49%). The "permissive" physicians' certificates accounted, however, for 62.3% of all days lost as shown in Table 9–3. This table also shows the percentage proportion of days lost as a result of booking off by three absence-duration categories.

The difference in distribution is significant at the 5% level (chi-squared, 2 degrees of freedom). If the number of certificates issued by each group is taken into account and standardized, the "permissive" physicians' certificates would have accounted for 2473 days, the other physicians' certificates for 1553 days, respectively 61.4% and 38.6%. This is a significant difference.

As the data shown above concern different groups of individuals, which may be considered to have had a possible influence on the results, a further survey was done to exclude such influence.

The "permissive" physicians whose certificates are reflected in Tables 9–2 and 9–3

TABLE 9–1.—COMPARISON OF CERTIFICATES ISSUED BY SINGLE PHYSICIANS FOR WHITE EMPLOYEES OVER A PERIOD OF 2 YEARS

	PERMISSIVE PHYSICIANS	STRICT PHYSICIANS
(certificates) =	114	159
tendance certificates	0%	1.8%
-3-day spells	24%	62.2%
-6-day spells	37%	20.1%
-14-day spells	39%	15.9%
edian duration	5 days	3 days
ode (duration)	5 days	2 days
verage duration	5.6 days	3.7 days
tal days booked off/100 certificates	555 days	375 days

TABLE 9–2.—COMPARISON OF CERTIFICATES ISSUED BY A GROUP OF "PERMISSIVE" PHYSICIANS AND ALL OTHER PHYSICIANS COMBINED FOR AFRICAN AND COLORED EMPLOYEES OVER A PERIOD OF 4 MONTHS (JUNE–SEPTEMBER, 1973)

	PERMISSIVE PHYSICIANS	ALL OTHER PHYSICIANS
n (certificates) =	761	731
Attendance certificates	0.4%	3.4%
1–3-day spells	57.5%	83.5%
4–6-day spells	40.4%	10.8%
7–14-day spells	1.7%	2.3%
Median duration	3 days	2 days
Mode (duration)	2 days	1 day
Average duration	3.3 days	2.1 days
Total days booked off/100 certificates	331 days	208 days

TABLE 9–3.—TOTAL CERTIFICATES, DAYS BOOKED OFF AND PERCENTAGE PROPORTION OF DAYS LOST FOR ABSENCE DURATIONS FOR A GROUP OF "PERMISSIVE" PHYSICIANS COMPARED WITH ALL OTHER PHYSICIANS COMBINED (JUNE–SEPTEMBER, 1973)

	PERMISSIVE PHYSICIANS (2)	ALL OTHER PHYSICIANS (10)	TOTALS
n (certificates) =	761 (51.0%)	732 (49.0%)	1493 certificates
Total days booked off	2521 (62.3%)	1523 (36.7%)	4044 days
Days			
Certified 0–3	36.0%	67.0%	1927 days
Off sick 4–6	58.0%	24.0%	1828 days
Percentage			
proportion 7–14 days	6.0%	9.0%	289 days
	100.0%	100.0%	4044 days

resigned from the panel on October 1, 1973. The medical files of 129 individuals who had been registered with these physicians while in the service of the company from at least 6 months prior to the starting date of the survey (October 1, 1972) were scrutinized. All these individuals changed to other physicians in October, 1973. The first period of observation was 1 year under "permissive" physicians; the second period was 1 year under other physicians. That the population under study was a relatively stable one is shown by the fact that 70 of these employees still were in the company's service in August, 1977 whereas the other 59 had left the company at varying points in time, but only after April 1, 1975 (6 months after the closing date of this survey). Only 1 employee was over 50 years of age; only 5 had underlying chronic disease that may have accounted for repeated absence (Table 9–4, Nos. 1, 3, 4, 7 and 11).

The system of certification used in the practice of the "permissive" physicians was as follows.

When a patient reported sick at the sur-

TABLE 9–4.—COMPARISON OF SICKNESS-ABSENCE OF 13 INDIVIDUALS WHO HAD MORE THAN 5 ABSENCE PERIODS IN 1972–1973 ("PERMISSIVE" PHYSICIANS) WITH 1973–1974 (OTHER PHYSICIANS)

NO.	ABSENCE P/A 1972/73	ABSENCE P/A 1973/74	DAYS CERTIFIED P/A 1972/73	DAYS CERTIFIED P/A 1973/74	REMARKS
1	6	3	13	1	
2	7	3	13	3	
3	7	2	20	6	4× "lumbago" (72/73)
4	7	2	21	2	2× alcotest+ (72/73)
5	6	5	30	9	
6	7	6	35	19	
7	7	5	19	8	
8	8	4	37	7	2× alcotest+ (72/73)
9	9	2	37	1	5× "gastritis" (72/73)
10	7	3	18	4	
11	6	5	30	9	
12	6	4	23	7	
13	6	2	18	2	
TOTALS	89 absences	46 absences	314 days	78 days	
Average	6.6 absences	3.5 absences	24 days	6 days	per man
			3.9 days	1.7 days	per absence

gery, the receptionist would fill in a certificate form, entering personal data, the date of consultation and the date from which the patient had not been at work (on 80% of all certificates studied). The physician, after seeing the patient, then would fill in the date that he would return to work and a diagnosis and sign the certificate without stipulating that "the patient informed me that he had been ill from such and such a date." Certificates were also, reportedly, issued on a request via telephone by either the patient or a relative.

The two "permissive" physicians issued 385 certificates during period A (October 1, 1972–1973) to the same people who received 347 certificates from 10 other physicians (10% less) during period B (October 1, 1973–1974). Only 16 certified absences of longer than 7 days were recorded over the 2 years out of the total of 732 certificates. This would make it acceptable to consider the data presented in Figure 9–1 as representing sickness-absence behavior rather than morbidity.

The scatter diagram (Fig 9–1) shows the distribution of 129 individuals by the number of absences they incurred during the period that they were under the care of the "permissive" physicians (X = 1972–1973) as against the period that they were under the care of other physicians (Y = 1973–1974). For example, of the 16 people who had had 5 absences during 1972–1973 (X axis), 2 had the same number in the following year (Y axis), 3 had more absences (2 × 6, 1 × 7) and 11 had fewer absences (3 × 4, 4 × 3, 3 × 2 and 1 × 0).

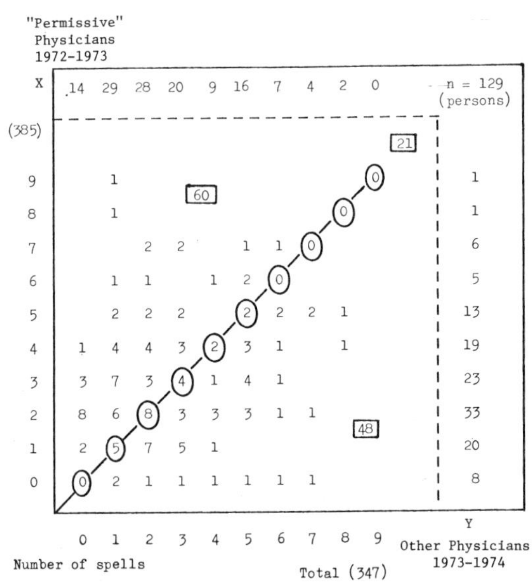

Fig 9–1.—Distribution by number of absences in 1972–1973 and 1973–1974.

In summary, 60 (46.5%) men had fewer absences in 1973–1974 than in 1972–1973, 21 (16.3%) men had the same number of absences and 48 (37.2%) men had more periods of sickness-absence. The difference in distribution by number of periods in 1972–1973 ("permissive" physicians) compared with 1973–1974 (other physicians) is significant at the 5% level (chi-squared, 9 degrees of freedom).

If sickness-absence behavior is considered a semiconstant personality trait resulting in a fairly consistent absenteeism pattern (external factors remaining unchanged), the 13 individuals who had more than 5 absences during the first period are of special interest (people with more than 9 absences were excluded). As the only discernible factor that had changed was the certifying physician, this variable appears to have been of determining influence. Nearly all 13 individuals had an appreciably lower absence frequency in the year under "other" physicians' care, as shown in Table 9–4. This group, as a whole, had significantly ($p < 0.05$) lower absence rates during the second period.

The differences in absence frequency, days lost per man and number of days lost per absence are obvious. These 13 men had had 1.9 times as many periods of absence in 1972–1973 as in 1973–1974, resulting in a 4 times higher loss of days than in 1973–1974.

There were, however, also 13 individuals who had more than 5 absences during the second period when they were under the care of "other" physicians. Of these, 6 were suffering from chronic or recurrent conditions (avascular necrosis of femur head, 7

TABLE 9–5.—CERTIFICATES WITH RETROACTIVE MARKING OFF OF WORKDAYS ISSUED BY "PERMISSIVE" PHYSICIANS OVER 1 WEEK IN 1973

				DIAGNOSES			
	CERTIFICATES	WORKDAYS BOOKED OFF	RETROACTIVE (WORKDAYS)	GASTRO-ENTERITIS	BACKACHE, FIBROSITIS	FLU	OTHERS
Monday	n = 6	15	1 × 3d	1	2	2	1
Tuesday	n = 20	67	13 × 1d 3 × 3d	4	5	6	5
Wednesday	n = 8	21	3 × 1d 2 × 2d	1	3	3	1
Thursday	n = 10	20	1 × 3d 3 × 1d	—	3	4	3
Friday	n = 7	14	1 × 1d	—	4	—	3
TOTAL	n = 51	137 d	39 d	6	17	15	13

periods as against 3 in 1972–1973), cardiovascular disease (2 persons, 7 periods and 6 periods as against, respectively, 0 and 2 in 1972–1973), bronchial asthma (9 as against 4 periods in 1972–1973), recurrent bronchitis (7 as against 2 periods in 1972–1973), or tuberculosis (7 as against 0 in 1972–1973). One employee was over 60 years of age (6 as against 2 periods in 1972–1973). The other 6 individuals taken together showed 31 absences in 1973–1974 as against 24 in 1972–1973. No explanation can be offered for this except that 2 of them were examined repeatedly in the hospital (total 8 periods of absence) with negative results.

When the 6 invalid persons are excluded, the differences in absence frequency rate for the others (5.1 in 1973–1974 as against 4 in 1972–1973) and days lost per absence (2.5 in 1973–1974 as against 4.2 in 1972–1973) do not appear to militate against the conclusion that the certifying physicians constituted the most important influencing factor on sickness absenteeism for the group of 129 individuals as a whole in 1972–1973 ("permissive" physicians).

The data presented above suggest that the physicians regarded as "permissive" were, in fact, more liberal in allowing days off by certification for minor complaints (subjective syndromes).

The hypothesis that these physicians attracted more individuals to their practice who were inclined to seek repeated absences (sanctioned by medical certificates) because the physicians concerned reportedly were "easier" than others was not subjected to statistical analysis. There is, however, a clear indication that this was the case in the data shown in Table 9–3. The group of "permissive" physicians represented only 2 physicians who looked after the employees concerned whereas "all other physicians" represented 4 physicians in individual practices and 6 others who were partners of a group practice (10 in all). The 2 "permissive" physicians had issued 761 certificates as against 732 issued by the other 10 during the same period of 4 months.

For sick pay purposes, the days marked off by physicians on their certificates before the actual consultation date were ignored. Such certificates, however, throw some light on certification habits, especially if the stipulation that "the patient had informed the physician that he was sick on those days" was not mentioned on the certificates. This was the case on 51 certificates collected from the "permissive" physicians over a period of 1 week (August 13 to August 17, 1973) (Table 9–5).

A striking feature of this retroactive certification is that 13 of 20 certificates issued on Tuesday "covered" the Monday before and another 3 certificates even "covered" the Friday before the consultation date.

SUMMARY AND CONCLUSION

Sickness-absence may be categorized as attributable to objective or to subjective illness syndromes or to a mixture of these. Objective syndromes generally result in medium to long periods of absence, subjective syndromes to short-term absences of only a few days, with a great degree of freedom for the patient to decide when he will be absent and when he will return to work.

The literature supports indications that there is an iatrogenic influence on the duration of longer-term sickness-absences. The role of the certifying physician in short-term absences has received less attention. A study of certification patterns of physicians regarded as "permissive" showed a striking disparity in distribution of absence durations, days lost, average absence duration and proportion of certificates issued compared with controls. A similar disparity was evident when a group of employees had changed physicians, confirming that an iatrogenic factor may contribute to sickness-absence.

Even though the findings of a small survey in one locality obviously may not be generalized, a conclusion that medical students should be taught the value, importance and ethics of medical certification of sickness-absence seems warranted. In a wider sense, they should be trained for the social role a physician has to fulfill in addition to his traditional medical role.

REFERENCES

1. de Kock van Leeuwen, J. A. C.: Verzuimgeneigdheid by dienstplichtige militairen in vredestyd. M.D. Thesis, N.I.P.G. Verhandelingen XXX, Leiden, The Netherlands, 1952.
2. Felton, J. S.: Organization and operation of an occupational health program. Occup. Health Inst. Publication U.S.A., Industrial Medical Association, 1964.
3. Gadourek, I.: Absences and well-being of workers. Health Research T.N.O., Van Gorcum-Assen., The Netherlands, 1965.
4. Grossmark, F. B., and Shares, P.: A study of certification in general practice, Practitioner 199:354, 1967.
5. Hogerzeil, H. H. W.: Arbeidsongeschiktheid en medisch-sociaal beleid, Ned. Tijdschr. Soc. Geneeskd. 50:538, 1972.
6. Howe, H. F.: Organization and operation of an occupational health program—Part I, J. Occup. Med. 17:360, 1975.
7. Linden, V.: The distribution of sickness absence in a working population, Acta Sociomed. Scand. 1:81, 1969.
8. Moss, N. H., Schwegman, C. W., and Dohan, F. C.: Surgical convalescence, JAMA 165:322, 1957.
9. Philipsen, H.: Afwezigheid wegens Ziekte. Ph.D. Thesis, N.I.P.G./T.N.O., Wolters-Noordhoff-Groningen, The Netherlands, 1968.
10. Proceedings of the Symposium on Absence from Work Attributed to Sickness (1968) Gardner, W. (ed.), updated edition, October, 1977. Research Panels Society of Occupational Medicine, London, England.
11. Report of the Committee on Abuse of Social Security Benefits (Chapter 9), Cmnd. 5228. Her Majesty's Stationery Office, London, 1973.
12. Robb, D. F.: Medical certification in "The economics of general practice," Supplement of Practitioner, July, 1967.
13. Taylor, P. J.: Individual variations in sickness absence, Br. J. Ind. Med. 24:169, 1967.
14. Tordoir, W. F., v.d. Klaauw, M. M., and van Manen-Boekestein, C. M. J.: Gezondheidszorg en Langdurig Arbeidsverzuim, Ned. Tijdschr. Soc. Geneeskd. 54:249, 1976.
15. Mets, J. T.: Absenteeism in a motor car manufacturing plant—a contribution to the study of absence behaviour and medically certified absence from work in South Africa. Dissertation, University of Pretoria, 1979.

10 / Rotational Shift Work

CHARLES M. WINGET, Ph.D., and JOSEPH LaDOU, M.D.

SHIFT WORK, which began during World War I and proliferated during World War II, has become a way of life for approximately 19% of the U.S. labor force.[20] The very high cost of capital equipment and the demands of the world market have forced industry to operate 24 hours a day. Moreover, industries whose products require continuity of a technologic process, such as steel, petroleum and pulp and paper production, operate on 3-shift, 24-hour schedules. For different reasons, public services, including utilities, police and fire protection and the military, must adhere to shift schedules. The functions of health service organizations and clinical and research laboratories also constrain them to utilize shift work schedules. It is estimated that more than 16 million persons in the United States work and live according to some type of shift scheduling.[20]

These individuals live in an abnormal time frame. They sleep when most of the community is awake, they breakfast when others are dining, they have time to play only when most of society is working. They are forced to adapt their times of sleep and leisure to family and community if they wish to spend time with their wives and children or maintain a semblance of social life. But these sociological pressures create dissatisfaction in the worker and restrict his ability to adapt to his abnormal work schedule.

Attempting to cope with this problem, management has tended more and more to favor rotational shift work, in which the individual works a certain percentage of his time on the day shift, a certain percentage on the evening shift and a certain percentage on the night shift. But this type of shift work scheduling imposes physiologic and emotional stresses on the individual that frequently are debilitating.

CIRCADIAN PERIODICITY

The problems that occur with rotational shift work arise because most human physiologic systems function according to rhythms, and these rhythms can be easily disturbed. Jürgen Aschoff, an authority in the field of biologic rhythms, has stated:

> It is well known even to the layman that each day the body temperature reaches a highest value toward the evening and a low point early in the morning. Since this phenomenon was described by Gierse in 1842, numerous clinical and physiological studies have shown that there is apparently no organ and no function of the body which does not exhibit a similar daily rhythmicity. Whether we measure, hour by hour, the number of dividing cells in any tissue, the volume of urine excreted, the reaction to a drug, or the accuracy and speed with which arithmetical problems are solved, we usually find that there is a maximum value at one time of day and a minimum value at another.[6]

Body temperature fluctuates according to a rhythm; the endocrine system fluctuates according to a rhythm; the flow of urine is rhythmic; and the cardiovascular, hematopoietic, respiratory and autonomic nervous systems all exhibit rhythmic patterns.[30]

The rhythms of most human physiologic systems and organs approximate a 24-hour pattern and consequently have been termed "circadian rhythms" (from the Latin *circa dies,* meaning "about a day").[49] These rhythms are entrained (synchronized) with the 24-hour period by periodic factors in the environment that are known as Zeitgebers (from the German meaning "time-givers"). The alternation of light and dark and, to a lesser degree, changes in environmental temperature are important Zeitgebers for animals.[97] Light is also an important Zeitgeber for man and is responsible for the entrainment of a large number of human rhythms—for example, the plasma level of 17-hydroxycorticosteroid.[66, 92] On the other hand, it has been claimed that prolonged darkness causes the rhythms in some functions to disappear[97] and changes almost immediately the rate of increase or decrease.[105] Social communication may also be a significant factor in entraining human physiologic rhythms.[7]

When the phase of a Zeitgeber is shifted—for example, when the light-dark cycle is shifted as it is during rotational shift work or experimentation—the physiologic rhythms either shift with the Zeitgeber or become desynchronized. Moreover, when the internal rhythms become desynchronized from the external environment, they also tend to become desynchronized from each other. Thus, the body temperature rhythm, when out of phase with the light-dark cycle, may run according to one time schedule while the endocrine system runs according to another. This phenomenon is demonstrated by the variations that have been observed in the time required for the various systems to resynchronize when the light-dark cycle is returned to normal. When resynchronizing to a 12-hour shift, the EEG rhythm resynchronizes within 5 days and the respiratory rate rhythm within 11 days whereas the potassium excretion rate rhythm requires more than 25 days to return to normal.[8]

Changes in the Zeitgebers do not seem to adversely affect workers who are assigned to a particular shift more or less permanently because their internal rhythms adjust to the new schedule over time, and their systems are not called on to readapt periodically.[30] The worker on a rotational shift work program, however, must adapt each time that his schedule changes. Unfortunately, the internal rhythms, once disturbed, do not adapt readily to the new schedule, nor do they readapt with ease when the worker is returned to his former schedule. In rotational shift work, just as the individual's rhythms are beginning to entrain to the new routine, he is switched to a different schedule. This repeated shifting is very debilitating, and organizations that utilize it can be faced with the problem of workers whose health, work performance, safety awareness and emotional status are at a low ebb.

CIRCADIAN RHYTHMS IN SHIFT WORKERS

Under normal conditions, humans sleep during the dark phase of the light-dark cycle and are awake and active during the light phase. In individuals on shift work, the sleep-work cycle is desynchronized from the light-dark cycle. This inversion of the primary Zeitgeber—light—and the attendant sleep reversal are primary problems in rotational shift work.[52]

Many investigators have sought to determine man's adaptability to this inversion, but most have been concerned with work performance, satisfaction with shift work and preference for one shift over another. Less emphasis has been given to studying changes in human physiologic rhythms that occur during rotational shift work. Although much remains to be done in this area, considerable information is available from the many studies conducted on physiologic rhythms in general, including body temperature,[9, 16, 25, 58, 111, 114, 116, 117, 126] neuroendocrine rhythms,[28, 29, 79, 126] EEG and sleep rhythms,[65, 126] excretory rhythms[27, 126] and heart rate.[16, 22, 30, 63, 91, 123]* The findings of these and related studies are applicable to

*For purposes of brevity, only representative studies are referenced.

the problem of desynchronization during rotational shifting.

One of the most serious effects of shifting the sleep-wake schedule from night to day is the fatigue that generally occurs because of the reversal. It stems from two causes. First, a prolonged stress (such as a change in the sleep period) in itself can induce fatigue. Second, it is atypical to sleep during the light phase, as has been demonstrated by sleep EEGs,[126] and sleep at an atypical time often is shortened or otherwise disturbed.[115] The result is fatigue during the waking hours.

Individuals differ greatly in their ability to adapt to a radical change in the sleep-wake cycle. Some adapt very readily, exhibiting an inversion of the physiologic and psychological rhythms that parallels the sleep-wake inversion.[8] Others adapt very slowly or not at all.

Psychological factors also play an important part in the ability of the worker to adapt to the inverted schedule. Despite the fact that the longer a person remains on an inverted sleep-wake cycle the better he will adapt, psychological factors must be taken into account in selecting persons for rotational shift work. Psychological stresses, such as not having enough time with the family because of conflicting schedules or being unable to participate in a social function, can disrupt the individual's adaptation to his new schedule.

Östberg,[93] as the result of a recent study, suggested that the individual's ability to adapt to shift work may depend on his personality make-up. Over a year-long period, he observed 37 computer operators and output handlers who worked on rotating 8-hour shifts beginning at 0800, 1600 and 2400 hours. Measurements were made during the morning, evening and night shifts and included oral body temperature, sleep performance, physical fitness, time estimation ability and food intake. From his findings, Östberg concluded that "morning" people (those who are alert and active early in the day) showed the greatest difficulty in adapting to the shift system, and that "night" people (those who are most alert and function most effectively during the dark hours) experienced the least difficulty in adapting to rotational shift work. He also found that adaptation to the night shift (2400–0800 hours) was the most difficult.

A number of investigators have studied the incidence of illness among shift workers.[1,2,11,19,35,39,72,88,109,112,119] Although some have reported that gastrointestinal and emotional illnesses were more prevalent among shift workers, others have concluded that shift workers suffered no more, and perhaps even fewer, illnesses than day workers. Taylor[109] has suggested, however, that these findings could have resulted from the small size of the groups studied and the higher than average job satisfaction among the workers.

In a recent study, Walker and De la Mare[122] reviewed the causes of absence from work for 4 calendar days or more by fixed-shift and day workers. The subjects were matched in terms of age, sex and job classification insofar as possible. Factors studied were cause of absence and number of days absent. The investigators concluded that fixed-shift workers were absent from work for health reasons more often than day workers. The primary causes, they determined, were respiratory problems and digestive disorders.

There is a wide difference of opinion concerning the optimal timing for rotating shifts. At one end of the scale are those who believe that shifts should be rotated at no less than 2-month intervals; at the other are those who advocate rotation every day, with some even advocating that shifts be advanced by 30 minutes every day. Murrell[89] and Andlauer and Fourrel[5] concluded that workers on rapid shift rotation suffered fewer health difficulties than those who were shifted weekly. Gavrilescu and coworkers,[44] on the other hand, found that workers adapted poorly and exhibited difficulties in the adjustment of their rhythms even during rotation every 2 days. Others have concluded that the biologic rhythm of body temperature begins to invert only from the third night of work, thus implying that night work should last no longer than 48 hours.[21]

Åkerstedt and colleagues[3] have undertaken a number of studies on the effects of rotational shifting and have suggested that rapid rotation may be better than slow rotational shifting insofar as the health and mental and social well-being of the worker is concerned. Although they concluded that permanent night workers adapted reasonably well to the night shift[95] (supporting the results of earlier studies), they found that workers who interchanged day and night shifts, even at 1-week intervals, did not adapt well to the night shift.[4] They believed that Teleky's suggestion[111] that shifts be rotated infrequently would appear to be questionable because slow rotation would result in constant desynchronization. Taylor,[110] in a later study, also suggested that workers on rapidly rotated shifts experienced fewer problems.

The merits of rapid rotational work shifting, however, have not been finally demonstrated.[21]

Physiologic responses to rotational shift work, as indicated earlier, have not been explored exhaustively, and much work remains to be done in this field. With the work that has been accomplished to date, however, it is possible to determine the problems that may occur during intermittent work shifting.

Most research on rotational shift work has been concerned with nonphysiologic factors such as employee output. Wyatt and Marriott[129] studied the output of three factories that rotated their shifts on a weekly, biweekly and monthly basis. When the workers were shifted every other week, performance did not improve until the second week after they returned to the day schedule. Even longer was required when the shifts were rotated on a monthly basis. Absenteeism also increased with each succeeding week on the night shift and decreased proportionally during the day shifts. Most of the workers interviewed during this study said that they preferred the day shift, and those on the night shift complained more frequently of fatigue. When questioned, 42% said that they were unable to sleep properly while on the night shift, 62% had difficulty adapting to changed mealtimes and 23% believed that they could not adapt to a new shift in less than 6 days.

The preference of workers for various shifts and their reactions to permanent shift work versus rotational shifting have been investigated.[32, 33] Most workers were not concerned about which shift they served on as long as they were assigned to that shift on a more or less permanent basis. Thus, regularity of the work schedule was the primary consideration.

Walker[121] studied the results in one steel plant that changed from a fixed 3-shift system, with breaks at weekends, to a system in which work schedules were shifted every 8 weeks. The change was made at the workers' request and was accompanied by a reduction in working hours from 45 to 42 hours per week and a 20% increase in pay. Consequently, the change was weighted toward a favorable response from the workers. Not surprisingly, all workers preferred the new system, and 50% claimed that they slept better.

As with physiologic rhythms in rotational shifting, many sociological and operational areas remain to be investigated more thoroughly.

PROBLEMS RESULTING FROM ROTATIONAL SHIFT WORK

Industries that utilize systems of rotational shift work use a variety of formulas for shifting their employees. The system most commonly used is to shift them every week, following a weekend rest period. Those who have studied the physiologic effects of intermittent work shifting consider this arrangement to be the least satisfactory of any devised.

Teleky,[111] after considerable and careful study in this field, recommended that schedules not be shifted more frequently than once a month. When rotated at shorter intervals, the employee's internal rhythms barely begin to entrain to one schedule before he is shifted to another.[88] The problems that can result from this situation include:

Impairment of physical health.
Emotional and behavioral problems.
Sleep difficulties.
Altered response to medication.
Decrements in work performance.
Safety awareness.

Any one or a combination of these problems can result in absenteeism, decreased productivity, social disorganization and poor safety records.

Health

A number of physiologic disorders and conditions have been found to exhibit circadian variations and consequently can be exacerbated when individuals are subjected to rotational shift work at too rapid a rate. The problem areas are diabetes mellitus; respiratory, cardiovascular and renal disorders; and epilepsy.

DIABETES MELLITUS.—Periodic variations in the metabolites in diabetes mellitus have been observed, including 24-hour rhythms in the excretion of citric acid and beta-hydroxybutyric acid and the production of ammonia in the kidney.[86] Möllerström,[80–85] who has conducted extensive research on the circadian rhythms of carbohydrate metabolism in diabetes mellitus, has suggested that the timing and dosage of insulin administered to patients with severe diabetes mellitus should be correlated with the rhythm of beta-hydroxybutyric acid excretion.

Insulin/glucose ratios have also been determined to be higher in the morning than they are in the afternoon,[43] and plasma glucose values in diabetics are significantly higher in the morning than at night.[42] Some investigators have further suggested that fasting plasma triglyceride levels may indicate the degree of circadian variation in plasma glucose.[54,70,108] But others maintain that fasting blood sugar in patients treated with insulin is not a reliable indicator of circadian variations in blood sugar.[70]

Serial electrocardiograms of diabetics over a 24-hour period sometimes show changes in the T wave and ST segment; these changes usually are considered to be indicative of coronary insufficiency.[56]

The existence of metabolic rhythms in diabetics and the possibility that they are associated with patterns of sleep, meal-taking and work suggest that individuals with this disease should not depart from their regular routines. Rotational shift work is particularly hazardous for them, since changes in insulin/glucose and plasma glucose values could result in imbalance and decreased insulin effectiveness. Undiagnosed or potential diabetics face the same possibility.

RESPIRATORY, CARDIOVASCULAR AND RENAL DISORDERS.—Abnormalities in the vital capacity rhythm have been noted in individuals suffering from asthma, pulmonary tuberculosis and heart disease.[36,38,73] In some cases, the rhythm has completely inverted during illness and returned to normal following recovery.[37] In other respiratory ailments, such as chronic bronchitis and emphysema, forced vital capacity and forced expiratory volume declined during night to a minimum at 0600 hours and rose again during the morning.[64] The forced expiratory volume rhythm has also been observed in healthy subjects.[48,120]

Hemoptysis, cerebral hemorrhage, pulmonary edema and cardiac asthma are believed to occur more frequently at night.[60,61] Circadian variations have also been observed in the blood pressure of hypertensive individuals,[71, 74, 78] and these variations may play some role in the frequency with which cerebral infarctions occur at night.[34, 113] Hypertensive individuals also exhibit significantly greater variations in plasma volume than do their nonhypertensive counterparts.[31] On the basis of these and other findings,[13–15, 46, 59, 98] it would seem advisable for hypertensive individuals and those with cardiac disorders to avoid rotational shift work programs.

Persons suffering from renal disorders are also poor prospects for intermittent shift work because the flow of urine and excretion of metabolites follow a circadian pattern. A high output of urine during the night hours has long been accepted medically as an indication of physiologic disorder. Furthermore, when renal problems occur, the other circadian rhythms may also be disturbed.[75, 76]

EPILEPSY.—Epileptic individuals, like diabetics, face particular problems during rotational shift work because epileptic attacks follow a rhythmic pattern with regard to the time of day when attacks occur.[62] Epileptics can be categorized into three groups: those subject to nocturnal seizures, those affected primarily during the day and those equally prone to attack at either time. Individuals in the night and day groups respond to the beginning and end of the sleep period in a diametrically opposite manner, the nocturnal group having attacks at the beginning of the sleep period and the diurnal group at the end.[47]

In a study of 110 epileptic patients, Griffiths and Fox[47] noted that the incidence of seizures rose steadily from 0300 hours and reached a very marked peak between 0600 and 0700 hours. The second highest incidence occurred between 2200 and 2400 hours. Bercel[10] found that night shift workers tend to experience seizures at the appropriate diurnal sleep time.

It has also been suggested that the time of seizure may be related to variations in corticosteroid levels,[41, 50] and corticosteroid rhythms, as we have seen, can be desynchronized when the light-dark cycle is shifted.[66, 92]

Emotional and Behavioral Problems

Changes in circadian rhythms frequently are associated with emotional and psychiatric disorders. Persons suffering from emotional disturbances have exhibited distinct variations in their circadian rhythms, particularly the excretion of metabolites.[40, 67] Schizophrenic patients, for example, have shown marked changes in the urine excretion and sleep-wakefulness rhythms.[45, 55, 100] In fact, the onset of schizophrenic behavior appears to be characterized by prolonged periods of wakefulness.[58]

Individuals who are subject to depression and emotional problems should be considered carefully before being assigned to rotational shift work. The danger here lies in the possibility that this type of shifting may place too great a stress on persons who under other circumstances might be able to cope with their emotional problems. To cite an extreme example, in a study in which the subjects were phase-shifted under careful experimental conditions, an apparently "normal" subject completed the experiment and not long thereafter committed suicide.[26] Subjects in other phase-shifting experiments in which the light-dark cycle was altered experienced a deep sense of depression and hopelessness within 72 hours after a phase shift.[26]

Sleep Difficulties

As indicated earlier, the body does not adjust readily when the sleep period is reversed from night to day. During such a change, sleep stages are altered noticeably, as has been observed consistently in the EEGs of research subjects.[8, 57, 58, 115, 124, 126] Although the individual may sleep for an adequate number of hours, the altered rhythm of his sleep leaves him unrefreshed, listless and vaguely uncomfortable. These conditions may result partly from the lowering of adrenal hormone levels that occurs when customary sleep time is reversed.[125, 127] During such a reversal, both the temperature pattern and the brain waves exhibit abnormalities, and neither has been observed to return to normal in less than 2 weeks. Consequently, workers who are shifted more frequently than every 3 weeks to a month will be continually deprived of the health-giving, normal patterns of sleep, and decrements in performance and safety awareness inevitably follow.

Effects of Medication

The effectiveness of various medications and human responses to them follow 24-hour rhythmic patterns. An oral dose of an antihistamine preparation will last 15–17 hours when administered at 0700 hours but only 6–8 hours when given at 1900 hours.[101] Similarly, both metyrapone and dexamethasone are more effective when administered at midnight,[69, 90] and digitalis has twice the impact when taken at night.[106] Glucocorticoids, on the other hand, are more effective and have fewer side effects when administered early in the day.[104, 107] Medications for diabetes mellitus[68] and epilepsy[68] also exhibit circadian variations, as do aspirin,[68] cold remedies,[68] barbiturates[103] and appetite suppressants.[102]

Work Performance and Safety Awareness

Research on performance and safety records of shift workers has correlated time of day with decrements in these areas. Investigators have also established that performance is closely related to disturbances in circadian rhythms.[99]

Browne[17, 18] determined that teleprinter switchboard operators in a large communication center exhibited a distinct circadian variation in performance. In his studies, delay in responding to calls was used as the criterion for performance effectiveness. Over a 3-month period, operator performance was noted to improve between 0900 hours and noon, remain fairly constant until 1700 hours and decline rapidly thereafter. The time of day was also determined to have a greater effect than did the pressure of the work load.

Bjerner and coworkers[12] investigated the number of errors made by workers during meter reading and computation to gain further insight into the circadian aspects of performance. The workers studied were required to read meters measuring such information as temperature, gas consumption and gas pressure, and to record their readings and computations in a ledger every hour. After examining 175,000 ledger entries, the investigators found that decrements in performance followed a circadian pattern. Errors reached a high peak at 0300 hours and a lesser one at 1500 hours. Changes in shifts at 0600, 1400 and 2200 hours had little effect on the pattern of error making. When the workweek was shortened, the number of errors decreased but the temporal pattern remained the same.

Similarly, industrial accidents seem to occur according to a 24-hour frequency,[77] the greatest number happening between 2200 and 0200 hours.

Performance is closely correlated with the body temperature rhythm. Colquhoun and associates,[25] in a study of young naval personnel on rotating and stabilized shift work, determined that body temperature is a predictor of performance efficiency. The findings were reinforced by later work, from which it was concluded that the optimal solution for achieving performance efficiency during night work would be a fixed night shift with all members living more or less permanently on an inverted sleep-work routine.[23]

Toulouse and Pieron[114] discovered that a number of individuals who had worked as night watchmen for several years had completely inverted body temperature rhythms, highs occurring in the morning and lows in the afternoon or evening. The implications of this finding are evident when we realize that performance is optimal when body temperature is high and minimal when it is low.

Teleky[111] compared the body temperature rhythms of nurses on intermittent night duty with those of bakery workers on various shift arrangements. The nurses worked from 2000 to 0800 or 0900 hours for 1 month in every 3 or 4 months. The bakery workers, on the other hand, varied from working on a fixed night shift to alternating shifts every other day. The nurses exhibited only a slight trend toward body temperature inversion during the first week on night duty, and none had a completely inverted curve by the end of the fourth week. Two of the bakery workers on a fixed night shift had completely inverted body temperature curves, and a third had his maximal body temperature at 0200 hours. Thirteen of them were accustomed to night work but also worked periodically on the day shift for 2-week intervals. The body temperature rhythms of 9 of this group inverted completely within 5 days after night work began, with the maximum occurring at 0700 hours. Three had maximal readings at 0200 hours. Only 1 showed no indication of body temperature inversion. When these workers returned to day work, their body temperature curves reverted to normal even more rapidly than they had inverted.

Similar findings have been reported by Bonjer,[16] Van Loon[116] and Wojtczak-Jaroszowa and Banaszkiewicz.[128]

It has been suggested that plasma corticosteroid concentration is associated with alertness.[49] Migeon and co-workers[79] noted that the normal corticosteroid rhythm persisted in nurses who had been on night duty for 6 months and in night watchmen; they observed a pattern very similar to that of subjects on day work, the usual decline beginning at about 0800 hours. Perkhoff and colleagues,[96] on the other hand, claimed that the rhythm of plasma 17-hydroxycorticosteroids could be reversed within 5–10 days after the sleep-work cycle was reversed. The subjects in their study changed their sleeping time to 0800–1600 hours. The phase of the plasma corticosteroid rhythm also shifted by 8 hours and attained a maximal concentration at 1600 hours. The amplitude of the rhythm was very low compared with that usually observed in day workers. Conroy[28] found that the rhythm can adapt in night workers who are on a fixed schedule as opposed to those on rotating shifts.

In a later study, Conroy[29] compared the circadian rhythms of 11-hydroxycorticosteroid plasma concentration in day and night workers at a light-engineering company with those of night workers in a newspaper printing plant. The engineers worked under a rotational shifting program whereas the newspaper employees were on night duty permanently. The engineering shift workers exhibited a greater variety of patterns and more irregularities in their plasma corticosteroid rhythms than did the newspaper workers. The investigators concluded, however, that an individual's suitability for rotational shift work could not be determined solely on the basis of the plasma corticosteroid rhythm.

Hale and his associates[51] found that rotational shift work induced upward physiologic displacement in the nocturnal excretion of epinephrine, norepinephrine, 17-hydroxycorticosteroids, urea and potassium, all of which are symptomatic of nonspecific stress.

In assessing the outlook for satisfactory performance and alertness during rotational shift work, it may become necessary to consider both the adrenal and body temperature rhythms. The former has been demonstrated to affect alertness[94, 118] and the latter can be easily and painlessly obtained.

PREPARATION OF EMPLOYEES FOR ROTATIONAL SHIFT WORK

Most bodily functions and systems are circadian in nature and therefore can be disturbed when day is reversed to night. On a fixed-shift system, the body adapts over time and the individual continues with the arrangement more or less permanently, with no particular problems. Under rotational shift work, however, the body is called on to adapt and readapt continually. Healthy, well-adjusted individuals can experience physiologic disorientation and desynchronization as well as impaired performance and alertness. Individuals who suffer from diseases such as diabetes mellitus and epilepsy or from psychological and emotional problems are subject to even greater difficulties because of the changes that occur in their internal rhythms.

The optimal solution would be for all shift work to be scheduled on a fixed basis, but not all companies and organizations will want to operate that way and will opt for rotational shift work. In so doing, they have responsibilities to their employees to ensure their health and safety. At the same time, companies will wish to ensure their own productivity and safety programs.

The major concern is with scheduling shifts. In this regard, management should schedule employees so that their physiologic rhythms (biologic clock) can adapt and stabilize satisfactorily before being required to readapt. Thus, shifts should not be rotated rapidly; they should be so arranged that the employee spends at least 3 weeks to 1 month on the same shift.

The second concern of management should be to carefully evaluate employees before they are assigned to rotational shift work programs to determine whether they will be seriously affected by the program, either physically or emotionally. This assessment can be accomplished through medical testing consistent with the findings of the research accomplished to date.

The third activity that management must be concerned with is to instruct those individuals who are cleared for the program on the problems they could face and how to cope with them.

We offer the following suggestions for screening and preparing employees for rotational shift work:

Screen out individuals who will face health hazards or emotional problems. (Accomplish with interviews and tests.)

Screen out employees required to take any medication, such as insulin, whose rhythm can be affected by reversal of the day-night cycle. (Accomplish through interviews, using knowledge of the drugs that are time-oriented.)

Determine whether employees have difficulty sleeping under normal conditions. (Tests can be made with small EEG monitoring devices recently developed.) Anyone who has radical sleep problems should not be considered for the program.

Assess the performance and alertness outlook of prospective shift work employees. (Temperature recording curves and urine excretory surveys can be used.)

Prepare all accepted employees for the problems that they may face during rotational shifting and instruct them in how to cope with those problems. With regard to the latter, we offer the following suggestions for coping:

Perform the most important tasks as soon after waking as possible.

Avoid working with power tools or driving a vehicle when feeling sleepy or disoriented.

Eat the largest meal of the day as soon as possible after waking. Decrease caloric intake slightly and avoid overloading the system with food.

Decrease intake of salt, coffee, beer, wine and hard liquor.

Use only prescribed medications and inform the plant medical adviser of the drugs being taken.

CONCLUSIONS

Night work, when more or less permanent, does not present serious problems to workers. Problems occur, however, during rotational shift work because of the disturbance of the internal bodily rhythms by the inversion of the light-dark cycle and the rapid disruption of this cycle during the rotational process. Organizations that utilize rotational shift work can ensure the health and safety of their employees and their own productivity by carefully screening all individuals assigned to the program and preparing them for the problems that they may face.

REFERENCES

1. Aanonsen, A.: Medical problems of shift work, Ind. Med. Surg. 28:422–427, 1959.
2. Aanonsen, A.: *Shift Work and Health* (Olso: Norwegian Monographs on Medical Science, 1964).
3. Åkerstedt, T., et al.: *Shift Work and Well-Being*. Reports from The Laboratory for Clinical Stress Research, Karolinska Institute, Stockholm. No. 63b, 1977.
4. Åkerstedt, T., Patkai, P., and Dahlgren, K.: Field studies of shiftwork: II. Temporal patterns in psychophysiological activation in workers alternating between night and day work, Ergonomics 20:621, 1977.
5. Andlauer, P., and Fourrel, L.: Le travail en équipes alternantes, Rev. Fr. Travail, Oct.–Dec., 1965, pp. 35–50.
6. Aschoff, J.: Circadian rhythms in man, Science 148:1427, 1965.
7. Aschoff, J.: Human circadian rhythms in continuous darkness: Entrainment by social clues, Science 171:213, 1971.
8. Beljan, J. R., Rosenblatt, L. S., Hetherington, N. W., et al.: *Human Performance in the Aviation Environment,* final report, NASA Contract NAS2-6657, 1972.
9. Benedict, F. G.: Studies in body temperature. I. Influence of the inversion of the daily routine; the temperature of night workers, Am. J. Physiol. 11:145, 1904.
10. Bercel, N. A.: The periodic features of some seizure states, Ann. N.Y. Acad. Sci. 117:555, 1964.
11. Bjerner, B., and Swennsson, A.: Shift work and rhythm, Acta Med. Scand. (supp.)278: 102, 1953.
12. Bjerner, B. A., Holm, A., and Swennsson, A.: Diurnal variation in mental performance. A study of three shift workers, Br. J. Ind. Med. 12:103, 1955.
13. Bliss, E. L., Sandberg, A. A., Nelson, D. H., et al.: The normal levels of 17-hydroxycorticosteroids in the peripheral blood in man, J. Clin. Invest. 32:818, 1953.
14. Bloch, M.: Rhythmic diurnal variation in limb blood flow in man, Nature 202:398, 1964.
15. Board, F., Wadeson, R., and Persky, H.: Depressive effect and endocrine functions, Arch. Neurol. Psychiatry 78:612, 1957.
16. Bonjer, F. H.: Physiological aspects of shift work, Proc. Int. Consort. Occup. Health 13: 848, 1960.
17. Browne, R. C.: The day and night performance of teleprinter switchboard operators, Occup. Psychol. 23:121, 1949.
18. Browne, R. C.: The Day and Night Performance Rhythm in Industry, in *5th Conf. Soc. Biol. Rhythm* (Stockholm: Aco Print, 1961), pp. 61–64.
19. Bruusgaard, A.: An investigation of inquiry on health problems in shift work in the Norwegian paper industry, A.M.A. Arch. Ind. Hyg. 2:465, 1950.
20. Bureau of Labor Statistics, U. S. Dept. of Labor, Washington, D. C., 1975.
21. Carpentier, J., and Cazamian, P.: *Night Work* (Geneva: International Labour Organisation, 1977).
22. Chiles, W. D., Alluisi, E. A., and Adams, O. S.: Work schedules and performance during confinement, Hum. Factors 10:143, 1968.
23. Colquhoun, W. P.: Circadian rhythms, mental efficiency and shift work, Ergonomics 13:558, 1970.
24. Colquhoun, W. P. (ed.): Circadian Variations in Mental Efficiency, in *Biological Rhythms and Human Performance* (London and New York: Academic Press, 1971), Chap. 2, pp. 39–105.
25. Colquhoun, W. P., Blake, M. J. F., and Edwards, R. S.: Experimental studies of shift work. II. Stabilized 8-hour shift systems, Ergonomics 11:527, 1968.
26. Conference on Circadian Dysrhythmias, Ames Research Center, NASA, Moffett Field, Calif., March 3–4, 1975.
27. Conroy, R. T. W. L.: Circadian excretory rhythms in night workers, Br. J. Ind. Med. 27:356, 1971.
28. Conroy, R. T. W. L.: Circadian rhythm of 11-hydroxycorticosteroids in night workers, J. Physiol. 191:21, 1967.
29. Conroy, R. T. W. L.: Circadian rhythms in plasma concentration of 11-hydroxycorticosteroids in men working on night shift and in permanent night workers, Br. J. Ind. Med. 27:170, 1970.
30. Conroy, R. T. W. L., and Mills, J. N.: *Human Circadian Rhythms* (London: J. & A. Churchill, 1970).
31. Cranston, W. I., and Brown, W.: Diurnal variation in plasma volume in normal and hypertensive subjects, Clin. Sci. 25:107, 1963.
32. De la Mare, G., and Shimmin, S.: Preferred patterns of duty in a flexible shift working situation, Occup. Psychol. 38:203, 1964.
33. De la Mare, G., and Walker, J.: Shift working: The arrangement of hours on night work, Nature 208:1127, 1965.

34. Dickinson, C. J.: *Neurogenic Hypertension* (London: Blackwell, 1965).
35. Dirken, J. M.: Industrial shift work: Decrease in well being and specific effects, Ergonomics 9:115, 1966.
36. Dissmann, E.: Klinische Studien über den 24-Studen-Rhythmus und seine Störungen bei Lungentuberkulösen, Acta Tuberc. Scand. 21:204, 1947.
37. Dissmann, E.: Lungenblutung und 24-Studen-Rhythmus, Acta Tuberc. Scand. 24:277, 1950.
38. Dissmann, E.: Zur Frage von Eigenrhythmus und Grundrhythmus in den Tagesschwankungen der Vitalkapazität, Acta Med. Scand. 137:441, 1950.
39. Doll, R., Jones, F. A., and Buckatzsch, M. M.: *Occupational Factors in the Aetiology of Gastric and Duodenal Ulcers, with an Estimate of their Incidence in the General Population*. Special Report Series No. 276, Medical Research Council, London, 1951.
40. Elithorn, A., Bridges, P. K., Lobban, M. C., et al.: Observations on some diurnal rhythms in depressive illness, Br. Med. J. 2:1620, 1966.
41. Engel, R., Halberg, F., and Gully, R. J.: The diurnal rhythm in EEG discharge and in circulating eosinophils in certain types of epilepsy, Electroencephalogr. Clin. Neurophysiol. 4:115, 1952.
42. Faiman, C., and Moorhouse, J. A.: Diurnal variation in the levels of glucose and related substances in healthy and diabetic subjects during starvation, Clin. Sci. 32:111, 1967.
43. Freinkel, N., Mager, M., and Vinnick, L.: Cyclicity in the interrelationships between plasma insulin and glucose during starvation in normal young men, J. Lab. Clin. Med. 71:171, 1968.
44. Gavrilescu, N., et al.: Control-Board Shift Work Turning Every Two Days, in *15th International Congress on Occupational Health, Vienna, 19–24 September, 1966*, Vol. IV, pp. 103–106.
45. Gjessing, R.: Beiträge zur Kenntnis der Pathophysiologie der hatonen Erregung, mit kritischem Beginn und Abschluss, Arch. Psychiatry 104:355, 1936.
46. Goldman, R.: Studies in diurnal variation of water and electrolyte excretion: Nocturnal diuresis of water and sodium in congestive cardiac failure and cirrhosis of the liver, J. Clin. Invest. 30:1191, 1951.
47. Griffiths, G. M., and Fox, J. T.: Rhythm in epilepsy, Lancet 2:409, 1938.
48. Guberan, E., William, M. K., Walford, J., et al.: Diurnal variation of FEV in shiftworkers, Br. J. Ind. Med. 26:121, 1969.
49. Halberg, F.: Physiologic 24-hour periodicity: General and procedural considerations with reference to the adrenal cycle, Z. Vitam. Horm. Fermentforsch. 10:225, 1959.
50. Halberg, F., Engel, R., Halberg, E., et al.: Diurnal variations in amount of electroencephalographic paroxysmal discharge and diurnal eosinophil rhythm of epileptics on days with clinical seizures, Fed. Proc. 11:62, 1952.
51. Hale, H. B., Williams, E. W., Smith, B. N., et al.: Neuroendocrine and metabolic responses to intermittent night shift work, Aerosp. Med. 42:156, 1971.
52. Higgins, E. A., Chiles, W. D., McKenzie, J. M., et al.: *The Effects of a 12-hour Shift in the Wake-Sleep Cycle on Physiological and Biochemical Responses and on Multiple Task Performance,* Report FAA-AM-75-10, Federal Aviation Administration, Office of Aviation Medicine, Oklahoma City, Okla., 1975.
53. Hoagland, H., Pincus, G., Fred, E., et al.: Study of adrenocortical physiology in normal and schizophrenic men, Arch. Neurol. Psychiatry 69:470, 1953.
54. Hollister, L. E.: Successive trials of induced alimentary lipemia, Am. J. Clin. Nutr. 13:214, 1963.
55. Hoskins, R. G.: *The Biology of Schizophrenia*. The Thomas William Memorial Lecture, N.Y. Acad. Sci. (New York: Norton, 1946).
56. Kilinskii, E. L., and Egart, F. M.: Coronary circulation in patients with diabetes mellitus (diurnal variations in ECG patterns), Fed. Proc. (transl. supp.) 23:301, 1964.
57. Kleitman, N.: Sleep, Sci. Am. 187:34, 1952.
58. Kleitman, N.: *Sleep and Wakefulness* (Chicago: The University of Chicago Press, 1967).
59. Knapp, M. S., Keane, P. M., and Wright, J. C.: Circadian rhythm of plasma 11-hydroxycorticosteroids in depressive illness, congestive heart failure, and Cushing's syndrome, Br. Med. J. 2:27, 1967.
60. Kranzfeld, B.: Zur Frage über die physiologischen Tagesschwankungen der Thrombocytenzahl, Pfluegers Arch. Ges. Physiol. 210: 583, 1925.
61. Kroetz, C.: Ein Biologischer 24-Studen-Rhythmus des Blutkreislaufs bei Gesundheit und bei Herzschwäche, zugleich ein Beitrag zur tageszeitlichen Häufung einiger akuter Kreislaufstörungen, Munch. Med. Wochenschr. 87:314, 1940.

62. Langdon-Down, M., and Brain, W. R.: Time of day in relation to convulsions in epilepsy, Lancet 1:1029, 1929.
63. Lehmann, G.: Effect of Environmental Factors on Biologic Cycles and Performance of Work, in Schaefer, K. E. (ed.), *Man's Dependence on the Earthly Atmosphere* (New York: The Macmillan Co., 1962), pp. 381–387.
64. Lewinsohn, H. C., Capel, L. H., and Smart, J.: Changes in forced expiratory volumes throughout the day, Br. Med. J. 1:462, 1960.
65. Litsov, A. N.: On the question of dynamics of the electroencephalogram in the case of man during sleep under common and altered 24-hour regimes, Izv. Akad. Nauk, SSSR Ser. Biol. 4:521, 1970.
66. Lobban, M. C.,: Dissociation in Human Rhythmic Functions, in Aschoff, J. (ed.), *Circadian Clocks* (Amsterdam: North-Holland Publishing Co., 1965), pp. 219–227.
67. Lobban, M. C., Tredre, B., Elithorn, A., et al.: Diurnal rhythms of electrolyte excretion in depressive illness, Nature 199:667, 1963.
68. Luce, G. L.: *Body Time* (New York: Pantheon Books, 1971).
69. Martin, M. M., and Hellman, D. F.: Temporal variation in SU 4885 responsiveness in man: Evidence in support of circadian variation in ACTH secretion, J. Clin. Endocrinol. 24:253, 1964.
70. Maruhama, Y., Goto, Y., and Yamagata, S.: Diabetic treatment and the diurnal plasma triglycerides, Metabolism 16:985, 1967.
71. Masoni, A.: 24-hour rhythms of cardiovascular functions in normal and hypertensive subjects. Atti VII Conf. Intern. Soc. Stud. Ritm. Biol. Turin, Panminerva Med. 110:66, 1960.
72. McGirr, P. O. M.: Health Consideration, in *The Benefits and Problems of Shift Working*. PERA Symposium, Sec. 5, 1–6, 1966.
73. Menzel, W.: Der 24-Studen-Rhythmus des menschlichen Blutkreislaufes, Med. Kinderh. 61:1, 1941.
74. Menzel, W.: Klinische Ziele der Rhythmusforschung, Acta Med. Scand. (supp.) 307:107, 1955.
75. Menzel, W.: Periodicity in urinary excretion in healthy and nephropathic persons, Ann. N.Y. Acad. Sci. 98:1007, 1962.
76. Menzel, W.: Wellenlänge, Phasenlage und Amplitude in der Nierenrhythmik des Menschen, Acta Med. Scand. (supp.) 278: 95, 1953.
77. Menzel, W.: Zur Physiologie and Pathologie des Nacht- und Schichtarbeiters, Arbeitsphysiologie 14:304, 1950.
78. Menzel, W., Timm, R., and Herrnring, G.: Über den diagnostischen Wert der Tag-Nacht-Schwankungen des erhöhten Blutdruckes, Verh. Dtsch. Ges. Kreislaufforsch. 15:256, 1949.
79. Migeon, C. J., Tyler, F. H., Mahoney, J. P., et al.: The diurnal variations of plasma levels and urinary excretion of 17-hydroxycorticosteroid in normal subjects, night workers, and blind subjects, J. Clin. Endocrinol. 16:622, 1956.
80. Möllerström, J.: Das Diabetesproblem: Die Rhythmischen Stoffwechselvorgänge, Acta Med. Scand. (supp.) 147:1, 1943.
81. Möllerström, J.: Diurnal rhythm in severe diabetes mellitus. The significance of harmoniously-timed insulin treatment, Diabetes 3:188, 1954.
82. Möllerström, J.: Periodicity of carbohydrate metabolism and rhythmic functioning of the liver. Their significance in the treatment of diabetes with insulin, Arch. Intern. Med. 52:649, 1933.
83. Möllerström, J.: Some new observations and principles concerning diabetes research and their practical application to diabetic therapy, Acta Med. Upsalien 41:287, 1935.
84. Möllerström, J.: The treatment of diabetes with reference to the endogenous periodicity of the carbohydrate metabolism, Acta Med. Scand. (supp.) 59:145, 1934.
85. Möllerström, J.: Theoretical considerations and practical results in the management of diabetes, Acta Med. Scand. (supp.) 196:12, 1947.
86. Möllerström, J., and Sollberger, A.: The 24-hour rhythm of metabolic processes in diabetes: Citric acid in the urine, Acta Med. Scand. 160:25, 1958.
87. Morgan, B. B., Jr., Brown, B. R., and Alluisi, E. A.: Effects on sustained performance of 48 hours of continuous work and sleep loss, Hum. Factors 16:406, 1974.
88. Mott, P. E., Mann, F. C., McLoughlin, Q., et al.: *Shift Work, The Social, Psychological and Physical Consequences* (London: Cresset Press, 1965).
89. Murrell, K. F. H.: *Ergonomics: Man in His Working Environment* (London: Chapman and Hall; New York: Halsted Press, 1969).
90. Nichols, T., Nugent, C. A., and Tyler, F. H.: Diurnal variation in suppression of adrenal function by glucocorticoids, J. Clin. Endocrinol. 25:343, 1965.
91. Nowlin, J. B., Eisdorfe, C., Whalen, R., et

al.: Effect of exogenous changes in heart-rate and rhythm upon reaction-time performance, Psychophysiology 7:186, 1970.

92. Orth, D. N., and Island, D. P.: Light synchronization of the circadian rhythm in plasma cortisol (17-OHCS) concentration in man, J. Clin. Endocrinol. 29:479, 1969.

93. Östberg, O.: Interindividual differences in circadian fatigue patterns of shift workers, Br. J. Ind. Med. 30:341, 1973.

94. Patkai, P.: Interindividual differences in diurnal variations in alertness, performance, and adrenalin excretion, Acta Physiol. Scand. 81:35, 1971.

95. Patkai, P., Åkerstedt, T., and Pettersson, K.: Field studies of shiftwork: I. Temporal patterns in psychophysiological activation in permanent night workers, Ergonomics 20: 611, 1977.

96. Perkhoff, G. T., Eik-Nes, K., Nugent, C. A., et al.: Studies of the diurnal variation of plasma 17-hydroxycorticosteroids in man, J. Clin. Endocrinol. 19:432, 1959.

97. Pittendrigh, C. S.: Circadian rhythms and the circadian organization of living systems, Cold Spring Harbor Symp. Quant. Biol. 25:159, 1960.

98. Rabinovitch, I. M., and Strean, G.: Hemoglobin content of the red blood cells in relation to their surface area; preliminary report, Arch. Intern. Med. 34:124, 1924.

99. Radnot, M., Wallner, E., and Hoenig, M.: Die Wirkung des Lichtes und des Hydergin auf die Eosinophilen Leukocyten des Blutes, Wein. Klin. Wochenschr. 72:101, 1960.

100. Randrup, A., and Munkvad, I.: Changes in urine volume and diurnal rhythm caused by reserpine treatment of schizophrenic patients, Br. J. Psychiatry 112:173, 1966.

101. Reinberg, A., and Sidi, E.: Circadian changes in the inhibitory effects of an antihistaminic drug in man, J. Invest. Dermatol. 46:415, 1966.

102. Scheving, L. E.: Daily circadian rhythms in rats to *d*-amphetamine sulphate: The effect of blinding and continuous illumination on the rhythm, Nature 219:621, 1968.

103. Scheving, L. E., Vidral, D. F., and Pauly, J. R.: A circadian susceptibility rhythm in rats to pentobarbital sodium, Anat. Rec. 160:741, 1968.

104. Segre, E. J., and Kainber, E. L.: Therapeutic utilization of the diurnal variation in pituitary-adrenocorticol activity, Calif. West. Med. 104:363, 1966.

105. Sharp, G. W. G.: The effect of light on the morning increase in urine flow, J. Endocrinol. 21:219, 1960.

106. Sollberger, A.: *Biological Rhythm Research* (New York: Elsevier Publishing Co., 1965).

107. Soyka, L. F., and Saxema, K. M.: Alternate day steroid therapy for nephrotic children JAMA 192:225, 1965.

108. Sterky, G. C. G., Persson, B. E. H., and Larson, Y. A. A.: Dietary fats, the diurnal blood lipids and ketones in juvenile diabetics, Diabetologia 2:14, 1966.

109. Taylor, P. J.: Shift and day work. A comparison of sickness absence, lateness and other absence behaviour at an oil refinery from 1962 to 1965, Br. J. Ind. Med. 24:93, 1967.

110. Taylor, P. J.: The effects of shift work on worker health, Ind. Med. Surg. 42:13, 1973.

111. Teleky, L.: Problems of nightwork: Influences on health and efficiency, Ind. Med. Surg. 12:758, 1943.

112. Thiss-Evenson, E.: Shift work and health, Ind. Med. 27:493, 1958.

113. Toole, J. F.: Nocturnal strokes and arterial hypotension, Ann. Intern. Med. 68:1132, 1968.

114. Toulouse, E., and Pieron, H.: Le mechanisme de l'inversion chez l'homme du rhythme nycthermal de la temperature, J. Physiol. Pathol. Gen. 9:425, 1907.

115. Tune, G. S.: The human sleep debt, Sci. J. 4:67, 1968.

116. Van Loon, J. H.: Diurnal body temperature curves in shift workers, Ergonomics 6:267, 1963.

117. Van Loon, J. H.: The diurnal rhythm of body temperature in nightworkers, Acta Physiol. Pharmacol. Neerl. 8:302, 1959.

118. Vernikos-Danellis, J., Winget, C. M., and Hetherington, N. M.: Diurnal rhythms of the pituitary-adrenocortical response to stress effect of constant light and constant darkness. COSPAR, Plenary Meeting, 12th. Prague, Czechoslovakia, 1970.

119. Wade, L.: "Human relations" approach to sickness, absenteeism and other employee problems, Arch. Ind. Med. 12:592, 1955.

120. Walford, J., Lammers, B., Schilling, R. S. F., et al.: Diurnal variation in ventilatory capacity. An epidemiological study of cotton and other factory workers employed on shift work, Br. J. Ind. Med. 23:142, 1966.

121. Walker, J.: Frequent alternation of shift on continuous work, Occup. Psychol. 40:215, 1966.

122. Walker, J., and De la Mare, G.: Absence from work in relation to length and distri-

bution of shift hours, Br. J. Ind. Med. 28:36, 1971.

123. Webb, R. A., and Obrist, P. A.: The physiological concomitants of reaction time performance as a function of preparatory interval and preparatory interval series, Psychophysiology 6:389, 1970.

124. Webb, W. B., Agnew, H., Jr., and Williams, R. L.: Effects on sleep of a sleep period time displacement, Aerosp. Med. 42:152, 1971.

125. Weitzman, E. D., Fukushim, D., Nogeire, C., et al.: 24-hour pattern of episodic secretion of cortisol in normal subjects, J. Clin. Endocrinol. Metab. 33:14, 1971.

126. Weitzman, E. D., Goldmacher, D., Kripke, D., et al.: Reversal of sleep-waking cycle: Effect on sleepstage pattern and certain neuroendocrine rhythms, Trans. Am. Neurol. Assoc. 93:153, 1968.

127. Weitzman, E. D., Schaumburg, H., and Fishbein, W.: Plasma 17-hydroxycorticosteroid levels during sleep in man, J. Clin. Endocrinol. 26:121, 1966.

128. Wojtczak-Jaroszowa, J., and Banaszkiewicz, A.: Physical work capacity during the day and at night, Ergonomics 17:193, 1974.

129. Wyatt, S., and Marriott, R.: Night work and night shift changes, Br. J. Ind. Med. 10:164, 1953.

PART FIVE

The Chemical Working Environment

11 / Current Aspects of Solvent-Related Disorders

OLAV AXELSON, M.D., MONICA HANE, Ph.D., and CHRISTER HOGSTEDT, M.D.

EXPOSURE TO SOLVENTS occurs frequently in various types of industry and constitutes a potential health hazard to millions of workers throughout the world. In Sweden, a country of 8 million inhabitants, a recent trade union inquiry revealed that 270,000 workers considered solvent exposure to be a problem. Estimates of specified solvent exposure might be taken from some of the NIOSH (National Institute for Occupational Safety and Health) criteria documents, stating that 100,000 workers may have exposure to toluene in the United States and some 140,000 individuals may have a potential occupational exposure to xylene. In many trades, almost every worker is exposed, for example, painters, varnishers and carpet layers, although some recent developments have taken place in the use of water-based paints and glues. The degree of solvent exposure apparently varies considerably in the context of painting, varnishing and open degreasing operations. It has been shown that high exposures to styrene have occurred in the manufacturing of plastic boats, styrene constituting a component of the plastic as well as a solvent for the polyester resin. Although many processes require the evaporation of solvents and therefore are problematic from the hygienic point of view, it is also possible to apply work practices and to use equipment that minimize exposure, for example, in metal-degreasing operations (Figs 11-1–11-5), when the solvent is reutilized. It should be remembered, however, that even modern and well-functioning equipment needs cleaning, servicing and repair, and such work often will result in high but short-time exposure levels. Open handling of solvents and primitive degreasing operations are common in small automobile repair shops, etc., but also in many temporary jobs in the large and usually well-organized factories. Furthermore, it should be recognized that the hygienic concerns about solvents are also applicable in the context of exposure to anesthetic gases in operating theaters and also with regard to handling gasoline and jet fuel in distribution or in repairing equipment such as pumps and tanks.

SOLVENT EXPOSURE: MEDICAL EFFECTS

The acute, narcotic effects of solvents have been known for a long time and some of the industrial solvents have a history of use as general anesthetics (e.g., ether, trichloroethylene and even gasoline). Toxic effects on the blood and liver were early recognized as caused by benzene and carbon tetrachloride. Irritation of mucous membranes is another acute but usually less severe effect caused by, for example, styrene and isopropyl alcohol. Sometimes asthmatic conditions are associated with solvent exposure, usually depending on a nonspecific (nonallergic) hyperreactivity, often requiring that the worker change to another job.

Although case reports have indicated a

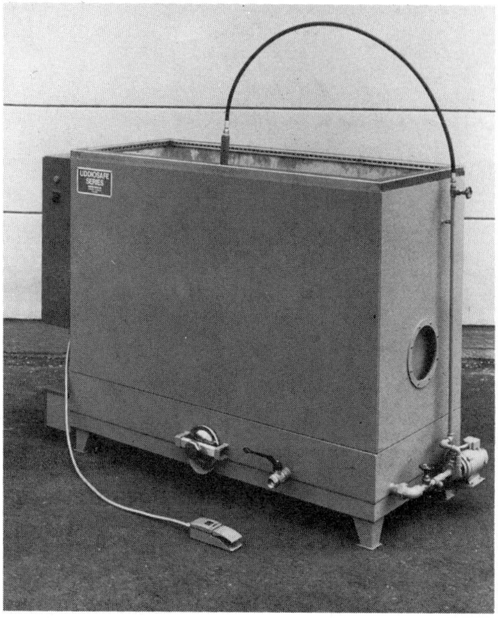

Fig 11–1.—Air-cooled vapor degreaser with spray lance. The ventilation air is also used for condensation of solvent vapor. No connection to tap water is necessary. (Courtesy of Uddeholm Co., Uddeholm, Sweden.)

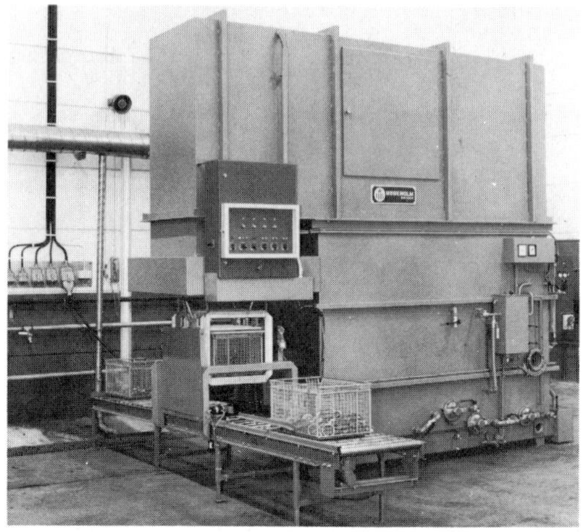

Fig 11–2.—Automatic cleaning machine for basket loads. Equipped with built-in still for cleaning in two boiling baths in countercurrent flow. Hood and slot exhaust ventilation for lowest possible workroom contamination. (Courtesy of Uddeholm Co., Uddeholm, Sweden.)

chronic effect of many solvents, comparatively little concern was given to this aspect until the 1970s, especially regarding the chronic neurotoxic effects. However, there is also an increasing interest in possible immunologic, carcinogenic, mutagenic and teratogenic effects of solvent exposure. Dermatologic problems are well known to be due to extraction of fat from the skin, but will not be considered in this chapter.

NEUROTOXIC EFFECTS

Experimental Studies

Although fairly well known, the acute effects of isolated short-time exposure to solvents have attracted an experimental interest during the past few years, resulting in better knowledge about the quantitative aspects of human solvent toxicology. By means of a uniform technique, Gamberale[22] has studied various commonly used solvents. Volunteers inhaled solvent vapors and the specific odors were masked by menthol. Exposure times of 1.5 hours were used and the uptake of the solvent was continually measured every 20 minutes; various psychological tests such as reaction time, short-term memory and single arithmetic items were measured and compared to the

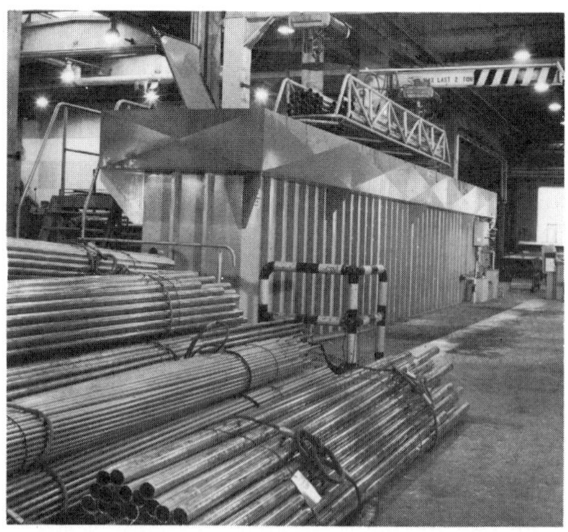

Fig 11–3.—Cool bath-vapor degreaser for large stainless steel tubes. (Courtesy of Uddeholm Co., Uddeholm, Sweden.)

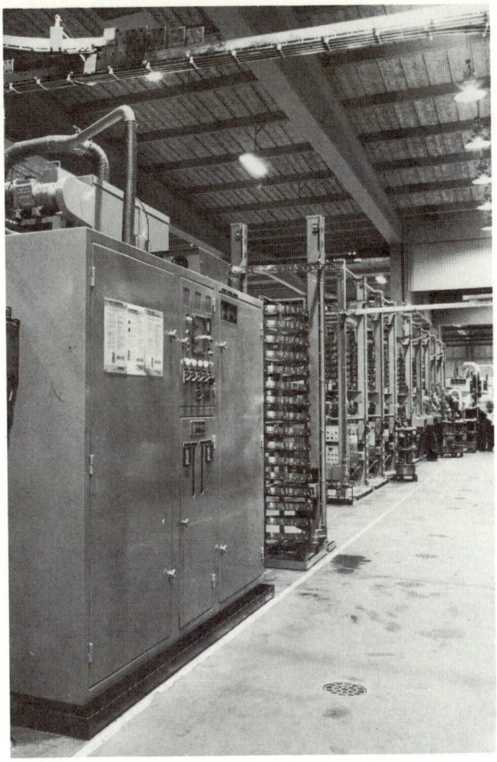

Fig 11–4.—Trichloroethylene degreaser with ultrasonics for cleaning all ball bearing rings in continuous line production. Cleaning cycle: vapor, ultrasonic rinse, spray, cooling and drying. (Courtesy of Uddeholm Co., Uddeholm, Sweden.)

results obtained without exposure. The overall result from these experiments seems to be that surprisingly low exposures will result in a significantly impaired performance; the results are briefly summarized in Table 11-1.

Similar studies have also been undertaken elsewhere and, according to one preliminary report, the results are fairly similar to those mentioned above[54] and, in particular, a prolonged reaction time seems to be a simple and reliable measure of the effect of solvent exposure.

It should also be recalled in this context that exposure to anesthetics bears on aspects similar to the industrial solvents. An American study[14] indicated decreasing perfor-

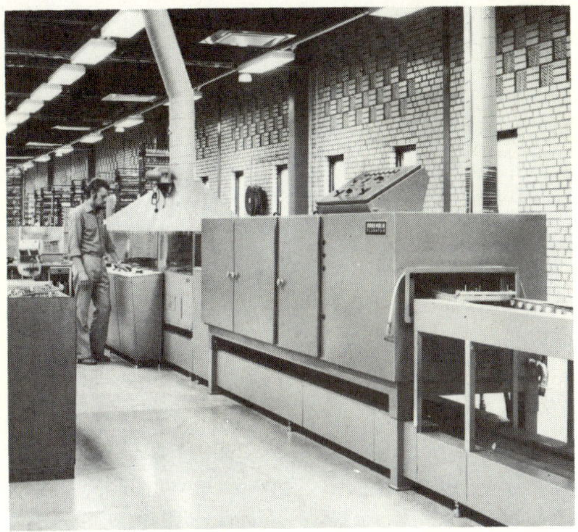

Fig 11–5.—Automatic machine for cleaning of printed circuit boards. The boards are cleaned from flux after soldering by brushing and spraying in three countercurrent stages. A built-in still continually feeds the cleaning chamber with regenerated solvent. Note exhaust system. (Courtesy of Uddeholm Co., Uddeholm, Sweden.)

mances on psychological tests about 2 hours after exposure to 50 ppm of nitrous oxide (N_2O), which is well below the concentrations that have been demonstrated in ordinary use in operating rooms where the operating personnel work all day. The psychological functions apparently most sensitive to anesthetics were visual perception and immediate memory, but lowered performances also were found on tasks that re-

TABLE 11–1.—MEANS OF CUMULATIVE UPTAKE OF SOLVENTS IN BLOOD AND TISSUES FOR GROUPS OF EXPERIMENTALLY EXPOSED SUBJECTS WHERE IMPAIRMENTS IN AT LEAST ONE PSYCHOLOGICAL FUNCTION HAVE BEEN DEMONSTRATED[3]

SOLVENT	UPTAKE (IN MG)	NUMBER OF SUBJECTS IN THE GROUP
Toluene	170	12
Methylchloroform	330	12
Styrene	590	12
White spirit (aromatic)	240	20
(aliphatic)	1055	
Methylene chloride	1145	14
Trichloroethylene	420	15

quired divided attention to simultaneous visual and auditory stimuli.

Population-based Studies

The evaluation of long-term effects of solvent exposure is associated with methodologic difficulties. Usually cross-sectional studies have been applied, i.e., the current disorders or complaints of an exposed group are referred to existing exposure levels. Consequently, the long-term effects might be overlooked, as those individuals who become more severely affected tend to have left the group of workers due to the symptoms or even because of disability or death. Thus, cross-sectional studies would easily underestimate the health hazard, and, therefore, negative results do not necessarily mean a safe work environment.

Another problematic aspect concerns the interpretation of isolated cases caused by work exposures. Medical knowledge at large as well as occupational health evaluations are to a great extent based on case reports, although there is a disputable basis for judgments about causal relationships. In the context of disorders due to solvent exposure, the evaluation of causability becomes even more uncertain, since the clinical symptoms sometimes are rather vague, i.e., tiredness, affect lability, irritability, memory disturbances, etc. Numerous cases with these symptoms possibly due to solvent exposure have been reported during several decades, and are reviewed by Browning.[13] However, similar cases still occur even in countries with an advanced industrial technology, to judge from recent reports and experiences in Sweden.[5]

The symptoms characterizing these cases usually are more or less in agreement with the so-called psycho-organic syndrome or neurasthenic syndrome.[10,41] Similar symptoms have also been found in workers with exposure to jet fuel, which chemically comes fairly close to the white spirit (kerosene) used in many paints. Thus, a recent study of Swedish aircraft factory workers revealed neurasthenic symptoms in 10 of 13 heavily exposed individuals and in 7 of 16 among those with less exposure. The exposure levels had been fairly high, amounting to 500–3100 ppm in earlier measurements. Low nerve conduction velocities and high vibration thresholds were also found in neurophysiologic examinations.[37] A similar study on another group of aircraft engine workers showed these consistent findings.[36]

Psychological Functional Impairments

The psycho-organic syndrome is characterized by a decreased ability to engage in abstract thinking whereas well-trained functions such as verbal understanding tend to be retained for a long time.[41] This discrepancy in intellectual functions is utilized for diagnosic purposes. Tests of verbal understanding are looked on as fairly stable tests ("hold tests") reflecting the original intellectual capacity of the individual, and performances on these tests are compared with performances on tests that require abstract thinking ("nonhold tests"). A lower performance on the nonhold tests than on the hold tests is used as an indicator of a functional impairment of the central nervous system.[63]

Several studies based on psychological testing have appeared during the 1970s, and the results from 8 Scandinavian studies of workers exposed to solvents are summarized in Table 11–2.

Hänninen[28] compared the performances on a battery of psychological tests of 50 carbon disulfide (CS_2) poisoned rayon-viscose workers with 50 rayon-viscose workers exposed to CS_2 but without clinical symptoms of poisoning and 50 workers not exposed to CS_2. There were large and statistically significant differences between the group means of the poisoned and the nonexposed group in most tests that required visual perception and cognition, perceptual speed, memory and psychomotor coordination.

TABLE 11–2.—SCANDINAVIAN STUDIES OF WORKERS OCCUPATIONALLY EXPOSED TO SOLVENTS

PSYCHOLOGICAL FUNCTION	EXPOSURE							
	CS_2	MIXTURE	MIXTURE	STYRENE	STYRENE	STYRENE	MIXTURE	JET FUEL
Vocabulary			–			–		
Cognition	–	–				–	+	
Visual perception and cognition	+	+	+			–	+	
Perceptual speed	+	+	+	+	+	+	–	+
Eye-hand coordination	+	+	+			+	+	–
Memory	+		+			–	+	–
Personality	+	–				+		
Reference	(28)	(39)	(11)	(26)	(23)	(40)	(29)	(36)

+ Indicates that at least one test measuring the psychological function at issue showed differences ($p < .05$) between exposed and nonexposed.
– Indicates that the psychological function was measured but did not result in significant differences.

There also were demonstrated differences in some variables from the Rorschach ink blot test, for example, diminished rational control and fewer emotional reactions among the poisoned. An exposed worker without clinical symptoms also showed impairment, although less severe.

Lindström[39] reported a study of a group of workers exposed to various common industrial solvents such as tri- and tetrachloroethylene, toluene, xylene and their mixtures. The methods applied were chosen among those used in the carbon disulfide (CS_2) study.[28] Significant differences were found between the exposed and the nonexposed in tests where visual perception and perceptual speed were supposed to be important functions and also in tests that presupposed psychomotor coordination whereas neither the variables from the Rorschach ink blot test nor the pure cognitive test revealed any significant differences. The occurrence of adverse effects from styrene on the central nervous system is supported by the findings of an increased prevalence of abnormal EEGs in exposed workers.[51]

A study of a random sample of union-affiliated house painters has also been reported.[11,27] The house painters were compared in a number of medical variables and psychological tests with a group of industrial workers having a corresponding age distribution. The groups proved to be on a par in relevant background variables, but the house painter group reported more subjective symptoms, such as fatigue, partial amnesia and diffuse chest pain. A simple health check did not show any correlates to the subjective complaints except for a somewhat lower hemoglobin concentration among the house painters. However, the house painter group had significantly lower mean scores on a test measuring the visual perception-cognition factor and on a test of psychomotor coordination than did the reference group of industrial workers. The house painter group also had significantly lower performances than expected on a memory test and the reaction time test.

Götell et al.[26] described complaints of workers manufacturing products of styrene-modified, glass fiber-reinforced polyester plastics, where exposure levels amounted to 100–300 ppm. Symptoms of gastritis and other complaints from the gastrointestinal tract, tiredness and sleep disturbances, memory problems and irritation of the eyes were common. The most exposed subgroup showed significantly prolonged simple reaction time compared to an age-matched control group both in the morning and in the afternoon. Prolonged reaction times along with a greater deterioration over a period of 10 minutes and a greater irregularity of responses among workers exposed to styrene were also demonstrated by Gamberale et al.[23]

Styrene workers have also been studied by Lindström et al.[40] A cumulative dose of exposure was expressed as the product of the duration of exposure (years) and the mean mandelic acid concentration (a specific method for determination of mandelic acid now is available[18]) in the urine during 5 consecutive weeks before the examination. A multiple regression analysis between cumulative dose and the test variables yielded a multiple correlation of 0.53 with the variables latency-time in the Rorschach ink blot test and performance on two tests measuring eye-hand coordination and age whereas age alone showed a correlation of 0.27.

Behavioral effects of long-term exposure to a mixture of organic solvents have been studied by Hänninen et al.,[29] who compared a group of car painters with an age-matched control group in a number of psychological tests. The exposed group consisted of 102 car painters from 27 car repair garages, chosen from all the car painters in Helsinki (total: 166). The nonexposed reference group was chosen from the employees of the Finnish State Railways, with ages of the subjects matched within 2 years. About half of the group consisted of engineers and the other half of locomotive assistants. Workplace air solvent concentrations were measured in 6 randomly selected car repair garages. The mean solvent concentrations in the breathing zone of 40 workers are presented in Table 11–3.

TABLE 11–3.—MEAN SOLVENT CONCENTRATIONS IN THE BREATHING ZONE OF CAR PAINTERS[29]

SOLVENT	MEAN CONCENTRATION (ppm)
Toluene	30.6
Xylene	5.8
Butyl acetate	6.8
White spirit	4.9
Methyl isobutyl ketone	1.7
Isopropanol	2.9
Ethyl acetate	2.6
Acetone	3.1
Ethanol	2.9

The average of the percentages was 31.8% of the Finnish threshold limit value (TLV) for solvent mixtures.

The test battery included tests of intelligence, memory, psychomotor performance and personality. In addition to the comparison of the mean results, two discriminant function analyses were done. In one, only the performance test variables were used, but in the other, personality variables were included. The results indicated impairments in psychomotor performance, as well as personality changes in the exposed group. Impairments in visual intelligence and verbal memory and a reduction of emotional reactivity were the central features of the adverse effects of solvent exposure. The possible role of the differences in the initial intelligence levels was checked with a separate comparison of the test results of 33 pairs of exposed and nonexposed subjects who were matched for age and for their intelligence level, measured during the military service at young age. Psychological tests were also used in the aforementioned study of workers with exposure to jet fuel.[36] The results indicated that the exposed workers had greater problems on tasks that required attention, perceptual speed and fast reactions.

Since various authors have used other methods and based the choice of tests on different theories of the structure of the intellectual capacity, comparative results from these studies are difficult. The classification of tests in Table 11–2 is based on a factor analysis made by Sjöborg and Frömark[52] of a test battery that was constructed to cover all the intellectual factors used in the Scandinavian studies, referred to in the table. Tests measuring vocabulary rarely gave discrepancies between exposed and nonexposed individuals as did the cognitive tests in which the component of visual perception was supposed to be of minor importance. Tests requiring a good ability to recognize figures and patterns, either tests requiring intellectual manipulation of the perception or tests where perceptual speed is supposed to be the most important factor, have indicated a difference between the exposed and the nonexposed individuals in almost all of these studies. Also eye-hand coordination tests tend to be more difficult for those with exposure than for the nonexposed controls. These tests are based on gripping and handling tiny pieces, for example, picking up needles with tweezers. Differences between exposed and nonexposed individuals have also been revealed by various types of memory tests, for example, to reproduce a specific pattern after watching it for a few seconds, to recall numbers or a story rich in details. Also the Rorschach ink blot test showed differences between individuals with and without exposure; for example, fewer emotional reactions among workers exposed to solvent.

All psychological tests require a combination of sensory and perceptual functions, cognitive processes and motor responses; i.e., the test material has to be perceived, intellectually treated in some way or another and a response, for example, to write down a chosen symbol, has to be given.

The classification of tests according to a factor analysis is based on the type of function that is most important for the variation of performance indicated by the test score. A lowered performance, as has been demonstrated for several groups occupationally exposed to solvents, on a test where the most important factor is the intellectual handling of the material does not necessarily mean that the intellectual function is influenced; i.e., the lowered performance might rather be due to reduced perceptual ability. These matters have to be studied further to reach a better understanding of the type of behavior effect that is caused by solvents.

It might be summarized that despite different methods in the various studies of the effects of solvent exposure, the results are fairly consistent; i.e., there seems to be an impaired performance on tests where visual perception, memory and motor functions are important.

Most of the studies referred to have been undertaken at least 24 hours after the latest exposure, which means that the effects should be of either a subacute or a chronic character. However, all these studies have been of the cross-sectional type, perhaps underestimating the actual hazards due to solvent exposure.

CHRONIC NEUROPSYCHIATRIC DISORDERS

Few studies are available that elucidate the severeness of the disorder due to solvent exposure. However, clinical experience indicates that more or less severe or disabling symptoms might occur. A case-referent (case-control) study in a disability pension register in Sweden[6] revealed that painters, varnishers and carpet layers, i.e., workers with considerable exposure to solvents, had a relative risk of about 1.8 to suffer from neuropsychiatric disorders in comparison to other skilled workers in various trades with some connection with construction work. To judge from this study, encompassing only 1 of the Swedish counties, about 3–4% of all neuropsychiatric disorders in men 36–65 years of age, severe enough to be considered as contributing to a sick-pension, might have a relationship to solvent exposure, or about 100 individuals per million employed men of the population in a highly industrialized country such as Sweden.[7] Such estimates are very uncertain, however, but might be justified as a crude attempt to quantitate the hazard in this particular respect.

Symptoms of neuropathy should be watched for among individuals exposed to solvents and have been observed particularly in the context of exposure to *n*-hexane and mixtures[31, 56] and methyl-*n*-butyl ketone[9, 34] but to some degree also among jet fuel workers.[37] Vague symptoms such as tingling and pricking sensations and even restless legs should be carefully noticed as indicating neuropathies when examining individuals exposed to solvents, but such findings usually are rare. However, neurophysiologic measurements of the nerve conduction velocity, particularly in slow motor fibers, might reveal abnormalities.[50]

OTHER CHRONIC EFFECTS

Carcinogenicity, Teratogenicity and Mutagenicity

Carcinogenicity, teratogenicity and mutagenicity are other aspects to be considered besides the neurotoxic effects from solvent exposure. The induction of angiosarcoma of the liver through exposure to vinyl chloride brought up these aspects, as did the increasing knowledge about metabolic pathways, since not only vinyl chloride but also other organic substances, for example, solvents, have been found to metabolize through epoxides. Thus, this transformation seems to occur in the metabolism of benzene, styrene and trichloroethylene. To some degree, a ring epoxidation also takes place in the metabolism of toluene and xylene.[17] It might be recalled that benzene rather early was recognized as a cause of aplastic anemia whereas toluene and xylene do not appear to induce the severe hematopoietic injury associated with benzene exposure.[24] Today, there also is rather convincing evidence of the leukemogenic effect from benzene.[1, 62]

Extensive studies based on proportional mortality[42] and case-control data,[61] respectively, have indicated an excess cancer mortality among painters with regard to malignancies of the respiratory system and the stomach. However, since the exposure pattern is complex for these painters, it is not clear if the indicated cancer hazard is referable to solvent exposure or other agents such as paint pigments from removal of old paint or paint-spraying operations.

In the middle of the 1970s there was reported from the National Cancer Institute[45] an increased frequency of hepatocellular cancer in mice (males only got a significantly increased frequency of this tumor) that were fed trichloroethylene through gastric intubation. Furthermore, trichloroethylene was found to possess mutagenic activity in bacterial test systems after microsomal activation[25]; this observation is not surprising in view of the probable epoxidation in the metabolism of this compound.[12] Consequently, there now also is an urgent need to determine the character and strength of a possible cancer hazard to man. However, a recent epidemiologic study[4] comprising 518 men with exposure to trichloroethylene did not show any excess of cancer or otherwise deviating mortality pattern, but the size of this study does not permit definite conclusions with regard to the possible carcinogenic effect of trichloroethylene on man. Presently, it seems reasonable, however, that this solvent should not constitute a very serious cancer hazard to man at low exposures, but further studies are urgently needed and might quickly change the view suggested here.

Similarly, as for trichloroethylene, there also is a current concern with regard to cancer hazards and teratogenic effects from styrene as probably metabolized through an epoxide.[46] Recently, malformations were reported in chickens as due to styrene and its metabolite, styrene epoxide,[59] and mutagenic activity has also been found in bacterial test systems.[60] It is disturbing that good exposure data from the 1950s and 1960s are lacking and, presumably, only small groups are available for studies. However, in a Finnish case-control study,[32] maternal exposure to styrene, together with other aromatic and aliphatic solvents, was associated with an increased occurrence of central nervous system defects in newborn children.

A Czechoslovakian report[38] has suggested a relationship between various types of solvent exposure and sacral agenesis. There is also some support for this suggestion in animal experiments, since xylene seems to exert a teratogenic effect in chick embryos.[38] This also is in some consistency with the observation of chromosomal aberrations in printers exposed to toluene[20] and hospital laboratory personnel,[21] who also might have an increased risk of spontaneous abortions.[55] It should be recalled here that exposure to anesthetics, some of them halogenated aliphatics of the solvent type, has been found associated with a high frequency of spontaneous abortions (see reference 33 for an overview). These anesthetics are also related to the freons, used as propellants, as solvents and in foaming processes; for example, in producing polyurethane plastics. The high exposure tolerances to freons, as applied in most countries, therefore might turn out to be hazardous as knowledge increases through further studies. Some rather recently introduced anesthetics are polyhalogenated ethers and their structual similarity to recognized carcinogens such as bischloromethylether, bischloroethylether and chloromethylmethylether has been a matter of some concern.[15] Further aspects of the potential health hazards of halogenated hydrocarbons, particularly with regard to mutagenicity, can be found elsewhere.[19]

OTHER TYPES OF DISORDERS

Kidney disorders also seem to have relationships to solvent exposure. During recent years there have appeared case reports as well as epidemiologic studies with regard to a possible correlation between solvent exposure and glomerulonephritis. Recently, a Swedish study[48] has been reported and seems to indicate a relationship between solvent exposure and glomerulonephritis just as has been found by others.[8,64] It is not clear at present, however, if the nephrotoxic effect from solvents is due to a long-time and low-grade exposure or if it is merely exerted through high-level but short-time exposures or through specific solvents. Nor is it sufficiently elucidated which other factors—heredity, infections, etc.—might influence these effects. It is of some interest in this context that aromatic solvents seem to decrease serum complement levels.[53]

Hepatotoxicity from certain solvents must not be overlooked. In particular, carbon tetrachloride has long been known to cause severe hepatic damage a couple of days after exposure and there also are some case reports indicating a later development of cirrhosis and hepatic tumors.[35] Carbon tetrachloride use nowadays is banned, severely restricted or substituted for, but there also might be liver toxic effects from some other chlorinated solvents; reciprocal potentiation from alcohol and solvents such as trichloroethylene and isopropyl alcohol[16,49,58] deserves attention. Therefore, the possibility of liver cirrhosis caused not only by alcohol but sometimes by a combination of alcohol abuse and solvent exposure must be considered.

Lens changes recently have been reported among Finnish car painters as probably caused by solvent exposure.[47] This observation has some support from animal studies, since cataracts have been induced by exposure to alkylaromatics.[44]

Finally, it might also be recalled that solvent exposure, namely, with regard to carbon disulfide, has been associated with cardiovascular disease in the rayon-viscose industry.[30,43,57] This probably is a rather specific effect for carbon disulfide, but little attention has been paid to the possibility that other solvents might cause cardiovascular disorders. There are apparent problems, however, in the epidemiologic evaluation of such effects with regard to the frequent exposure to solvents as well as the high background morbidity from cardiovascular diseases in industrialized countries.

VAPOR DEGREASING: PRINCIPLES

Appropriate engineering controls to prevent and/or minimize solvent exposure should be utilized.

Vapor degreasing is a method of removing soluble soils and other entrapped soils from metals and nonporous objects.

Solvents used in this process are trichloroethylene, 1,1,1-trichloroethane, perchloroethylene, methylene chloride and trichlorotrifluoroethane.

In its simplest form (as shown in Fig 11–1), a solvent vapor degreaser is a tank with a heat source to boil the solvent, a vapor zone, a condenser, a freeboard zone and a slot exhaust ventilation at the top of the tank.

The articles to be cleaned are lowered into the solvent vapor zone. The hot vapor condenses onto the cool parts, dissolving oil and grease, and provides a continual rinse in clean solvent condensate. As the condensed solvent drains from the parts, it carries away soluble and insoluble soil and returns to the boiling liquid sump. The work is held in the vapor zone until it reaches vapor temperature, at which time condensation stops. The load then is withdrawn from the vapor and dries almost immediately in the freeboard zone of the degreaser.

The slot exhaust ventilation ensures that the TLV for the solvent (30 ppm for trichloroethylene in Sweden and 100 ppm in the United States) is not exceeded.

The vapor treatment often is augmented by mechanical action, such as spraying with clean solvent condensate (see Fig 11–2). Cleaning also can be performed by immersion of boiling solvent (see Fig 11–3) or immersion in cool solvent agitated by ultrasonics (see Fig 11–4), brushing, etc. (see Fig 11-5). The process is a safe, rapid and economical procedure for preparing dry and clean articles for subsequent finishing or fabricating.

REFERENCES

1. Aksoy, M., Erdem, S., and Dincol, G.: Types of leukemia in chronic benzene poisoning. A study in thirty-four patients, Acta Haematol. 55:65, 1976.
2. Åstrand, I.: Uptake of solvents in the blood and tissues of man: A review, Scand. J. Work Environ. Health. 1:199, 1975.
3. Åstrand, I., and Gamberale, F.: Effects on humans of solvents in the inspiratory air. A method for estimation of uptake, Environ. Res. 15:1, 1978.
4. Axelson, O., Andersson, K., Hogstedt, C., Holmberg, B., Molina, G., and de Verdier, A.: A cohort study on trichloroethylene exposure and cancer mortality, J. Occup. Med. 20:194, 1978.
5. Axelson, O., Hane, M., and Hogstedt, C.: Case reports on chronic psycho-organic syndrome in house painters (English summary), Lakartidningen 73:317, 1976.
6. Axelson, O., Hane, M., and Hogstedt, C.: A case-referent study on neuropsychiatric disorders among workers exposed to solvents, Scand. J. Work Environ. Health 2:14, 1976.
7. Axelson, O., Hane, M., and Hogstedt, C.: A case-referent study on neuropsychiatric disorders among workers exposed to solvents—a review and some further aspects. International symposium of the control of air pollution in the working environment, Stockholm, 6–8 September, 1977, International Labour Office, 1977.
8. Beirne, G., and Brennan, J.: Glomerulonephritis associated with hydrocarbon solvents, Arch. Environ. Health 25:365, 1972.
9. Billmaier, E., et al.: Peripheral neuropathy in a coated fabrics plant, J. Occup. Med. 16:665, 1974.
10. Bleuler, M.: *Lehrbuch der Psychiatrie* (Berlin: Springer-Verlag, 1969).
11. Blume, J., Hane, M., Sundell, L., and Ydreborg, B.: Mental function changes among house painters (English summary), Lakartidningen 72:702, 1975.
12. Bonse, G., Urban, T., Reichert, D., and Henschler, D.: Chemical reactivity, metabolic oxirane formation and biological reactivity of chlorinated ethylene in the isolated perfused rat liver preparation,

Biochem. Pharmacol. 24:1829, 1975.

13. Browning, E.: *Toxicity and Metabolism of Industrial Solvents* (Amsterdam: Elsevier Publishing Co., 1965).
14. Bruce, D., and Bach, M.: Effects of trace concentrations of anesthetic gases on behavioral performance of operating room personnel. Washington, D.C., Dept. HEW Publication No. (NIOSH) 76:169, 1976.
15. Corbett, T.: Cancer and congenital anomalies associated with anesthetics, Ann. N.Y. Acad. Sci. 271:58, 1976.
16. Cornish, G., and Adefuin, J.: Ethanol potentiation of halogenated aliphatic solvent toxicity, Am. Ind. Hyg. Assoc. J. 27:57, 1966.
17. De Bruin, A.: *Biochemical Toxicology of Environmental Agents* (Amsterdam: Coronel University, 1976).
18. Engström, K., and Rantanen, J.: A new gas chromatographic method for determination of mandelic acid in urine, Int. Arch. Arbeitsmed. 3:163, 1974.
19. Fishbein, L.: Industrial mutagenes and potential mutagenes. I. Halogenated aliphatic derivates, Mutat. Res. 32:267, 1976.
20. Forni, A., Pacifico, E., and Limonta, A.: Chromosome studies in workers exposed to benzene or toluene or both, Arch. Environ. Health 22:373, 1971.
21. Funes-Cravioto, F., et al.: Chromosome aberrations and sister-chromatid exchange in workers in chemical laboratories and a rotoprinting factory and in children of women laboratory workers, Lancet 2:322, 1977.
22. Gamberale, F.: Behavioral effects of exposure to solvent vapors, Arbete och Hälsa, 1975:14, Stockholm: Arbetarskyddsverket, 1975.
23. Gamberale, F., Lisper, H., and Anshelm-Olson, B.: The influence from styrene on reaction ability in plastic boat industry (English summary), Arbete och Hälsa, 1975:8, Stockholm: Arbetarskyddsverket, 1975.
24. Gerarde, H. W.: *Toxicology and Biochemistry of Aromatic Hydrocarbons* (New York: Elsevier Publishing Co., 1960).
25. Greim, H., Bonse, G., Radwan, Z., Reichert, D., and Henschler, D.: Mutagenicity in vitro and potential carcinogenicity of chlorinated ethylenes as a function of metabolic oxirane formation, Biochem. Pharmacol. 24:2013, 1975.
26. Götell, P., Axelson, O., and Lindelöf, B.: Field studies on human styrene exposure, Work Environ. Health 9:76, 1972.
27. Hane, M., Axelson, O., Blume, J., Hogstedt, C., Sundell, L., and Ydreborg, B.: Psychological function changes among house painters, Scand. J. Work Environ. Health 3:91, 1977.
28. Hänninen, H.: Psychological picture of manifest and latent carbon disulphide poisoning, Br. J. Ind. Med. 28:374, 1971.
29. Hänninen, H., Eskelinen, L., Husman, K., and Nurminen, M.: Behavioral effects of long-term exposure to a mixture of organic solvents, Scand. J. Work Environ. Health 2:240, 1976.
30. Hernberg, S., Nurminen, M., and Tolonen, M.: Excess mortality from coronary heart disease in viscose rayon workers exposed to carbon disulphide, Work Environ. Health 10:93, 1973.
31. Herskowitz, A., Ishii, N., and Schaumburg, H.: *n*-Hexane neurophathy, N. Engl. J. Med. 285:82, 1971.
32. Holmberg, P. C.: Central-nervous-system defects in children born to mothers exposed to organic solvents during pregnancy, Lancet 2:177, 1979.
33. IARC Monographs Vol. II: Cadmium, nickel, some epoxides, miscellaneous industrial chemicals and general considerations on volatile anaesthetics. Lyon: International Agency for Research on Cancer, 1976, p. 285.
34. Johnson, B., Setzer, J., Lewis, T., and Anger, K.: Effects of methyl *n*-butyl ketone on behavior and the nervous system, Am. Ind. Hyg. Assoc. J. 38:567, 1977.
35. Johnstone, R. T.: *Occupational Medicine and Industrial Hygiene* (St. Louis: The C. V. Mosby Company, 1948).
36. Knave, B, Anshelm-Olson, B., Elofsson, S., Gamberale, F., Isaksson, A., Mindus, P., Persson, H., Struwe, G., Wennberg, A., and Westerholm, P.: Long-term exposure to jet fuel. II. A cross-sectional epidemiological investigation on occupationally-exposed industry workers with special reference to the nervous system, Scand. J. Work Environ. Health 4:19, 1978.
37. Knave, B., Persson, H., Goldberg, M., and Westerholm, P.: Long-term exposure to jet fuel. An investigation on occupationally exposed workers with special reference to the nervous system, Scand. J. Work Environ. Health 2:152, 1976.
38. Kučera, J.: Exposure to fat solvents: A possible cause of sacral agenesis in man, J. Pediatr. 72:857, 1968.
39. Lindström, K.: Psychological performances of workers exposed to various solvents, Work Environ. Health 10:151, 1973.
40. Lindström, K., Härkönen, H., and Hern-

berg, S.: Disturbances in psychological functions of workers occupationally exposed to styrene, Scand. J. Work Environ. Health 2:129, 1976.

41. Mayer-Gross, W., Slater, E., and Roth, M.: *Clinical Psychiatry* (3d ed.; London: Baillière, Tindall & Cassel, 1969).
42. Milham, S.: Occupational mortality in Washington state, 1950–1971, Vol. III. Washington, D.C., U.S. Dept. HEW, 1976.
43. Mowé, G.: Coronary heart disease and occupational exposure to carbon disulfide. Abstract of the II International Symposium on Toxicology of Carbon Disulfide, Banja Koviljaca, Yugoslavia, May 25–28, 1971. Eds. Dusan Djuric et al., Beograd, Institute of Occupational and Radiological Health, 1971.
44. Nau, C. A., Neal, J., and Thornton, M.: C_9-C_{12} fractions obtained from petroleum distillates, Arch. Environ. Health 12:383, 1966.
45. NCI: Carcinogenesis bioassay of trichloroethylene. CAS No. 79-01-6 National Cancer Institute Tech. Rep. Series No. 2, Feb., 1976, U.S. DHEW Publ. No. (NIH) 76-802, Washington, D.C.
46. Ohtsuji, H., and Ikeda, M.: The metabolism of styrene in the rat and stimulatory effect of phenobarbital, Toxicol. Appl. Pharmacol. 18:321, 1971.
47. Raitta, C., Husman, K., and Tossavainen, A.: Lens changes in car painters exposed to a mixture of organic solvents, Albrecht von Graefes Arch. Klin. Exp. Ophtalmol. 200:149, 1976.
48. Ravnskov, U., Forsberg, B., and Skerfving, S.: Glomerulonephritis and exposure to organic solvents, Acta Med. Scand. 205:575, 1979.
49. Schüttmann, W.: Zur Frage der Leberschädigung durch beruflichen Kontakt mit Triklorätylen, Dtsch. Z. Verdau Stoffwechselkr. 30:43, 1970.
50. Seppäläinen, A. M.: Applications of neurophysiological methods in occupational medicine: A review, Scand. J. Work Environ. Health 1:1, 1975.
51. Seppäläinen, A. M., and Härkönen, H.: Neurophysiological findings among workers occupationally exposed to styrene, Scand. J. Work Environ. Health 2:140, 1976.
52. Sjöborg, A., and Frömark, A.: Standardisering av ett psykologiskt testbatteri för beteendetoxikologiska undersökningar (Standardization of a battery of psychological tests to be used in behavioral toxicological studies). Information from Psykotekniska Institutet No. 93, 1977.
53. Smolik, R., Grzybek-Hryncewicz, K., Lange, A., and Zatónski, W.: Serum complement level in workers exposed to benzene, toluene and xylene, Int. Arch. Arbeitsmed. 31:243, 1973.
54. Stokholm, J., and Cohr, K.: Akutte subjektive og objektive reaktioner på 7 timers exposition for mineralist terpentin (Acute subjective and objective reactions after 7 hours exposure to mineral turpentine). Abstract to the 26 Nordic Occupational Hygiene meeting, Helsinki, October 24–26, 1977. Helsinki: Institute of Occupational Health, 1977, pp. 35–36.
55. Strandberg, M., Sandbäck, K., Axelson, O., and Sundell, L.: Spontaneous abortions among women in hospital laboratory, Lancet 1:384, 1978.
56. Taheuchi, Y., Mabuchi, C., and Tagaki, S.: Polyneuropathy caused by petroleum benzene, Int. Arch. Arbeitsmed. 34:185, 1975.
57. Tiller, J., Schilling, R., and Morris, J.: Occupational toxic factor in mortality from coronary heart disease, Br. Med. J. 4:407, 1968.
58. Traiger, G., and Plaa, G.: Chlorinated hydrocarbon toxicity. Potentiation by isopropyl alcohol and acetone, Arch. Environ. Health 28:276, 1974.
59. Vainio, H., Hemminki, K., and Elovaara, E.: Styrens och styrenoxids toxicitet för utvecklande kycklingembryo. (The toxicity of styrene and styrene oxide on developed chick embryos). Abstract to the 26 Nordic Occupational Hygiene Meeting, Helsinki, October 24–26, 1977. Helsinki: Institute of Occupational Health, 1977, p. 25.
60. Vainio, H., Pääkkönen, R., Rönnholm, K., Raunio, V., and Pelkonen, O.: A study on the mutagenic activity of styrene and styrene oxide, Scand. J. Work Environ. Health 2:147, 1976.
61. Viadana, E., Bross, I., and Houten, L.: Cancer experience of men exposed to inhalation of chemicals or to combustion products, J. Occup. Med. 18:787, 1976.
62. Vigliani, E.: Leukemia associated with benzene exposure, Ann. N.Y. Acad. Sci. 271: 143, 1976.
63. Zimmerman, I., and Woo-Sam, J.: *Clinical Interpretation of the Wechsler Adult Intelligence Scale* (New York: Grune & Stratton, 1973).
64. Zimmerman, S., Groehler, K., and Beirne, G.: Hydrocarbon exposure and chronic glomerulonephritis, Lancet 2:199, 1975.

12 / Diagnostic and Health Care Aspects of Workers Exposed to Solvents

CHRISTER HOGSTEDT, M.D., MONICA HANE, Ph.D., and OLAV AXELSON, M.D.

INDIVIDUAL diagnostic recognition of solvent-induced disorders must be based on careful history taking and psychological testing. Symptoms such as increased fatigue, neurasthenia, depressive complaints and impaired memory should be specifically elicited. Neurophysiologic and neuroradiologic examinations might be useful but usually would require rather advanced effects to provide any valuable information. Electroencephalographic tracings usually are nonspecific, but some support for a psycho-organic syndrome might be obtained from an abnormal electroencephalogram.[20] Computerized tomography of the brain may be of increasing diagnostic value in the near future, particularly if some degree of cerebral atrophy is suspected. Sometimes it is difficult to rule out other possible causes of a psycho-organic syndrome, such as alcoholism, hereditary presenility, generalized arteriosclerosis, cerebrovascular disorders and earlier encephalopathy, electroconvulsive therapy and "solvent sniffing," as well as exposure to lead, mercury, etc.

ASSESSMENT OF EXPOSURE

The work exposure exploration is as important as the medical examination for the recognition of a psycho-organic syndrome due to solvent exposure. The nature of the exposure, its duration and intensity should be taken into account. Sometimes it might be valuable to calculate exposure-hours per year, thereby adjusting for outdoor painting and wallpapering, which is the task of painters in some countries. Work load should also be considered as apparently strongly influencing the amount of solvent absorption.[1] Sometimes records of exposure measurements are available or biologic monitoring might have been undertaken; for example, determinations of mandelic acid in the urine of workers exposed to styrene and trichloroacetic acid in the urine in the case of trichloroethylene exposure, etc. Certain further aspects of determining solvent exposure will be discussed.

Various countries have different regulations and/or criteria for occupational diseases that govern views taken with regard to compensation. However, if the findings in the clinical examination and the results from psychological testing, as outlined here, are consistent with a psycho-organic syndrome, and if there has been a considerable known exposure to solvents, it might be reasonable to support an occupational insurance claim. According to available estimates,[4] about half of the disabling neuropsychiatric disorders among solvent workers can be attributed to solvent exposure. Therefore, the diagnosis of a solvent-induced psycho-organic syndrome is difficult to assess, and the etiology of solvent exposure has to be established through exclusion of other possible etiologies and not only through the presence of more or less typical examination findings.

Consistent findings, not only in clinical examinations and psychological testing but also in neurophysiologic examinations, strengthen the suggestion of a solvent-induced condition. Methods for examinations of polyneuropathy have been described by Seppäläinen[20] and others.[3]

HEALTH SCREENING PROCEDURES

The desirability of prevention and early detection of solvent-induced ill health, along with the large number of solvent-exposed workers, calls for screening procedures that make health examinations reasonably effective and inexpensive. Attempts have been made to construct self-administered questionnaires for primary screening. In this specific situation, a high sensitivity is desirable to avoid overlooking relevant symptoms. High sensitivity tends to give a considerable number of "falsely positive" individuals. However, these individuals may be excluded by ordinary clinical procedures. The examining of "falsely positive" individuals is not too cumbersome in view of the benefits of not having to examine everybody in a solvent-exposed population.

A screening questionnaire for neuropsychiatric symptoms is illustrated in Table 12–1, which—in translation from Swedish—gives 16 questions primarily based on common Scandinavian experiences[3] and then further elaborated through a validation procedure.[14] Thus, the wording of the questions was repeatedly revised to obtain a correlation between the information from the questionnaire and the physician's evaluation from an interview with the solvent-exposed worker.[14] This questionnaire was also sent to about 250 solvent-exposed workers (house painters, car painters and metal degreasers) and 200 non-exposed workers (electricians and postmen), randomly chosen from local Swedish trade union registers. More than 90% of the questionnaires were completely answered and returned. Exposed workers showed symptoms such as abnormal fatigue, depression, memory disturbances, unclear chest pains, etc., more often than the postmen, and significant differences were obtained in most of the questions after standardization for age.

The possibility of suggestive effects is difficult to definitely rule out, but no apparent tendencies were noted in working with these groups. Furthermore, those questions indicating serious neurologic disturbances (e.g., buttoning and unbuttoning) showed no differences, which might be taken as an indication of absence of suggestive effects, since, then, there would have been at least some correlation in the answers to these questions and to those merely reflecting psychological functional changes.

A final step in the validation procedure was to send the questionnaire once more to those two thirds of the samples who had returned the questionnaire within 3 weeks. The correlation between number of symptoms marked at the first and at the second time was about 0.90 for both exposed and non-exposed workers, indicating a fairly good reliability of the questionnaire. Fifteen questions that had elicited strong statistical differences between the exposed and non-exposed groups were included in the final version of this screening questionnaire. A 16th question was added to check for possible suggestive effects when the questionnaire is used in group surveys.

Based on the 90th percentile for the number of symptoms among the non-exposed workers, a tentative recommendation has been made that young solvent-exposed men (less than 28 years of age) indicating more than 4 symptoms in the 16 questions and those 28 years of age or older indicating more than 6 symptoms should be seen by a physician. If the physician confirms the symptoms of solvent-induced effects, further clinical examinations, with neurologic and

TABLE 12–1.—RESULTS OF A VALIDATED QUESTIONNAIRE OF SOLVENT-EXPOSED AND NON-EXPOSED MALE WORKERS

QUESTION	EXPOSED WORKERS (N = 229)	NON-EXPOSED WORKERS (N = 173)	χ^2
1. Are you abnormally tired?	31	6	37.0
2. Do you have palpitations of the heart even when you don't exert yourself?	13	5	6.3
3. Do you often have painful tingling in some part of your body?	28	10	16.4
4. Do you often feel irritated without any particular reason?	34	13	22.8
5. Do you often feel depressed without any particular reason?	21	6	15.0
6. Do you often have problems with concentrating?	28	9	20.7
7. Do you have a short memory?	49	30	12.4
8. Do you often perspire without any particular reason?	20	10	6.5
9. Do you have any problems with buttoning and unbuttoning?	1	1	0.5
10. Do you generally find it hard to get the meaning from reading newspapers and books?	22	7	16.5
11. Have your relatives told you that you have a short memory?	42	24	13.7
12. Do you sometimes feel an oppression in your chest?	34	12	25.5
13. Do you often have to make notes about what you must remember?	28	11	16.9
14. Do you often have to go back and check things you have done such as turned off the stove, locked the door?	39	16	23.1
15. Do you have a headache at least once a week?	27	14	10.0
16. Are you less interested in sex than what you think is normal?	11	1	12.8

NOTES: These questions give the percentage of symptoms among solvent-exposed male workers (a random sample from the local trade union of painters and car painters and workers exposed to solvents in the metal industry) and non-exposed male workers (a random sample of electricians and postmen). The groups were stratified for age and the chi-squares calculated according to the Mantel-Haenszel formula.
χ^2 (1 df) > 3.84; the p-value < 0.05 (two-tailed).

psychological tests, are recommended to reach a diagnosis.[15]

BATTERY OF PSYCHOLOGICAL TESTS

Collaborative work between various groups of Swedish psychologists has resulted in a battery of 13 psychological tests that have been standardized on an unselected Swedish population.[21] Since the battery has been used in many studies of workers exposed to various solvents that are in progress in Sweden, there is a fair amount of data to be used as reference material also when the battery is used for individual diagnostic and health checkups. Presently, the battery is used in several departments of occupational medicine throughout Sweden.

The classification of tests is based on a factor analysis carried out on a sample of 99 subjects at the age of 16 and pupils in the last class of the compulsory school, thus reflecting the unrestricted variation in every variable. The first factor included tests of vocabulary, i.e., the type of tests regarded to be less influenced in case of diffuse organic brain damage.[17] The second factor included tests in which both visual perception and cognitive processes are supposed to be important. The third factor covered tests in which the cognitive components are supposed to be of minor importance, and the score is mainly based on perceptual speed. The fourth factor consisted of tests that require eye-hand coordination, called psychomotor tests. The memory tests did not come out as a separate factor in the factor analysis due to reduced variation but nevertheless could be grouped together. The test battery is briefly described below. When nothing else is marked in the description of the test, there is a time limit given for administrative reasons, but the performance is, to a very small extent, influenced by speed.

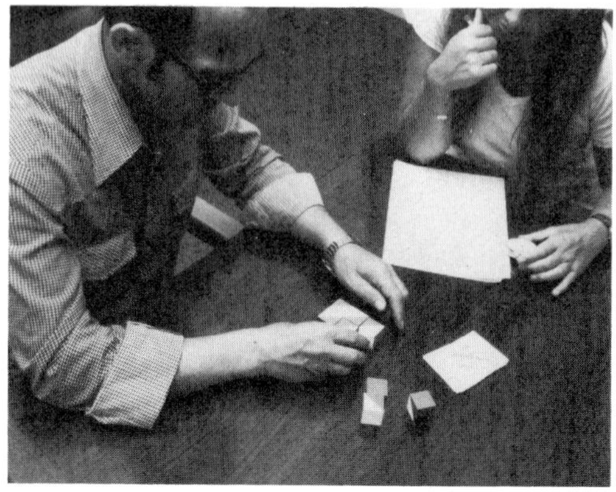

Fig 12–2.—Block (see text).

Vocabulary

Synonyms—The task is to find the synonym of a given key word among five alternatives. The test includes 30 items.[9]

Opposites—The task is to find the opposite of a given key word among five alternatives. The test includes 30 items.[8]

Visual Perception/Cognition

Figure classification (Fig 12–1)—Every item consists of 5 geometric figures. Four figures have a common characteristic and the task in all of the 30 items is to mark the one that does not belong to the group.[9]

Block (Fig 12–2)—The test material consists of 16 cubes. One side is red, one side is white and one side is divided into a white and a red triangle. The other sides of the cubes are blue and yellow. The task is to put these cubes in accordance with different patterns shown on cards. Only patterns in white and red are used. The first 4 patterns are based on 4 cubes, the next 2 patterns on 9 cubes and the last pattern on 16 cubes. Both speed and correctness are evaluated.[9, 25]

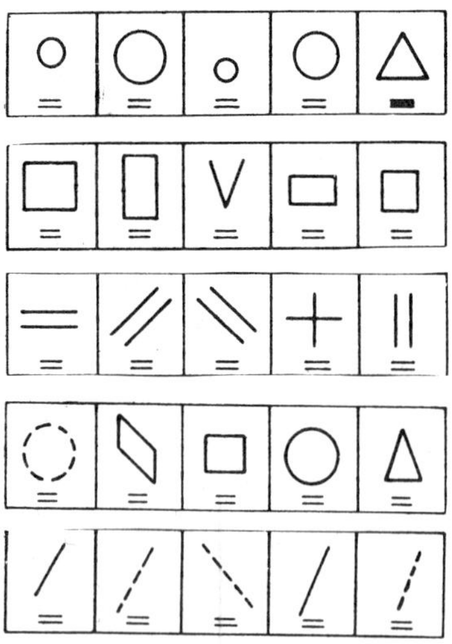

Fig 12–1.—Figure classification (see text). Five out of 30 items are shown.

Unfolding (Fig 12–3)—Each of the 10

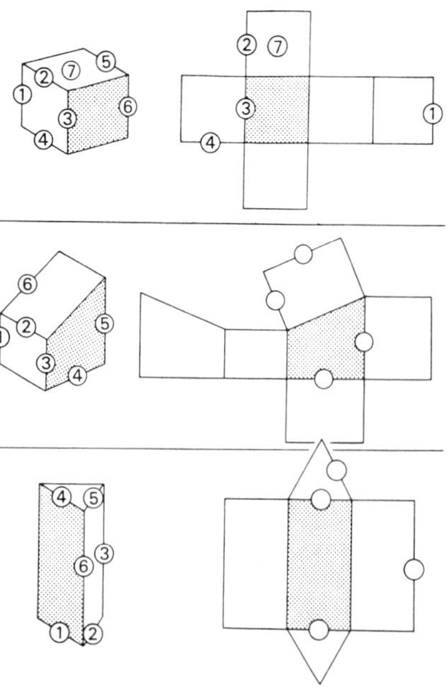

Fig 12–3.—Unfolding (see text).

items consists of a picture of a folded figure drawn in three dimensions and the same figure unfolded into two dimensions. On the folded figure, the sides and edges are numbered. The task is to transfer the numbers from the three-dimensional figure to the two-dimensional one.[8]

Visual gestalt (configuration) ability test (Fig 12–4)—Each item consists of a consecutive succession of 4 pictures. The first one in the succession is a very fragmentary one and the last an almost complete picture. Every picture in the succession is shown for 7 seconds and the task is to identify the picture as quickly as possible. The test has three parts with 14 items in each.[21]

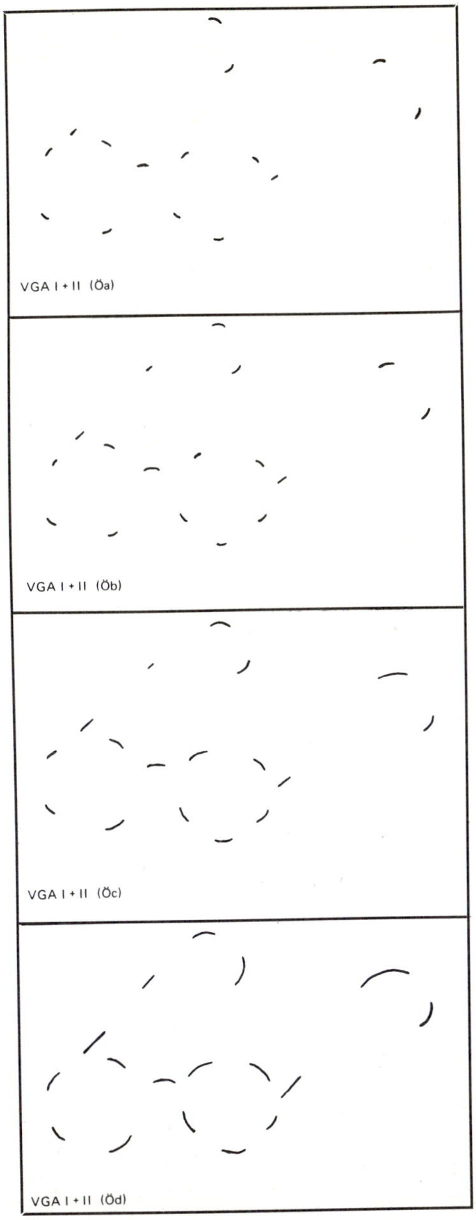

Fig 12–4.—Visual gestalt (configuration) ability test (see text).

Perceptual Speed

Digit symbols (Fig 12–5)—Each digit (1–9) is given a special symbol shown on the top of the test sheet. The task is to write the correct symbol under the digits when given in random order as quickly as possible. The score is based on performance in 90 seconds.[25]

Dots (Fig 12–6)—The test consists of 6 parts, and every part consists of 8 lines with groups of 3, 4 or 5 dots. The task is to mark all groups that consist of 4 dots as quickly as possible. Speed and accuracy are evaluated and also deviation in speed and accuracy between different parts of the test, which might be an indicator of fluctuation in vigilance.[21]

The same number (Fig 12–7)—The test includes 3 pages with 30 columns on each page. Every column consists of 8 numbers with 3 digits. The task is to underline all

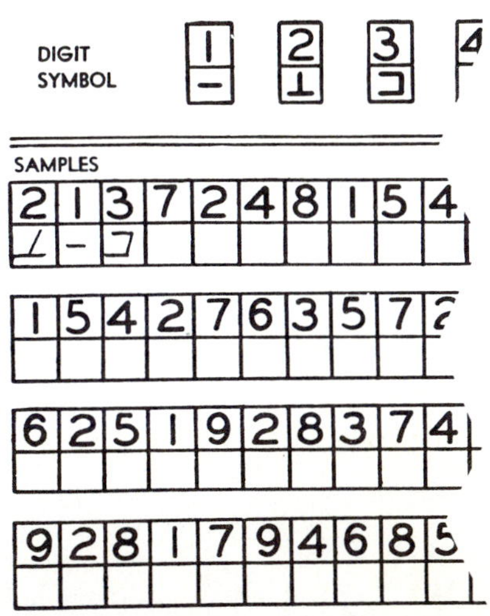

Fig 12–5.—Digit symbols (see text).

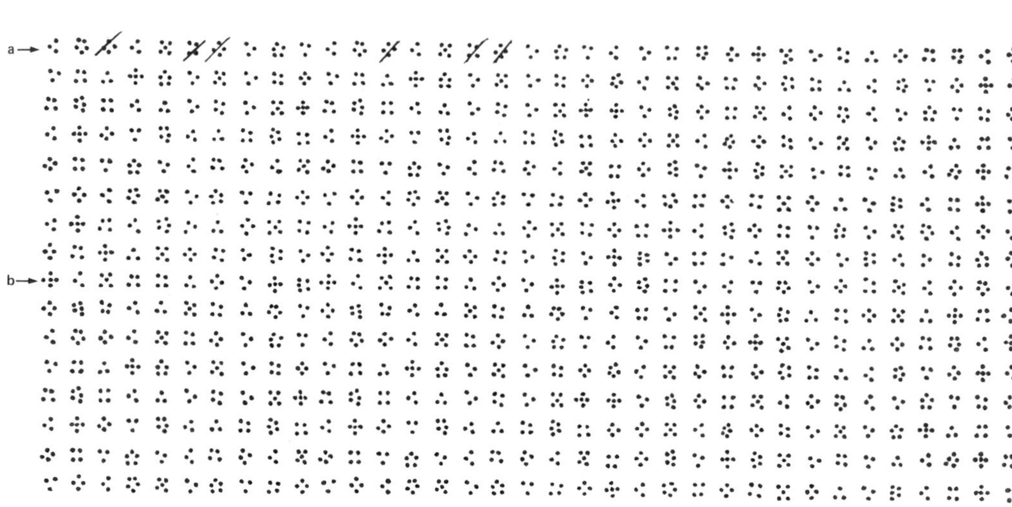

Fig 12–6.—Dots (see text).

numbers that correspond to the number given at top of each column.[8]

Eye-Hand Coordination

The bolt test (Fig 12–8)—The task is to take a bolt and a needle from two separate boxes, put the bolts in holes on a T bar and lock them with the needles as quickly as possible. The performance is scored every 30 seconds up to 3 minutes.[23]

Pins (Fig 12–9)—The task is to quickly move pins from a wooden plate to holes in a T bar by means of a pair of tweezers. The performance is scored every 30 seconds up to 90 seconds.[23]

729	346	412	145	834
639	518	536	173	834
639	518	536	173	834
729	346	812	145	630
746	824	579	451	874
719	346	412	165	834
729	316	732	374	283
321	346	647	145	534

Fig 12–7.—The same number (see text).

Cylinders (Fig 12–10)—The test consists of 2 wooden plates with 60 holes in each plate. In one plate, the holes are filled with

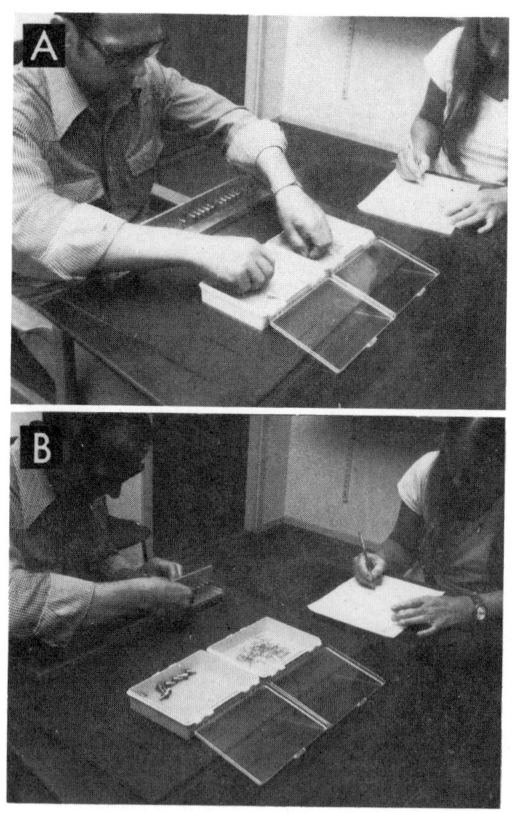

Fig 12–8.—The bolt test (see text).

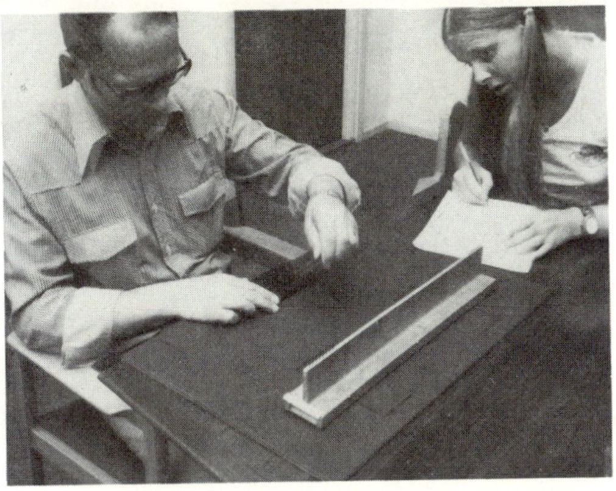

Fig 12–9.—Pins (see text).

easily graspable cylinders, and the task is to move the cylinders from one plate to another as fast as possible, first with one hand and then with the other.[13]

Memory

Benton visual retention test—The test consists of 10 drawings with geometric figures. Each drawing is shown for 10 seconds, and the task is to reproduce the drawing immediately after its removal. Both the number of errors (more than one error can be made in each item) and the number of entirely correct reproductions are scored.[5]

Auditory perception and retention—The test consists of a tape-recorded short story with a lot of details. The tape is presented to the subject, who afterward is asked 14 multiple-choice questions about the content of the text.[21]

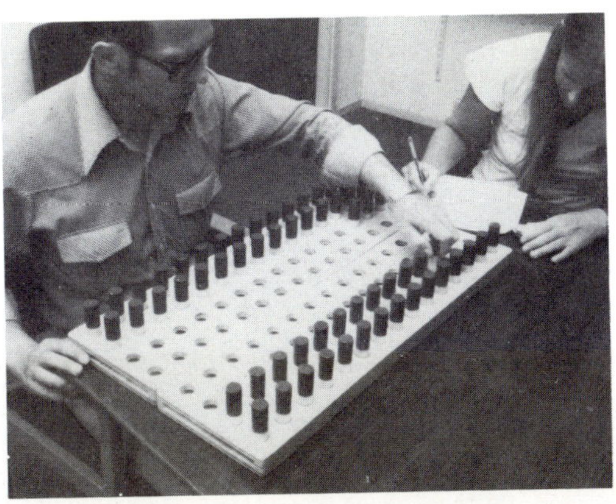

Fig 12–10.—Cylinders (see text).

"Impaired memory" is a frequent subjective symptom among workers exposed to solvents (see reference 6 and Table 12–1), but the memory tests do not always correlate with the symptoms. "Memory," however, is a very broad concept including several different functions, and it is very plausible that the memory tests used cover only a limited part of the memory functions. Attempts have been made to construct relevant memory tests, which should make it possible to distinguish between changes caused by pathologic processes and the normal individual variability of memory performance,[7] but these need further development.

Hitherto, the effects of solvents were looked on as a weakening of the normal psychological function and thus indicated by a difference in means between the exposed subjects and the nonexposed referents. Furthermore, the most sensitive tests to demonstrate mean differences have been chosen, although more specific changes might be found among less sensitive tests, i.e., demonstrable only after more serious deterioration, heavier exposure, etc.

Health checkups concerning other effects from solvents—Although this chapter deals primarily with the neuropsychiatric disorders resulting from long-time solvent exposure, a few comments are devoted to other effects. Thus, there usually is little to gain in checking blood or liver status except when exposure takes place to benzene, carbon tetrachloride and perhaps some of the aromatics, for example, styrene. Nevertheless, such tests usually are included in a health checkup program for solvent workers. Glomerulonephritis is a fairly rare disease that sometimes results from solvent exposure, but a simple measurement of proteinuria is convenient and inexpensive. Health checkups for painters may also include other measurements such as lead and chromium in blood or urine when exposure takes place to pigments in addition to solvents, as for many spray painters.

MONITORING SOLVENT EXPOSURE

Technical hygienic methods, as well as biologic monitoring, might be used for the control of solvent exposure; i.e., solvent concentrations in the air might be measured or, alternatively, reliance might be placed on determinations of solvent metabolites in the urine of the exposed workers. It is not the purpose of this chapter to delineate and describe methods for air measurements of solvents, but it might be briefly recalled that mixtures of various solvents are difficult to measure. A commonly used technique is the adsorption of solvents on activated charcoal, and this method is preferable for its simplicity and the possibility of sending the charcoal tubes to remote laboratories for the analyses. However, it has been found that alcohols are difficult to dissolve from charcoal,[12] and exposure to such solvents, therefore, might be underestimated. There are other problems as well, especially in storing the exposed tubes.[19] Moreover, technical hygienic monitoring is resource demanding, since hygienists usually cannot follow more than a few workers with measurements through the shift.

Biologic monitoring may be convenient and preferable whenever possible. A contributing factor to this preference is that the *work load greatly influences the amount of solvent uptake,* as demonstrated in experimental studies.[1] It also was found that the solvent uptake in connection with various work loads might be fairly different for various types of solvents. For example, methylene chloride is taken up to a much lesser degree than toluene and styrene.

Biologic monitoring might be based on either a metabolite in the urine or on determination of the compound itself in alveolar air.

It has been suggested that the ratio between the alveolar air concentration and the concentration in ambient air be taken as a measure of the uptake.[2] This method requires a number of samples over the workday, however, and might be somewhat uncertain if there is a great variation in the solvent concentration over the day (as would be the metabolite determinations). Nevertheless, this method of monitoring seems to be better than utilization of alveolar air samples at the end of the workday and during the following 12–16 hours. Such sampling requires the comparison of the measured concentrations in the alveolar air to so-called decay curves. In our experience, we have found it difficult to calculate average exposures from workplaces by means of decay curves. It also is theoretically disturbing that any combination of work time and exposure level tends to result in its own curve. Moreover, the body fat mass probably tends to greatly influence such decay curves.[10]

The utilization of metabolites in urine, for example, trichloroacetic acid in case of exposure to trichloroethylene and mandelic acid as a result of styrene exposure, has the advantage of permitting simple sampling methods. However, for most of the solvents, the knowledge is comparatively incomplete with regard to the relationship between exposure levels and metabolites in urine, nor is there sufficient knowledge about the effects—for example, disturbances in physiologic variables in relation to metabolite concentrations in urine. Although trichloroacetic acid in the urine has been widely used as a measure of trichloroethylene exposure, there still is considerable uncertainty about the relationship. It is somewhat disturbing that there is a delay of about 24 hours before trichloroacetic acid appears in the urine.[18]

Styrene is another solvent for which the metabolite, mandelic acid in the urine, has been utilized as a measure of exposure. At low levels, there have been some difficulties, however, due to the background excretion of mandelic acid as measured through nonspecific methods, but specific methods for mandelic acid now are available.[11, 22]

The relationship of biologic effects and concentrations of metabolities in urine, as well as other aspects of biologic monitoring of solvents and other industrial chemicals, can be found elsewhere.[16, 24, 26] It seems that further efforts should be made to improve the methods, both with regard to the relationship between air concentrations and metabolites and concerning physiologic effects of solvents at various metabolite concentrations. Presently, the authorities tend to establish standards based on air concentrations, and, therefore, the relationship between air concentrations and metabolites in urine is of the greatest interest from the compliance point of view. But it might be more relevant, and perhaps more demanding, to create tolerance limits in respect to metabolites or blood and tissue concentrations of solvents in direct relation to their physiologic effects.

REFERENCES

1. Åstrand, I.: Uptake of solvents in the blood and tissues of man: A review, Scand. J. Work Environ. Health 1:199, 1975.
2. Åstrand, I., and Gamberale, F.: Effects on humans of solvents in the inspiratory air: A method for estimation of uptake, Environ. Res. 15:1, 1978.
3. Axelson, O. (ed.): Responsregistrering vid lösningsmedelsexposition (Registration of responses to solvent exposure). Summary from a Scandinavian meeting in Örebro, April 15–16, 1975. Örebro: Yrkesmedicinska kliniken 1975.
4. Axelson, O., Hane, M., and Hogstedt, C.: A case-referent study on neuropsychiatric disorders among workers exposed to solvents, Scand. J. Work Environ. Health 2:14, 1976.
5. Benton, A.: *The Revised Visual Retention Test* (Ames, Iowa: The State University of Iowa, 1963).
6. Blume, J., Hane, M., Sundell, L., and Ydreborg, B.: Mental function changes among house painters (English summary), Lakartidningen 72:702, 1975.
7. Chalupa, B.: Examination of the defects of memory caused by poisoning with some kinds of industrial poisons, (Czech, Russian and English summaries), C. Psychologie 2:356, 1958.
8. Deltabatteriet (Delta-battery): *Manual* (Stockholm: Psykologiförlaget AB, 1970).
9. Dureman, I., Kebbon, L., and Österberg, E.: *Manual till DS-Batteriet (Manual to the DS-Battery)* (Stockholm: Skandinaviska Testförlaget, 1971).
10. Engström, J., and Bjurström, R.: Exposure to methylene chloride. Content in subcutaneous adipose tissue, Scand. J. Work Environ. Health 3:215, 1977.
11. Engström, K., and Rantanen, I.: A new gas chromatographic method for determination of mandelic acid in urine, Int. Arch. Arbeitsmed. 33:163, 1974.
12. Fracchia, M., Pierce, L., Graul, R., and Stanley, R.: Desorption of organic solvents from charcoal tubes, Am. Ind. Hyg. Assoc. J. 38:144, 1977.
13. Gammabatteriet (Gamma-battery): *Manual* (Stockholm: Psykologiförlaget AB, 1976).
14. Hane, M., Hogstedt, C., and Sundell, L.: Neuropsychiatric symptoms among solvent-exposed workers—a questionnaire for screening (English summary), Lakartidningen 77:439, 1980.
15. Hogstedt, C., Hane, M., and Axelson, O.: Organic solvents in occupational health—a review (English summary), Nord föret halsov 1:44, 1978.
16. Lauwerys, R.: Biological criteria for selected industrial toxic chemicals: A review, Scand. J. Work Environ. Health 1:139, 1975.
17. Mayer-Gross, W., Slater, E., and Roth, M.: *Clinical Psychiatry* (3d ed.; London: Baillière, Tindall & Cassel, 1969).
18. Müller, G., Spassorski, M., and Henscher, D.: Trichloroethylene exposure and trichloroethylene metabolites in urine and blood, Arch. Toxicol. 29:335, 1972.
19. Saalwaechter, A. T., McCammon, C. S., Jr., Roper, C. P., and Carlberg, K. S.: Performance testing of the NIOSH charcoal tube technique for the determination of air concentration of organic vapors, Am. Ind. Hyg. Assoc. J. 38:476, 1977.
20. Seppäläinen, A. M.:. Applications of neurophysiological methods in occupational medicine: A review, Scand. J. Work Environ. Health 1:1, 1975.
21. Sjöborg, A., and Frömark, A.: Standardisering av ett psykologiskt testbatteri för beteendetoxikologiska undersökningar (Stan-

dardization of a battery of psychological tests to be used in behavioral toxicological studies). Information from Psykotekniska Institutet, No. 93, 1977.

22. Slob, A.: A new method for determination of mandelic acid excretion at low level styrene exposure, Br. J. Ind. Med. 30:390, 1973.
23. Balkprovet (T-bar test): *Manual* (Stockholm: Psykologiförlaget AB, 1967).
24. Vesterberg, O.: General aspects on biotransformation and elimination of organic compounds in connection with occupational exposure, Int. Arch. Occup. Environ. Health 35:89, 1975.
25. Wechsler, D.: *Manual for Wechsler Adult Intelligence Scale* (New York: Psychological Corporation, 1955), p. 110.
26. Zielhuis, R. L.: Biological monitoring. Guest lecture given at the 26th Nordic Symposium on Industrial Hygiene, Helsinki, October, 1977, Scand. J. Work Environ. Health 4:1, 1978.

13 / Occupational Health Aspects of Pesticides: Clinical and Hygienic Principles

GEORGE NAGLE, M.P.H., MARY ANN WOODBURY, M.C.H., and CARL ZENZ, M.D.

WITH WORLD-WIDE, ceaseless demand for foodstuffs, control of vegetation, crop preparation, storage (of seeds and edibles), shipment and distribution from the field into the home there are parallel research, production, formulating and packaging, storage, shipment and distributing, supplying and application of an array of pesticides, creating a chain of events with potential occupational health impact. A general overview is presented here, emphasizing occupational medical and hygienic principles applicable to selected substances and major groups of compounds in common use. Frequently overlooked are chemical measures applied world-wide for disease control in fish, fowl, wild game and livestock of all varieties. Occupational exposures may occur inadvertently with these working groups as well as for growers, harvesters, packagers, handlers and sellers of flowers. Environmental considerations are beyond the scope of this chapter, and the reader is referred to the references.

The continuing need for crop protection and the control of disease-spreading rodents and pests is clear. In areas where mechanization and an integrated scientific approach to agriculture are well established, the farmer wants more crops of better quality, based largely on consumer ("societal") demands. In other areas where populations expand faster than agriculture, the question becomes not only one of the quality of foods and fibers produced but of life itself. For this reason, the regulatory restraints imposed on the use of agricultural crop protection agents in one country may be inappropriate for the same product's use in another part of the world.

Currently, each government sets its own policies for use, based on each country's own needs and priorities. Regulatory uniformity is being discussed by agricultural experts and government officials as the world-wide agricultural community attempts to establish common standards of safety in handling, safety in use and environmental considerations.

The use of chemical compounds for protecting crops is not a twentieth century innovation. Actually, chemical crop protection predates Biblical times, when farmers used sulfur to control mildew. Nicotine was widely used in France as early as 1690 to kill lace bugs, and in the United States in the 1860s, arsenic-based compounds were used to control the potato beetle.

Since the early 1940s, when organic insecticides were first introduced, thousands of new compounds have been developed to help farmers control the pests that destroy their crops.

The United States Federal Insecticide, Fungicide and Rodenticide Act (FIFRA) defines a pesticide as:

1. "Any substance or mixture of substances intended for preventing, destroying, repelling or mitigating any pest (insect, rodent, nematode, fungus, weed, other forms of terrestrial or aquatic plant or animal life or viruses, bacteria or other microorganisms, except microorganisms on or in man or other living animals), which the administrator of the Environmental Protection Agency (EPA) declares to be a pest, and
2. "Any substance or mixture of substances intended for use as a plant regulator, defolient or desiccant."[28]

There are approximately 1500 active ingredients in common use registered by the EPA. In addition, there are numerous pesticide active ingredients that are registered on an experimental basis only or that are produced in the United States for export only. Pesticides are an extremely diverse group of substances with a wide potential for a variety of toxic effects. These substances range in acute toxicity from the lethal at low doses, such as strychnine, to the edible in relatively large quantities, such as sodium chloride. With many pesticides, the possibility of dermal exposure with subsequent absorption through the skin may present a greater problem to workers than does exposure through inhalation. However, it must be emphasized that both routes of absorption may occur concomitantly. Some of the compounds have been known to produce carcinogenic, teratogenic, mutagenic and neurotoxic effects, as well as alterations of reproductive processes or functions in experimental animals and in man. Early-used pesticides were materials of natural origin, such as the salts of arsenic, copper, lead, mercury and zinc, leading into the era of the synthetic organic pesticides, which began with the discovery of the insecticidal activity of DDT in 1939. Research continued to develop a wide variety of other synthetic pesticides and there are now more than 40,000 registered pesticide compounds in the United States.[93] More than 3 billion kg of pesticide active ingredients were produced in 1974 in this country. Of this vast total, about 1.6 billion kg were herbicides, 1.3 billion kg insecticides and the remainder fungicides. Domestic industrial capacity increased by 12% in 1976 and 7% in 1978, and this trend is expected to continue. Approximately 90% of present-day pesticides are organic compounds, with insecticides consisting primarily of the organochlorine compounds, the organophosphate compounds and the carbamate compounds. Fumigants include the halogenated hydrocarbons and certain inorganic gases. The herbicides include the amides, arsenicals, carbamates and thiocarbamates and substituted ureas. Fungicides include thiocarbamates, phthalimides and organotin compounds. A listing of significant pesticides with corresponding chemical identities and main uses is found in the Glossary at the end of the chapter. Often overlooked is the well-known compound called "creosote," a preservative long known for its ability to kill both fungi and boring insects likely to infest wood. Creosote is a mixture of phenols derived from wood or bituminous coal by distillation and used principally as a wood preservative. In the United States, more than 0.5 billion kg of creosote are produced annually, an amount nearly equaling that of the snythetic organic pesticides produced. The inorganic pesticides, which account for the remaining 10% of production, include calcium arsenate, lead arsenate, arsenic acid, borate sulfur and sodium chloride.

Most insecticides are synthesized from other chemicals, and it is during these beginning stages where occupational exposure can occur. These materials have been classified according to the chemical vernacular as the "chlorinated hydrocarbons" (DDT being the most well known of this group) and "organophosphate compounds" (parathion, as a chief example) and marketed under a host of trade and generic names—Abate, azinphosmethyl (Guthion), carbophenothion (Trithion), chloropyrifos (Dursban), demeton (Systax), Diazinon, dicapthon (DiCaptan), etc. A special class is termed "carbamates." Among these are the well-known carbaryl (Sevin), aldicarb

(Temik), carbofuran (Furadan), fometanate HCl (Carzol), metalkamate (Bux) and methomyl (Lannate).

As mentioned earlier, the inorganic arsenicals were among the earliest insecticides used throughout the world: lead arsenate, "Paris green" and sodium arsenite (these will be discussed briefly). Certain other well-known chemicals, because of their inherent toxic nature, have been used as "fumigants," usually in areas that can be safely sealed off and any human contact scrupulously restricted. Typical fumigants are:

Cyanides: Acrylonitrile, calcium cyanide (Cyanogas), hydrogen cyanide, etc. (see Chapter 14).

Halogens: Methyl bromide and sulfuryl fluoride (Vikane).

Phosphines: Aluminum phosphide (Celphos, Phostoxin).

Herbicides, commonly called "weed-killers," are produced in large quantities to control growth of weeds and other undesirable plants in lawns, along highways, railroads, airports, etc. Factory occupational exposures are overshadowed by exposures during private use. Prominent herbicides are: endothal (dicarboxylic acid derivative), diquat and paraquat (quaternary ammonia derivatives).

The organic acids and some of their common derivatives are: cacodylic acid, dichlorophenoxyacetic acid (2,4-D), DSMA, MSMA (sodium methanearsonate), Silvex (2,4,5-TP), fenuron TCA (Urab) and monuron (Telvar).

Rodenticides constitute another major class: Diphacinone (Diphacin), Fumarin, Pival (Pivalyn), PMP (Valane) and warfarin.

Manufacturers usually operate integrated chemical synthesis plants and may produce many other chemical products in addition to pesticides. The work force normally includes chemists, engineers, managers, skilled chemical operators, pipefitters, electricians, laborers, truck drivers and warehouse workers.

Manufacturing includes pretreatment of reactants (change of size, temperature and state), reaction, purification and post-treatment of products (change of size and state). Raw materials for manufacture are delivered in bulk by pipeline, railroad car, barge, tank trucks, etc., or may be produced in-plant, often as by-products of other reactions. Manufacturers may produce several pesticide active ingredients at a single plant, which usually consists of several separate but interconnectable production areas or subplants. A subplant contains the equipment necessary for carrying out all the unit processes and operations, such as reaction, distillation, filtration and mixing, which are necessary to synthesize a product from raw materials. Subplant equipment may include mills, screens, hoppers, tanks, reactors, absorption columns, cooling towers, stills, filters, centrifuges, dryers, etc. Process monitoring, sampling and analyses are performed to determine temperatures, pressures, flowrates, densities and composition changes in order to control the chemical reactions. The production of pesticides involves complex chemical processes, including chlorination, alkylation, nitration, phosphorylation, sulfonation and bromination.

Pesticide formulating establishments generally are smaller than manufacturing establishments. Employees may include engi-

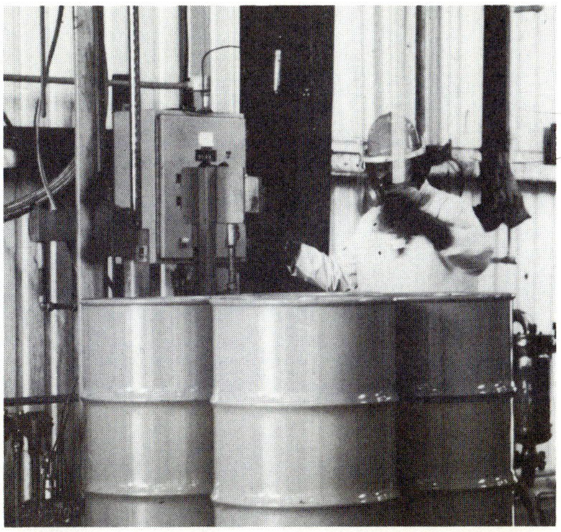

Fig 13–1.—Filling drums—the end stage of the manufacturing process.

neers, chemists, operators and laborers. There are major variations among formulators both in size and in operating practices. Seventy-one per cent of all formulating establishments employ less than 20 employees. Only 6% of all establishments employ more than 100 employees, but these larger plants dominate total production. Formulators with 100 or more employees account for 56% of production whereas formulators with fewer than 20 employees account for only 12.5% of all production.[92, 93]

A formulating operation generally is less complex than a manufacturing operation. Usually, a formulator receives concentrated active ingredients from a manufacturer and dilutes them with various nonpesticidal materials known as "inerts." The term "inert" refers to the effect of the substance on the target organism relative to the effect of the pesticide on that organism. However, as with any chemical, a toxic effect can be obtained with any inert at some dose, and many so-called inerts are more toxic to man than the term would lead one to believe. The formulating process may also include physical or chemical treatment to yield particular product forms: dust, powder, wettable powder, granule, pellet, emulsifiable concentrate, encapsulated or aerosol. Further processing may be done by wholesalers, retailers, repackagers or end users. With a few exceptions, formulating is a simple process varying in type according to the desired end product.

The preparation of dust and powder pesticide formulations entails dispensing from hoppers, screening for size and mixing with flour, silica, sulfur, lime, gypsum, talc or clay in a hammer mill, roller mill or other type of mill. Granule formulating consists of dispensing and sizing the inert (e.g., clay, vermiculite, ground corncobs, diatomaceous earth), dissolving or melting the pesticide in a tank and then spraying the pesticide onto the inert in a mixer.

Frequently overlooked when evaluating exposure is the potential role of the vehicle. In the laboratory, new products can be dissolved in a variety of solvents. In the field, however, the delivery medium is mainly water, so one of four basic formulations is used: emulsifiable concentrates, wettable powders, dusts or granular materials. However, solvents or mixtures of solvents can be used to a limited degree. Primarily, these are hydrocarbons such as diesel oil, gasoline, kerosene, xylene, with or without water, and "wetting" or "dispersing" agents.

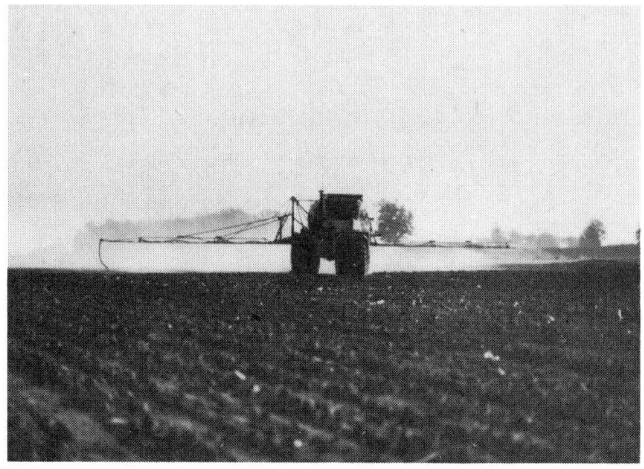

Fig 13–2.—Large-scale agricultural pesticide application using pressurized spraying.

Occupational exposures are not limited to the pesticide manufacture and formulation operations already described. The American Public Health Association (1979) estimates that, almost daily, nearly 1,275,000 U.S. farm workers are exposed to pesticides. This estimate does not take into account children (preschool and older) who work part or full time, nor does it consider wives of "migrant workers" who join their husbands in field work, often while pregnant and continuing work as long as possible before delivery.

Various physical and chemical properties of materials present during the manufacture and formulation of pesticides significantly affect the magnitude and/or subsequent effects of exposure. The following sections describe possible routes of exposure and certain physical, chemical and toxicologic properties.

AERIAL SPRAYING

Gribetz et al.[41] determined the physiologic and subjective effects of heat stress in the cockpits of agricultural spray pilots. Nine pilots flying for a large Israeli aerial spray company were studied. The pilots' daily work load was demanding (early work hours, 4–5 hours flight time, 10–15 takeoffs and landings, several hundred 180° turns, frequent passes under telephone and power lines) and included exposures to noise, vibrations, gravitation forces and various pesticides in addition to heat. The heat stress produced in the cockpits exceeded the heat exposure threshold limit value (TLV) for continual heavy work (25° C) 10 out of 10 times and was sustained for periods of up to 3½ hours. The heat stress exceeded TLVs for continual moderate work (26.7° C) 7 out of 10 times.

Cockpit air cooling was suggested as a necessary measure for preventing heat stress in hot climates. The need for appropriate filter technologies to prevent pesticide exposure during flight was noted as well as precautionary cockpit monitoring for pesticides and carbon monoxide. An unresolved question was whether conventional threshold standards for heat exposure are appropriate for spray pilots. (Standards are based on the prevention of symptoms more gross than the subtle psychomotor changes in pilot performance.) Heat and dehydration, together with other hazards (g-forces, organophosphates), are hypothesized to produce fluid loss, peripheral vasodilatation and blood pressure drops, and decreased threshold exposures to all these hazards may pose an insidious danger. Therefore, engineering and other measures to prevent heat stress and dehydration should rank high as part of a comprehensive program to protect health and performance levels of agricultural spray pilots.[36]

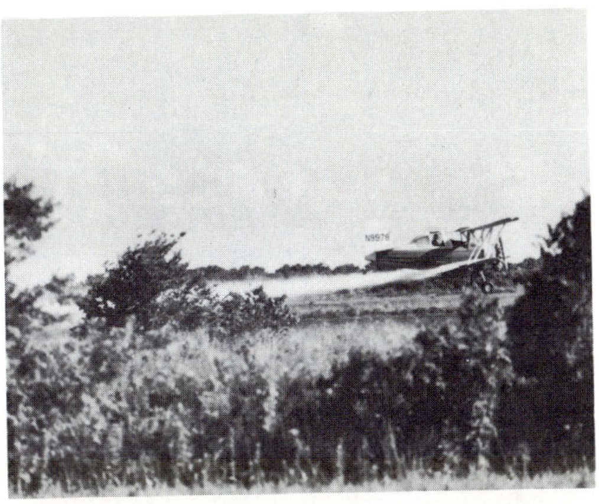

Fig 13–3.—Aerial application. Hazards involved include mixing and loading of the chemicals, fatigue and heat stress—frequently overlooked in assessing work exposures.

Workers assigned as "flagmen" during aerial application are especially vulnerable to overspray and contamination. Suitable respiratory protective equipment and clothing are required. (Preferably, other means for directing aerial applications should be used.)

INHALATION EXPOSURES

The inhalation of pesticide dusts, vapors, mists and gases may represent a significant occupational hazard.

In pesticide operations, dusts are generated by the mechanical agitation of solid material, such as milling or grinding. Note that fine dusts can be generated as a result of dry sweeping or vehicle traffic over an area contaminated with "coarser" material.

Dust hazards may involve the formulation of wettable powders, granules or baits. The "finer" the solid material the greater is the potential problem of workplace emissions and subsequent contamination of the general work area.

Retention of particles within the lungs depends on many factors: size, shape, hydroscopicity, density, reactivity and inhalation process (nasal or oral). Hayes[47] speculated that in the absence of specific information on a particulate, it can be assumed that about 25% of inhaled material would be exhaled, about 50% would be deposited in the upper respiratory passages and subsequently swallowed and about 25% would be deposited in the lower respiratory passages. Even dusts too large to be considered "respirable" may present a potential hazard due to deposition in the throat, with subsequent ingestion.

Volatility of the material affects the environmental concentration and thus is a significant factor in respiratory exposure. Vapor pressures of pesticides vary from nonvolatile materials such as DDT and dieldrin to compounds with extremely high vapor pressures such as methyl bromide and dichlorvos. Some fumigants such as phosgene and ethylene oxide are gases at standard temperature and pressure.

For all pesticides, both the aerosol (dust or mist) and vapor/gas component of the total potential inhalation exposure must be considered.

DERMAL EXPOSURE

Employees frequently experience dermal exposure to pesticides, with subsequent absorption through the skin. The rate at which a pesticide is absorbed through the skin is determined by the nature of the compound, the condition of the skin and external factors, such as temperature. The most rapid and complete absorption occurs with pesticides that have some solubility in both water and lipid.[131]

Skin absorption for a specific pesticide is also related to the area of skin exposed, duration of exposure and the region exposed. Different areas of the human skin absorb chemicals at different rates. Maibach and co-workers[76] determined that the parathion absorption rate was significantly higher for the scrotal skin, axilla, head and neck areas than for the hands or arms.

The degree and rate of skin absorption may be increased if the skin barrier is injured due to washing with solvents, irradiation and thermal/chemical burns.[48] Other factors include increased circulation of blood through the dermis of the skin and sweat rate.

Fine powders tend to be absorbed more readily than coarse powders for equivalent contact. Hayes[48] found that very finely ground technical dieldrin was absorbed as readily as dieldrin applied to the skin in solutions. In contrast, coarsely ground dieldrin powder was not as well absorbed.

INGESTION EXPOSURE

Oral exposures may occur through accidental splashing of liquid pesticide into the mouth, by smoking/eating with pesticide-contaminated hands or with accidentally contaminated food or smoking materials, by rubbing the mouth area with contaminated hands and by swallowing inhaled material that either entered the upper respiratory tract or was swept up by ciliary action into the trachea.

The degree of hazard is related to the extent of absorption of the specific pesticide for the specific portion of the gastrointestinal system involved.

OCULAR EXPOSURE

Ocular exposure usually is a result of accidental spills/splashes. Acute local effects may be produced on the eye or associated structure (eyelids, conjunctiva) in the absence of systemic effects.

During the past decade, the possibility of visual impairment following chronic pesticide exposure has gained importance. Ishikawa et al.[56,57] reported ocular disease attributed to chronic organophosphate pesticide exposure. In 1977, the Japanese government restricted the use of parathion, EPN and TEPP[58] and the Japanese Ministry of Public Welfare set forth standards for ocular conditions stemming from these pesticides. Plestina and Piukovic-Plestina,[105] noted the lack of published information on ocular effects and conducted a study of workers engaged in pesticide formulation for 5 years or longer. Sixty-three workers were divided into three groups according to pesticide exposure. The ophthalmologic data sought included measurement of corneal curvature, visual acuity, accommodation and focusing, intraocular pressure, visual fields, dark adaptation, color vision and retinal fields. Pupillary size and reaction were not recorded. Group A consisted of 31 workers selected according to the length of time each worker had been engaged in pesticide production. All of them were well-trained permanent staff, mostly involved in the production of pesticide emulsions.

Initially, working conditions of those occupationally exposed to pesticides were rather poor, but they improved gradually. The active ingredients produced were predominantly, but not exclusively, anticholinesterase compounds, consisting mainly of different types of dimethoxy- and diethoxyphosphates, thiophosphates and carbamates. A few compounds were chlorinated hydrocarbons or herbicides. Workers had no fixed working place, and a system of irregular rotation was introduced to equalize exposure. Usual working time was 8 hours a day, 5 days a week for 9–10 months a year. However, overtime work was quite common, particularly when seasonal production had to be increased. A regular monitoring of cholinesterase activity showed an association between overtime work and decreased blood cholinesterase activity.

Among 12 workers in Group B, 7 were engaged for more than 5 years in pesticide application, largely in public health programs, but also in disinfestation of food stores. Two workers were pilots who applied pesticides in agriculture, and those remaining supervised pesticide production. Common factors for all workers in this group were irregular exposure, good protective measures and good working conditions. All this accounted for a considerably milder exposure than for workers in Group A. Again, the active materials were predominantly anticholinesterase compounds, except for the pilots, who were equally exposed to different fertilizers and herbicides. Blood cholinesterase activity data, monitored over a long period, did not reveal any toxicologically meaningful pattern of enzyme inhibition. Similarly, other routine biochemical and hematologic tests required by clinicians at their periodic medical checkups were normal.

Group C, a group of 20 subjects, was formed to serve as control. The workers were recruited among those of similar socioeconomic status as for the two preceding groups. They were matched by age and habits, but had no closer contact with pesticides than the general population. They worked either in internal transport or in the storage of end products that were not insecticides. Thus, except by sex, the three groups were matched as closely as possible.

Plestina and Piukovic-Plestina's main findings in these workers were a decreased dark adaptation, a mild constriction of peripheral visual fields (3–4%) and slightly more conjunctival injection. In this report, as noted in others, "highly" exposed and "heavily" exposed terms are not defined. In the United States, optic atrophy or other visual sequelae from work exposures to organophosphate pesticides has not been observed.[84]

CHLORINATED HYDROCARBON COMPOUNDS

Summaries of the salient toxicologic aspects of the most representative chlorinated hydrocarbon compounds are set forth: DDT(1,1-bis(*p*-chlorophenyl)2,2,2-trichloroethane) was first used in 1947 and gained world-wide acceptance in malaria eradication programs but now is banned in most countries. A brief background description can serve as reference to other related "chlorinated hydrocarbon" insecticides with somewhat similar chemical structures.

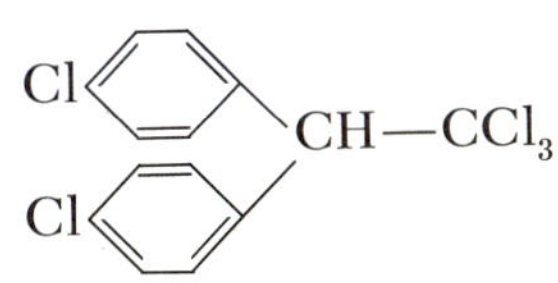

The 1979 American Conference of Governmental Industrial Hygienists (ACGIH)

VELSICOL

MATERIAL SAFETY DATA SHEET

Revised 12/21/77 *"Essentially Similar" to U. S. Department of Labor Form, OSHA-20, Rev. May '72*

SECTION I IDENTIFICATION OF PRODUCT

MANUFACTURER'S NAME	EMERGENCY TELEPHONE NO.
Velsicol Chemical Corporation	(312) 670-4500

ADDRESS
341 E. Ohio Street, Chicago, Illinois 60611

TRADE NAME AND SYNONYMS
BANVEL Tech. Dicamba

CHEMICAL NAME AND SYNONYMS
2-methoxy-3, 6-dichlorobenzoic acid

CHEMICAL FAMILY	MOLECULAR FORMULA
Organic herbicide	$C_8H_6Cl_2O_3$

SECTION II HAZARDOUS COMPONENTS OF MIXTURES

COMPONENT	%	THRESHOLD LIMIT VALUE (UNITS)	COMPONENT	%	THRESHOLD LIMIT VALUE (UNITS)

Technical Banvel

Acute oral LD_{50} (rats) 1707 mg/kg
Acute dermal LD_{50} (rabbits) 200 mg/kg
Acute inhalation $LD_{50} > 9.6$ mg/l (4-hour exposure)
Not a skin irritant but extremely irritating and corrosive to the eye

SECTION III PHYSICAL DATA

BOILING POINT (°F.)			SPECIFIC GRAVITY (H_2O=1) 30°C (86°F)	1.565
VAPOR PRESSURE (mm Hg)	100°C (212°F)	3.75 x 10	PERCENT VOLATILE BY VOLUME(%)	
VAPOR DENSITY (AIR=1)		7.64	EVAPORATION RATE (______=1)	
SOLUBILITY IN WATER		0.5%	Melting Point °F (90°-100°C)	194-212
APPEARANCE AND ODOR	Light tan granular solid—practically odorless.			

SECTION IV FIRE AND EXPLOSION HAZARD DATA

FLASH POINT	FLAMMABLE LIMITS BY VOLUME (%)	LOWER	UPPER
Does not flash.			

FIRE-EXTINGUISHING MEDIA
Fog or water spray, foam, carbon dioxide.

SPECIAL FIRE-FIGHTING PROCEDURES Wear full protective clothing, self-contained breathing apparatus. Use water spray to keep containers cool. Heat from fire can cause decomposition with the evolution of toxic and irritating fumes.

UNUSUAL FIRE AND EXPLOSION HAZARDS

(SEE OTHER SIDE)

96.30-030

Fig 13-4.—A sample material safety data sheet, which has widespread use throughout industry. *(Continued.)*

SECTION V HEALTH HAZARD DATA

THRESHOLD LIMIT VALUE
Has not been established.

EFFECTS OF OVEREXPOSURE
Nonspecific. Severe eye injury can occur.
"Skin irritation may occur when handling finely ground material."

EMERGENCY AND FIRST AID PROCEDURES
EYE CONTACT: Flush with water for at least 15 minutes; get prompt medical attention.
SKIN CONTACT: Wash with mild soap and water.
INGESTION: Induce vomiting, saline emetic; call a physician.
INHALATION: Remove to fresh air.

SECTION VI REACTIVITY DATA

STABILITY	UNSTABLE		CONDITIONS TO AVOID
	STABLE	XX	

INCOMPATIBILITY *(Materials to avoid)*

HAZARDOUS DECOMPOSITION PRODUCTS Thermal decomposition may yield HCl, organochloride products, carbon monoxide, carbon dioxide.

HAZARDOUS POLYMERIZATION	MAY OCCUR		CONDITIONS TO AVOID
	WILL NOT OCCUR	XX	

SECTION VII SPILL OR LEAK PROCEDURES

STEPS TO BE TAKEN IN CASE MATERIAL IS RELEASED OR SPILLED
Contain spill, sweep and collect in drums; follow by thoroughly washing down with detergent and water. Collect washings; do not allow in drainage ditches or sewers.

WASTE DISPOSAL METHOD
Controlled incineration, designated landfill, or disposal in accordance with applicable local, state and federal regulations.

SECTION VIII SPECIAL PROTECTION INFORMATION

RESPIRATORY PROTECTION *(Specify type)*
Low levels—MESA/NIOSH-approved chemical cartridge respirator for pesticides.

VENTILATION	LOCAL EXHAUST	SPECIAL
	MECHANICAL *(General)*	OTHER

PROTECTIVE GLOVES
Rubber gloves or the equivalent.

EYE PROTECTION
Chemical goggles.

OTHER PROTECTION EQUIPMENT
Shower, daily change of clothing.

SECTION IX SPECIAL PRECAUTIONS

PRECAUTIONS TO BE TAKEN IN HANDLING AND STORING
Store in area away from seed fertilizers, insecticides or fungicides.

OTHER PRECAUTIONS
Treat as with any pesticide. Self-contained breathing apparatus and protective clothing should be available in case of severe fire.

The information presented herein, while not guaranteed, was prepared by technically knowledgeable personnel and to the best of our knowledge is true and accurate. It is not intended to be all-inclusive and the manner and conditions of use and handling may involve other or additional considerations.

Fig 13–4 *(cont.).*

threshold limit value (TLV) for DDT is 1 milligram per cubic meter (mg/m^3) of air for an 8-hour time-weighted average (TWA).*

As an insecticide, DDT proved to be cheaper and much more effective against many insect species than the previously used natural insecticides. Although its acute toxicity to mammals and man was low (because of its low water solubility, its low vapor pressure and lack of reactivity with oxygen), it had a long persistence following spraying or dusting. DDT was found to accumulate in the environment as well as being deposited in the lipids of mammals, birds, fish and other creatures. It was determined that, under certain conditions, DDT proved to be carcinogenic in several strains of animals.[89]

With heavy exposure to DDT dust, eye and skin irritation can result. At chronic high absorbed doses for man, the central nervous system is affected, causing paresthesias and tremors. With sufficient exposure (usually occurring with accidental ingestion of 10 mg/kg or greater), convulsions have occurred in some persons within 2–3 hours after ingestion. Clinically, excessive and chronic exposure is characterized by malaise, headache, dizziness, paresthesias of the tongue, face and lips, a feeling of apprehension, tremors and sometimes confusion. Severe intoxication may result in convulsions, and ingestion of very large doses induces vomiting. Fortunately, recovery occurs in most cases within 24 hours, with few residual effects. Chronic poisoning in man has not been reported.

Laws et al.[72] reported on the clinical evaluation and laboratory findings of 31 workers exposed to an equivalent of 3.6–18 mg daily over a period of 21 years without evidence of hepatotoxicity. An increased activity of hepatic microsomal enzymes was noted, but no apparent evidence of reduction of general health. Earlier investigations by Laws et al.[73] involving a study of 20 workers exposed to DDT for a period of 11–19 years, with a daily intake of 18 mg per person, demonstrated the isomers and metabolites of DDT in fat range from 38 to 647 ppm (compared with an average of 8 ppm for the general population). DDE (1,1-bis[p-chlorophenyl]-2,2-dichloroethylene) is the major excretory product in workers exposed to DDT.[23]

The hepatocarcinogenicity of DDE has been shown and confirmed in various strains of mice by chronic oral feeding studies, and liver cell tumors were found in both sexes of the experimental animals (mice), with metastases to the lung.[54]

Methoxychlor

Methoxyclor, another much-used insecticide that is closely related to DDT, is a solid with main exposure through inhalation. It is a substance of low toxicity with no reported effects in humans. The substitution of the methoxy groups for chlorine, as noted in the formula below, decreases considerably the toxicity of methoxychlor. Thus, whereas the oral LD_{50} for DDT in male rats is about 200 mg/kg, the oral LD_{50} for methoxychlor in rats is about 5000 mg/kg.

The TLV for methoxychlor is 10 mg/m^3.

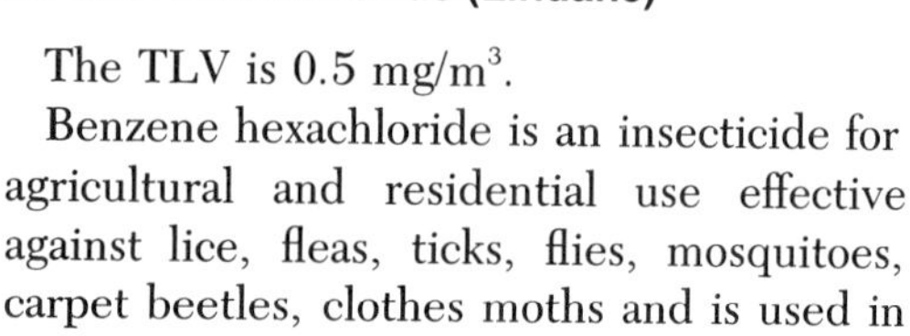

Benzene Hexachloride (Lindane)

The TLV is 0.5 mg/m^3.

Benzene hexachloride is an insecticide for agricultural and residential use effective against lice, fleas, ticks, flies, mosquitoes, carpet beetles, clothes moths and is used in Kwell shampoo and spray for body lice.

BHC, 1, 2, 3, 4, 5, 6-hexachlorcyclohexane has six isomers, with the γ-isomer noted to

*Hereinafter to be stated as "TLV," and "parts per million" as "ppm" and parts per billion as "ppb."

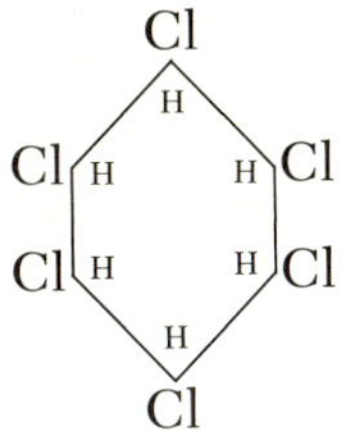

have insecticidal properties (since 1942) and named "lindane" in honor of Van der Linden, discoverer of four isomers. Lindane has a fumigant action, as it is about 100 times more volatile than DDT. The insecticidal toxicity of BHC is based chiefly on the content of its most toxic components, the γ-isomer, which is about 50–10,000 times more potent than the other isomers. The isomers have different toxic actions, with the γ- and α-isomers acting as central nervous system stimulants and the β- and δ-isomers being CNS depressants. Occupational exposures may occur by inhalation and skin absorption, rarely by ingestion. Exposure to the vapor causes eye, nose and throat irritation, and continued exposure can cause nausea and headache.

In Sweden, Kolmodin-Hedman and her co-workers[69] studied groups of workers who used lindane and DDT in various concentrations during several types of agricultural activities between 1974 and 1977. Different methods of treatment were observed: dipping, spraying in a spray tunnel and spraying on fields. Also, exposure in connection with handling of the treated plants was studied and the concentration of the substances in the air above treated plants was measured. Exposures were determined as concentrations in the air, as a result of both personal and stationary air sampling. The uptake was measured as the plasma concentration of the substances. Exposures varied a great deal, but the concentration of lindane or DDT in air never was higher than one-half of the TLV value. On the whole, no uptake of DDT (increased DDT in plasma) could be demonstrated. Working with lindane gave a small and variable but significant increase of the lindane concentration in plasma, which disappeared very rapidly when exposure was stopped. The concentration of lindane in plasma never was so high as to cause alteration of liver enzyme function. No symptoms related to exposure were found.

Further studies by Kolmodin-Hedman et al.[70] involved workers who treated pine and fir trees with an emulsion containing 1% lindane. Ten persons packed these plants for 2 days indoors. After packing for 2 days, their plasma levels of lindane were 1.2–25.7 ng/ml. Plasma levels decreased to half the initial value in 3–5 days. Planting resulted in plasma levels of lindane of 0.2–22.3 ng/ml at the end of the first week. Despite continued planting, the lindane levels decreased to 0.2–3.5 ng/ml at the end of the second week. Symptoms were not noted with higher frequency in a group of planters exposed to lindane compared to a group of planters who worked with unprepared plants, and symptoms did not correlate with higher plasma levels of lindane.

In another investigation, Kolmodin-Hedman et al.[71] studied 11 workers who treated pine and fir trees with a solution containing 1% lindane. Eight workers packed plants for 1 week and 60 persons thereafter planted them for 1–2 weeks. Exposure to dry lindane powder resulted in a plasma lindane level of 44.0 and 28.0 ng/ml, respectively. The packing personnel had plasma levels of 10.5±6.8 mg/ml. After 1 month, the high values had declined and were about 1 ng/ml. The investigators thought that plasma levels exceeding 10 ng/ml might induce liver microsomal enzyme changes.

Lindane has been suspected to cause aplastic anemia, but reports have not been conclusive in humans. Fatalities have occurred following accidental ingestion (estimated fatal oral dose 150 mg/kg), with severe convulsions, respiratory distress and cyanosis.[46]

Dieldrin

The TLV is 0.25 mg/m^3.

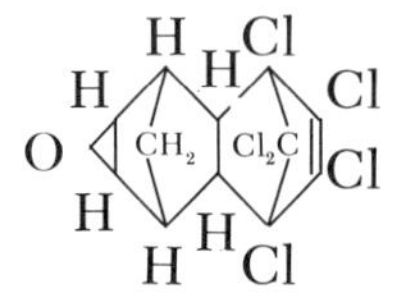

Among the chlorinated cyclodienes, dieldrin is the most frequently used pesticide. Main occupational exposure may occur through inhalation, skin absorption and ingestion. Dieldrin is considered a convulsant and has been known to cause liver cancer in mice.[55,101] Early symptoms of overexposure include malaise, increased sweating, headache, dizziness, nausea, vomiting and, with high exposures, myoclonic jerking of the extremities. Clonic and tonic convulsions, which may be followed by coma, have occurred. Brown et al.[14] reported case studies of 5 workers who had been exposed to aldrin-dieldrin and were found to have suffered one or more convulsive seizures and/or myoclonic limb movements. They noted that the blood concentration of dieldrin during the acute phase ranged from 16 to 62 µg/100 gm of blood. The analysis of blood for dieldrin concentration may assist in estimating the extent of absorption following exposure.

Aldrin

The TLV is 0.25 mg/m^3.

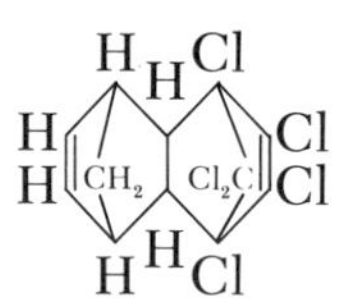

This insecticide is an odorless, white crystalline solid readily absorbed through the skin and by inhalation. Noteworthy is that it is rapidly metabolized into dieldrin, and, in cases of acute poisoning, these compounds can produce generalized convulsions. In the same report by Brown et al.,[14] the 5 workers were exposed to aldrin concentrations up to 8.5 mg/m^3. Other early symptoms of aldrin intoxication resemble those of dieldrin.[59]

Chlordane

The TLV is 0.5 mg/m^3.

(See Chapter 3 for background discussion.)

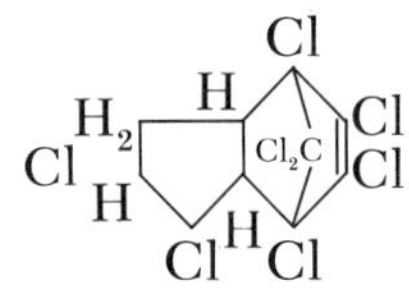

Technical chlordane is an amber-colored viscous material. Occupational exposures may occur chiefly through skin absorption and/or inhalation. Early symptoms of overexposure are coughing, blurred vision, confusion, ataxia and delirium. Accidental or suicidal ingestion causes abdominal pain, nausea, vomiting and diarrhea. Severe overexposure causes irritability, tremor, convulsions and death. Derbes et al.[24] described the case of a worker who had spilled a 25% chlordane suspension on his clothing, with convulsions occurring 40 minutes later and death shortly thereafter (the contaminated clothing was not immediately removed). Ingestion of 6 gm (100 mg/kg) in a suicide attempt resulted in severe mouth burns, severe gastritis, diffuse pneumonia, anuria, convulsions and mania, with death occurring after 9½ days.

Endrin

The TLV is 0.1 mg/m^3.

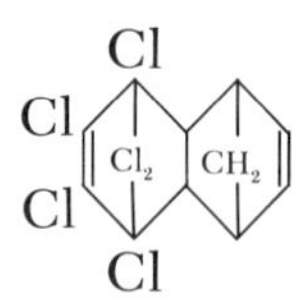

In addition to use as an insecticide, endrin is also utilized as an aviacide and rodenticide and is readily absorbed through the skin and by inhalation and ingestion. Its chief toxic effect is as a convulsant; in humans, early effects of acute intoxication are sudden epileptiform convulsions, lasting for several minutes, which can occur from 30 minutes up to 10 hours following overexposure. Coble et al.[20] described dysrhythmic changes, often preceding convulsions, and showed that removal from exposure generally results in a normal electroencephalogram within 1–6 months. In most cases, recovery is rapid, but anorexia, lethargy, weakness, headache and dizziness may persist for 2–4 weeks. Jager[59] reported that in less severe cases of endrin intoxication, the main complaints were headache, dizziness, abdominal distress, nausea, vomiting, insomnia and occasionally slight mental confusion. Many fatalities have occurred from ingestion of endrin, usually from accidental intake of bread made with contaminated flour. Such cases result in sudden onset of convulsions, with serum endrin levels of 0.053 ppm 30 minutes after the convulsion and 0.083 ppm after 20 hours. A high incidence of fetal organogenesis was reported in golden hamsters fed single doses of 2.5 mg/kg of endrin. Ottolenghi et al.[101] reported congenital anomalies and growth retardation in offspring, and rats fed a diet of 100 ppm of endrin for 2 years developed degenerative changes.[59]

Heptachlor

The TLV is 0.5 mg/m^3.

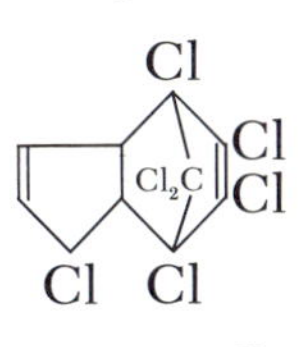

Heptachlor is chemically closely related to chlordane but is considered to be more toxic than chlordane. Occupational exposures by inhalation, dermal and oral exposures are possible, with toxic responses in man similar to those of chlordane and the other chlorinated insecticides. Following feeding of 90 mg/kg in rats, convulsions have been noted, with effects occurring within 30–60 minutes. Necropsy revealed liver necrosis in the rats, and repeated applications of 20 mg/kg solution to the skin of rats revealed a toxic cumulative action. Heptachlor was tested for carcinogenicity by oral administration in rats. The hepatocarcinogenicity found was not reproducible in other experiments with similar dose ranges. Rats fed a diet containing 6 mg/kg heptachlor developed cataracts after 4$^1/_2$ and 9$^1/_2$ months of feeding.[82]

Toxaphene

The TLV is 0.5 mg/m^3.

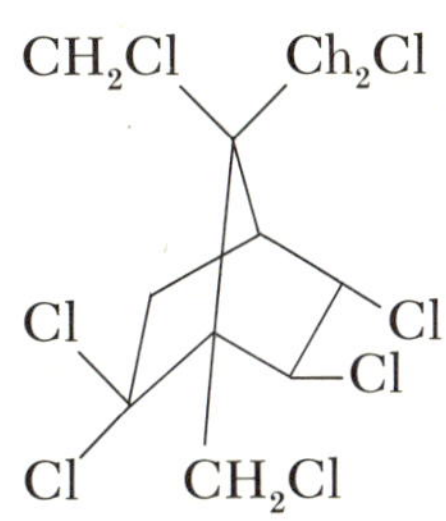

This yellow, wax-like compound is prepared by chlorinating bicyclic terpene-camphene to contain up to 69% chlorine. In 1976, toxaphene production in the United States amounted to more than 50 million kg, with about 85% for use on cotton crops. Other major uses are on cattle and swine, on soybeans, corn, wheat and peanuts. Substantial amounts also are used for lettuce, tomatoes and other food crops. Standard commercial formulation is a dust containing 20% toxaphene, and emulsifiable concentrates contain up to 1 kg toxaphene per liter; oil solutions are 90% toxaphene and wettable powders are 40% toxaphene. Toxaphene also is mixed with other insecticide chemicals for a variety of uses. Toxaphene is highly toxic to most fish species and was added to open waters at levels between 0.5 and 0.2 ppm to destroy unwanted fish.

Strobane is a substance similar to toxaphene, prepared by chlorinating camphene and pinene to contain 65% chlorine, and is also widely used, as it is inexpensive, with a residue effect. Exposure may occur through inhalation, skin absorption and, rarely, by accidental ingestion. Moderate skin irritation has been reported, but there have been few occupational exposures. Waraki[130] described 2 cases of pneumonitis in sprayers. Nonfatal poisonings by ingestion have shown symptoms of nausea, mental confusion, "jerking" of arms and legs and convulsions. The estimated accidental fatal oral dose in man is 2–7 gm, with severe effects within 1/2 hour after ingestion and frequent, violent convulsions and a rapid cyanosis.

There are no specific tests for toxaphene poisoning. Prompt application of soap and water for skin decontamination is recommended. If severe toxaphene poisoning is recognized, convulsions must be controlled by administration of intramuscular or intravenous sodium phenobarbital or diazepam.

Analysis and evaluation of data from bioassay studies by the National Cancer Institute revealed that, under test conditions, toxaphene was carcinogenic to male and female mice, causing cancers of the liver. Development of cancerous and noncancerous tumors in the thyroid glands of male and female rats suggested, but did not establish conclusively, that toxaphene was carcinogenic in rats as well.[124] (It is to be noted that this substance has been used for more than 32 years.)

As discussed for lindane and extensively studied and reported by Kolmodin-Hedman et al., organochlorine pesticides can be determined in blood by gas chromatography, with plasma levels providing a satisfactory measurement of total body burden. This has been demonstrated in man and in laboratory animals for *p,p'*DDT, lindane, dieldrin and endrin. Jager[59] states that the threshold level in the blood below which no signs or symptoms of intoxication occur is at 0.20 μg/ml for dieldrin. Brown et al.[14] placed the threshold level for dieldrin in the blood at 0.15 μg/ml.

ORGANOPHOSPHATES

This group of insecticides is classified according to a common mode of toxic action, related to the inhibition of the enzyme cholinesterase, so that, as a group, these substances are called "cholinesterase inhibitors." However, the toxicity of the various organophosphate compounds can vary widely, ranging from the highly toxic, such as TEPP (tetraethylpyrophosphate) with an LD_{50} of 1 mg/kg, to compounds with a low order of acute toxicity, such as Abate with an LD_{50} of more than 8 gm/kg. Nearly all of the organophosphate insecticides are readily absorbed by inhalation, ingestion and through intact skin.

Occupationally, the most common exposures occur during manufacture, packaging, handling during shipping, storage and formulating for actual use in homes and agricultural settings. There is a great similarity of symptoms and signs of overexposure to the organophosphate insecticides that are caused by the inactivation or inhibition of the enzyme cholinesterase, resulting in an accumulation of acetylcholine at synapses in the peripheral nervous system. The developmental sequence of systemic effects can vary with the route of entry. Although acute toxicity usually is rapid in onset, symptoms may be delayed up to 12 hours. With inhalation overexposure, respiratory and ocular effects appear, initially usually within minutes. It has been noted that skin absorption is more frequent with increased workplace temperatures.

For simplification of the discussion of the toxic responses, the organophosphate compounds may be considered as a group, the first or mild symptoms and signs developing as anorexia, headache, dizziness, weakness, anxiety, tremors of tongue and eyelids, miosis and impairment of visual acuity. With moderate exposure, symptoms and signs are increased sweating, nausea, excess salivation, lacrimation, abdominal cramps, vomiting, a slow pulse and muscle tremors. With severe overexposure, pinpoint and nonreactive pupils develop, along with respiratory difficulty, diarrhea, pulmonary edema, cyanosis, loss of sphincter control, convulsions, coma and heart block. Following severe intoxication by any route, the excess acetylcholine at the neuromuscular junctions of skeletal muscles is the cause of the weakness, easily aggravated by exertion, along with muscle fasciculations leading to eventual paralysis with the most serious consequence, that of respiratory muscle paralysis. Central nervous system effects include dizziness, slurred speech, ataxia, confusion, Cheyne-Stokes respiration, convulsions, coma and loss of reflexes. There are multiple cardiovascular responses, including fall in blood pressure and cardiac irregularities, and a complete heart block may occur. Fortunately, complete recovery usually occurs within a week, but there is an increased susceptibility to the effects of the anticholinesterase chemicals, in some persons persisting up to several weeks following exposure. Occupational exposure concentrations insufficient to produce symptoms following single exposures can readily result in the onset of symptoms with continued daily exposures. It is emphasized that *a worker who has recovered from the acute phase of intoxication remains hypersusceptible for up to several weeks*. Any of the anticholinesterase compounds inactivate cholinesterase by phosphorylation of the active site of the enzyme to form dimethylphosphoryl enzyme. In the subsequent 24–48 hours after exposure there is a process termed "aging" of conversion to the monomethylphosphoryl enzyme. This so-called aging is of clinical importance, since during the treatment of organophosphate intoxication, the cholinesterase reactivators, such as pralidoxime (2-PAM, Protopam) chloride, are ineffective after "aging" has occurred.[61, 92]

DIAGNOSTIC TEST PROCEDURES.—Two types of cholinesterase are clinically significant: true acetylcholinesterase, found principally in the nervous system and the red blood cells, and the pseudo- or butyrylcholinesterase, found in the plasma, the liver and the nervous system. Both types are inhibited by the organophosphate compounds, *but the level of depression of the red blood cholinesterase is a more reliable indicator of clinically significant reduction of cholinesterase activity*. Verification of organophosphate intoxication may be determined from laboratory evidence of the amount of depression of red blood cell cholinesterase activity to a level considerably below pre-exposure levels—that is, a reduction of at least 50%, or much lower. The measurement of the enzyme cholinesterase is very difficult and usually not done. The activity (hydrolytic capacity) of the enzyme is usually measured. With each method for estimating cholinesterase activity of blood there can be an associated difference of normal values and reporting units. The laboratory report of cholinesterase determinations must state the units involved along with the appropriate normal range for that laboratory. The clinically usually acceptable normal range of red blood cell cholinesterase activity (by the Michel method) in delta pH per hour is 0.39–1.02 for men and 0.34–1.10 for women. The normal range of the enzyme activity in delta pH per hour of plasma is 0.04–1.63 for men and 0.24–1.54 for women. There is regeneration of cholinesterase primarily by the synthesis of new enzyme, which takes place at the rate of approximately 1% per day.

Average baseline values of erythrocyte and plasma ChE (cholinesterase) activity determined for healthy nonexposed men and women are given in Table 13–1. The value

TABLE 13–1.—MEAN BASELINE VALUES OF ERYTHROCYTE AND PLASMA CHOLINESTERASE IN MEN AND WOMEN (ΔpH/HR)

	Men	Women
Erythrocyte Cholinesterase		
Mean	0.861	0.843
Plasma Cholinesterase		
Mean	0.953	0.817

for average red blood cell (RBC) ChE activity for men is drawn from Wolfsie and Winter.[133] The value for women is obtained by multiplying the average RBC ChE activity figure for men by the ratio of mean ΔpH/hr for women to mean ΔpH/hr for men derived from the data of Rider et al.[109] The use of the data of Wolfsie and Winter allows for the increased packing and possible contamination of RBCs by plasma ChE. Plasma ChE values were selected from Rider et al., since their larger data base probably provides a closer approximation of the true population mean of normal values for plasma ChE activity. For the same reason, their data provide the most reliable women/men ratio for RBC ChE activities. The data of Wolfsie and Winter and Rider et al. are presented in Table 13–2.

TREATMENT.—Depending on the compounds involved and the occupational factors occurring at the time of exposure, treatment may be directed to simple removal from exposure in mild or suspected cases or to the most severe clinical intoxication requiring hospitalization and intensive care with special antidotal measures. Initially, it is of utmost importance to rapidly decontaminate the exposed worker. It is an important reminder that persons undertaking decontamination must be protected with proper work clothes and gloves to avoid contaminating themselves, as well as having had prior education as to how to respond to such events. Contaminated work clothing, including shoes and socks, must be removed quickly, followed by thorough washing with soap and water or detergent and generous amounts of water, preferably under a shower or even submersion, if available, in the field.[93] The hair should be shampooed and fingernails and toenails should be cleaned as well. Contaminated articles of clothing must be placed in plastic bags, marked as contaminated and disposed of properly. It is wise and preferable to transport the sick worker to the nearest facility, making note of the substances that may have caused the illness. Because of the danger of pulmonary complications and the possible need for artificial respiration, care must be given to the removal of excess secretions and provision made for a patent airway. Anticonvulsant medication may be necessary, and, if cyanosis has been overcome, atropine should be given intravenously in doses of 2–4 mg. (This amount of atropine is about 10 times the amount ordinarily administered for other medical conditions in which atropine is used.) This dose may be repeated at 5–10-minute intervals until signs of atropinization appear—a dry, flushed skin, a tachycardia as high as 140 beats per minute and pupillary dilation. A mild degree of such atropinization should be maintained for at least 48 hours. Doses of pralidoxime (2-PAM, Protopam) chloride as

TABLE 13–2.—NORMAL VALUES FOR CIRCULATING CHOLINESTERASES IN HEALTHY NONEXPOSED PERSONS*

SUBJECTS	ERYTHROCYTE CHOLINESTERASE Activity (ΔpH/Hr)			PLASMA CHOLINESTERASE Activity (ΔpH/Hr)			REFERENCE
	Range	Mean	SD	Range	Mean	SD	
400 men	0.58–0.95	0.766	0.081	0.52–1.39	0.953	0.187	109†
400 women	0.56–0.94	0.750	0.082	0.38–1.25	0.817	0.187	109†
255 men	0.554–1.252	0.861	0.091	0.408 1.652	0.912	0.112	133‡

*Method of Michel.[83]
†Ranges, means and standard deviations in this study are estimates based on data extrapolated to age 40; ranges reflect elimination of highest 1% and lowest 1% of values.
‡Analytic method modified for smaller blood sample.

a cholinesterase reactivator can be given in doses of 1 gm intravenously at a rate not in excess of 500 mg/min to complement the action of the atropine. (After an hour, a second dose, 1 gm, may be given if muscle weakness has not improved.) Treatment with 2-PAM is effective if given within 24 hours after intoxication. *Avoid morphine, theophylline, aminophylline, barbiturates and phenothiazines!* Blood samples for cholinesterase tests should be drawn in 10 ml quantities in heparinized tubes, preferably before the 2-PAM is given. In addition, urine *p*-nitrophenol may verify or indicate exposure. To reiterate: speed in initiating therapy is essential; *no* atropine is to be given to a cyanotic person; oral atropine never is used and atropine prophylaxis *is not condoned!* Cholinesterase levels of 30–50% of normal indicate exposure, although symptoms in some individuals may not appear until the level falls to 20% or less. The worker whose cholinesterase falls to or below 40% of the pre-exposure baseline must be removed from further exposure until the activity returns to within 80% of the pre-exposure baseline.

Hayes[46–48] noted that measurement of cholinesterase activity and pesticide metabolite determination in urine yield complementary findings, since metabolite excretion occurs rapidly whereas enzyme activity recovers slowly. Cholinesterase activity determination integrates the effects of exposure during a long time interval (several weeks) whereas metabolite measurement gives information on very recent exposure.[75]

Some selected and widely used organophosphate compounds follow (see Glossary for a more comprehensive listing).

Parathion (0, 0-diethyl-0-*p*-nitrophenyl thiophosphate)

This is a widely used acaricide/insecticide. In its liquid form, it has a high boiling point and low vapor pressure. It is supplied as a dust or as a liquid for further dilution before spraying. Overexposure in the factory or in the field may result from inhalation or skin contact.

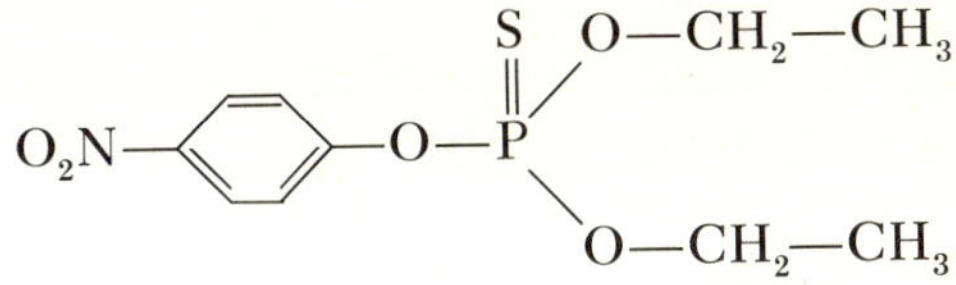

The minimal lethal oral dose of parathion for man has been estimated to range from less than 10 mg up to 125 mg. Arterberry et al.[5] observed and reported findings in 115 workers exposed to parathion under various conditions, the majority excreting significant amounts of *p*-nitrophenol in the urine whereas those with heavier exposures had a measurable decrease in blood cholinesterase. One of its metabolites, paraoxon, is the active inhibitor of cholinesterase.

Measurement of urinary *p*-nitrophenol excretion has been found to be a reliable index of parathion exposure, even more sensitive as an absorption index than a decrease in blood cholinesterase activity. A biologic threshold of 100 μg/l in urine has been proposed. This may provide a high margin of safety, as excretion rates of more than 100 μg/l have been found in sprayers exposed to parathion without symptoms of intoxication, according to Wolfe et al.[132]

Some clinicians have thought that absorption of parathion can be tolerated without illness and with little or no reduction in cholinesterase activity as long as the concentration of *p*-nitrophenol in urine does not rise much above 2 mg/l. However, poisoning has been reported by Arterberry et al.[5] in which the *p*-nitrophenol excretion was lower than 2 mg/l (0.9, 0.57 and 1.6 mg/l[47, 96]).

Methyl Parathion

The TLV is 0.2 mg/m^3

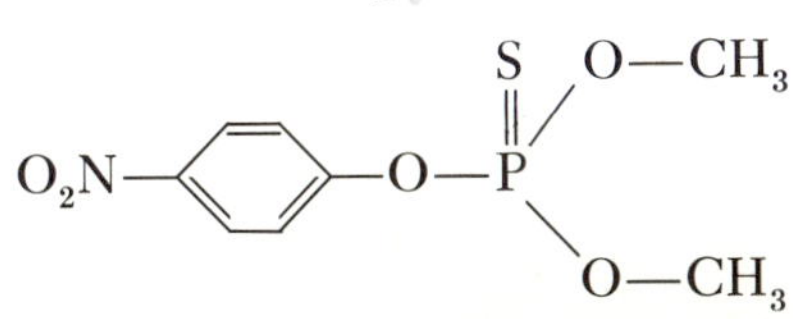

Methyl parathion itself is not a strong cholinesterase inhibitor, but one of its metabolites, methyl paraoxon, is an active cholinesterase inhibitor and inactivates cholinesterase to those compounds mentioned earlier. The minimal lethal oral dose for adults appears to be less than 1.84 gm, and data from human intoxication from this compound are not detailed enough to identify the range between the doses producing initial symptoms and those severe or fatal.[95]

Roan et al.[110] found the determination of ethyl or methyl parathion in serum samples by gas chromatography to be more sensitive than urine *p*-nitrophenol measurements. Several other anticholinesterase pesticides are amenable to analysis by unsophisticated techniques. Measurement of these metabolites may indicate a biochemical test of exposure, but insufficient human data exist for the proposal of credible biologic threshold limit values for most of these metabolites, and additional studies are needed for exposed worker evaluation.

Malathion

The TLV is 10 mg/m^3.

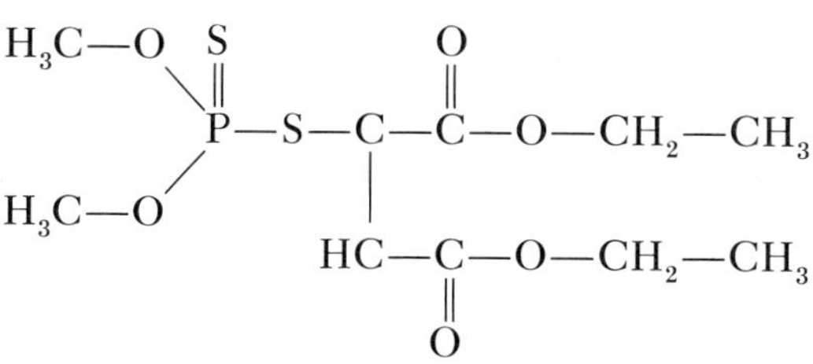

This colorless to light amber liquid insecticide is of a relatively low order of toxicity when compared to the other organophosphates. Although malathion has only a mild direct inhibitory action on cholinesterase, one of its metabolites, malaoxon, is an active inhibitor, and both malathion and malaoxon are rapidly detoxified by the liver esterases and other organs. This apparent rapid metabolism is the main reason for the lower toxicity of this compound. Malaoxon otherwise inactivates cholinesterase in the toxic sequence similar to the other organophosphates described. Relative safeness of malathion to man has been demonstrated repeatedly. Culver et al.[21] studied a group of workers with average exposure of 3.3 mg/m^3 for 5 hours (maximum of 56 mg/m^3), finding that the cholinesterase levels in the blood were not significantly lowered, and no worker exhibited signs of cholinesterase inhibition. Golz,[34] using a controlled human exposure to malathion in which 4 men were exposed 1 hour daily for 42 days to 85 mg/m^3, found moderate nasal irritation and conjunctivitis but no cholinergic symptoms and signs. Nonlethal intoxication occurring in agricultural workers usually has been the result of gross exposures with concomitant skin absorption.[94] Nearly all reported fatalities from malathion have been through ingestion. Milby[85] reported that malathion has caused skin sensitization, and dermatitis may occur under conditions of heavy field use.

Baker et al.[8] described an epidemic of malathion intoxication, estimated to have affected 2800 workers in the Pakistan malaria-control program, that was attributed to a combination of poor pesticide-handling techniques among spray team workers and to increased concentrations of toxic by-products in two of the three pesticide formulations used (isomalathion and *o,o,s*-trimethyl phosphorodithioate). Cholinesterase depression in field personnel was greatest in those using the pesticide brands with the highest concentrations of isomalathion and other malathion degradation products. Workers with greatest dermal exposure to malathion (spraymen and mixers) were more severely affected than supervisors. Cholinesterase activities were highest on Monday and fell during the week, reflecting cumulative effects of repeated exposures. Proscription of use of the contaminated pesticide and special instructions in pesticide-handling techniques halted the epidemic.

Dermal absorption from excessive skin contact during spraying and mixing operations was the primary route of pesticide uptake; respiratory exposure was relatively unimportant, according to the authors, who estimated the average daily dermal exposure for spraymen to have been 330 mg of malathion (applying measured exposure rates to a body surface area of 1.75 m^2) and the percutaneously absorbed dose to have been 26 mg/day (based on 8% absorption of the pesticide). Baker et al. observed the cholinesterase depression and illness at this exposure level to be consistent with controlled studies, which found the minimal effective dose of malathion to range from 24 to 48 mg/day. Carriers and surfactants used in the manufacture of malathion water-dispersible powders were believed to be important in the formation of isomalathion and other toxic components in powders held under tropical storage conditions. A comprehensive training and medical surveillance program was developed to prevent recurrence of pesticide toxicity during the next spray season.

Mevinphos (Phosdrin) $(CH_3O)_2PO_2(CH_3)C{=}CHC(O)OCH_3$

The TLV is 0.01 ppm.

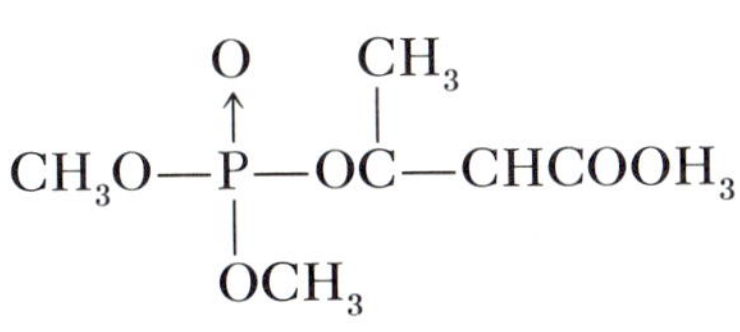

Holmes et al.[51] described 2 cases of moderate intoxication to this insecticide, with urinary excretion of dimethylphosphate, a metabolite of mevinphos, as late as 50 hours after exposure. Therefore, this metabolite present in urine may be useful in estimating absorption.

EPN (0-ethyl-0-*p*-nitrophenyl phenylphosphonothioate)

The TLV is 0.5 mg/m^3.

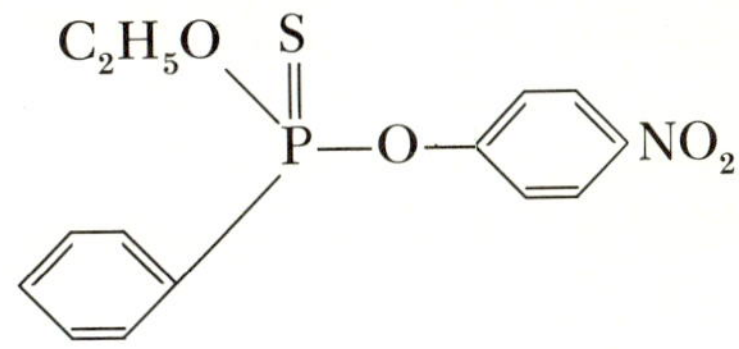

This parathion analogue differs somewhat, as it has a direct carbon-phosphorus link and is less volatile than parathion. EPN is used as an acaricide and insecticide for orchard pests and some soil insects and is relatively toxic to mammals, with an acute oral LD_{50} in rats of 8–36 mg/kg.[48,61] EPN is suspected of delayed neurotoxicity, based on experimental evidence in chickens.[92]

Demeton

Demeton is known commercially as Systox and is a mixture of two isomers having a strong mercaptan odor. This systemic insecticide is highly toxic to mammals (oral LD_{50} in rats of 2–12 mg/kg) and has a long residual life within plants.

$$(C_2H_5O)_2\overset{\overset{\displaystyle O}{\|}}{P}{-}S{-}CH_2CH_2{-}S{-}CH_2CH_3 \quad \leftarrow \text{Thiol isomer}$$

$$(C_2H_5O)_2\overset{\overset{\displaystyle S}{\|}}{P}{-}O{-}CH_2CH_2{-}S{-}CH_2CH_3 \quad \leftarrow \text{Thiono isomer}$$

The used mixture consists of 65 parts thiono and 35 parts thiol isomers. At least 4 fatal, several severe, nonfatal and several mild cases of demeton poisoning have been reported.[46]

Dichlorvos

The TLV is 1 mg/m^3.

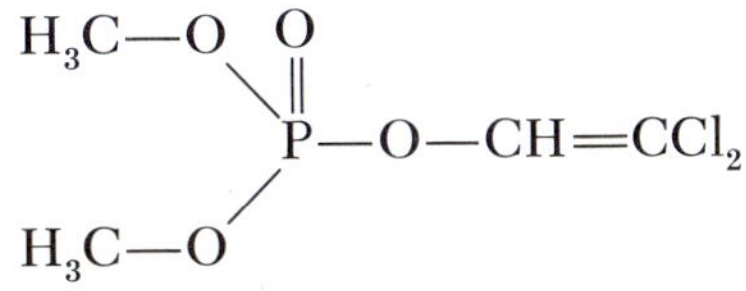

This substance has a much higher vapor pressure than most other similar chemicals, with an extremely high toxicity for many insects but presenting little hazard to man from inhalation. Dichlorvos is applied as a film to plastic strips that may be suspended in the room or areas to be cleared of flying insects as a space fumigant commonly known as "s-strips" and is very effective against flies and mosquitoes, the insects being killed by exposure to the substance.[8]

Naled (1,2-dibromo-2,2-dichloroethyl dimethyl phosphate)

The TLV is 3 mg/m^3.

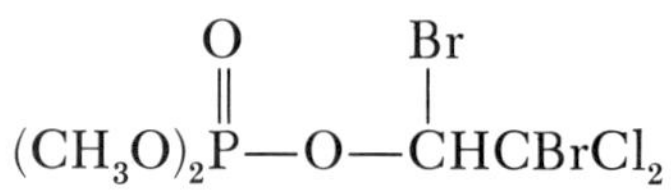

This compound is essentially a dibrominated dichlorvos, acting as a contact insecticide. The acute oral lethal dose (LD_{50}) to rats is about 430 mg/kg, relatively low compared to parathion but greater than malathion. Edmundson and Davies[27] described dermatitis in 9 of 12 women who were cutting tops of unflowered chrysanthemum plants which had been sprayed with naled. The dermatitis involved the exposed skin of the face, neck and hands, apparently from exposure within 2 hours after plant spraying. It is known that naled hydrolyzes within 2 hours, simplifying control of contact exposures by allowing time before cutting plants.

Ronnel

The TLV is 10 mg/m^3.

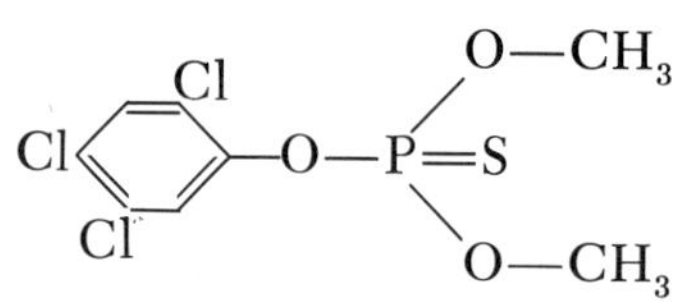

This white crystalline powder is a weak cholinesterase inhibitor used in animal feed to kill external as well as internal parasites and actually is used as a systemic insecticide in livestock care. Occupational exposure occurs mainly by inhalation, not by skin absorption and rarely by ingestion. It is a weak cholinesterase inhibitor affecting primarily the pseudocholinesterases of the blood plasma rather than the erythrocyte acetylcholinesterase. McCollister et al.,[79] using humans as subjects, evaluted the primary skin-irritating and skin-sensitizing potential of ronnel. Fifty subjects received 3 applications per week for 3 weeks of gauze saturated with a 10% suspension of ronnel in sesame oil without significant effects on the skin. Application of small amounts of powder into the eyes of rabbits produced slight discomfort and transient conjunctival irritation, subsiding in 48 hours. The LD_{50} for the rat is about 3000 mg/kg and presumably, therefore, ronnel is one of the least toxic insecticides to man.

Tetraethylpyrophosphate: $(C_2H_5)_4P_2O_7$

The TLV is 0.004 ppm.

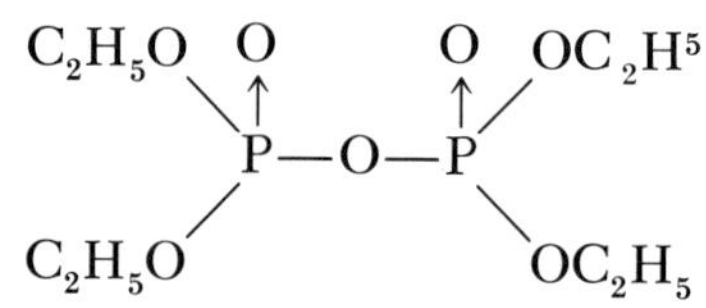

Commonly known as TEPP, this colorless, odorless liquid is a widely used insecticide and may be systemically absorbed via inhalation, skin or ingestion. Quinby and Doornink[106] reported mild intoxication in 15 people exposed to a dust of 1% TEPP, the predominant symptoms being shortness of breath occurring after breathing dust-laden air for 30 minutes. Symptoms subsided rapidly when exposure was terminated.

Ten cases of possible organophosphate pesticide poisoning in florists exposed to pesticide residues on cut flowers were reported by Morse et al.,[87] who conducted a prospective random-sample survey to determine residual pesticide levels on flowers imported into Miami, Florida. Sampling of flowers imported into Miami on 3 days in January, 1977 showed that 18 (17.7%) of 105 lots contained pesticide residue levels up to 5 ppm and that 3 lots had levels up to 400 ppm. Twenty quarantine workers in Miami and 12 commercial florists exposed to contaminated flowers were clinically examined. Occasional nonspecific symptoms compatible with possible organophosphate exposure were noted, but no abnormalities in plasma or red blood cell cholinesterase levels were found. This study documents a previously unrecognized potential source of occupational pesticide exposure, and the authors suggest that safety standards should be set for residue levels on cut flowers.

Carbamates

Carbamates are derivatives of carbamic acid (CO_2NH_3), differing from the chlorinated hydrocarbon and organophosphate insecticides by the absence of chlorine and phosphorus. Work exposures may occur from inhalation, skin absorption and, rarely, ingestion. Clinically, toxic responses are similar to those of the organophosphates, as carbamates are anticholinesterase agents with the characteristic of having rapid reversibility of inhibition of the enzyme. Typical of this class of insecticides is carbaryl, commonly sold under the trade name Sevin. It has a low mammalian toxicity with a wide spectrum against nearly 150 insect species. Carbaryl dusts at 2–5% concentrations are used to kill fleas on dogs and cats (except puppies and kittens under 4 weeks old). With DDT restricted in the United States, carbaryl dust is one of the insecticides useful to control the rat flea in murine typhus control programs and also wild rodent fleas in rural plague control. Sprays and dusts have been applied in adult mosquito control.

The TLV is 5 mg/m^3.

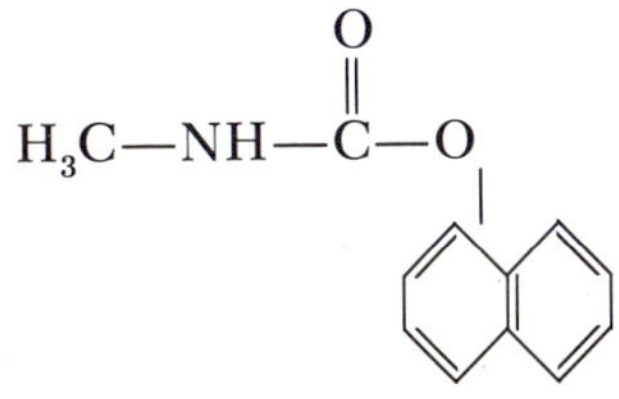

Because carbaryl is metabolized rapidly, monitoring of exposure and measurements of the cholinesterase levels may not indicate the true magnitude of occupational exposure, which can be clinically misleading. Best and Murray[11] studied 59 workers exposed to concentrations ranging from 0.23 to 31 mg/m^3 during a 19-month period, noting that there were no symptoms or signs of anticholinesterase activity. In the most heavily exposed workers, relatively large amounts of 1-naphthol, a metabolite of carbaryl, were excreted in the urine and the blood cholinesterase activity was only slightly depressed. They concluded that an excretion level of total 1-naphthol significantly above 500 μg/100 ml of urine indicated absorption and metabolism of carbaryl. Concentrated solutions may produce skin irritation and systemic intoxication. Oral administration of carbaryl to guinea pigs during organogenesis was teratogenic at dose levels of 300 mg/kg and in beagle dogs in doses of 25 mg/kg (see Chapter 2 for details). Because of the rapidly reversible inhibition of cholinesterase, 2-PAM and other oxine reactivators are not used in treatment of carbaryl intoxication.[91]

Other carbamates are methomyl (Lannate), propoxur (Baygon) and carbofuran (Furadan); the mode of action is identical to carbaryl. The TLVs for methomyl, propoxur and carbofuran are 2.5 mg/m^3, 0.5 mg/m^3 and 0.1 mg/m^3, respectively.

Nonanticholinesterase Effects

There is evidence that many organophosphate compounds can inhibit enzyme systems other than cholinesterase. Tri-ortho-cresyl phosphate (TOCP), for example, inhibits an enzyme contained in nerve cells, and this inhibition can initiate a sequence of events that may end with loss of function and structural changes in affected nerve fibers. The physiologic function of this enzyme is not known but, because of the delayed neurotoxicity that follows its inhibition, it has become known as neurotoxic esterase.[65]

Roberts[114] reported evidence for other

nonanticholinesterase actions of organophosphate compounds from the observation that mipafox and leptophos, when given to rats for 35 days at dose levels of 5 mg/kg and 10 mg/kg, respectively, reduced the dopamine level in the corpus striatum. The functional changes associated with a reduction in striatal dopamine include akinesia, rigidity and tremor in man and in experimental animals, and this action may contribute to the ataxia found in experimental and occupational exposures to certain organophosphate compounds such as mipafox and leptophos.

Another region of the brain with both cholinergic and adrenergic synapses is the optic tectum, where a change in the balance between acetylcholine and dopamine could lead to various visual and perceptual defects. Neurophysiologic evidence for this has been found in pigeons experimentally exposed to a single dose of mevinphos of 0.1 mg/kg. These effects assume importance for *spray pilots* and others whose work requires coordination of visual and motor skills. When atropine is used to suppress the acute anticholinesterase effects of organophosphate exposure, it may also cause central neurologic disturbances, particularly when given in large doses.[114]

Axonal degeneration followed by degeneration of myelin sheath cells in peripheral nerves and, in some cases, degeneration of tracts within the spinal cord have been observed as a result of prolonged exposure to such organophosphate compounds as tri-o-cresyl phosphate, mipafox[12] and leptophos.[134] Demyelination was the probable explanation seen in poisoning caused by tri-o-cresyl phosphate.[64]

It is known that some fluoro-organophosphate compounds cause delayed neurotoxicity.[2, 3, 60, 113] Hexane[134] and other hydrocarbon solvents have caused polyneuropathy.[18, 135] Simplified methods of electromyography (EMG) have been developed, using surface electrodes to stimulate the ulnar nerve and to record action potentials from the adductor muscle of the thumb.[18] These methods are not specific for organophosphorus compounds or for anticholinesterase effects but may detect subtle and early changes in nerve and muscle function. EMG has been used to evaluate exposure of workers to several organophosphate pesticides.[60, 120]

Mevinphos, an organophosphate, was administered to male volunteers by Verberk and Salle[129] with a dose of 25 μg/kg daily for 28 days, comparing findings with a control group. A 7% decrease in slow fiber motor nerve conduction velocity and a 38% increase in Achilles tendon reflex force were found after exposure. No effect on neuromuscular transmission was observed and the red blood cell cholinesterase depression was 19%.

To determine if cholinesterase inhibition might affect neuromuscular transmission in exposed workers, Stålberg et al.[120] utilized electromyography to study 11 men commercially applying insecticides. All were spraymen, working daily with solutions of 4% lindane, 0.2% pyrethrum, 0.125% piperonylbutoxide, 2.5% malathion or 2% bromophos in kerosene with intermittent exposure to 0.5% diazinon and dursbane. The workers' employment periods varied between 1 and 24 years. All were equipped with routine protective devices such as respirators, boots, overalls and gloves and all were examined clinically, neurophysiologically, along with measurements of blood cholinesterase activity. They formed their own reference group, since measurements were also made after 1–4 weeks of non-exposure (pre-exposure values). Measurements following exposure generally were made within 1–24 hours after a period of spray work, with exposure values taken during spring and pre-exposure values after summer vacation. Blood samples for cholinesterase activity and analysis were taken immediately before each EMG investigation. Cholinesterase activity of plasma and erythrocytes was determined with a gasometric technique using whole blood samples with activity expressed in microliters of carbon dioxide evolved in 30 min/50 μl blood or simply b_{30}.

Slight changes in plasma cholinesterase activity were not correlated with disturbed neuromuscular transmission in the subjects.

Lower sensory nerve conduction velocities after work in 7 subjects was found, with average reduction for the group small (3%) but statistically significant ($p = 0.05$). Reduced conduction velocity usually is a sign of neuropathy, which was thought might be present in some of the workers. The increased jitter values seen in some recordings were thought to indicate an uncertain impulse transmission in reinnervation structures (nerve sprouts, immature motor endplates[63]) but did not relate to acute exposure and preceding denervation due to neuropathy, as suggested by Stålberg et al.

Stålberg and his co-investigators indicated that a peripheral neuropathy could cause a reduced surface action potential, for example, due to reduced excitability (demyelination) or axonal degeneration and concluded that the slight neurophysiologic abnormalities found in this investigation were unrelated to a lowered cholinesterase activity.

Persisting electroencephalogram (EEG) changes in men following exposure to the organophosphate ester Sarin were reported by Duffy,[26] who recorded brain wave activity of 67 workers exposed at least once, but not in the preceding year, and described a significant difference from that of 26 workers who had no prior exposure to Sarin. The brain waves of the unexposed workers also differed significantly from those of 38 exposed workers who had 3 or more exposures within the preceding 6 years, but excluding the most recent years, according to Duffy. Worker exposure levels were not given. Activity in the beta range was greater in the exposed workers than in the nonexposed, being the chief difference between the observed groups. However, Duffy stated that the exposed group revealed a greater number of EEGs with decreased alpha activity, increased epochs of slow activity and deviation of background activity with faster or slower rhythms, which did not have clear diagnostic value, as the electroencephalographer's interpretations were at a level of chance, only 49.5%.

Sarin (Isopropyl Methylphosphonofluoride)

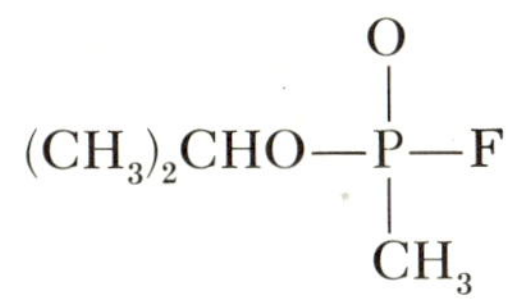

Tabun (not in use)

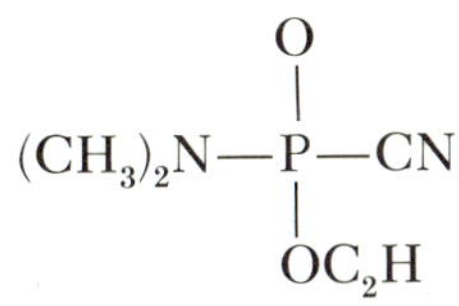

Sarin is the most toxic of the "nerve gases." It is related to tabun and both are extremely active cholinesterase inhibitors, much more severe in activity than parathion. The lethal dose for man is estimated to be 0.01 mg/kg.

Other Clinical Aspects of Organophosphate and Carbamate Insecticides—A Reiteration

Depression of plasma and/or erythrocyte cholinesterase is considered a good index of the absorption of cholinesterase-inhibiting pesticides (organophosphate esters, *N*-methyl or *N*-dimethyl carbamate esters). Selection of the enzyme activity to be determined (red blood cell or plasma) depends on the relative affinity of the pesticide for both enzymes; there is interindividual variability in blood cholinesterase activity, and it is important to compare exposure values with pre-exposure levels, with a 50% reduction in activity dictating removal of the worker from continued exposure. Cholinesterase enzyme determinations are sufficiently sensitive and specific for monitoring programs (if pre-exposure activities are known); problems can occur with inadequate sample preservation before analyses and urinary metabolites may be sought. Various techniques available for measuring these enzymes have been reported, but it must be pointed out that the *inhibition* of the *enzymes by free active pesticides can occur during blood storage;* the cholinesterase activity may not indicate the true activity in vivo. Carbamylated cholinesterases and some phosphorylated cholinesterases can be reactivated during storage, and *further inhibition or partial recovery after sampling* must be recognized in determining conditions of assay.[86]

Serum activity is within normal ranges in patients manifesting myasthenia gravis, bronchial asthma, epilepsy, hyperthyroidism, hypertension and diabetes mellitus.

In addition to the organophosphate and carbamate compounds, depression of serum cholinesterase activity is produced by suxamethonium and certain other substances. Short-term depression: adrenaline, antipyrine and antipyrine derivatives, amidone and isoamidone, antimalarial drugs, atropine, barbiturates, caffeine, chloroform, codeine, Dilaudid, ether, folic acid, morphine, para-aminobenzoic acid, phenothiozine derivatives, physostigmine, procaine hydrochloride, prostigmine, quaternary ammonium compounds, quinine, sulfanilamides, tetraethylammonium chloride, theobromine, theophylline, thiamine and vitamin K. Long-term depression: alkyl fluorophosphates. Other factors affecting these levels may be impairment of liver function, certain anemias, malnutrition and pregnancy. Howard et al.[53] observed 6 healthy young women before and during pregnancy, noting a significant fall in plasma cholinesterase activity in the first 3 months of normal pregnancy. There was some evidence of return to normal pre-pregnancy levels in later pregnancy. No hypothesis was suggested to account for this phenomenon, although it seems possible that it may be the result of altered liver enzyme synthesis. None was exposed to organophosphates or other cholinesterase depressants. The percentage fall ranged from 17.7 to 46.4, but values returned to normal later in pregnancy. These findings introduce another important variable into the routine biologic monitoring of female workers exposed to anticholinesterase compounds, complicating assessment of the significance of depressions of cholinesterase activity in relation to exposure to organophosphates and similar compounds.

To re-emphasize: The important difference in the toxicology between *organophosphate* and *carbamate* insecticides is that the organophosphate compounds almost *irreversibly* phosphorylate the acetylcholinesterase whereas the *carbamates cause reversible* carbamylation of the enzyme. In man, organophosphate exposure can cause depression of plasma cholinesterase to persist for 1–3 weeks; red blood cell depression can persist up to 12 weeks. With carbamate poisoning, plasma and red blood cell cholinesterase may be depressed, but usually return to normal within a few hours after exposure.[86]

A summary of emergency medical treatment for acute insecticide poisoning is given in Table 13–3.

HERBICIDES

Herbicides are compounds intended for killing plants or interrupting their normal growth, for example, the elimination of dandelions in lawn grasses.

The chlorophenoxy herbicides are one well-known class of herbicides, including 2, 4, 5-T(2, 4, 5-trichlorophenoxyacetic acid and 2,4-D (2,4-dichlorophenoxyacetic acid).

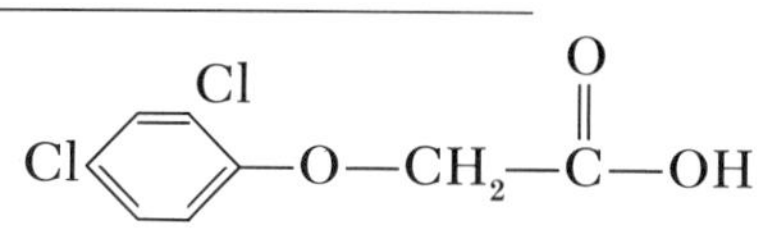

2,4-D

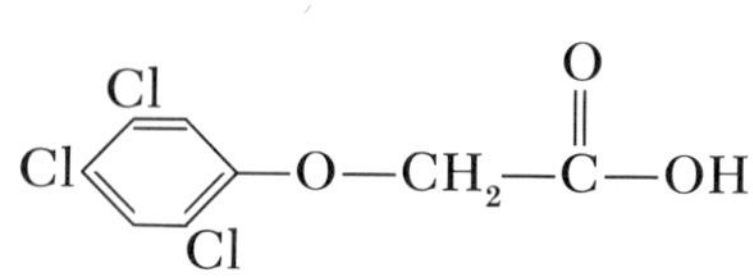

2,4,5-T

TABLE 13-3.—A Summary of Emergency Medical Treatment for Acute Insecticide Poisoning (Some typical compounds)

ORGANOPHOSPHATES (Irreversible Cholinesterase Inhibitors)	CARBAMATES (Reversible Cholinesterase Inhibitors)	CHLORINATED HYDROCARBONS
chlorpyrifos (Dursban) diazinon dichlorvos (Vapona, DDVP) dimethoate (Cygon) fenthion (Baytex, Entex) rabon (Gardona) malathion methyl parathion parathion naled (Dibrom) ronnel (Korian) trichlorfon (Dipterex)	carbaryl (Sevin) dimetilan landrin propoxur (Baygon)	CNS depressant/stimulant aldrin—BHC chlordane—DDT dieldrin heptachlor—lindane mirex toxaphene In general, these act on the central nervous system to stimulate or depress, varying by compound
	Symptoms and Signs	
1. MILD—headache, dizziness, weakness, anxiety, miosis, impairment of visual acuity 2. MODERATE—nausea, salivation, lacrimation, abdominal cramps, vomiting, sweating, slow pulse, muscle tremors 3. SEVERE—diarrhea, pinpoint and nonreactive pupils, respiratory difficulty, pulmonary edema, cyanosis, loss of sphincter control, convulsions, coma and death	Constriction of pupils Salivation Profuse sweating Lassitude Muscle incoordination Nausea Vomiting Diarrhea Epigastric pain Tightness in chest	Typical onset—20 minutes to 4 hours Nausea Vomiting Restlessness Tremor Apprehension Convulsions Coma Respiratory failure Death DO NOT INDUCE EMESIS IF THE INGESTED POISON IS PRINCIPALLY A HYDROCARBON SOLVENT (e.g., kerosene)

Therapy

1. Support respiration. Keep airways clear. Use artificial respiration with oxygen if cyanosis is indicated. Death from pesticide poisoning usually is due to respiratory failure
2. Decontamination as indicated. Remove contaminated clothing. Wash skin, hair and fingernails with soap and water. Sponge with alcohol. Cleanse eyes. If ingested, lavage stomach with 5% sodium bicarbonate if person is not vomiting. Protect first aid and medical personnel!!
3. Draw 5 ml heparinized blood for cholinesterase determination. Save samples of first urine and first/early vomitus for possible laboratory analysis
4. Consult insecticide label under "ACTIVE INGREDIENTS" for specific chemicals involved
5. When mixtures of organophosphates and chlorinated hydrocarbons are involved (e.g., endrin and methyl parathion), give specific treatment for organophosphates first and indicated support therapy and decontamination

ANTIDOTE	ANTIDOTE	TREATMENT
1. Adults: After cyanosis is overcome, use atropine sulfate, 2–4 mg intravenously. Repeat doses at 5–10-minute intervals until signs of atropinization appear. Maintain for 24 hours or longer if necessary 2. Children: Atropine sulfate in proportion to body weight: approx. 0.05 mg/kg 3. Support atropine treatment with 2-PAM (pralidoxime chloride) (Protopam Chloride, Ayerst) a. Adult dose: 1 gm, slowly, intravenously b. Infants: 0.25 gm, slowly, intravenously NOTE: Contraindicated are morphine, aminophylline, theophylline, phenothiazine tranquilizers and barbiturates	1. Adults: After cyanosis is overcome, use atropine sulfate, 2–4 mg intravenously. Repeat dose at 5–10-minute intervals until signs of atropinization appear. Maintain for 24 hours or longer if necessary 2. Children: Atropine sulfate in proportion to body weight: approx. 0.05 mg/kg NOTE: 2-PAM is contraindicated in carbamate insecticide poisoning. Also avoid morphine, aminophylline, theophylline, phenothiazine tranquilizers and barbiturates	1. Gastric lavage with 2–4 l tap water. Catharsis with 30 gm (10 oz) sodium sulfate in 1 cup of water 2. Barbiturates in appropriate dosages repeated as necessary for restlessness or convulsions 3. Avoid oils, oil laxatives and epinephrine (adrenalin). Do not give stimulants 4. Give calcium gluconate (10% in 10-ml ampules) intravenously every 4 hours

FOR SPECIFIC INFORMATION: CALL NEAREST POISON CONTROL CENTER

Enormous quantities of 2,4,5-T and 2,4-D (in excess of 6,000,000 kg annually) are produced and used throughout the world. The materials are formulated as emulsifiable concentrates for air or ground spray applications.

During the manufacture of 2,4,5-T, the 2,4,5 trichlorophenol intermediate can react with itself to produce TCDD (2,3,7,8-tetrachlorodibenzopara-dioxin). Although 2,4,5-T and 2,4-D have essentially low toxicity for animals and man, TCDD is one of the most toxic compounds known.

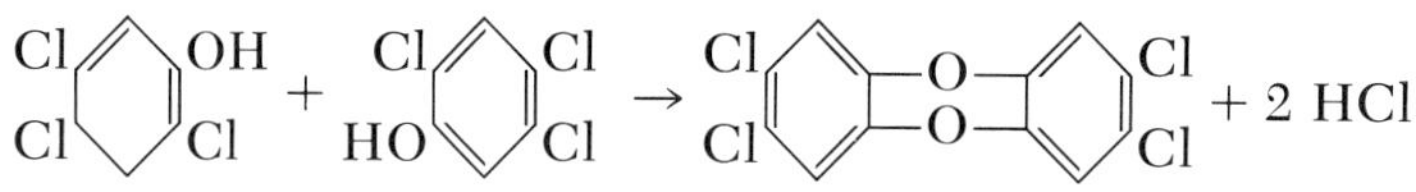

TCDD

The intense toxicity of TCDD, called "dioxin," was underscored in 1976 in an accident in the ICMESA factory producing 2,4,5-trichlorophenol (used to make the bactericide hexachlorophene. as well as the herbicide 2,4,5-T). The reactor vessel heat-regulating valves failed, with safety valve blowout, exhausting an estimated 10% of the contents into the external plant atmosphere, forming a huge cloud reported to contain some 500 kg 2,4,5-T and 2 (or more) kg of TCDD. An area about 5 kilometers long and 700 meters wide was contaminated in the nearby town of Seveso (population 17,000) 20 km north of Milan, Italy. Of the 14 workers in the plant, or who entered the area shortly thereafter, 13 had abnormal liver function tests, but normal ones within 2 weeks. Some workers developed mild chloracne. The entire plant was contaminated by TCDD, and inadvertently production was resumed in some areas. Within 6 months, 79 chloracne cases were noted, especially in maintenance workers. Evacuation of a large segment of the community was ordered, involving hundreds of people of all ages. About 2000 persons were exposed to TCDD, 300 treated for skin disorders; more than 1100 animals were killed by direct exposure (up to 225 ng TCDD per gm of tissue were found in dead rabbit livers). Occupational health services were initiated to observe the 60 plant workers and a large-scale epidemiologic program was enacted involving the 200,000 people in the area to investigate long-term effects.[29]

Because of the potential for contamination of the herbicide 2,4,5-T and Silvex, the EPA in April, 1979 suspended use for crops used for human food, around aquatic areas and recreational areas and around homes. In the United States, current allowed use is only on pastures, rangelands, rights of way and for rice crops. In the late 1970s, more than 2,000,000 kg was used in the United States for commercial weed control and more than 1,000,000 kg on pastures and rangelands.

2,4-D is a systemic herbicide widely used for control of broadleaf weeds in cereal crops and sugar cane and on turf, pastures and non-croplands. It is also used to control the ripening of bananas and citrus fruits, to delay preharvest dropping of some fruits and is used in some countries as a fungicide for the control of Alternaria rots when lemons are to be held for storage.

2,4-D was used to defoliate jungle areas in South Viet Nam, where it was a component of "Agent Orange" (a 50:50 mixture of the *n*-butyl esters of 2,4-D and 2,4,5-T, containing up to 30 mg/kg TCDD). About 40 million liters of "Agent Orange" were sprayed in South Viet Nam between 1965 and 1971 for defoliation or crop destruction.

2,4,5-T was banned in Italy in 1970 and also banned in the Netherlands and Sweden. The 1979 ACGIH TLV for 2,4,5-T is 10 mg/m^3 for an 8-hour TWA.

The 1979 ACGIH TLV for 2,4-D is 10 mg/m^3 for an 8-hour TWA. The corresponding standard in West Germany is also 10 mg/m^3, and the acceptable ceiling concentration in the USSR[107] is 1 mg/m^3.

Occupational Exposure

2,4,5-T dust is a slight skin irritant, but it and 2,4-D may cause dermatitis on prolonged skin contact. Occupational exposure to phenoxy acids (2,4-D and 2,4,5-T) has been studied in forestry work with 4 tractor spraymen spraying a 2% emulsion in water and the phenoxy acid levels in the breathing zone of the subjects determined by Kolmodin-Hedman et al.[69a] The phenoxy acid levels in plasma and urine were determined by electron capture gas chromatography and the air samples analyzed by UV-spectrophotometry and thin-layer chromatography. The air levels of phenoxy acids ranged between 0.1 and 0.2 mg/m^3, with occasional higher levels (about 1 mg/m^3) obviously due to contamination of the impinger flash by larger droplets. Plasma and urine levels were followed during a week of exposed work and for 36 hours after exposure. Plasma levels ranged from the detection limit up to 0.1–0.2 μg/ml. The levels varied due to intermittent exposure. After exposure, these levels declined to near the detection limit overnight. Mean urinary levels of phenoxy acids were (2,4-D and 2,4,5-T, respectively) 8 and 4.5 μg/ml, ranging from 3 to 14 μg/ml for 2,4-D and 1 to 11 μg/ml for 2,4,5-T in the afternoon of the day of exposure. In a second investigation, the mean 24-hour excretion in urine was 9 mg of 2,4-D and around 1 mg of 2,4,5-T. Urinary elimination was rapid. Absorption seemed to be caused by inhalation and dermal exposure, but the conditions did not allow an assessment of the relative importance of these channels of uptake. Improved hygienic conditions are suggested to decrease exposure. None of the subjects reported clinical symptoms except 1, who had slight irritation of the eyes after direct contact with the spray liquid. In control subjects with a low and indirect exposure, no 2,4-D and 2,4,5-T could be detected in plasma or urine. The authors concluded that exposure to 2, 4-D and 2,4,5-T could best be followed by measurement of the phenoxy acid levels in the urine, with sampling preferably made in the afternoon of an exposed working day or within a day following exposure. The lowest detectable concentration in urine of 2,4-D and 2,4,5-T is 0.05 μg/ml. A variety of toxicologic effects have been reported in workers engaged in manufacturing 2,4,5-T and 2,4-D. Chloracne, liver disorders, neurologic and behavioral changes and signs of porphyria cutanea tarda are among the more frequently reported clinical findings.

Chloracne, one of the common and prominent features of TCDD exposure, is characterized by inclusion cysts, comedones and pustules, with scarring of the skin, more often on the face but on other areas of the body as well. Blepharoconjunctivitis and irritation of other mucous membranes have been noted. The chloracne may be preceded by erythematous and edematous skin. Latency between exposure and the appearance of signs of chloracne ranges from a few weeks to several months, according to May.[77]

Chloracne and liver impairment, formerly thought to be caused by the chlorophenols, were shown to be due to TCDD, but the actual cause of certain other findings, particularly the neurologic ones, may also be from other substances, such as 2,4-D or chlorophenols. Chloracne affected 60 workers at the 2,4,5-T factory of the Dow Chemical Company in Midland, Michigan in 1964.[29]

Eleven of 29 subjects with features of chloracne working in a 2,4-D and 2,4,5-T-producing factory of the Diamond Alkali Company, Newark, New Jersey also showed increased uroporphyrin excretion. In 3 cases, a diagnosis of porphyria cutanea tarda was unquestionable; 2 of these had raised serum glutamic oxaloacetic transaminase levels. Many of the workers, regardless of uroporphyrinuria, had hirsutism, hyperpigmentation, increased skin fragility and vesiculobullous eruptions on exposed areas of skin.[13, 29]

Similar findings were described by Jirásek et al.,[62] who reported 76 cases of chloracne between 1965 and 1968 in a factory in Czechoslovakia producing 2,4,5-T and pentachlorophenol. These effects were attributed to TCDD. Fifty-five patients were submitted to medical follow-ups for more than 5 years. Four deaths were observed, 2 of which were from bronchogenic carcinomas. Some of the workers had symptoms of porphyria cutanea tarda, uroporphyrinuria, abnormal liver tests (bilirubin, serum glutamic oxaloacetic transaminase, serous glutamic pyruvic transaminase and bromosulphthalein) and liver enlargement. The majority of workers were reported to have "severe neurasthenia" and "depressive syndrome." In 17, signs of peripheral neuropathy, notably in the lower extremities, were confirmed by electromyographic studies. More than half showed increased blood cholesterol and total lipids. In 1949, an accident occurred at the 2,4,5-T-producing factory of the Monsanto Chemical Company in Nitro, West Virginia; 228 people were affected. Symptoms included chloracne, melanosis, muscle aches and pain, fatigue, nervousness and intolerance to cold.[29]

Czeizel and Király[22] studied the frequency of chromosome aberrations in the peripheral blood lymphocytes of 76 workers at a Budapest chemical factory producing herbicides and in 33 controls. Thirty-six workers had been exposed to 2,4,5-trichlorophenoxyethanol (TCPE) and 26 to Buvinol, a combination herbicide containing TCPE and 2-chloro-6-ethylamino-4-isopropylamino-1,3,5-triazine (atrazine); 14 had never been engaged in herbicide production or use. The TCDD contamination of the final products was said to be less than 0.1 mg/kg and generally not more than 0.05 mg/kg. The frequency of chromatid-type and unstable chromosome aberrations was found to be statistically significantly higher in the factory workers, whether they had been directly exposed in herbicide production or not. The aberrations were more frequent among workers preparing Buvinol and TCPE than in other factory workers, but the difference was significant only for the chromatid-type effect.

Hardell and Sandström[42] investigated workers engaged as herbicide applicators in northern Sweden and found a number of patients with soft tissue sarcomas and previous exposure to phenoxyacetic acids. Due to this observation, a matched case-control study was performed with consideration for exposure to chlorophenols included. The results showed that exposure to phenoxyacetic acids or chlorophenols gave an approximately sixfold increase of the risk for this type of tumor. They considered it most unlikely that the results were influenced by uncontrolled confounding factors or other defects in the validity of the study. A specific evaluation of the effect of separate chemical substances was not possible, as nearly all exposed persons were also exposed to chlorinated dioxins, including their most potent form, 2,3,7,8-tetrachlorodibenzo-*p*-dioxin (TCDD). They were not able to determine if the carcinogenic effect was exerted by these compounds or by impurities such as chlorinated dibenzodioxins and dibenzofurans that in almost all cases were part of the commercial preparations used. The authors suggested that the increased risk for this type of tumor after exposure to phenoxyacetic acids or chlorophenols may be caused by the pure chemical substances, impurities in the commercial preparations or a combination of both.

Axelson and Sundell[6] studied a cohort of Swedish railway workers exposed to a variety of herbicides, finding a significant twofold excess of all cancers observed in exposed workers, as compared to the Swedish national average. The situation was difficult to evaluate because of the combined exposure of many workers to more than one herbicide. Most of the excess, however, seemed to be due to exposure to 3-amino-1,2,4-triazole (amitrole); within the subgroups that had been exposed to phenoxy acids (2,4-D and/or 2,4,5-T), only a small difference was detected: 5 cancers at all sites observed versus 2.8 expected. The authors state that the use of 2,4-D and 2,-4,5-T probably had been higher than that they could trace.

Thiess and Goldmann[125] traced 4 cancer deaths (1 lung carcinoma at 54 years, 2 gastric carcinomas at 64 and 77 years and 1 colonic carcinoma at 70 years) out of 15 deaths occurring in a cohort of 53 workers exposed accidentally to TCDD at the BASF factory in Ludwigshafen, West Germany in 1953.

There are reports describing the occurrence of cancer in workers exposed to TCDD. Jirásek et al.[62] followed 55 subjects of a cohort of 78 exposed workers for 5–6 years: 4 deaths were observed, 2 of which were from bronchogenic carcinoma at 47 and 59 years. Smoking history was not reported and no causal conclusion was drawn. However, if 1965 WHO lung cancer mortality rates for Czechoslovakia were applied to the age structure of the whole cohort of 78 workers, the expected number of lung cancer deaths in 5 years would be only 0.12.

Recently, chemical processes for 2,4,5-trichlorophenol production that do not cause TCDD to be formed have been inaugurated so that production of these herbicides is free from the TCDD hazard. The herbicide Dalapan (2,4-dichloropropionic acid) is a substitute herbicide having a low toxicity for animals and man.

In addition TCDD-contaminated pesticides, several other types of pesticides and their intermediates have been associated with chloracne. Chlorinated naphthalenes, diphenyls, diphenyl oxides, azoxybenzenes and chlorinated dibenzofurans have been implicated in producing chloracne and hyperpigmentation of the skin.

Paraquat (1,1′-dimethyl-4,4′-bipyridilium dichloride)

The TLV is 0.5 mg/m^3.

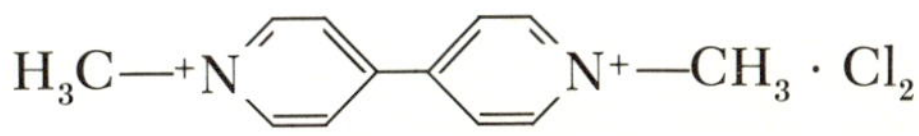

Paraquat has world-wide use in killing leafy plants, in harvesting cotton (by spray) in order to desiccate the leaves to defoliate the plants, making the cotton bolls easier to be picked mechanically. In use in field applications, paraquat is rapidly decomposed and inactivated by the action of sunlight. The sale and use of paraquat is carefully regulated in most countries and generally is formulated as a 20% solution that is sprayed on the desired areas. The solutions often contain surfactants as wetting agents and ordinarily are mixed or added to the spray shortly before use. Paraquat is applied on large areas by aerial spraying. It gained prominence in 1978 when used to destroy marijuana crops in Mexico, causing much concern to users of marijuana, but actual paraquat toxicity was ruled out by a CDC investigation.[104, 121]

Although paraquat had been studied mainly in laboratories since 1933, reports on occupational intoxication had not been made until the 1960s, when this compound was introduced for agricultural use. The first report of intoxication to paraquat was due to accidental ingestion in 2 young men who consumed a small quantity of paraquat concentrate mistakenly thought to contain an alcoholic beverage. Death occurred within several days from a rapidly developing and progressive fibrosis of the lungs.[104] These examples, along with laboratory animal studies, revealed that paraquat by ingestion was extremely toxic and rapid in action, producing irreversible lung damage even though elimination in the urine was quite rapid.

Vaziri et al.[127] studied 3 patients with paraquat poisoning, 2 due to suicidal ingestion (a 56-year-old woman ingested a "large cup" of paraquat, a 16-year-old male a "mouthful", a 17-year-old male a "mouthful" by accident). Renal function studies revealed acute renal failure observed in all 3 cases. The glomerular filtration rate improved for 2 patients who survived 3 weeks, illustrating the reversible nature of paraquat-induced acute renal failure. A mild-to-moderate transient proteinuria was observed during the first and second weeks following paraquat ingestion. Renal glucosuria, marked amino aciduria and increased fractional excretion of phosphorus, sodium and uric acid were observed. These findings, which have not been described previously in man, are indicative of proximal tubular dysfunction and parallel observations previously made in experimental animals.

Symptoms that have been displayed by agricultural workers subjected to excessive periods of paraquat spray exposure are related to local irritation and include nosebleed, upper respiratory and buccal mucous membrane inflammation, cough, headache, eye irritation, skin irritation and damaged fingernails with transverse bands of nail discoloration; other lesions were loss of nail surface, ridging, gross nail deformities and, in some, loss of the nail.[122] These signs of overexposure should be sufficient indicators for removal of the worker from the area and prevention of further overexposure. Although absorption via healthy skin is thought to be minimal, injured skin, i.e., abraded, small lacerations, etc., can enhance absorption and contamination of scrotal skin must be avoided.

EXPERIMENTAL TOXICOLOGY.—Ingestion of paraquat by laboratory animals produces signs of poisoning similar to those described for man, which include oral and pharyngeal irritation in addition to pulmonary and possible renal complications.

Carefully controlled skin exposure studies, which eliminate the possibility of ingestion, failed to demonstrate any signs of lung toxicity. However, a 20% decrease in body weight was reported in the paraquat-treated animals. Acute dermal exposure to paraquat concentrate has produced mild erythema, hyperkeratoses and desquamation in rats and rabbits. The effects were diminished when typical field spray concentrations were used.[19]

Prolonged exposure to respirable paraquat spray has been demonstrated to produce pulmonary congestion and edema in rats.[19] The reaction is immediate, resulting in the development of chemical pneumonitis in the form of congestion and edema. This does not resemble the syndrome seen following ingestion. Discoloration, swelling and clouding of renal tissue in rats subjected to paraquat aerosol inhalation indicated that the herbicide may be partially absorbed by this route. It must be noted that agricultural sprays have much larger particles and, therefore, do not reach the aveoli.

Investigations have been conducted on the possible hazard from dust from paraquat-treated soils. Rats, mice, guinea pigs and rabbits were exposed to a dust cloud containing 500 ppm paraquat at a level of 10 gm/m^3, of which 0.25 gm/m^3 was respirable. No effects were noted.

Two-year feeding studies were conducted in mice using 9, 25, 50 and 75 ppm paraquat cation in the diet without evidence of carcinogenic activity. Paraquat was tested to determine if dominant lethal gene formation occurred in mice. No mutagenic properties were demonstrated. However, certain antifertility effects were noted in mice administered 17.3 mg paraquat cation/kg orally. There was a decreased percentage of pregnancies in treated mice. No differences were found between control and treated animals regarding the number of fetal deaths.[19]

No teratologic effects have been reported from dietary intake of paraquat in experimental animals.[103] A three-generation, two-litter reproduction study on rats sustained on diets containing 30 and 100 ppm paraquat cation demonstrated that the compound did not influence the growth or fertility of the treated animals or their offspring, nor were any teratogenic effects noted.

An extensive report on the toxicology of paraquat, diquat and morfamquat was published by Pasi[103] in 1978.

CLINICAL. —Paraquat can be determined in urine and dialysate. However, the technique is lengthy and requires ion-exchange resins not generally available. In emergencies, paraquat levels should be determined, but treatment should not be delayed. Obtain a 100-ml urine sample and/or a dialysate sample and store under refrigeration until arrangements for analysis are made.* The Chevron Chemical Company's Environmental Health Group has prepared a valuable document describing paraquat poisoning, signs and symptoms, along with treatment.[102]

Urea Derivatives

Certain urea derivatives are commonly used as herbicides. Some of these are monuron (Monurex, Telvar), diuron (Di-on, diurex, Karmex) and others.

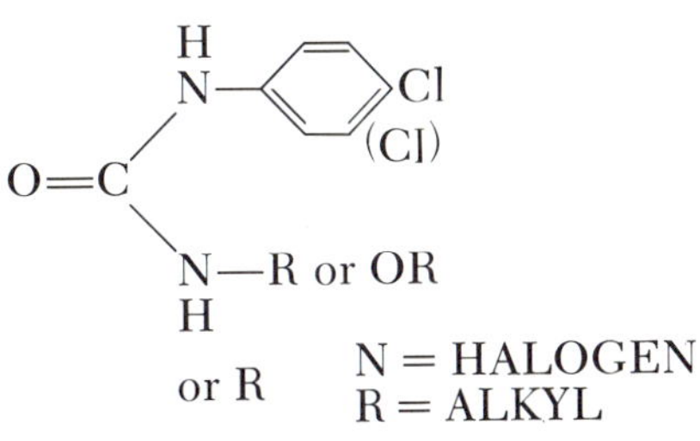

Some uracil compounds are bromacil (Borea, Hyvar X, Hyvar X-2), terbacil (Sinbar) and others. Triazines: atrazine (Atarex, Atranex, Primatol A, etc.) and a host of other trade names. Occupational exposures to these compounds rarely have produced adverse effects, and most have been skin irritation following prolonged contact.

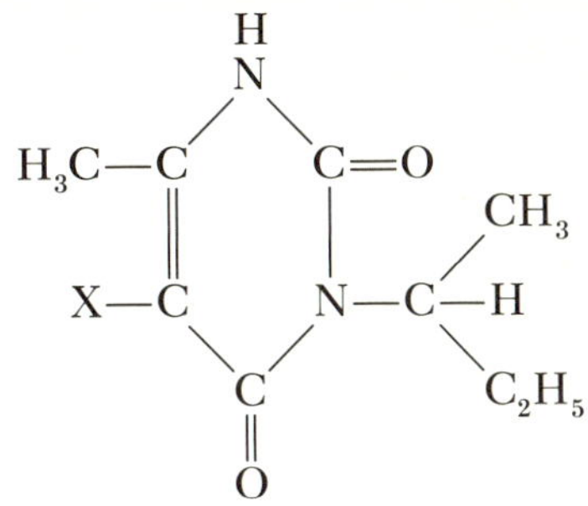

Although certain newer herbicides show low systemic toxicity in laboratory animals, most are irritating to the skin, eyes and the upper respiratory system. The acetanilids and acetamides have demonstrated severe skin sensitization reactions. Application formulations include petroleum distillates. Selected products are alachlor (Lasso), allidochlor (Randox), chloropropham, propachlor (Ramrod) and propanil (Stam, Propanex).

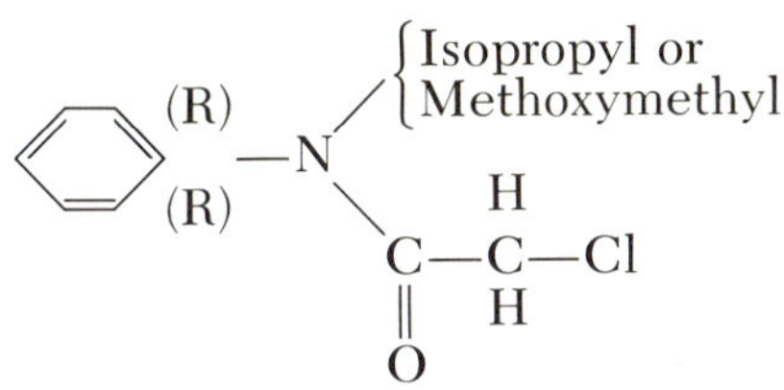

FUNGICIDES

Fruit trees, vegetable crops and ornamentals, as well as germinating seeds, are subject to fungal attack unless protected. There are several classes of fungicides in common use. Sulfur, the earliest chemical used, still is available in a wettable powder or sold as "lime-sulfur" and is relatively nontoxic to man.

Fungicides include forms of copper and sulfur, mercury, complexes of cadmium, iron, manganese and zinc, along with a variety of organic compounds (common examples are disulfiram, ferbam, nabam, ziram and zineb). Use of certain metallic compounds, especially mercurials, now is for-

*The Chevron Chemical Company will perform urine and dialysate analysis for paraquat at no cost. Arrangements for this service can be made by telephoning the Chevron Poison Information Center—(415) 233–3737.

bidden in many countries because of their toxicity.

Wood preservatives include three classes: creosote (evaporates slowly, insoluble in water), certain metallic salts (injected as water solution into wood) and other chemicals (inorganic solvents).

Creosote

This is an oily distillate obtained from either coal or wood tar and is a mixture of more than 150 compounds. Coal-tar creosote or creosote oil is used mainly as a wood preservative to protect against fungi, shipworms and termites. About 100 million kg are used in the United States to pressure-impregnate building lumber, factory floor blocks, pilings and telephone poles.

Creosote is highly toxic to wood-destroying organisms and has a low rate of evaporation. NIOSH has recommended a 0.1 mg/m^3 permissible limit for an 8-hour TWA exposure.

Creosote can be absorbed through the skin and is extremely irritating to human skin. Vapors can produce an intense burning sensation of the mucous membranes of the eyes and upper respiratory system. Eye injuries include conjunctivitis, keratitis and corneal scarring. To be noted is that treated wood retains creosote for more than 25 years; therefore, caution is advised in handling and sawing old creosoted lumber (much heat is generated from saw cutting teeth, increasing vapor production as well as throwing off much dust and particles of wood, easily lodging on skin and in clothing and creating inhalation exposure hazards and danger to the eyes). Suitable clothing and eye protection are necessary as well as wash-up facilities for workers. Other than conservative therapy and prevention of secondary skin infection there is no satisfactory treatment for creosote irritation.

Pentachlorophenol

The TLV is 0.4 mg/m^3.

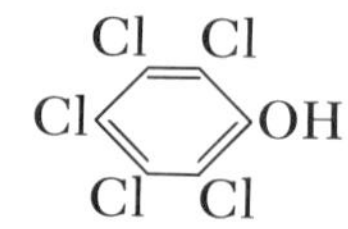

This compound is used as a fungicide and for slime control in the manufacture of paper pulp. It is also used in the United States for agricultural seed treatment, as a wood preservative against termites, molds and against wood-boring insects. Pentachlorophenol is used as a preharvest defoliant and a general herbicide. It is readily absorbed through the skin and by inhalation. Other nonpesticide uses include processing of glues, oils, leather, paints and textiles, and it has been incorporated into certain shampoos.

Exposure can cause irritation to the eyes and upper respiratory system, and prolonged skin exposure causes an acneiform dermatitis. Hyperpyrexia and an increase in metabolic rate have been shown in humans following systemic absorption. Human exposure to dust or mist concentrations of 1 mg/m^3 or more causes discomfort in the nose and throat, along with violent sneezing and coughing. As little as 0.3 mg/m^3 has caused nose irritation, but workers have become inured to concentrations up to 2.4 mg/m^3. Because this substance easily penetrates intact skin and the systemic concentration is cumulative, fatalities have been reported. Symptoms of intoxication are anorexia, sweating, weight loss and weakness, as well as headache, dizziness, nausea, vomiting, dyspnea and chest pain. Body temperature has been observed as extremely high, and death has occurred as early as 3 hours after onset of symptoms, with risk of serious intoxication increased during hot weather, according to Bergner et al.[10] Acneiform dermatitis has been reported with chronic low-level dermal exposures in 10 workers engaged in production of this compound for 5–10 months. Also, widely disseminated skin eruptions were noted by Baader and Bauer[7] in their case reports describing small and large furuncles and brown pigmentation. Some workers were reported to develop severe bronchitis. More than a year following cessation of exposure, all but 1 worker showed signs of extensive acne and 4 still complained of bronchitis. Urinary pentachlorophenol analysis may prove helpful in diagnosis, but knowledge and history of work exposure to the substance is required.

In a plant manufacturing pentachlorophenol, Glauser[33] described "a complete plant study" of 305 workers, emphasizing use of the blood chemistry profile ("SMA 24"), and noted 45 workers with "2 or more abnormalities" with low-level exposures to pentachlorophenol. Glauser reported exposures to be within the TLV, although no measurements were presented. There were no clinical illnesses, no chloracne, and BUN and creatinine levels and renal clearances were normal. Eight of 145 nonexposed workers had similar abnormal findings. The workplace was improved by engineering controls.

A strongly acidic phenol, pentachlorophenol is mainly excreted unchanged in human urine. Urinary concentrations of pentachlorophenol above 10 mg/l may be considered an indicator of excess absorption. Tetrachlorohydroquinone is also excreted in the urine of workers exposed to pentachlorophenol.[1]

Copper Compounds

Copper (cupric) sulfate is used as an algicide and fungicide. This substance is a relatively nontoxic chemical; reports of irritation or other toxic effects from occupational exposure are lacking. Copper 8-hydroxyquinoline is a greenish yellow crystalline powder used as a fungicide in the treatment of textiles, but also used in paper and wood preservation and in agriculture. There is no established TLV.

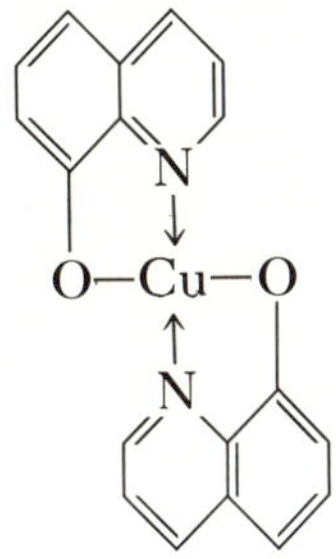

It is found in many interior paints as a protection against fungus where mercurial compounds cannot be used because of their toxicity. In the United States it is approved for use as a fungicide on wooden containers that may have contact with food products, beverage boxes, field crates, hampers, pallets and wooden containers for fruits and vegetables. The minor uses include incorporation into plastics and paper. Generally, it is used in liquid concentrates or pastes, containing from 0.25% to 10% of the main material and 5–30% in pastes. With liquid concentrate use, copper 8-hydroxyquinoline may be used in combination with 17% pentachlorophenol and 2.5% tetrachlorophenol. Other uses are for textile treatment of fabrics, webbing and cordage, rope and threads and fishing nets. No occupational health problems resulting from exposure have been reported.

Ferbam

The TLV is 10 mg/m^3

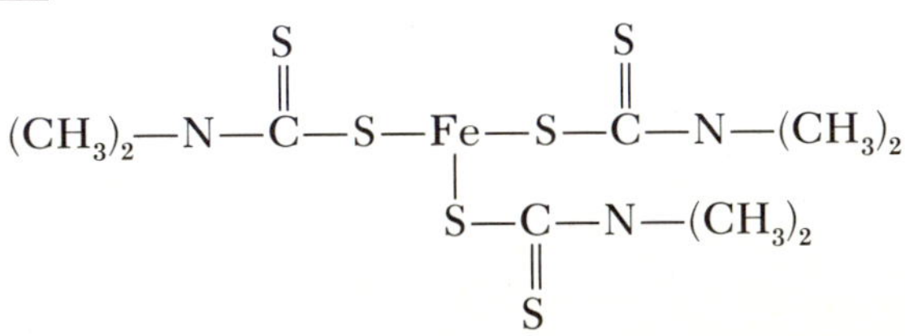

In humans, the dust is irritating to the eyes and respiratory tract; it can cause dermatitis in individuals sensitized to sulfur compounds. Large oral doses cause gastrointestinal disturbances. Ten of 20 rats died from a diet containing 0.5% ferbam for 30 days; there was a slight and ill-defined tendency toward anemia. At autopsy there was no evidence of a regularly appearing tissue injury; minor abnormalities of the lung, liver, kidney and bone marrow were observed in a few animals.[50]

Thiram

The TLV is 5 mg/m^3.

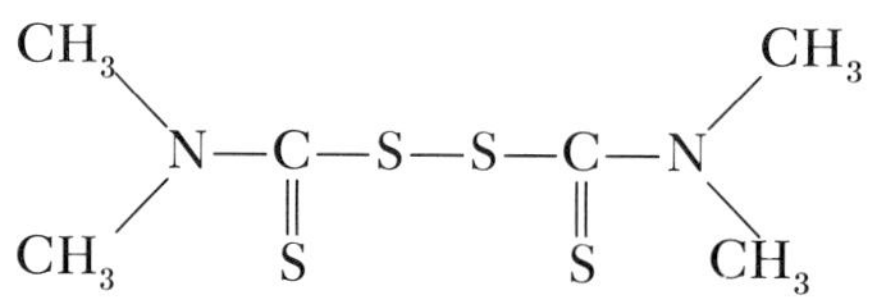

Thiram (tetramethylthiuram disulfide) dust is an irritant to the respiratory tract, eyes and skin and causes sensitization dermatitis. Thiram was teratogenic (skeletal malformations) in hamsters given a single oral dose of 250 mg/kg during the period of organogenesis and in mice given oral doses of 5–30 mg/animal daily between days 6 and 17 of pregnancy.[111, 115] In exposed humans, sensitization dermatitis in the form of eczema has occurred on the hands, forearms and feet.[116] Ingestion of ethanol by workers exposed to thiram has caused a rapid skin response of a nonallergic nature characterized by flushing, erythema, pruritus and urticaria (see Chapter 14).

FUMIGANTS

A fumigant is a substance or mixture of substances that produces a gas, vapor, fume or smoke intended to destroy insects, bacteria or rodents.

Fumigants may be solids, volatile liquids or substances already in the gaseous state. They may be used to disinfect the interiors of buildings, objects and materials that can be enclosed so as to retain or entrap the fumigants.

Other chemicals used as insecticides and as fumigants are acrylonitrile, calcium cyanide (cyanogas), carbon disulfide, carbon tetrachloride, dichlorobenzene, ethylene dibromide, ethylene dichloride, hydrogen cyanide, naphthalene and sulfur dioxide. Since these substances are widely used in industry for other purposes and occupational exposures are common, a more detailed discussion for selected compounds will be found in Chapter 14.

Methyl Bromide ($BrCH_3$)

The TLV is 15 ppm.

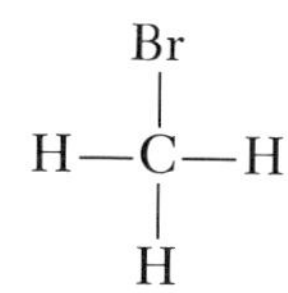

Methyl bromide is also known as bromyl methane, Embafume, isobram and monobromomethane, and at room temperatures and normal pressures, it is a colorless gas, liquefying at 3° C, used chiefly as a fumigant-insecticide. It also is used as a rodenticide and in the synthesis of other chemicals and dyes. Because of its rapid action and significant toxicity, methyl bromide must be handled with special care. The vapor is more than 3 times as dense as air, and sometimes pockets of the gas may collect in low spots as well as poorly ventilated places. Occupational exposures may occur during fumigation of warehouses, storage areas, railroad cars, buildings, etc. Methyl bromide is used for preservation of flour, cereals, rice, grain, seeds, dates and nuts. Methyl bromide is commercially packed, compressed to a liquid, in various sized metal containers for ease in handling and storage. The main routes of absorption are through inhalation and the skin. Contact with either the gas or liquid may induce eye irritation, and dry, scaling and itching dermatitis may result from chronic but less concentrated exposures. The gas can act as a pulmonary irritant and also as a neurotoxin; high concentrations cause pulmonary edema and convulsions; chronic exposures have caused peripheral neuropathy.[49] Human intoxication arises from accidental occupational exposures and during use as a fumigant. The onset of toxic symptoms often is delayed, having a latency period of from 30 minutes to several hours. Initial symptoms may include malaise, headache, nausea, vomiting, visual disturbances and, in some cases, eye irritation, dizziness and tension tremors of the hands. Tremors may progress to twitchings and, in some instances, to convulsions. Greenburg[40] reported convulsions of the jacksonian type, first restricted to one extremity but gradually spreading to the entire body. Severe exposure has caused pulmonary edema, and tubular damage to the kidneys has been reported in fatal cases. Concentrations estimated to have caused human fatalities have ranged from 8000 ppm for a few hours' exposure to 60,000 ppm for shorter exposures. Hine[49] has reported that those who have recovered from severe intoxications have had persistent central nervous system defects, including vertigo, anxiety, depression, hallucinations and inability to concentrate.

Kantarjian and Shaheen[68] reported that 8 of 14 workers repeatedly exposed to the vapor (concentration unmeasured) for 3 months developed peripheral neuropathy, but all recovered within 6 months after exposure ceased. Hine[49] observed that the determination of bromide in human blood for the purpose of estimating degree of exposure has been inconsistent. Blood bromide levels are not recommended for routine monitoring of occupational exposure.

Verberk et al.[128] studied 33 men employed in soil disinfection inside greenhouses using only methyl bromide, applied from fumigating tubes (23 workers) or from cans (10 men). Slight electroencephalographic changes were found in 10 workers and a small increase in serum transaminases was found that could not be related to bromine concentration in the blood.

Workers dispensing methyl bromide, checking on concentration or using the compound must wear approved respiratory protective equipment and must not work alone. Periodic medical examinations are advisable for employees regularly working with methyl bromide, with emphasis on the respiratory and neurologic systems.

All contaminated clothing must be promptly removed and the contaminated skin should be rapidly and thoroughly washed (*special admonition:* methyl bromide can penetrate ordinary rubber gloves; therefore, adequate protective equipment [polyvinyl alcohol, neoprene or nitrile latex composition] and instructions must be provided in advance to all workers). Special therapy must be directed to prevent acidosis, pulmonary edema, bronchial spasm, respiratory paralysis and/or kidney failure.

Sulfuryl Fluoride

The TLV is 5 ppm.

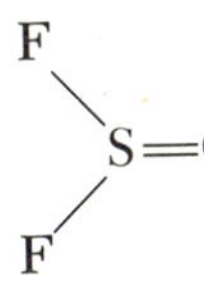

Sulfuric oxyfluoride, trade name Vikane (SO_2F_2), is a colorless, odorless gas used as an insect fumigant, with occupational exposure occurring by inadvertent inhalation. This compound is a central nervous system depressant and a pulmonary irritant. Taxay[123] described findings in a worker exposed to an unknown concentration of a mixture of sulfuryl fluoride and 1% chloropicrin for 4 hours who developed nausea, vomiting, abdominal pain, pleuritis with diffuse rhonchi and paresthesia of the right leg, all rapidly subsiding after pulmonary exposure. The exact role of the sulfuryl fluoride was not known, but the cyanotic symptoms are those expected of chloropicrin overexposure. Limited other human exposure has been reported; by analogy, its toxicity has been derived from animal studies. High but unspecified concentrations of the gas to exposed animals caused signs of narcosis and, in some animals, tremors, convulsions and pulmonary edema; with repeated exposure, lung and kidney damage was found. Animal exposures of 1000 ppm for 3 hours or to 15,000 ppm for 6 minutes was fatal to less than 5% of animals tested. The oral LD_{50} for rats and guinea pigs was 100 mg/kg. There are no special tests, and strict work controls to prevent exposure are necessary.

Phosphine Fumigants

The phosphine fumigants are aluminum phosphide (Celphos, delicia, phostoxin). These compounds are highly toxic on inhalation; the main target organs are the lungs. Phosphine (PH_3), a colorless gas, is an insecticide fumigant also known as hydrogen phosphide, phosphorated hydrogen and phosphorus trihydride. Phosphine has a fishy or garlic-like odor, detectable at about 2 ppm, but this odor threshold does not provide sufficient warning of toxic exposure. The 1979 ACGIH TLV for phosphine is 0.3 ppm for an 8-hour TWA exposure. Jones et al.[66] described findings in workers engaged in wheat fumigation with aluminum phosphide who were exposed intermittently to concentrations up to 35 ppm but averaging below 10 ppm and who complained of nausea, vomiting, diarrhea, chest tightness, cough, headache and dizziness, but no evidence of cumulative effects was noted. Harger and Spolyar[43] reported that single severe exposures caused similar symptoms and signs, as well as excessive thirst, muscle pains, chills, sensation of pressure in the chest, dyspnea, syncope and stupor, and, in some cases, dizziness and staggering gait. Since 1900, 59 cases of phosphine poisoning, with 26 deaths, have been reported, and the most frequently seen effect was marked pulmonary edema. If it is known that phosphine has been inhaled, immediate hospitalization is recommended for observation for up to 72 hours to guard against delayed onset of pulmonary edema. There are no specific tests for use in diagnosis.

ARSENICALS (INORGANIC)

The TLV for arsenic and compounds (as arsenic) is 0.5 mg/m^3 for an 8-hour TWA. The TLV for arsenic trioxide (as arsenic) is 0.05 mg/m^3 for an 8-hour TWA.

$$O{=}As{-}O{-}As{=}O$$

Arsenic Trioxide

$$K{-}O{-}As{=}O$$

Potassium Arsenite

$$Cu{-}(O{-}\overset{\overset{\displaystyle O}{\|}}{C}{-}CH_3)_2 \;\bullet\; Cu_3{-}(As\ O_2)_2$$

Copper Acetoarsenite
(Paris green)

Inorganic arsenicals, long used as insecticides, include lead arsenate, Paris green and sodium arsenite. (In addition to use as insecticides, these arsenicals have been used for control of worms in cattle, goats, sheep and other animals.) All are highly toxic when inhaled or ingested; keep in mind that if inhalation occurs, simultaneous ingestion of accumulated inhaled material in the mucous secretions from the upper respiratory system may enter the gastrointestinal system by normal swallowing of the mucus. Prolonged overexposure to lead arsenate can cause arsenic and/or lead intoxication. With acute intoxication, symptoms and signs of arsenic intoxication usually predominate. With chronic exposure to lead arsenate, symptoms of lead poisoning may occur. The effects of acute arsenic poisoning are nausea, vomiting, diarrhea, inflammation and ulceration of the mucous membranes and kidney damage. Chronic effects of arsenic poisoning are increased pigmentation and keratinization of skin, patchy dermatitis and epidermoid carcinoma.[90] Ingestion rarely is encountered during occupational exposure, but symptoms may occur 30 minutes to many hours after ingestion. In addition to those symptoms mentioned earlier there may be bloody diarrhea later; colicky pains in the abdomen, thirst, dizziness, dehydration, muscle cramps and cyanosis may occur as well as toxic effects leading to delirium and convulsions. Eventually, marked weakness, shock, muscle paralysis, liver and kidney damage and death due to circulatory failure occur. Diagnosis of arsenic intoxication requires an accurate history of the substances inhaled or ingested. Analysis of urine has indicated a great variation in levels of excreted arsenic. Some studies have reported that 0.7–1.0 mg/1 in the urine of exposed workers may be considered an indication of exposure. However, dietary factors may confound these urinary levels of arsenic, as certain seafoods, especially shellfish, are high in arsenic content. The analytic procedures for arsenic are difficult to perform, and not all laboratories can perform such analyses. If severe arsenic intoxication is diagnosed, BAL (British anti-Lewisite compound) is valuable in treatment (promptly administered BAL intramuscularly as a 10% solution in vegetable oil). Recommended dosage schedule is[86]:

	Mild Poisoning	*Severe Poisoning*
Days 1 and 2	2.5 mg/kg q6h × 8 doses	3.0 mg/kg q4h × 12 doses
Day 3	2.5 mg/kg q12h × 2 doses	3.0 mg/kg q6h × 4 doses
Succeeding 10 days	2.5 mg/kg q24h × 10 doses	3.0 mg/kg q12h × 20 doses

CAUTION: *Dimercaprol* can cause troublesome side effects (hypertension, tachycardia, nausea, headache, paresthesias and pain, lacrimation, sweating, anxiety and restlessness). Although usually not so severe as to handicap treatment, these manifestations may require antihistaminic therapy for adequate control.

The NIOSH has designated arsenic and its compounds as human carcinogens, and has recommended restricting employee arsenic exposure to the lowest level that can be reliably measured (0.002 mg/m^3 for a 15-minute duration). No increase of urinary arsenic above the "background" level (100 μg/l) is to be permitted. Arsenic determination in hair is considered unreliable for monitoring worker exposure, since it is difficult to distinguish between externally deposited arsenic and that systemically incorporated.

RODENTICIDES

Rodenticides are preparations intended for the control of rats, mice, gophers, porcupines and closely related animals (such as rabbits). Rodenticide chemicals include Pival, warfarin, ANTU, sodium fluoroacetate, strychnine and thallium.

Warfarin

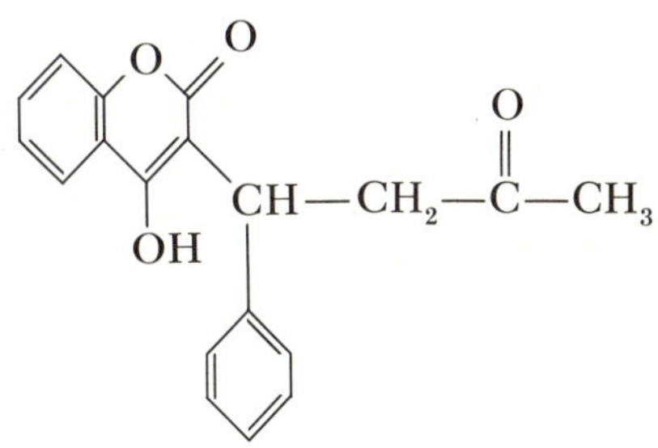

Warfarin ($C_{19}H_{16}O_4$) is a colorless, odorless and tasteless crystalline-like substance, most commonly absorbed into the body by inhalation and skin absorption. Its usefulness as a rodenticide is its inherent ability to cause hypoprothrombinemia and vascular injury, resulting in hemorrhages. Warfarin is known to suppress the liver formation of prothrombin and other factors essential for blood clotting. A marked reduction of prothrombin activity of the blood also occurs as well as dilatation and engorgement of blood vessels, with an increase in capillary fragility. There is a latency period of several days following absorption, and acute ingestion reveals hemorrhage or depression of plasma prothrombin. Fristedt and Sterner[31] reported a farmer who had skin exposure of a 0.5% solution of warfarin over a period of 24 days and developed gross hematuria 2 days following the last contact with the solution. He developed spontaneous hematomas on the arms and legs. Within 4 days, other effects were noted, such as epistaxis, hemorrhages of the palate and mouth and bleeding from the lower lip. After appropriate treatment, normal blood findings occurred.

Flint[30] reported a potentially dangerous drug interaction between cimetidine (trademark name Tagamet in the United States) and warfarin (Coumadin, Panwarfarin and others). Of 17 patients stabilized on warfarin, their prothrombin time increased by 20% when 1 gm daily of cimetidine, a drug used to treat peptic ulcers, was added to the drug regimen. With increasing prescribing of cimetidine, those following workers stabilized on warfarin must be warned to watch for early signs of bleeding (easy bruising, bleeding gums, dark stool, etc.).

Pival

The TLV is 0.1 mg/m^3.

Pival, 2-pivalyl-1,3-indandione ($C_{14}H_{14}O_3$), a yellow powder, also labeled Pindone, Pivalyl Valone and Triban, is commonly used as a rat killer. Pival is a vitamin K antagonist, inhibiting prothrombin formation, resulting in hemorrhages. In rats, ingestion of a single large dose causes death due to multiple internal hemorrhages. There have been no reports of effects in man. If accidental ingestion occurs, the symptoms and signs are anticipated to be similar to those caused by warfarin, which may include hematuria, spontaneous hematomas on the arms and legs, epistaxis, bleeding from the lips, punctate hemorrhages from mucous membranes, abdominal and back pain, vomiting, blood in the feces, petechial rash and abnormal blood findings, such as increased prothrombin time and blood plasma, blood in urine and feces and hypochromic and microcytic anemia. Hypoprothrombinemia may be treated with vitamin A_1 or parenteral injections of aquamephyton or similar products—20–40 mg, repeatable every 4 hours until the prothrombin time returns to normal.[52]

ANTU

The TLV is 0.3 mg/m^3.

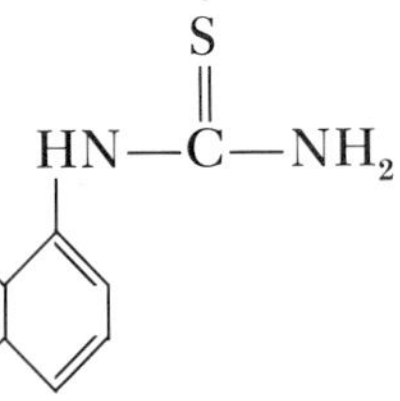

ANTU (alpha-naphthyl-thiourea) is a blue or grayish rodenticide powder, and exposure may occur by inhalation but most commonly by ingestion; occupational exposures are rare. ANTU dust may cause pulmonary edema and pleural effusion in animals. Accidental ingestion in humans has shown that the lethal dose is about 4 gm/kg. Intoxication in man has been reported in 1 case, by accidental ingestion involving 80 gm of a rat poison containing 30% ANTU. Signs were vomiting, dyspnea, cyanosis and pulmonary rales, without evidence of pleural effusion, the pulmonary signs clearing on supportive therapy.[78]

Sodium Fluoroacetate

The TLV is 0.05 mg/m^3.

Sodium fluoroacetate (CH_2FCOON_a) is a fine white rodenticide powder, commonly known as Compound 1080, fluoroacetic acid or sodium monofluoroacetate. Exposure may occur through inhalation, skin absorption and ingestion. This is one of the most acutely toxic substances known to man, causing convulsions and ventricular fibrillation. The lethal oral dose in humans has been estimated to be 5 mg/kg. Fluoroacetate is metabolized to fluorocitrate, inhibiting the oxidation of acetate in the tricarboxylic acid cycle. On accidental poisoning, symptom onset may occur within 30 minutes or up to 2 hours, with central nervous system effects noted as apprehension, tingling sensation of the nose, numbness of the face, facial twitching, vomiting, auditory hallucinations and, in severe instances, epileptiform convulsions. There are no special tests to detect this compound in man. Rigid precautions and instructions must be used in handling this compound.[44, 45]

Strychnine

The ACGIH TLV is 0.15 mg/m^3.

Strychnine ($C_{21}H_{22}N_2O_2$), a white crystalline powder, is commonly used as a poison bait for the larger animals. Human exposure may occur through inhalation but more commonly by accidental ingestion. Strychnine is a poison well known to act as a potent and long-lasting convulsant. The human lethal oral dose has been estimated to vary between 100 and 120 mg. Symptoms following ingestion may occur within 10–30 minutes and include stiffness of face and neck muscles, exaggerated reflexes and excitability. Convulsions may ensue rapidly along with cyanosis. Without prompt treatment, convulsions may be followed by an asphyxic death. If it is known that strychnine has been swallowed and the person is conscious, vomiting may be induced unless convulsions are imminent. Treatment consists of supportive therapy, such as artificial resuscitation, oxygen and endotracheal intubation. Convulsions may be controlled with diazepam or sodium phenobarbital given intravenously or intramuscularly. Sensory stimulation must be reduced by keeping the poisoned subject in a quiet, warm and darkened room, with hospital observation imperative.[35]

THALLIUM COMPOUNDS

The TLV for soluble thallium compounds is 0.1 mg/m^3.

The thallium salts have had longstanding use as a rodenticide and may be inhaled or absorbed through the skin, with most common poisonings occurring through accidental ingestion. Toxic effects are primarily on the nervous system, but occupational exposures are rare and usually have not been fatal.

Thallium salts are used less frequently in the United States because of the known severe toxicity. Richeson[108] studied 15 workers who had handled organic thallium salt solutions over a 7½ year period, finding that 6 workers presented some form of thallium intoxication, the chief complaints being abdominal pain, fatigue, weight loss, pain in the legs and nervous irritability. Three workers displayed albuminuria and 1 had hematuria. Thallium may be detected in the urine but is not a conclusive indicator of true systemic absorption. There is no good form of treatment; therefore, exposure prevention is mandatory.

NATURALLY OCCURRING INSECTICIDES

Nicotine

The TLV is 0.5 mg/m^3.

Nicotine — 1-methyl-2-(1 pyridyl)pyrrolidine—is a liquid insecticide with high toxicity and rapid action ($C_{10}H_{14}N_2$). Route of entry is by inhalation, skin absorption and ingestion. Nicotine causes a transient stimulation, followed by depression or paralysis of the central nervous system; it also directly stimulates smooth muscle. Many fatal human cases of nicotine intoxication have occurred, usually as a result of accidental or suicidal ingestion of nicotine insecticides. Nicotine is readily absorbed through the skin; in fatal cases of intoxication, death nearly always occurs within 1 hour and has occurred within 1 minute. The fatal adult dose is about 60 mg. Symptoms include nausea, salivation, abdominal pain, vomiting, diarrhea, cold sweat, headache, dizziness, disturbed hearing and vision, confusion, weakness and incoordination. Initially, respiration is deep and rapid, blood pressure is elevated and the pulse is slow; intense vagal stimulation may cause transient cardiac standstill or paroxysmal atrial fibrillation; the pupils generally are constricted. Excitation of the central nervous system results in tremor and sometimes clonic-tonic convulsions. As central nervous system depression ensues, the pupils dilate, the blood pressure falls and the pulse becomes rapid and often irregular; faintness, prostration, dyspnea and paralysis of respiratory muscles are followed by death.[39] Recovery usually occurs if the victim survives 1–4 hours. Skeletal system malformations occurred in the offspring of pregnant mice injected subcutaneously with nicotine between days 9 and 11 of pregnancy.[99]

Pyrethrum

The TLV is 5 mg/m^3.

Pyrethrum is an insecticide obtained from flowers of the genus *Chrysanthemum* and is used as a dusting powder. Pyrethrum dust causes dermatitis and occasionally sensitization. In animals, effects of intoxication are excitation, convulsions, muscle fasciculations and tetanic paralysis. The chief effect in humans from exposure to pyrethrum is dermatitis. The usual lesion is a mild erythematous dermatitis, with vesicles, papules in moist areas and intense pruritus; a bullous dermatitis may develop. In a study of workers engaged in processing pyrethrum powder, 30% had erythema, skin roughening and pruritus, which subsided on cessation of exposure. One of these workers had an anaphylactic type of reaction; shortly after entering a dust-laden room, the facial skin turned red and the person felt a sensation of burning and itching; the cheeks and eyes rapidly became swollen; the pruritus became severe. The entire condition disappears in 2 days after removal from exposure. Some persons exhibit sensitivity similar to pollinosis, with sneezing, nasal discharge and nasal stuffiness. A few cases of asthma due to pyrethrum mixtures have been reported; some of the individuals involved had a previous history of asthma, with allergy to a wide spectrum of substances.[17]

Rotenone

The TLV is 5 mg/m^3.

Rotenone is the active constituent of the cube and derris plants and several other leguminous plants. It is highly toxic to insects but presents a relatively low hazard to mammals, making it a widely used insecticide. It is about one-half as toxic as pyrethrum. Rotenone dust affects the nervous system and causes convulsions in animals. Animals repeatedly fed derris powder (the botanical source containing 9.6% rotenone) at levels from 312 to 4000 ppm developed focal liver necrosis and mild kidney damage. Of 40 female rats given daily intraperitoneal injections of rotenone in sunflower oil of 1.7 mg/kg for 42 days, more than 60% developed mammary tumors 6–11 months after the end of treatment; most of the tumors were mammary adenomas and one was a differentiated adenocarcinoma; none of the control animals had tumors when examined 19 months after treatment.[37] The lethal oral dose in humans is estimated to be 0.3–0.5 gm/kg. In humans, inhalation of dust is suspected to cause pulmonary irritation. Symptoms of absorption in humans (inferred mostly from animal studies) may include numbness of oral mucous membranes, nausea, vomiting and abdominal pain. There may be muscle tremors, incoordination, clonic convulsions and stupor. The dust is irritating to the eyes and skin.

MISCELLANEOUS REPELLENT INSECTICIDES

Dibutyl Phthalate

The TLV is 5 mg/m^3.

Dibutyl phthalate ($C_{16}H_{22}O_4$) is used as the active ingredient in many insect repellents applied to the skin; it is also used as a plasticizer. Extensive experience with dibutyl phthalate as an insect repellent has shown that it is relatively nonirritating to the skin, eyes and mucous membranes. Aerosols from heated dibutyl phthalate may cause irritation of the eyes and upper respiratory tract. In one report of a human case, accidental ingestion of 10 gm of this compound by a chemical operator produced nausea and dizziness, with lacrimation, photophobia and conjunctivitis, but recovery was prompt and uneventful. Animal experiments to determine dermal and oral toxicity of dibutyl phthalate showed that extremely high doses were required to produce toxic effects. Dibutyl phthalate was found to be teratogenic by intraperitoneal injection in female rats.[118]

Dimethyl phthalate ($C_{10}H_{10}O_4$) is also used as a skin-applied insecticide, but is slightly more irritating to the eyes and mucous membranes.

PRINCIPLES FOR CONTROLLING WORKPLACE HEALTH HAZARDS

The foundation for a comprehensive occupational health program is the continuing effort to ensure that workers, line and staff managers appreciate the impact of their actions on the over-all health/safety performance of the organization. The successful program must integrate both industrial hygiene and medical aspects with other functions at all levels of the organization. One means of integration involves the formation of a "health and safety committee" composed of workers, line and staff facility managers and occupational health professionals (nurse, physician, safety engineer, industrial hygienist, etc.)

The basic industrial hygiene principles involving the recognition, evaluation and control of potential health hazards in the workplace are directly applicable to pesticide-handling situations (for specific details, refer to Fundamentals of Industrial Hygiene, National Safety Council[100]). Several specific items require additional emphasis.

Care must be taken to ensure that all potential routes of employee exposure to pesticides are evaluated and controlled.

A great majority of the pesticides can be readily absorbed through intact skin. In many cases where various routes of exposure have been quantified, skin absorption has much greater potential for exposure than inhalation. Therefore, care must be taken to minimize frequency and duration of skin contact with these materials. Impervious protective clothing must be used whenever skin contact is likely. Suitable work clothing must be provided, with the employer responsible for its laundry. Contaminated work clothing can be cleaned at the facility or sent outside to a contract industrial laundry that has been informed of the potential hazards. Routine washing of hands, face and neck prior to breaks, lunch, etc. must be emphasized. Mandatory daily showers at the end of the work shift are required. Showers should be immediate for unplanned situations where overt overexposures can occur (spills, leaks, etc.).

Many pesticides also have significant oral toxicity and this route of exposure must be considered. Storage or consumption of food/cosmetics/smoking materials must not occur in unsanitary areas or work areas potentially contaminated with pesticides.

In most instances of pesticide manufacture, formulation or use, several chemicals are present and therefore additive or synergistic toxic effects always must be considered. Also, the presence of many different chemicals and the use of the same equipment require care to be taken to eliminate significant cross-contamination from one product to another and identify all containers as to contents.

Housekeeping procedures must be effective. Routine periodic decontamination procedures for both work area and general area (lunchroom, locker room, quality control labs, offices) should be initiated. Wet mopping or vacuum cleaning with a vacuum designed for handling toxic dusts is preferable to dry sweeping to minimize contamination. Swipe testing to evaluate the degree of surface contamination may be an important component of an over-all contamination evaluation program.

Effective control ultimately is composed of considering the health implications of a seemingly infinite number of details. This consideration can and should transcend "typical" industrial hygiene concerns and impact on related areas.

The potential health hazards associated with the performance of typical maintenance activities (welding, abrasive blasting, solvent cleaning) can be drastically increased if the equipment is potentially contaminated with a pesticide. The problem is further compounded if the work is being performed by an outside contractor.

Emergency planning for fires, explosions, spills and leaks is mandatory if employees and the surrounding community are to be protected from untoward health effects. In this regard, a National Agricultural Chemicals Association brochure, "Pre-Fire Planning and Guidelines for Handling Agricultural Chemical Fires" is very informative.[87a]

Effective 24-hour-a-day security prevents the entry of unauthorized personnel (vandals, juveniles, etc.) into areas where chemicals are stored or handled.

Environmental aspects of occupational exposures must be considered. Air-cleaning devices should be utilized on all exhaust ventilation systems. Waste materials, including empty containers, must be permanently disposed of in an environmentally secure manner.

Employee training should be designed to influence employee behavior to comply with appropriate work practices. Such training should be conducted for all newly hired persons and periodically for all employees.

Training should include the following areas:

1. Qualitative and quantitative identification of materials handled (Fig 13–4).
2. Potential risks of overexposure.
3. Description of signs and symptoms that might occur.
4. The importance of industrial hygiene and biologic monitoring and notification of test results.
5. Description of work practice controls, including personal protective equipment (respirators, gloves, etc.).
6. First aid and emergency training.

The medical aspects of the occupational health program should parallel the ongoing industrial hygiene activities, since both are vital for a successful program. Preplacement medical examinations are important because they:

1. Establish a baseline for each employee's health status.
2. Identify pre-existing illnesses or other conditions so that individuals can be placed in occupational settings consistent with their health and other physical capabilities.
3. Provide a data base for determining incidence and prevalence of any adverse effects stemming from the job.

The preplacement evaluation should include a comprehensive medical, family, occupational history and reproductive history, if indicated. The physical examination should be complete, and at the time of the examination, the employer should provide the physician with a description of the employee's prospective job and identification of any hazards that might be encountered. The physician should order appropriate tests based on this information and the results of the physical examination. After a review of the type of work and any potential exposure, clinical tests such as urinalysis, pulmonary function, chest x-ray, liver enzyme determinations and complete blood count (CBC), other tests may be carried out at the discretion of the responsible physician, but these tests need not be done routinely.[136] At the same time, a judgment of the worker's ability to use negative- and positive-pressure respirators may be made (see Chapter 14). If the person will be or has been exposed to the ChE-inhibiting pesticides as indicated in Table 13–1, red blood cell (RBC) ChE activity shall be measured for determination of a pre-exposure baseline.

"Pre-exposure baseline" for the RBC ChE is defined as the mean of two ChE activity determinations, each of which is derived from a separate sample of blood taken at least 1 day apart after a period of at least 60 days without known exposure to any ChE-inhibiting compounds. If the determinations produce values differing by more than 15%, additional determinations on new samples must be performed until successive tests do not differ by more than 15%.

"Working baseline" for the ChE is defined as the mean of two ChE activity determinations, each of which is derived from a separate sample of blood taken at least 1 day apart and differing by no more than 15%, or the arithmetic mean of normal values for an appropriate control population of adults for that laboratory, whichever is higher. A "working baseline" is determined only for an individual whose work history does not permit a pre-exposure baseline to be determined as specified in this section.

"Mean or normal values" is defined as the arithmetic mean of ChE activities for healthy adults as determined by the laboratory's experience with repeated analyses.

Periodic examinations shall be made available on at least an annual basis and shall include at least:

1. Interim medical and work histories.
2. Physical examination as described.

Periodic measurement of RBC ChE activity shall be made available to workers exposed to organophosphate insecticides at more frequent intervals, depending on hygienic surveys. These intervals may be as frequently as every day or may be increased after 3 weekly determinations to testing as frequently as every 8 weeks, based on the decision of the responsible physician after consideration of the following for each employee:

A. The degree of workplace contamination.
B. The toxicity of the pesticides to which the employee may be exposed.
C. The potential duration and concentration of the pesticide exposure.
D. The state of health of the employee.
E. The results of previous ChE determinations.
F. The extent of ongoing workplace improvements.

Each employee shall be given a copy of the results of his initial periodic test and of any special ChE test results as soon as possible after the test and an interpretation.

The scope of the examination is to be determined by the physician designated as the medical advisor for that plant. Community medical relationships must not be overlooked, and results of the examinations and attendant studies, whether clinically positive or negative, may be forwarded to the employee's personal physician. During examinations, applicants or employees found to have medical conditions such as skin disease, chronic lung disease or abnormalities of the central or peripheral nervous system that could be directly or indirectly aggravated by exposure to pesticides shall be counseled as to the possible increased risk of impairment of their health from working with certain substances. Employees should be further counseled about reproductive effects that have been noted in male workers and in laboratory animals involving certain pesticides, pointing out that the significance to humans of the effects in laboratory animals are not fully known but that they do indicate that exposure should be minimized, particularly in men and women of reproductive age. As has been discussed in preceding chapters, residues of some organochlorine (OC) and carbamate pesticides have been found in human breast milk. The NIOSH recommends that complete examination, including all findings, shall be offered to all employees within 1 month after employment ends. All medical and hygienic records should be kept for at least 30 years.

One of the most important responsibilities

of an agricultural chemicals manufacturer is to provide correct instructions on how to handle and apply the products. The information must be readily available, easy to understand (in the language of the farmer or pest control operator) and must contain the necessary educational elements. It is imperative that these products be handled properly and that the correct dosages be applied. This means that the user must know the sensitivity and compatibility of his crop and the proper dosage of the crop-protection product and to follow the recommendations of the manufacturer to prevent potentially harmful effects in workers.

In the United States, for example, wherever compounds that may present significant hazards are used for weed or insect control, persons responsible for applying these products must pass written examinations and be certified by state or federal authorities to handle these materials.

Grateful appreciation is given to Harvey V. Davis, Ph.D., for advice and encouragement.

GLOSSARY: COMMON PESTICIDES

COMMON NAME	CHEMICAL NAME	MAIN USES
Abate	0,0-dimethyl phosphorothioate 0,0-diester with 4,4′-thiodiphenol	insecticide
acrylonitrile	acrylonitrile	fumigant
alachlor	2-chloro-2′-6′ diethyl-*N*-(methoxy-methyl)-acetanilide	herbicide
aldrin	1,2,3,4,10,10-hexachloro-1,4,4a,5,8,8a-hexahydro-1,4,-endoexo-5,8-dimethanonaphthalene	insecticide
allidochlor	*N,N*-diallyl-2-chloroaceteamide	herbicide
aluminum phosphide	aluminum phosphide	insect fumigant
Amiben	amino-2,5-dichlorobenzoic acid	herbicide
amitrole	3-amino-1,2,4-triazole	herbicide
ammonium sulfamate	ammonium amidesulfate	herbicide
ANTU	alpha-naphthyl-thiourea	rodenticide
atrazine	2-chloro-4-ethylamino-6-isopropylamine-s-ariazine	herbicide
azinphosmethyl	0,0-dimethyl S[4-oxo-1,2,3-benzotriazin-3, 4 methyl] phosphorodithioate	fungicide
Azodrin	3-hydroxy-*N*-methyl-cis-crotonamide dimethyl phosphate	insecticide
Baygon	0-isopropoxyphenyl methyl carbamate	insecticide
benomyl	methyl-1-(butylcarbamoyl)-2-benzimidazole-carbamate	fungicide
benzene hexachloride	1,2,3,4,5,6-hexachlorocyclohexane (mixture of isomers)	insecticide
Bidrin	3-hydroxy-*N,N*-dimethyl-cis-crotonamide dimethyl phosphate	insecticide
Binapacryl	2-sec-butyl-4,6-dinitrophenyl-3-methyl-2-buteneate	insecticide
borax	sodium biborate	fungicide, herbicide
Brassicol	pentachlorophenol	fungicide
bromacil	5-bromo-3-*sec*-butyl-6-methyluracil	herbicide
bromophos	0-(4-bromo-2,5-dichlorophenyl)-0,0-dimethylphosphorothioate	insecticide, acaricide
bromoxynil	4-hydroxy-3,5-dibromobenzonitrile	herbicide
butylate	S-ethyl diisobutylthiocarbamate	herbicide
Buvinol	mixture of TCPE and atrazine	herbicide
cacodylic acid	dimethylarsinic acid	herbicide, defoliant
calcium arsenite	mono-calcium arsenite	insecticide
calcium cyanide	calcium carbimide	herbicide
carbaryl	1-naphthyl-*N*-methylcarbamate	insecticide
carbofuran	2,3-dihydro-2,2-dimethyl-7-benzofuranyl methyl carbamate	insecticide, nematocide
carbon tetrachloride	CCl_4	fumigant
carbophenothion	S-((*p*-chlorophenylthio) methyl)-0,0-diethyl phosphorodithioate	acaricide, insecticide

GLOSSARY: COMMON PESTICIDES (*cont.*)

COMMON NAME	CHEMICAL NAME	MAIN USES
Carzol	*N,N*-dimethyl, N′-(2-methyl-4 chlorophenyl)-formanidine	acaricide, insecticide
CDAA	*N,N*-diallyl-2-chloroacetamide	herbicide
chlordane	1,2,4,5,6,7,8,8-octachlor-2,3,3a,4,7,7a-hexahydro-4,7-methanoindane	insecticide
chlorophyrifos	0,0-diethyl 0-(3,5,6-trichloro-2-pyridyl)-phosphorothioate	insecticide
chlorprophan	isopropyl *m*-chlorocarbanilate	herbicide
Chlorthion	0,0-dimethyl 0-(3-chloro-4-nitrophenyl) phosphorothioate	insecticide
copper-8-hydroxy-quinoline	copper (II) 8-quinolinol	fungicide
copper sulfate	cupric sulfate pentahydrate	fungicide, algicide
cryolite	sodium hexafluoroaluminate	insecticide
cube (root)	rotenone	insecticide
2,4-D	2,4-dichlorophenoxyacetic acid	herbicide
dalapan	2,2-dichloropropionic acid, sodium salt	herbicide
DBCP	1,2-dibromo-3-chloropropane	soil fumigant for nematode control
DDA	bis (chlorophenyl) acetic acid (degradation product of DDT)	
DDE	1,1-bis (*P*-chlorophenyl)-2,2-dichloroethylene (degradation product of DDT)	
DDT	1,1,1-trichloro-2,2-bis (chlorophenyl) ethane	insecticide
DEF	S,S,S,-tributylphosphorotrithioate	defoliant
demeton	mixture of 0,0-diethyl S(and 0)-[2-(ethylthio) ethyl] phosphorothioates	insecticide
Dexon	sodium [4-(dimethylamino)phenyl] diazenesulfonate	soil fungicide, seed treatment
Diazinon	0,0-diethyl 0-(2-isopropyl-4-methyl-6-pyrimidyl) phosphorothioate	insecticide
dicamba	3,6-dichloro-0-anisic acid	herbicide
dicapthon	0-(2-chloro-4-nitrophenyl)-0,0-dimethyl phosphorothioate	insecticide
dichlone	2,3-dichloro-1,4-naphthoquinone	fungicide, herbicide
dichloropropene	1,3-dichloropropylene	soil fumigant, herbicide, insecticide, fungicide, nematocide
dichlorvos (DDVP)	0,0-dimethyl-2,2-dichlorovinyl phosphate	insecticide
dicofol	4,4′-dichloro-alpha-(trichloromethyl)-benzhydrol	insecticide
dieldrin	1,2,3,4,10,10-hexachloro-6,7-epoxy-1,4,4a,5,6,7,8,8a-octahydro-1,4-endoexo-5,8-dimethanonaphthalene	insecticide
dimethoate	0,0-dimethyl S-(*N*-methylcarbamylmethyl) phosphorodithioate	systemic acaricide, insecticide
dinitrocresol	4,6-dinitro-0-cresol	insecticide, herbicide
diphacinone	2-diphenylacetyl-1,3 indandione	rodenticide
diquat	1,1′-ethylene-2,2′-dipyridinium dibromide	herbicide, desiccant
disulfiram	bis(diethylthiocarbamoyl) disulfide	fungicide
disulfoton	0,0-diethyl S-[2-(ethylthio) ethyl]phosphorodithioate	insecticide
diuron	3-(3,4-dichlorophenyl)-1,1-dimethylurea	herbicide
DMPA	0-(2,4-dichlorophenyl)0′-methyl-*N*-isopropylphosphoroamidothioate	fly larvicide
DN-111	dicyclohexylamine salt of 2-cyclohexyl-4,6-dinitrophenol	insecticide
DNBP (dinitrobutylphenol)	2,4-dinitro-6-sec-butylphenol	herbicide, insecticide
DNOC	2-methyl-4,6 dinitro phenol	herbicide
2,4-DP (dichlorprop)	2-(2,4-dichlorophenoxy) propionic acid	herbicide
DSMA	disodium methanearsonate	herbicide
endosulfan	6,7,8,9,10,10-hexachloro-1,5,5a,6,9,-9a-hexahydro-6,9-methano-2,4,3-benzodioxathiepin-3-oxide	insecticide

GLOSSARY: COMMON PESTICIDES *(cont.)*

COMMON NAME	CHEMICAL NAME	MAIN USES
endothall	7-oxabicyclo (2,2,1)heptane-2,3 dicarboxylic acid, sodium salt	herbicide
endrin	1,2,3,4,10,10-hexachloro-6,7-epoxy-1,4,4a,5,6,7,8,8a-octahydro-1,4-endo-endo-5,8-dimethanonaphthalene	insecticide
EPN	0-ethyl-0-*p*-nitrophenyl phenylphosphonothioate	insecticide
EPTC	S-ethyl-*n,n*-dipropylthiocarbamate	herbicide
ethion	0,0,0′,0′-tetraethyl S,S′-methylenebisphosphorodithioate	insecticide
ethylene dibromide	1,2-dibromoethane	fumigant, nematocide
ethylene dichloride	1,2-dichloroethane	insecticide
ethylene oxide	ethylene oxide	herbicide
ethyl formate	ethyl formate	fumigant
fenthion	0,0-dimethyl [0-4-(methylthio)-m-tolyl] phosphorothioate	acaricide, insecticide, bird control
fenuron	3-phenyl-1,1-dimethylurea	herbicide
ferbam	ferric dimethyldithiocarbamate	fungicide
Fumarin	3(a-acetonylfurfuryl)-4-hydroxycoumarin	rodenticide
Fumazone	1,2-dibromo-3-chloropropane	soil fumigant, nematocide
Haloxon	0,0-di-(2-chloroethyl)-0-3-chloro-4-methyl-coumarin-7-yl) phosphate	anthelmintic
heptachlor	1,4,5,6,7,8,8-heptachloro-3a,3,7,7a-tetrahydro-4,7-endo-methanoindene	insecticide
hydrogen cyanide	hydrocyanic acid	insect fumigant
Kepone	decachlorooctahydro-1,3,4-metheno-2H-cyclobuta(cd)pentalene-2-one	insecticide
lead arsenate	diplumbic hydrogen arsenate	insecticide, fungicide
leptophos	0-(4-bromo-2,5 dichlorophenyl)-0-methylphenylphosphonothioate	insecticide
lime sulfur	30% calcium polysulfide and various small amounts of calcium thiosulfate plus water and free sulfur	acaricide, fungicide, insecticide
lindane	gamma isomer of 1,2,3,4,5,6-hexachlorocyclohexane of 99%	insecticide
linuran	3-(3,4-dichlorophenyl)-1-methoxy-1 methylurea	herbicide
malathion	S-[1,2-bis(ethoxycarbonyl) ethyl] 0,0-dimethyl phosphorodithioate	insecticide
maneb	manganese ethylene bisdithiocarbamate	fungicide
MCPA	4-chloro-2-methyl-phenoxyacetic acid	herbicide
MCPB	4-chloro-2-methylphenoxy butyric acid	herbicide
MCPP	2-(4,chloro-2-methyl-phenoxy) propionic acid	herbicide
Merphos	tributyl phosphorotrithioite	defoliant
metaldehyde	metaldehyde	insecticide
metalkamate	mixture of m-(ethylpropyl) phenyl methylcarbamate and m-(1-methylbutyl) phenyl carbamate in approximate ratio of 1:3	insecticide
methomyl	S-methyl-*N*-((methyl carbamoyl) oxy) thioacetimidate	insecticide, nematocide
methoxychlor	1,1,1-trichloro-2,2-bis (*p*-methoxyphenol) ethane	insecticide
methyl bromide	bromomethane	fumigant
methyl chloride	chloromethane	aerosol propellent
methyl formate	methyl formate	insect fumigant
methyl parathion	0,0-dimethyl 0-*p*-nitrophenyl phosphorothioate	insecticide
Methyl Trithion	S-[[(*p*-chlorophenyl) thio] methyl] 0,0-dimethyl phosphorodithioate	insecticide
mevinphos	methyl 3-hydroxy-alpha-crotonate dimethyl phosphate	insecticide
mipafox	*N,N′*-diisopropylphosphorodiamidicfluoride	insecticide
mirex	dodecachlorooctahydro-1,3,4-metheno-2H-cyclobuta[Cd] pentalene	insecticide
monuron	3-(*p*-chlorophenyl)-1,1-dimethylurea	herbicide
Morestan	6-methyl-2-oxo-1,3-dithio(4,5-b)quinoxaline	acaricide, fungicide
MSMA	monosodium methanearsonate	herbicide
nabam	disodium ethylene bisdithiocarbamate	fungicide
naled	1,2-dibromo-2,2-dichloroethyl dimethyl phosphate	insecticide
naphthalene	naphthalene	insecticide

GLOSSARY: COMMON PESTICIDES *(cont.)*

COMMON NAME	CHEMICAL NAME	MAIN USES
neburon	3-(3,4-dichlorophenyl)-1-methyl-1-*n*-butylurea	herbicide
Nemacide	0-(2,4-dichlorophenyl)-0,0-diethyl ester of phosphorothionic acid	insecticide
nicotine	1-methyl-2-(1 pyridyl)pyrrolidine	insecticide
ovex	*p*-chlorophenyl *p*-chlorobenzene-sulfonate	insecticide
paradichlorobenzene	*p*-dichlorobenzene	insect fumigant
paraquat	1,1′-dimethyl-4-4′dipyridylium cation	herbicide
parathion	0,0-diethyl-0-*p*-nitrophenyl phosphorothioate	acaricide, insecticide
paris green	copper acetoarsenite	insecticide
Patoran	4-(4-bromophenyl)-1-methyl-1′-methoxyurea	herbicide
pentachlorophenol	pentachlorophenol	herbicide, wood preservative, molluscicide
Perthane	1,1-dichloro-2,2-bis (*p*-ethylphenyl) ethane	insecticide
petroleum oils		acaricide, insecticide, herbicide
phorate	0,0-diethyl S-[(ethylthio)methyl] phosphorodithioate	insecticide
phosphamidon	2-chloro-2-diethylcarbamoyl-1-methylvinyl dimethyl phosphate	insecticide
pindone	2-pinaloyl-1,3-indandione	rodenticide, insecticide
piperonyl butoxide	butyl carbitol (6-propyl piperonyl)ether	insecticide synergist
Pival	2-pivalyl-1,3 indandione	rodenticide
PMA	phenylmercuric acetate	fungicide, herbicide
propachlor	2-chloro-*N*-isopropylacetanilide	herbicide
propanil	3′,4′-dichloropionanilide	herbicide
propylene dichloride	1,2-dichloropropane	fungicide, herbicide, insecticide, nematocide, soil fumigant
propylene oxide	propylene oxide	insecticide synergist
pyrazon	5-amino-4-chloro-2-phenyl-3 (2H) pyriadazione	herbicide
pyrethrins	the active insectidicial constituents of pyrethrum	insecticide
pyrethrum	dalmation insect flowers	insecticide
red squill	inner bulb scales of *Urquinea maritima*	rodenticide
ronnel	0,0-dimethyl 0-(2,4,5-trichlorophenyl)-phosphorothioate	insecticide
rotenone	the primary active compound of derris and cube roots	insecticide
Ruelene	4-tert-butyl-2-chlorophenyl methyl methylphosphoramidate	insecticide
ryania	powdered stemwood of *Ryania speciosa*	insecticide
sabadilla	ground seeds of sabadilla containing veratrine, a complex mixture of alkaloids	insecticide
sarin	isopropylmethyl phosphonofluoridate	nerve gas
Silvex	2-(2,4,5-trichlorophenoxy)propionic acid	herbicide
Simazine	2-chloro-4,6-bis(ethylamino)-5-triazine	herbicide
Smithion	0,0-dimethyl 0-(4-nitro-m-tolyl) phosphorothioate	insecticide, space fumigant
sodium arsenite	sodium meta-arsenite	herbicide, insecticide, poison bait ingredient
sodium chlorate	sodium chlorate	herbicide (desiccant)
sodium fluoroacetate	sodium monofluoroacetate	rodenticide
sodium *N*-methyldithiocarbamate	sodium *N*-methyldithiocarbamate	fungicide, herbicide, nematocide
Strobane	terpene polychlorinates	insecticide
strychnine	nux vomica alkaloid	rodenticide; used in poison baits for birds, moles and other rodents
sulfur (brimstone)	sulfur	acaricide, fungicide
sulfuryl fluoride	sulfuryl fluoride	insecticide, fumigant
2,4,5-T	2,4,5-trichlorophenoxyacetic acid	herbicide
tabun	dimethylamidoethoxyphosphoryl cyanide	nerve gas
tartar emetic	antimony potassium tartrate	herbicide
2,3,6-TBA	2,3,6-trichlorobenzoic acid	herbicide
TCA	sodium trichloroacetate	herbicide

GLOSSARY: COMMON PESTICIDES *(cont.)*

COMMON NAME	CHEMICAL NAME	MAIN USES
TCPE	2,4,5-trichlorophenoxyethanol	herbicide
TDE (DDD)	2,2-bis (*p*-chlorophenyl)-,1-dichloroethane	insecticide
Telodrin	isobornyl thiocyanoacetate	insecticide
telone	mixed dichloropropenes	insecticide
Temik	2-methyl-2(methylthio)propionaldehyde 0-(methyl carbamoyl)oxime	insecticide, acaricide, nematocide
TEPP	tetraethyl pyrophosphate	insecticide
terbacil	3-tert-butyl-5-chloro-6-methyluracil	herbicide
tetradifon	*p*-chlorophenyl 2,4,5-trichlorophenyl sulfone	insecticide
thallium sulfate	thallium sulfate	insecticide, rodenticide
thiram	tetramethylthiuram disulfide	fungicide, animal repellent
TME	0,0,S-trimethyl phosphorodithioate	by-product of malathion
toxaphene	chlorinated camphene	insecticide
trichlorfon	0,0-dimethyl (1-hydroxy-2,2,2-trichloro-ethyl) phosphonate	systemic insecticide
2,4,5-trichlorophenol	sodium 2,4,5-trichlorophenate	fungicide
trifluralin	a,a,a-trifluoro-2,6-dinitro-*N*,*N*-dipropyl-*p*-toluidine	herbicide
Valone	2-isovaleryl-1,3 indandione	rodenticide
warfarin	3-(1′-phenyl-2′-acetylethyl)-4-hydroxycoumarin	rodenticide
white arsenic	arsenic trioxide	animal dip, herbicide, ingredient in insect baits
zectran	4-dimethylamino-3,5-xylyl *N*-methylcarbamate	pesticide for control of snails and slugs
zinc white	zinc oxide	ingredient in animal remedies
zineb	zinc ethylene bisdithiocarbamate	fungicide
Zinophos	0,0-diethyl 0-2-pyrazinyl phosphorothioate	insecticide, fungicide, nematocide
Ziram	zinc dimethyldithiocarbamate	fungicide

REFERENCES

1. Ahlborg, U. G., Lindgren, J. E., and Mercier, M.: Metabolism of pentachlorophenol, Arch. Toxicol. (Berl.) 32:271, 1974.
2. Aldridge, W. N., Bares, J. M., and Johnson, M. K.: Studies on delayed neurotoxicity produced by some organophosphorus compounds, Ann. N.Y. Acad. Sci. 160:314, 1969.
3. Aldridge, W. N., and Johnson, M. K.: Side effects of organophosphorus compounds: Delayed neurotoxicity, Bull. WHO 44:259, 1971.
4. Arsenic, medical and biological effects on environmental pollutants. National Academy of Sciences, Washington, D.C., pp.216–223, 1977.
5. Arterberry, J. D., et al.: Exposure to parathion—measure by blood cholinesterase level and urinary *p*-nitrophenol excretion, Arch. Environ. Health 3:476, 1961.
6. Axelson, O., and Sundell, L.: Herbicide exposure, mortality and tumor incidence. An epidemiological investigation on Swedish railroad workers, Scand. J. Work Environ. Health 11:21, 1974.
7. Baader, E. W., and Bauer, H. J.: Industrial intoxication due to pentachlorophenol, Ind. Med. Surg. 20:286, 1951.
8. Baker, E. L., et al.: Epidemic malathion poisoning in Pakistan malaria workers, Lancet 1:31, 1978.
9. Berg, G. L. (ed.): *Farm Chemicals Handbook* (Willoughby, Ohio: Meister Publishing Company, 1977).
10. Bergner, H., et al.: Industrial pentachlorophenol poisoning in Winnipeg, Can. Med. Assoc. J. 92:448, 1965.
11. Best, E. M., Jr., and Murray, B. L.: Observations on workers exposed to Sevin insecticide: A preliminary report, J. Occup. Med. 10:507, 1962.
12. Bidstrup, P. L., Bonnel, J. A., and Beckett, A. G.: Paralysis following poisoning by a new

organic phosphorus insecticide (mipafox), Br. Med. J. 1:1068, 1953.

13. Bleiberg, J., Wallen, M., Brodkin, R., and Applebaum, I. L.: Industrially acquired porphyria, Arch. Dermatol. 89:793, 1964.
14. Brown, V. H. K., Hunter, C. G., and Richardson, A.: A blood test diagnostic exposure to aldrin and dieldrin, Br. J. Ind. Med. 21:283, 1964.
15. Brown, V. K.: Solubility and solvent effects as rate-determining factors in the acute percutaneous toxicities of pesticides, Soc. Chem. Ind. Monogr. 29:93, 1968.
16. Bullivant, C. M.: Accidental poisoning by paraquat: Report of two cases in man, Br. Med. J. 1:1272, 1966.
17. Casida, J. E. (ed.): *Pyrethrum—the Natural Insecticide* (New York: Academic Press, 1973), pp. 123–142.
18. Cavanaugh, J. B.: Peripheral neuropathy caused by chemical agents, Crit. Rev. Toxicol. 2:365, 1973.
19. Clark, D. G., et al.: The toxicity of paraquat, Br. J. Ind. Med. 23:126, 1966.
20. Coble, Y., et al.: Acute endrin poisoning, JAMA 202:153, 1967.
21. Culver, D., et al.: Studies of human exposure during aerosol application of malathion and chlorthion, A.M.A. Arch. Ind. Hyg. 13:37, 1956.
22. Czeizel, E., and Király, J.: Chromosome Examinations in Workers Producing Klorinol and Buvinol, in Bánki, L. (ed.), *The Development of a Pesticide as a Complex Scientific Task* (Budapest: Medicina, 1976), pp. 239–256.
23. Davies, J. E., et al.: An epidemiologic application of the study of DDE levels in whole blood, Am. J. Public Health 59:435, 1969.
24 Derbes, V. J., et al.: Fatal chlordane poisoning, JAMA 158:1367, 1955.
25. Drenth, H. J., et al.: Neuromuscular function in agricultural workers using pesticides, Arch. Environ. Health 25:395, 1972.
26. Duffy, F. H.: Long-term effects of pesticides on the brain—a new finding. Annual Meeting of the Society for Occupational & Environmental Health, December 10–13, 1978, Washington, D.C.
27. Edmundson, W. F., and Davies, J. E.: Occupational dermatitis from naled—a clinical report, Arch. Environ. Health 15:89, 1967.
28. Federal Insecticide, Fungicide and Rodenticide Act ("Federal Environmental Pesticide Control Act of 1972"); amended, 1978, United States Environmental Protection Agency, Office of Pesticide Control Programs, Washington, D. C.
29. Firestone, D.: The 2,3,7,8-tetrachlorodibenzo-para-dioxin problem: A review, in Ramel, C. (ed.), Chlorinated Phenoxy Acids and Their Dioxins: Mode of Action, Health Risks and Environmental Effects, Ecol. Bull. 27 (Stockholm) pp. 39–52, 1977.
30. Flint, A.: Cimetidine and oral anticoagulants, Br. Med. J. 2:1367, 1978.
31. Fristedt, B., and Sterner, N.: Warfarin intoxication from cutaneous absorption, Arch. Environ, Health 11:205, 1965.
32. Gage, J. C.: Toxicity of paraquat and diquat aerosols generated by a size-selective cyclone: Effect of particle size distribution, Br. J. Ind. Med. 25:304, 1968.
33. Glauser, S. C.: Early reversible health effects from pentachlorophenol. Annual Meeting of the Society for Occupational & Environmental Health, December 10–13, 1978, Washington, D. C.
34. Golz, H.H.: Controlled human exposures to malathion aerosols, A.M.A. Arch. Ind. Hyg. 19:516, 1959.
35. Goodman, L. S., and Gilman, A.: *The Pharmacological Basis of Therapeutics* (5th ed.; New York: The Macmillan Publishing Company, 1975), pp. 359–361, 365–366.
36. Gordon, M., et al.: Recommendation for prevention of flight crashes resulting from factors impairing performance of agricultural spray pilots. An outline statement of medical policy. Civil Aviation Authority, Ministry of Transportation, Israel, 1978.
37. Gosalvez, M., and Merchan, J.: Induction of rat mammary adenomas with the respiratory inhibitory rotenone, Cancer Res. 33:3047, 1973.
38. Gosselin, R. E., Hodge, H. C., Smith, R. P., and Gleason, M. N.: *Clinical Toxicology of Commercial Products* (4th ed.; Baltimore: Williams & Wilkins, 1976), Sect. II, pp. 225–227.
39. Gosselin, R. E., et al.: *Clinical Toxicology of Commercial Products* (4th ed.; Baltimore: Williams & Wilkins, 1976), Sect. III, pp. 168–171.
40. Greenburg, J. O.: The neurological effects of methyl bromide poisoning, Ind. Med. 40:27, 1971.
41. Gribetz, B., et al.: Heat stress exposure of aerial spraying, Aviat. Space Environ. Med. 5 (no. 1), Jan. 1980.
42. Hardell, L., and Sandström, A.: Case con-

trol study: Soft tissue sarcomas and exposure to phenoxyacetic acids or chlorophenols. Annual Meeting of the Society for Occupational & Environmental Health, December 10–13, 1978, Washington, D. C.

43. Harger, P. N., and Spolyar, L. W.: Toxicity of phosphine, with a possible fatality from this poison, A. M. A. Arch. Ind. Hyg. 18:497, 1958.
44. Harrisson, J. W. E., et al.: Acute poisoning with sodium fluoroacetate (Compound 1080), JAMA 149:1520, 1952.
45. Harrisson, J. W. E., et al.: Fluoroacetate (1080) poisoning, Ind. Med. Surg. 21:440, 1952.
46. Hayes, W. J., Jr.: Clinical Handbook on Economic Poisons. Public Health Service Publication No. 476, Government Printing Office, Washington, D. C., pp. 47–50, 71–73, 1963.
47. Hayes, W. J., Jr.: Studies on exposure during the use of anticholinesterase pesticides, Bull. WHO 44:277, 1971.
48. Hayes, W. J., Jr.: *Toxicology of Pesticides* (Baltimore: Williams & Wilkins, 1975).
49. Hine, C. H.: Methyl bromide poisoning, J. Occup. Med. 11:1, 1969.
50. Hodge, H. C., et al.: Acute and short-term oral toxicity tests of ferric dimethyldithiocarbamate (ferbam) and zinc dimethyldithiocarbamate (ziram), J. Am. Pharm. Assoc. 41:662, 1952.
51 Holmes, J. H., et al.: Short-term toxicity of mevinphos in man, Arch. Environ. Health 29:84, 1974.
52. Holvey, D. N. (ed.): *The Merck Manual of Diagnosis and Therapy* (12th ed; Rahway, N. J.: Merck & Co., Inc., 1972), p. 1627.
53. Howard, J. K., East, N. J., and Chaney, J. L.: Plasma cholinesterase activity in early pregnancy, Arch. Environ. Health 33: 2775, 1978.
54. International Agency for Research on Cancer: IARC Monographs on the Evaluation of the Carcinogenic Risk of Chemicals to Man. Vol. 5, Some Organochlorine Pesticides, Lyon, France, pp. 90–124, 1974.
55. International Agency for Research on Cancer: IARC Monographs on the Evaluation of the Carcinogenic Risk of Chemicals to Man. Vol. 5, Some Organochlorine Pesticides, Lyon, France, pp. 25–38, 125–156, 1974.
56. Ishikawa, S.: Chronic optico-neuropathy due to environmental exposure of organophosphate pesticides (Saku disease). Clinical and experimental study, Nippon Ganka Gakkai Zasshi 77:1835, 1973.
57. Ishikawa, S.: Eye injury by organic phosphorus insecticides (preliminary report), J. Ophthalmol. 15:60, 1971.
58. Ishikawa, S.: Optico-autonomic-peripheral Neuropathy due to Chronic Organophosphate Pesticide Intoxication, in *Proceedings of 22d International Congress on Ophthalmology* (Paris: Masson, 1976).
59. Jager, K. W.: *Aldrin, Dieldrin, Endrin and Telodrin—An Epidemiological and Toxicological Study of Long-Term Occupational Exposure* (Amsterdam: Elsevier Publishing Company, 1970), pp. 78–87, 217–218, 225–234.
60. Jager, K. W.: Organophosphate exposure from industrial usage, electroneuromyography in occupational medical supervision of exposed workers. Paper presented at the E.P.A. seminar on "Pesticide induced delayed neurotoxicity," February 19–20, 1976.
61 Jager, K. W., Roberts, D. V., and Wilson, A.: Neuromuscular function in pesticide workers, Br. J. Ind. Med. 27:273, 1970.
62. Jirásek, L., et al.: Acne chlorina, porphyria cutanea tarda and other manifestations of general intoxication during the manufacture of herbicides, I. Cesk. Dermatol. 49:145, 1974.
63. Johnson, M. K.: A phosphorylation site in brain and the delayed neurotoxic effect of some organophosphorus compounds, Biochem. J. 111:487, 1969.
64. Johnson, M. K.: Organophosphorus esters causing delayed neurotoxic effect. Mechanism of action and structure/activity studies, Arch. Toxicol. (Berl.) 34:259, 1975.
65. Johnson, M. K.: The delayed neuropathy caused by some organophosphorus esters: Mechanism and challenge, Crit. Rev. Toxicol. 3:289, 1975.
66. Jones, A. T., et al.: Environmental and clinical aspects of bulk wheat fumigation with aluminum phosphide, Am. Ind. Hyg. Assoc. J. 25:376, 1964.
67. Kantantzis, G., et al.: Poisoning in industrial workers by the insecticide aldrin, Br. J. Ind. Med. 21:46, 1964.
68. Kantarjian, A. D., and Shaheen, A. S.: Methyl bromide poisoning with nervous system manifestations resembling polyneuropathy, Neurology 13:1054, 1963.
69. Kolmodin-Hedman, B., et al.: Yskesmedicinsk kontrol av berörd personal vid lindanresp DDT- behandling av barrträdsplantor, En jämförelse, Arbete och Hälsa: 7, Arbetarskyddsstyrelsen, 17184 Solna, Sweden, 1977.

69a. Kolmodin-Hedman, B., Erne, K., Håkansson, M., and Engqvist, A.: Kontrol av yrkesmässig exponering för fenoxisyror (2,4-D and 2,4,5-T). Arbete och Hälsa: 17, Arbetarskyddsverket, Stockholm, 1979.

70. Kolmodin-Hedman, B., Ny, V., Lidblom, A., and Swensson, A.: Försöksverksamhet med lindanbehandling av tall- och granplantor, Hösten, 1974 - Yrkeshygieniska Aspekter. Arbetarskyddsstyrelsen, Fack, 100 27 Stockholm. Arbete och Hälsa: 5, 1975.

71. Kolmodin-Hedman, B., Palmer, L., Götel, P., and Skerfving, S.: Plasma levels of lindane, p,ṕ-DDE and p,ṕ-DDT in occupationally exposed persons in Sweden, Work Environ. Health 10:100, 1973.

72. Laws, E. R., Jr., et al.: Long-term occupational exposure to DDT. Effect on the human liver, Arch. Environ. Health 27:318, 1973.

73. Laws, E. R., Jr., et al.: Men with intensive occupational exposure to DDT—a clinical and chemical study, Arch. Environ. Health 15:766, 1967.

74. Lindgren, S., Collste, P., Norlander, B., and Sjöqvist, F.: Gas chromatographic assessment of the reproducibility of phenazone plasma half-lives in young healthy volunteers, Eur. J. Clin. Pharmacol. 7:381, 1974.

75. Lores, E. M., Bradway, D. E., and Moseman, R. F.: Organophosphorus pesticide poisoning in humans: Determination of residues and metabolites in tissues and urine, Arch. Environ. Health 33:270, 1978.

76. Maibach, H. I., Feldmann, R. J., Milby, T. H., and Serat, W. F.: Regional variation in percutaneous penetration in man, Arch. Environ. Health 23:208, 1971.

77. May, G.: Chloracne from the accidental production of tetrachlorodibenzodiozin, Br. J. Ind. Med. 30:276, 1973.

78. McClosky, W. T., and Smith, M. I.: Studies on the pharmacologic action and the pathology of alphanaphthylthiourea (ANTU), J. Pharmacol., Public Health Reports 60:1101, 1945.

79. McCollister, D. D., et al.: Toxicological studies of O-O-dimethyl-O-(2,4,5-trichlorophenyl) phosphorothioate (Ronnel) in laboratory animals, Agricultural and Food Chemistry 7:689, 1959.

80. McGee, L. C.: Accidental poisoning by taxaphene, JAMA 149:1124, 1952.

81. Menz, M., et al.: Long-term exposure of factory workers to dichlorvos (DDVP) insecticide, Arch. Environ. Health 28:72, 1974.

82. Mestitzova, M.: On reproduction studies and the occurrence of cataracts in rats after long-term feeding of the insecticide heptachlor, Experientia 23:42, 1967.

83. Michel, H. O.: An electrometric method for the determination of red blood cell and plasma cholinesterase activity, J. Lab. Clin. Med. 34:1564, 1949.

84. Milby, T. H.: Does chronic exposure to organophosphate insecticide cause eye complications?, JAMA 236:1891, 1976.

85. Milby, T. H.: Prevention and management of organophosphate poisoning, JAMA 216:2131, 1971.

86. Morgan, D. P.: Recognition and management of pesticide poisoning. U. S. Environmental Protection Agency Office of Pesticide Programs, Washington, D. C., August, 1977.

87. Morse, D. L., Baker, E. L., and Landrigan, P. J.: Cut flowers: A potential pesticide hazard, Am. J. Public Health 69:1, 1969.

87a. National Agricultural Chemicals Association: Pre-Fire Planning and Guidelines for Handling Agricultural Chemical Fires, 1979.

88. National Institute of Occupational Safety and Health: Aldrin/Dieldrin—Special Occupational Hazard Review, NIOSH, Dept. of Health, Education, and Welfare, PHS, Center for Disease Control, 4676 Columbia Parkway, Cincinnati, Ohio, 1978.

89. National Institute of Occupational Safety and Health: Agricultural Chemicals and Pesticides—a subfile of the Registry of Toxic Effects, 1977.

90. National Institute of Occupational Safety and Health. Criteria for a recommended standard: Occupational Exposure to Inorganic Arsenic. U.S. Dept. of Health, Education, and Welfare, Washington, D.C., 105 p., 1973.

91. National Institute of Occupational Safety and Health. Criteria for a recommended standard: Occupational Exposure to Carbaryl. U.S. Department of Health, Education, and Welfare, Washington, D.C., 1976.

92. National Institute of Occupational Safety and Health. Criteria for a recommended standard: Occupational Exposure during the Manufacture and Formulation of Pesticides. U.S. Dept. of Health, Education, and Welfare (NIOSH), No. 78-174, 1978.

93. National Institute of Occupational Safety and Health. Health and Safety Guide for Pesticide Formulation. U.S. Dept. of Health, Education, and Welfare, PHS, Center for Disease Control, Division of

Technical Services, Cincinnati, Ohio, May, 1977.

94. National Institute of Occupational Safety and Health. Criteria for a recommended standard: Occupational Exposure to Malathion. U.S. Dept. Of Health, Education, and Welfare, Washington, D. C., 1976.

95. National Institute of Occupational Safety and Health. Criteria for a recommended standard: Occupational Exposure to Methyl Parathion. U.S. Dept. of Health, Education, and Welfare, Washington, D.C., 1976.

96. National Institute of Occupational Safety and Health. Criteria for a recommended standard: Occupational Exposure to Parathion. U.S. Dept. of Health, Education, and Welfare, Washington, D.C., 1976.

97. National Institute of Occupational Safety and Health. Pesticide Residue Hazards to Farm Workers. Proceedings of a Workshop, 1976.

98. Negberbon, W. O. (ed.): *Handbook of Toxicology* (Philadelphia: W. B. Saunders Company, 1957), Vol. III, p. 665.

99. Nishimura, H., and Nakai, K.: Developmental anomalies in off-spring of pregnant mice treated with nicotine, Science 127: 877, 1958.

100. Olishifski, J. B. (ed.): Fundamentals of Industrial Hygiene, 2d ed. National Safety Council, Chicago, Ill., 1979.

101. Ottolenghi, A. D., et al.: Teratogenic effects of aldrin, dieldrin and endrin in hamsters and mice, Teratology 9:11, 1974.

102. Paraquat Poisoning—A Physician's Guide. Chevron Environmental Health Center, San Francisco, California, 1975.

103. Pasi, A.: *The Toxicology of Paraquat, Diquat and Morfamquat* (Bern, Stuttgart, Vienna: Hans Huber Publishers, 1978).

104. Peaslee, C. H.: Spotlight on paraquat and marijuana, Laboratory Medicine for Practicing Physicians, pp. 29–31, July/August, 1978.

105. Plestina, R., and Piukovic-Plestina, M.: Effect of anticholinesterase pesticides on the eye and vision, CRC Crit. Rev. Toxicol. pp. 1–23, December, 1978.

106. Quinby, G. E., and Doornink, G. M.: Tetraethylpyrophosphate poisoning following airplane dusting, JAMA 191:95, 1965.

107. Ramel, C. (ed.): Chlorinated phenoxy acids and their dioxins. Mode of action, health risks and environmental effects. Report from a conference arranged by the Royal Swedish Academy of Sciences, Stockholm, Sweden, February 7–9, 1977.

108. Richeson, E. M.: Thallium poisoning, Arch. Neurol. 26:456, 1972.

109. Rider, J. A., Hodges, J. L., Jr., Swader, J., and Wiggins, A. D.: Plasma and red blood cell cholinesterase in 800 "healthy" blood donors, J. Lab. Clin. Med. 50:376, 1957.

110. Roan, C. C., Morgan, D. P., Cook, N., and Paschal, E. H.: Blood cholinesterases, serum parathion concentrations and urine P-nitrophenol concentrations in exposed individuals, Bull. Environ. Contam. Toxicol. 4:382, 1969.

111. Robens, J. F.: Teratologic studies of carbaryl, diazinon, norea, disulfiram, and thiram in small laboratory animals, Toxicol. Appl. Pharmacol. 15:152, 1969.

112. Roberts, D. V.: A longitudinal electromyographic study of six men occupationally exposed to organophosphorus compounds, Int. Arch. Occup. Environ. Health 38:221, 1977.

113. Roberts, D. V.: E.M.G. voltage and motor nerve conduction velocity in organophosphorus pesticide factory workers, Int. Arch. Occup. Environ. Health 36:267, 1976.

114. Roberts, D. V.: Theoretical and practical consequences of the use of organophosphorus compounds in industry, J. Soc. Occup. Med. 29:15, 1979.

115. Roll, R.: Tetratologische untersuchungen mit thiram (TMTD) an zwei Mausestammen, Arch. Toxikol. 27:173, 1971.

116. Shelly, W. B.: Golf-course dermatitis due to thiram fungicide, JAMA 188:415, 1964.

117. Silver, A.: A Biology of Cholinesterases, in Neuberger, A., and Tatum, E. L. (eds.), *Frontiers of Biology*, North-Holland Research Monographs (Amsterdam: North-Holland, 1974), Vol. 36.

118. Singh, A. R., et al.: Teratogenicity of phthalate esters in rats, J. Pharm. Sci. 61:51, 1972.

119. Spiotta, E. J.: Aldrin poisoning in man, A.M.A. Arch. Ind. Hyg. 4:560, 1951.

120. Stålberg, E., et al.: Effects of occupational exposure to organophosphorus insecticides on neuromuscular function, Scand. J. Work Environ. Health 4:255, 1978.

121. Surveillance Summary—Paraquat Contamination of Marijuana—United States. Center for Disease Control, Morbidity and Mortality Weekly Report 28:8, March 2, 1979.

122. Swan, A. A. B.: Exposure of spray operators to paraquat, Br. J. Ind. Med. 26:322, 1969.

123. Taxay, E. P.: Vikane inhalation, J. Occup. Med. 8:425, 1966.

124. Technical Background Information Report

on Carcinogenesis Bioassay of Toxaphene. National Institutes of Health, National Cancer Institute, Bethesda, Maryland, March 16, 1979.

125. Thiess, A. M., and Goldmann, P.: Über das Trichlorophenol - Dioxin - Ungall - geschehen in BASF AG vom 13, November, 1953, in Vortrag, auf dem IV. Medichem-Kongress, Haifa, 1977.

126. Vandekar, M., and Wilford, K.: The effect of cholinesterase activity of storage of undiluted whole blood sampled from men exposed to 7-isopropoxyphenyl methylcarbamate (OMS-33) Bull. WHO 40:91, 1969.

127. Vaziri, N. D., et al.: Nephrotoxicity of paraquat in man, Arch. Intern. Med. 139:2, 1979.

128. Verberk, M. M., Rooyakkers-Beemster, M., De Vlieger, M., and Van Vliet, A. G. M.: Bromine in blood, EEG and transaminases in methyl bromide workers, Br. J. Ind. Med. 36:59, 1979.

129. Verberk, M. M., and Salle, H. J. A.: Effects on nervous function in volunteers ingesting mevinphos for one month, Toxicol. Appl. Phamacol. 42:351, 1977.

130. Warraki, S.: Respiratory hazards of chlorinated camphene, Arch. Environ. Health 7:137, 1963.

131. Wills, J. H.: Percutaneous Absorption, in Montagna, W., Van Scott, J., and Stoughton, R. B. (eds.), *Pharmacology and the Skin* (New York: Appleton-Century-Crofts, 1972), Chap. 12, pp. 169–176.

132. Wolfe, H. R., Durham, W. F., and Armstrong, J. F.: Urinary excretion of insecticide metabolites: Excretion of paranitrophenol and DDA as indicators of exposure to parathion and DDT, Arch. Environ. Health 21:711, 1970.

133. Wolfsie, J. H., and Winter, G. D.: Statistical analysis of normal human red blood cell and plasma cholinesterase activity values, Am. Ind. Hyg. Assoc. J. 6:43, 1952.

134. Xintaras, C., et al.: NIOSH Survey of Velsicol Pesticide Workers—Occupational Exposure to Leptophos and Other Chemicals. DHEW (NIOSH) Publication No. 78 - 136, 1977.

135. Yamamura, Y.: *n*-Hexane polyneuropathy, Folia Psychiatr. Neurol. Jpn. 23:45, 1969.

136. Zenz, C.: The Occupational Physician, in Olishifski, J. B. (ed.), *Fundamentals of Industrial Hygiene* (Chicago: National Safety Council, 1979), pp. 827–860.

14 / Selected Potentially Hazardous Substances Commonly Encountered

CARL ZENZ, M.D., ERIC P. KINDWALL, M.D.,
KENNETH BRIDBORD, M.D., and FRANK L. MITCHELL, D.O.

WITH EXPANDING USES of new materials such as are found in adhesives, coatings (paints and finishes), a multitude of plastics and other synthetic entities, more workers are potentially exposed, at various levels of risk, often unintentionally. Those concerned with occupational health practices (preventive programs) should and must be aware of the more commonly encountered substances and have some knowledge of what is going on in the factories near them. The immense quantities of certain hazardous materials used are awesome. Indeed, some chemicals being produced and used for other processes range into and beyond millions to billions of kilograms each year; e.g., phosgene, used as an intermediate to make isocyanates, has an annual production in the United States in excess of 300 million kg; sodium hydroxide produced each year in the United States is more than 10 billion kg. In the smaller workshops particularly, points of concern may be found in processing and formulating, packaging, storage, shipping, reformulating, applications, maintenance work, laboratory testing, etc. Often overlooked is that these varied activities occur over geographically widely scattered areas and mainly involve small numbers or groups of workers. Despite technologic advances in the highly industrialized countries, some occupational exposures continue and are troublesome: exposures to carbon monoxide, hydrogen sulfide, other irritating agents such as acids and caustics, oxides of nitrogen, etc., all found in varying amounts in certain occupational settings. New methods of treatment are discussed and the principles and practices described in this chapter are applicable to many other occupational exposures.

Terms used to describe "exposure limits" are outlined in Table 14–1. The American Conference of Governmental Industrial Hygienists (ACGIH) publishes annually the threshold limit values for chemical substances and physical agents in the working environment and also prepares and publishes at appropriate intervals documentation of these values, which should be consulted for a better understanding of the TLVs.

The Appendix at the end of the book summarizes significant information such as health effect or effects that were considered in the derivation of the NIOSH reports and criteria documents. It should be noted that this summary is not intended to provide details of these publications, and reference to

Appreciation for assistance with this chapter is given Jay P. Bartlett, M.D., Louis S. Beliczky, M.S., Herbert E. Christensen, Sc.D., Ernest M. Dixon, M.D., Eugene H. Kremer, III, M.D., Robert N. Ligo, M.D., Eric Ortman, M.D., John A. Peterson, M.D., Donald M. Rowe, M.D., Joseph A. Solomayer, M.D., Shiro Tanaka, M.D. and Mary Ann Woodbury, M.C.H.

TABLE 14–1.—TERMS USED TO DESCRIBE OCCUPATIONAL EXPOSURE LIMITS (PPM)

MAC	Maximal Acceptable Concentration. The American National Standards distinguishes three different MACs*
MAC-TWA	Maximal Acceptable Concentration Time-Weighted Average is the time-weighted average concentration for protection of health assuming an 8-hour workday. Concentrations are restricted to be within the MAC-peak and Mac-ceiling concentrations described below
MAC-peak	Maximal Acceptable Concentration for Peaks in the highest concentration acceptable within a given time interval during an 8-hour workday. (Formerly Maximal Allowable Concentration)
MAC-ceiling	Maximal Acceptable Concentration for Ceiling is the highest concentration acceptable if the time-weighted average is within the MAC-TWA value
PEL	Permissible Exposure Limit. An employee's exposure to any material,* the name of which is not preceded by "C,"† in any 8-hour work shift of a 40-hour workweek shall not exceed the 8-hour time-weighted average given for that material
C	Ceiling. An employee's exposure to any material,†,‡ the name of which is preceded by a "C," shall at no time exceed the value given for that material. Acceptable ceiling concentrations as described in MAC-ceiling except for a time period and up to a concentration not exceeding the MAC-peak
TLV	Threshold Limit Values refer to time-weighted concentrations for a 7- or 8-hour workday and 40-hour workweek(§)
STEL	Short-Term Exposure Limit. Refers to the maximal concentration to which workers can be exposed in a 15-minute period(‖)

*American National Standards Institute, Inc., 143 Broadway, New York, New York 10018.
†"C" refers to ceiling as described after PEL. Different ceiling terms apply, depending on which materials are cited.
‡Material refers to the substances in Tables of Standards as shown in 29CFE 1910.1000 and Fed. Reg. 36, No. 105, May 29, 1971.
(§)Threshold Limit Values for Airborne Contaminants, ACGIH, Cincinnati, Ohio, 1968.
(‖)Threshold Limit Values for Chemical Substances in Workroom Air, ACGIH, Cincinnati, Ohio, 1977.

the full documents is recommended for those requiring elements of a recommended standard, work practices, sampling, analytic methods, engineering control measures and complete references. These documents have been published after critically evaluating all known and available medical, biologic, engineering, chemical and trade data and any other information that may be relevant to recommending a standard. Included as part of the standard is a permissible exposure level; i.e., the concentration of a substance in the occupational environment that will not cause adverse effects in exposed persons. Historical reports and extent of occupational exposures always have been part of the criteria documents. Since 1976, the NIOSH has incorporated animal and human data, if available, on the effects of reproduction, carcinogenicity, mutagenicity and teratogenicity. Attempts are made to correlate these adverse reactions with exposures and effects, where possible. For detailed discussions on pertinent substances, refer to Chapters 3 and 13.

Acrylamide

$$CH_2 = CHCONH_2$$

Synonyms for acrylamide include propenamide, acrylic amide and akrylamid. The terms "acrylamide" and "acrylamide monomer" are used in this document interchangeably. The major application for monomeric acrylamide is in the production of polymers as polyacrylamides. Polyacrylamides are used for soil stabilization, gel chromatography, electrophoresis, papermaking strengtheners, clarification and treatment of potable water and foods. Approximately 30 million kg of acrylamide were produced in 1974 in the United States. The NIOSH estimates that approximately 20,000 workers in the United States are potentially exposed to acrylamide.

Toxic manifestations of exposure to acrylamide involve both localized and systemic effects. Localized effects include peeling and redness of the skin of the hands and less often of the feet, numbness of the lower limbs and excessive sweating of the feet and hands. The systemic effects due to acrylamide intoxication involve central and peripheral nervous system damage manifested primarily as ataxia, weak or absent reflexes, a positive Romberg sign and loss of vibration and position senses.

Since skin contact with the substance may result in localized or systemic effects, the NIOSH recommends that medical surveillance be made available to all employees working in an area where acrylamide is stored, produced, processed or otherwise used, except as an unintentional contaminant in other materials at a concentration of less than 1% by weight. The present federal standard is 0.3 mg/m^3 as a time-weighted average concentration for up to a 10-hour workday, 40-hour workweek.

REFERENCE

Acrylamide

1. National Institute for Occupational Safety and Health. A Recommended Standard for Occupational Exposure to Acrylamide. U.S. Dept. of Health, Education, and Welfare, PHS, Center for Disease Control, NIOSH, Cincinnati, Ohio, 1976.

Acrylonitrile

Acrylonitrile is an explosive, flammable liquid having a normal boiling point of 77° C and a vapor pressure of 80 mm (20° C). The chemical structure of acrylonitrile, $CH_2{=}CHCN$, resembles that of vinyl chloride. Synonyms for acrylonitrile include acrylon, carbacryl, cyanoethylene, fumigrain, 2-propenenitrile, VCN, ventox and vinyl cyanide.

Almost ³/₄ of a billion kg of acrylonitrile are manufactured annually in the United States by the reaction of propylene with ammonia and oxygen in the presence of a catalyst.

The major use of acrylonitrile is in the production of acrylic and modacrylic fibers by copolymerization with methyl acrylate, methyl methacrylate, vinyl acetate, vinyl chloride or vinylidene chloride. Acrylic fibers, marketed under various trade names, such as Acrilan, Creslan, Orlon and Zefran, are used in the manufacture of apparel, carpeting, blankets, draperies and upholstery. Some applications of modacrylic fibers are synthetic furs and hair wigs.

Other major uses of acrylonitrile are manufacture of acrylonitrile-butadiene-styrene (ABS) and styrene-acrylonitrile (SAN) resins (used to produce a variety of plastic products), nitrile elastomers and latexes and other chemicals (e.g., adiponitrile, acrylamide). Acrylonitrile is also used as a fumigant. The U.S. Food and Drug Administration recently has banned the use of an acrylonitrile resin for soft drink bottles.

The NIOSH estimates that 125,000 persons are potentially exposed to acrylonitrile in the workplace. The acute toxic effects of acrylonitrile are similar to those from cyanide poisoning. Toxic effects of acrylonitrile inhalation that have been noted in animals include damage to the central nervous system, lungs, liver and kidneys. Embryotoxic effects in mice have also been reported. However, more recent evidence of acrylonitrile's chronic toxicity has caused a reassessment of the hazard to workers of acrylonitrile. In April, 1977, the Manufacturing Chemists Association reported interim results of 2-year feeding and inhalation studies (conducted by the Dow Chemical Company) of acrylonitrile in laboratory rats. By both routes of administration, acrylonitrile caused the development of central nervous system tumors and Zymbal gland carcinomas; no such tumors were seen in control animals. Exposure to 80 ppm of acrylonitrile also revealed an increased incidence of mammary region masses.

A preliminary epidemiologic study conducted by the E. I. Du Pont de Nemours & Company, Inc. of a cohort of 470 acrylonitrile polymerization workers from the company's Camden, South Carolina textile fibers plant indicates an excess risk of lung and colon cancer among workers with potential acrylonitrile exposure. A total of 16 cancer cases occurred between 1969 and 1975 among the cohort first exposed between 1950 and 1955; only 5.8 cancer cases would have been expected, based on Du Pont Company rates (excluding the cohort). Although the epidemiologic findings are preliminary in nature and may not alone provide definitive evidence of the carcinogenicity of acrylonitrile in man, when considered in light of the laboratory experiments demonstrating carcinogenicity in rats, a serious suspicion is raised that acrylonitrile is a human carcinogen. Thus, the NIOSH believes that acrylonitrile must be handled in the workplace as a suspected human carcinogen.

The current Occupational Safety and Health Administration (OSHA) standard for occupational exposure to acrylonitrile is an 8-hour time-weighted average of 20 ppm. However, in light of the new human information generated by Du Pont, as well as the animal data provided by MCA, the NIOSH believes that it would be prudent to handle acrylonitrile in the workplace as if it were a human carcinogen.

REFERENCE

Acrylonitrile

1. Acrylonitrile. NIOSH, Current Intelligence Bulletin No. 18, Dept. of Health, Education, and Welfare, PHS, Center for Disease Control, 4676 Columbia Parkway, Cincinnati, Ohio, July, 1977.

Ammonia

Ammonia (NH_3) is a colorless gas and is one of the most widely used industrial chemicals, ranking fourth in volume of production after sulfuric acid, lime and oxygen. Production in the United States is about 15 million metric tons. The principal uses of ammonia are direct-application fertilizer—26%; conversion to other chemical fertilizers—48%; fibers and plastics—8%; explosives and plastics—4%; animal feeds—3%; other uses—7%; losses—4%. It also is used in producing other chemicals, as a food additive, in detergents, in insecticides and as a major commercial refrigerant. No precise figure is available as to the extent of employee exposure to ammonia; however, the NIOSH estimates that 500,000 workers have potential exposure. Occupational exposure to ammonia may occur in a number of industries, including laboratories, nitriding furnaces, fertilizer manufacturing, explosives manufacturing, coke making, diazotype reproducing operations, commercial refrigerator repair and in various plants producing other materials mentioned earlier.

Ammonia vapor is a severe irritant to the eyes, respiratory tract and skin. Inhalation of concentrations of 2500–6500 ppm causes severe corneal irritation, dyspnea, bronchospasm, chest pain and pulmonary edema that may be fatal; production of pink, frothy sputum often occurs. Complications can include bronchitis or pneumonia; some residual reduction in pulmonary function has been reported. In a human experimental study that exposed 10 subjects to various vapor concentrations for 5 minutes, 134 ppm caused irritation of the eyes, nose and throat in most subjects and 1 person complained of chest irritation; at 72 ppm, several reported the same symptoms; at 50 ppm, 2 reported nasal dryness; and at 32 ppm, only 1 reported nasal dryness. In a survey of 8 workers in a blueprint shop, ammonia concentrations of 4–29 ppm caused "barely noticeable" to "moderate" eye irritation; no respiratory irritation was reported. Tolerance to usually irritating concentrations of ammonia may be acquired by adaptation, a phenomenon frequently observed among workers who became inured to the effects of exposure. No data are available on concentrations that are irritating to workers who are regularly exposed to ammonia and who presumably have a higher irritation threshold. Liquid anhydrous ammonia in contact with the eyes may cause serious eye injury or blindness; on the skin, it causes first and second degree burns that often are severe and, if extensive, may be fatal. Vapor concentrations of 10,000 ppm are mildly irritating to the moist skin and 30,000 ppm or greater cause a stinging sensation and may produce skin burns and vesiculation.

Wherever ammonia is used in quantity, respiratory equipment should be available for emergencies. Explosive concentrations of ammonia can be produced when the contents of a tank or a refrigeration system are released into an open flame, boiler fire or arc.

TREATMENT.—Prompt removal from exposure; if liquid splash has occurred, immediately flush eyes and skin with water. Consideration should be given to hospitalization and observation for 72 hours for delayed onset of pulmonary edema.

A TLV of 25 ppm has been selected to protect against irritation to eyes and the respiratory tract.

REFERENCES

Ammonia

1. American Conference of Governmental Industrial Hygienists: Ammonia. Documentation of the Threshold Limit Values for Substances in Workroom Air, 3d ed., Cincinnati, Ohio, 1974.
2. Exposure to Ammonia, Proposed Standards, Federal Register, 40:54684-54693, November 25, 1975.
3. Hygienic Guide Series: Anhydrous Ammonia, Am. Ind. Hyg. Assoc. J. 32:139, 1971.
4. National Institute for Occupational Safety and Health, U.S. Dept. of Health, Education, and Welfare: Criteria for a Recommended Standard . . . Occupational Exposure to Ammonia (NIOSH), U.S. Government Printing Office, Washington, D.C., 1974.

Benzidine-Derived Dyes

The National Occupational Hazard Survey (NOHS), conducted between 1972 and 1974 by the National Institute for Occupational Safety and Health, indicates that workers are occupationally exposed to Direct Black 38, Direct Brown 95 and Direct Blue 6 in a variety of industries, including: paper and allied products, petroleum and related industries, rubber and plastic products, leather and leather products, instrumentation and measuring devices and banking. In addition, the textile industry accounts for a substantial occupational exposure. It is estimated that 25% of the benzidine-derived azo dyes are applied to textiles, 40% to paper, 15% to leather and the remainder to other diverse applications.[3] The Color Index,[2] a reference by Great Britain's Society of Dyers and Colorists, reports the following uses for the three dyes.

Direct Black 38: Dyeing or staining of wool, silk, fibers for rope and matting, hog hair, cellulose, acetate, nylon and biologic stains.

Direct Brown 95: Dyeing or staining silk, cotton, acetate, cellulose, wood, nylon, leather, paper and certain plastics.

Direct Blue 6: Dyeing or staining silk, wool, cotton, nylon, leather, paper, biologic stains and writing inks.

Benzidine has been an important intermediate in dye production since its introduction to the dyestuff industry around 1890. In 1948, production of benzidine-derived dyes was 16 million kg, which accounted for 25% of all domestic dyes manufactured and almost all of the direct-class dyes. Domestic production of direct benzidine-derived dyes dropped to 6 million kg in 1971. Domestic production in 1978 was limited to 12 benzidine dyes. The latest domestic production figures for Direct Black 38 show 3 million kg in 1971, down to 1 million kg in 1975, which rose to 2 million kg in 1976. Direct Brown 95 showed an increased production to 300,000 kg in 1976, which was up from 200,000 kg in 1975 and 150,000 kg in 1974. Domestic production figures for Direct Blue 6 indicated that 150,000 kg were produced in 1973, which is the last available figure for that dye. In the general population, unspecified exposure levels to the three dyes are thought to occur through the use of retail packaged dyes for home dyeing and for home and school use in art and craft projects such as tie-dyeing or batik. The Art Hazards Project of the Center for Occupational Hazards, New York City, has reported that packaged dyes sold in supermarkets, variety stores and hardware stores are combinations of direct, acid and basic dyes, and thus may contain benzidine-derived dye components.[4] Two of these dyes, Direct Black 38 and Direct Blue 6, have been used in hair dyes.[11]

Caution is also indicated by preliminary

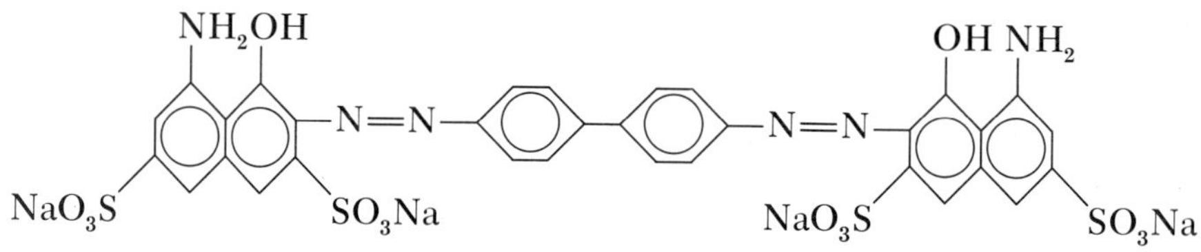

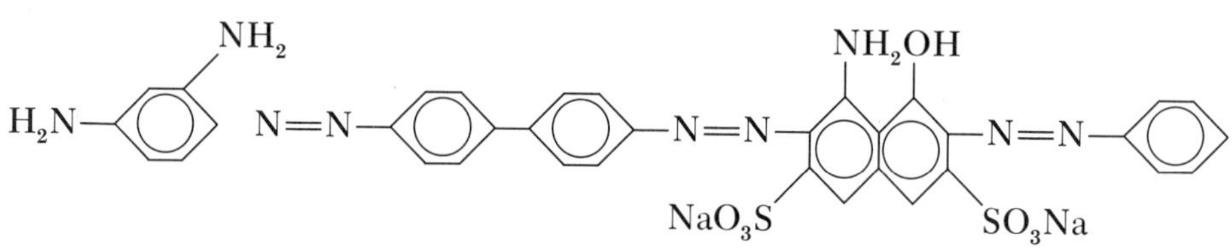

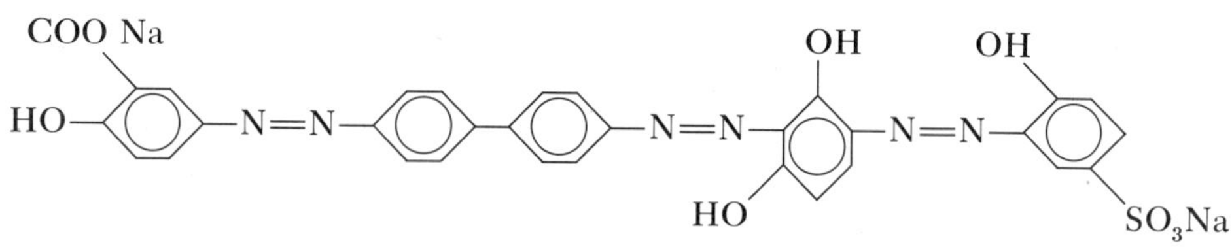

results from NIOSH field studies showing that humans working with these same dyes also excrete higher than expected levels of benzidine in their urine. Both laboratory and field studies indicate that these benzidine-derived dyes can be metabolized to benzidine, which is present in the urine of animals and humans. Based on the data from the short-term study, NCI scientists believe that a cancer-causing potential exists on exposure to the benzidine-derived dyes, most likely through the mechanism of metabolic conversion of the dyes to benzidine in the animal system.

NIOSH FIELD STUDIES

Preliminary results from NIOSH studies indicate the presence of benzidine or monacetylbenzidine (MAB), a metabolite of benzidine, in the urine of workers in 4 of 5 industrial facilities in which urine samples were collected. The facilities surveyed to date include 2 benzidine dye manufacturers, 2 textile-finishing companies and a leather tannery.

In one dye manufacturing plant, benzidine and MAB were found in all dye workers who worked solely with the finished dyes. Bulk benzidine-based dyes were quantitatively analyzed for residual free benzidine content, which ranged from less than 1 to 19 ppm. It was conservatively estimated that about 20 times more benzidine and up to 200 times more MAB were present in the urine of these dye workers than if they had been exposed only to the residual benzidine content in the dyes. The concentrations of benzidine found in the urine of these workers were significant fractions of those concentrations associated with a high incidence of bladder cancer as reported in the scientific literature. Among textile dyers included in the NIOSH study, 4 of 10 had benzidine or MAB present in their urine and all had elevated aromatic amine levels. No benzidine or MAB was detected in urine samples collected at a leather tannery where good work practices were observed. Although there was biologic variability in body burden tolerance and differences in metabolism among those studied, it appears likely that work practices and personal hygiene played a major role in minimizing exposure. Analyses of data from these NIOSH studies are ongoing. The relatively large particle size of the dry dye powders causes inhaled dyes to be deposited largely in the upper respiratory tract and then ingested. Prevention of worker inhalation or ingestion of these dyes would greatly reduce absorption into the body and subsequent benzidine exposure. A strong association relating human exposure to benzidine-based dyes with the subsequent development of bladder tumors was presented after a case-control mortality study of 200 bladder cancer patients in Japan.[14] The patients were found to have been predominantly kimono painters and dyers. The kimono painters had a habit of forming a point on their brushes by drawing the brush between their lips, which allowed for ingestion of the dyes. Several other case-control mortality studies indicate an increased risk of developing bladder cancer in the textile and leather industries, both large users of direct dyes. However, only a few references have been made concerning benzidine-derived dyestuffs. In Russia, a medical study concerning the early detection of bladder tumors among textile dyers using benzidine-derived dyes revealed an unusual incidence of bladder lesions, some of which were suggested as being of a precancerous nature. The greatest number of such lesions were found in those workers with the highest potential exposure to these dyes.[5]

The NIOSH recommends that it would be prudent to handle Direct Black 38, Direct Brown 95 and Direct Blue 6 in the workplace as if they were human carcinogens. Exposure to Direct Black 38, Direct Brown 95 and Direct Blue 6 should be limited to as few employees as possible, while minimizing workplace exposure levels. The area in which they are used should be restricted to only those employees essential to the process or operation.

EXPOSURE MONITORING

Initial and routine employee exposure surveys should be made by competent industrial hygiene and engineering personnel. These surveys are necessary to determine the extent of employee exposure and to ensure that controls are effective.

MINIMIZING EMPLOYEE EXPOSURE.—There are four basic methods of limiting employee exposure; none of these is a simple industrial hygiene or management decision and careful planning and thought should be used prior to implementation of any of them.

Product substitution.—The substitution of an alternative material with a lower potential health and safety risk is one method. However, extreme care must be used when selecting possible substitutes. Alternatives to Direct Black 38, Direct Brown 95 and Direct Blue 6 should be fully evaluated with regard to possible human effects. Unless the toxic effects of the alternative have been thoroughly evaluated, a seemingly safe replacement, possible only after years of use, may be found to induce serious health effects.

Contaminant controls.—The most effective control of Direct Black 38, Direct Brown 95 and Direct Blue 6, where feasible, is at the source of contamination by enclosure of the operation and/or local exhaust ventilation. If feasible, the process or operation should be enclosed with a slight vacuum so that any leakage will result in the flow of air into the enclosure. The next most effective means of control would be a well-designed local exhaust ventilation system that physically encloses the process as much as possible, with sufficient capture velocity to keep the contaminant from entering the work atmosphere. To ensure that ventilation equipment is working properly, effectiveness (e.g., air velocity, static pressure or air volume) should be checked at least every 3 months. System effectiveness should be checked soon after any change in production, process or control that might result in significant increases in airborne exposures to Direct Black 38, Direct Brown 95 and Direct Blue 6.

Employee isolation.—A third alternative is the isolation of employees. It frequently involves the use of automated equipment operated by personnel observing from a closed control booth or room. The control room is maintained at a greater air pressure than that surrounding the process equipment so that air flow is out of, rather than into, the room. This type of control will not protect those employees who must do process checks, adjustments, maintenance and related operations.

Personal protective equipment.—The least preferred method is the use of personal protective equipment. This equipment, which may include respirators, goggles, gloves and other devices, should not be used as the only means to prevent or minimize exposure during routine operations. Exposure to Direct Black 38, Direct Brown 95 and Direct Blue 6 should not be controlled with the use of respirators except during the time period necessary to install or implement engineering or work practice controls, or in work situations in which engineering and work practice controls are technically not feasible, or for maintenance, or for operations that require entry into tanks or closed vessels or in emergencies.

REFERENCES

Benzidine-Derived Dyes

1. Benzidine Derived Dyes—Current Intelligence Bulletin 24, Joint NIOSH/NCI, U.S. Dept. of Health, Education, and Welfare, PHS, Publications Dissemination, DTS, National Institute for Occupational Safety and Health, Cincinnati, Ohio, April 17, 1978.

2. Color Index, 1975, 3d Ed. The Society of Dyers and Colorists.
3. Environmental Protection Agency, 40 CFR Part 129, Benzidine: Proposed Toxic Pollutant Effluent Standards, Federal Register Vol. 41, No. 127, June 30, 1973.
4. Jenkins, C.: Dye Hazards Report, February, 1978. American Association of Textile Chemists and Colorists, Raleigh, North Carolina.
5. Korosteleva, T., Kljuckareu, B., Belokhuostave, A., and Ayzomyatnikov, A.: Immunological diagnosis in early stages of occupational cancer of the urinary bladder, Probl. Oncol. 19:2832, 1973.
6. Lubs, H.: The chemistry of synthetic dyes and pigments. American Chemical Society Monograph No. 127, Washington, D.C., 1952.
7. Synthetic Organic Chemicals: United States Production and Sales. U.S. International Trade Commission Report, Washington, D.C., 1973.
8. Synthetic Organic Chemicals: United States Production and Sales, U.S. International Trade Commission Report, Washington, D.C., 1974.
9. Synthetic Organic Chemicals: United States Production and Sales, U.S. International Trade Commission Report, Washington, D.C., 1975.
10. Synthetic Organic Chemicals: U.S. Tariff Commission, Report on Synthetic Organic Dyes. Series 6-2, 1948.
11. 13-Week Subchronic Toxicity Studies of Direct Blue 6, Direct Black 38, and Direct Brown 95 Dyes. National Cancer Institute. Carcinogenesis Technical Report. DHEW Publication #"NIH" 78-1358, 1978.
12. Synthetic Organic Chemicals: United States Production and Sales. U.S. International Trade Commission Report, Washington, D.C., 1971.
13. Venkataraman, K.: *The Chemistry of Synthetic Dyes* (New York: Academic Press, 1952), pp. 506–514.
14. Voshida, O., and Miyakaqa, M.: Etiology of Bladder Cancer: "Metabolic" Aspects, in Nakahara, W., Hirayama, T., Nishioka, K., et al. (eds.), *Analytic and Experimental Epidemiology of Cancer* (Baltimore: University Park Press, 1974), pp. 31–39.

Benzoyl Peroxide

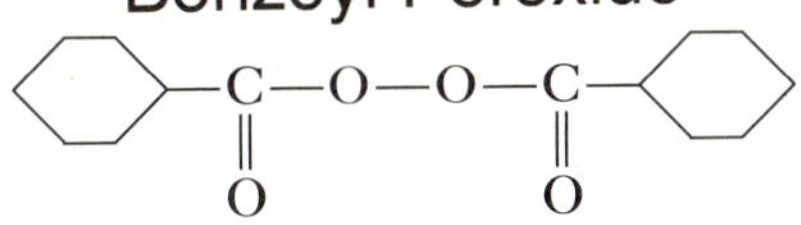

Benzoyl peroxide, also called dibenzoyl peroxide, is a flammable solid that may decompose explosively if subjected to excessive heat, friction or sudden shock. If benzoyl peroxide is exposed to temperatures of 75–80° C for prolonged periods, it becomes unstable and may decompose spontaneously. This type of sudden decomposition, a deflagration, is the rapid spreading of fire through a mass of reactive material. Such decomposition is accompanied by a 200-fold increase in volume and yields a dense white smoke consisting of benzoic acid, phenyl benzoate, terphenyls, biphenyls, benzene and carbon dioxide. The resulting biphenyls promote the further decomposition of benzoyl peroxide into products that can catch fire and ignite the remaining benzoyl peroxide.

Benzoyl peroxide is synthesized commercially by a reaction of benzoyl chloride, sodium hydroxide and hydrogen peroxide. Water, plasticizers, corn starch or other diluents are added to make the numerous commercial products containing benzoyl peroxide. Benzoyl peroxide has been produced commercially in the United States since 1927, 3 million kg being produced in 1975. It is used in a number of industrial processes, particularly in the manufacture of plastics. Benzoyl peroxide is a curing agent for silicone rubber, a source of free radicals in the resin cements used in dentistry, automobile body putty and roof bolting systems in the mining industry and an initiator in the synthesis of polyvinyl chloride. It is also a component of flour and cheese bleaches. In the early 1900s, benzoyl peroxide was used to bleach edible oils, but this practice now is rare. In the past, textiles and paper were also treated with it. In medicine, it is used in the treatment of acne and of decubitus ulcers. Formerly, it was applied in the treatment of poison ivy.

The NIOSH estimates that 25,000 workers in the United States are potentially exposed to benzoyl peroxide or its formulations. Occupations involving possible exposure to benzoyl peroxide are automobile body repair workers, bakers, benzoyl peroxide makers, cheese makers, dentists, dental assistants, flour-mill workers, miners, nurses, pharmaceutical products makers, pharmacists, physicians, plastic product makers, polyester makers, printers, silicone rubber makers, styrene makers and telephone repair workers.

Inhalation is the main route of exposure. Benzoyl peroxide dust causes both primary irritation and sensitization dermatitis. Application to the face as a lotion for the treatment of acne in 2 individuals caused facial erythema and edema; patch tests with benzoyl peroxide were positive. It may produce eye irritation and, if allowed to remain on the skin, inflammation. No systemic effects have been reported in man.[1,2] The 1979 TLV: 5 mg/m^3. The present federal standard for exposure to benzoyl peroxide in the workplace is an 8-hour TWA concentration limit of 5 mg/m^3, based on the 1968 ACGIH TLV.

REFERENCES

Benzoyl Peroxide

1. Eaglestein, W. H.: Allergic contact dermatitis to benzoyl peroxide—report of cases, Arch. Dermatol. 97:527, 1968.
2. Grant, W. M.: *Toxicology of the Eye* (2d ed.; Springfield, Ill.: Charles C Thomas, Publisher, 1974), pp. 183, 1196.
3. NIOSH Criteria for a Recommended Standard . . . Occupational Exposure to Benzoyl Peroxide. U.S. Dept. of Health, Education, and Welfare, PHS, Center for Disease Control, DHEW (NIOSH) Publication No. 77-166, June, 1977.

Benzyl Chloride (Chloromethylbenzene; Chlorotoluene)

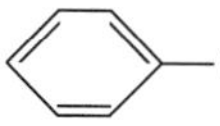

—CH_2Cl

Production of this substance is by the photochlorination of toluene. About 50 million kg of benzyl chloride is produced annually in the United States.

At present, an estimated 60–70% of the benzyl chloride manufactured in the United States is for the production of *n*-butyl benzyl phthalate, a plasticizer for the flexible vinyl polymers used in coatings and floor coverings. Benzyl alcohol, the manufacture of which accounts for 10–15% of the benzyl chloride output, is used as an adjunct in the dispersion, uptake and rate of fixation of dyes in the textile industry and to make specialized solvents. Another 10–12% of the benzyl chloride output is used to form a variety of quaternary ammonium compounds that are used as germicides, fungicides and sanitizers and in products such as hair conditioners, wetting agents, dispersing agents and emulsion paint preservatives. The remaining 5–10% of benzyl chloride production is used in the synthesis of such materials as benzyl acetate, benzyl cyanide, benzyl salicylate, benzyl butyrate and benzyl amines, many of which are prepared as batches. These products are used in the pharmaceutical, perfume, flavors and dye industries. Benzyl chloride is reported to be effective as an extreme-pressure lubricant, the lubricating property of which is attributed to a chloride film that forms condensation reactions, forming low molecular weight polybenzyl resins that are temperature and pressure stable and noncorrosive and have been proposed for use as hydraulic fluids, heat transfer fluids and heat-stable fuel. The NIOSH estimates that 3000 workers in the United States are potentially exposed to benzyl chloride. Occupations involving potential exposure to benzyl chloride are algicide makers, analytical chemists, benzyl alcohol workers, benzyl chloride workers, benzyl ester makers, butyl benzyl phthalate workers, disinfectant makers, drug makers, dye intermediate makers, dye makers, dyers, extreme-pressure lubricant makers and users, gasoline additive workers, germicide makers, motor fuel blenders, perfume makers, pharmaceutical workers, photographic developer makers, quaternary ammonium compound workers, resin makers, rubber makers, synthetic organic chemists, tannin makers and wetting-agent makers.[9]

Benzyl chloride vapor and aerosol may irritate the skin, eyes, nose and upper respiratory tract. The irritant properties provide sufficient warning such that employees do not voluntarily remain in areas of high (50 mg/m^3) concentrations. The odor of benzyl chloride, however, does not provide adequate warning of concentrations that may cause eye irritation. Direct contact of liquid benzyl chloride with the skin can cause burns.

Benzyl chloride has been demonstrated to be an extreme lacrimator and capable of causing lung edema.[8] It is believed that benzyl chloride, like other chlorinated hydrocarbons, is metabolized chiefly in the liver, thus causing liver and kidney damage in high concentrations. In addition, severe corneal damage with permanent disability has been caused by benzyl chloride liquid contacting the eye. Typical signs and symptoms from benzyl chloride exposure are irritation of the eyes and respiratory tract. Weakness, headaches, irritability, insomnia, anorexia and finger tremors may also occur. The TLV of 1 ppm for benzyl chloride has been established because of its irritating effect on the eyes.

In a test for mutagenicity, it was shown that benzyl chloride was slightly mutagenic when applied directly onto an open plate with strain TA100 of *Salmonella typhimurium*. However, when the test was repeated in a desiccator that would retain benzyl chloride vapor, it was reported that benzyl chloride was highly mutagenic.[3,5] It has also been shown that benzyl chloride is a primary carcinogen in rats, causing sarcomas at the point of subcutaneous injections, although no excessive tumors were reported from intraperitoneal injections of mice.[6,7] Although benzyl chloride is included in the suspected carcinogen list, there are no references involving humans.[1]

Medical surveillance shall be made available as outlined below to all employees occupationally exposed to benzyl chloride.

Exposure to benzyl chloride shall be controlled so that no employee is exposed to benzyl chloride at a concentration greater than 5.0 mg/m^3 determined as a ceiling concentration during any 15-minute sampling period.[4]

REFERENCES

Benzyl Chloride

1. Christensen, H. E., et al. (eds.): Suspected carcinogens, a subfile of the NIOSH toxic substances list. U.S. Dept. of Health, Education, and Welfare, PHS, Rockville, Maryland (DHEW Publication No. 74-117), 1975.
2. Documentation of threshold limit values. 3d edition. American Conference of Governmental Industrial Hygienists, Cincinnati, Ohio, p. 24, 1971.
3. McCann, J., et al.: Detection of carcinogens as mutagens: Bacterial tester strains with R factor plasmids, Proc. Natl. Acad. Sci. 72:979, 1975.
4. NIOSH Criteria for a Recommended Stan-

dard . . . Occupational Exposure to Benzyl Chloride. Dept. of Health, Education, and Welfare, PHS, Center for Disease Control, NIOSH, Robert A. Taft Laboratories, Cincinnati, Ohio. August, 1978.
5. Personal communication between S. Henson, Stanford Research Institute, and V. F. Simmon, Stanford Research Institute, Menlo Park, California, 1976.
6. Poirier, L. A., Stoner, G. D., and Shimpin, M. B.: Bioassay of alkyl halides and nucleotide base analogs by pulmonary tumor response in strain A mice, Cancer Res. 35:1411, 1975.
7. Preussman, R.: Direct alkylating agents as carcinogens, Food Cosmet. Toxicol. 6:575, 1968.
8. Smyth, H. F., Jr.: Improved communication—hygienic standards for daily inhalation, Am. Ind. Hyg. Assoc. Q. 17:129, 1956.
9. Technical Report—Survey of Benzyl Chloride: Extent of Exposure. U.S. Dept. of Health, Education, and Welfare, PHS, Center for Disease Control, NIOSH, DHEW Publication No. 78-160, Cincinnati, Ohio, February, 1978.

Boron Oxide

B_2O_3

Boron compounds are excellent fluxing materials used in welding, soldering and certain metal refining, alloying and high-temperature resistive refractories. Occupational exposure may occur by inhalation. Boron oxide aerosol is of low toxicity but is found to be irritating to the mucous membranes of animals. Repeated exposure of rats to an aerosol at a concentration of 470 mg/m^3 for 10 weeks caused only mild nasal irritation; repeated exposure of rats to 77 mg/m^3 for 23 weeks resulted in elevated creatinine and boron content of the urine in addition to increased urinary volume.[2] Conjunctivitis resulted when the dust was applied to the eyes of rabbits, probably the result of the exothermic reaction of boron oxide with water to form boric acid; topical application of boron oxide dust to the clipped backs of rabbits produced erythema that persisted for 2–3 days.[1,2] By analogy to effects caused in animals, prolonged exposure may cause nasal irritation; dust in the eyes may cause conjunctivitis and, on the skin, erythema. The 1979 TLV: 10 mg/m^3.

REFERENCES

Boron Oxide

1. American Conference of Governmental Industrial Hygienists: "Boron Oxide," Documentation of the Threshold Limit Values for Substances in Workroom Air (3d ed., 2d printing), Cincinnati, Ohio, p. 26, 1974.
2. Hampel, C. A., and Hanley, G. G.: *The Encyclopedia of Chemistry* (3d ed.; New York: Van Nostrand Reinhold Co., 1973).
3. Wilding, J. L., et al.: The toxicity of boron oxide, Am. Ind. Hyg. Assoc. J. 20:284, 1959.

Boron Trifluoride

Boron trifluoride, BF_3, is a colorless gas that is stable in dry atmospheres. At present, boron trifluoride is known to be produced as a specialty chemical by only one U.S. company, whose production figures are not available. Although the predominant use of boron trifluoride is as a catalyst, that is not its only use (*synthesis of:* saturated hydrocarbons, alcohols, olefins, ketones, ethers and sulfur compounds; *condensation of:* acid with olefin, acid with acetylene, acid with alcohol, nitrite with alcohol, amide with alcohol and aldols; *dehydration of:* alcohols, acids and ketones; *alkylation of:* paraffinic hydrocarbons, alkyl esters and aromatic hydrocarbons; *polymerization of:* ethylene, propylene, butylene, isobutylene, vinyl compounds, dienes and cyclic oxides; and for some epoxy resin curing). The magnesium industry utilizes the fire-retardant and antioxidant properties of boron trifluoride in casting and heat treating. Nuclear applications of boron trifluoride include neutron detector instruments, boron-10 enrichment and the production of neutron-absorbing salts for molten-salt breeder reactors. Boron trifluoride has also been identified as having insecticidal properties.[2] Employees with potential exposure to boron trifluoride include the initial manufacturers, magnesium founders, organic synthesizers, neutron detector instrument manufacturers and fumigant producers.[3] The NIOSH estimates that 50,000 employees are potentially exposed to boron trifluoride in the United States.

On contact with air, boron trifluoride gas immediately reacts with water vapor to form a mist that, at a high enough concentration, may provide a visible warning of its presence. Boron trifluoride gas is a severe irritant of the lungs, eyes and skin. Exposure of 6 animal species to 100 ppm for 30 days resulted in a high mortality rate. Exposure of animals to a concentration of 42 mg/m^3 (approximately 15 ppm) for an unspecified period was fatal in some cases; autopsy findings were pneumonitis and degenerative changes in the renal tubules. Repeated exposure of mice to 15 ppm for 30 days resulted in mortality of 19% due to pulmonary irritation; rats similarly exposed for 2 weeks developed hypoplasia of the teeth and deposition of fluoride up to 25 times normal levels, both in the incisors and in femoral epiphyses. Three species of animals repeatedly exposed to levels of 12.8, 7.7 or 3 ppm for periods up to 6 months developed pneumonitis and evidence of dental fluorosis; the higher concentrations caused deaths in guinea pigs. In man, the gas in high concentration produces burns of the eyes and skin similar to those caused by hydrogen fluoride but less severe. Workers exposed to concentrations of up to 90 mg/m^3 (approximately 32 ppm) for 10–15 years developed dryness of the nasal mucous membranes and epistaxis. No chronic effects have been observed in workers who were exposed to low concentrations at frequent intervals over a period of years.[1,5]

The present federal standard is a ceiling value of 1 ppm (3mg/m^3), which was based on the 1-ppm ceiling ACGIH TLV for boron trifluoride adopted in 1968.

In the absence of a suitable monitoring method, the NIOSH recommends that medical surveillance, including comprehensive preplacement and annual periodic examinations, be made available to all workers employed in areas where boron trifluoride is manufactured, used, handled or is evolved as a result of chemical processes. Engineering controls should be used to maintain boron trifluoride concentrations at the lowest feasible level. Air-supplied respirators should be used only in certain nonroutine situations or in emergency situations when air concentrations of boron trifluoride are sufficient to form a visible mist.

REFERENCES

Boron Trifluoride

1. Allied Chemical Corporation: Material Safety Data Sheet, Boron Trifluoride, Morristown, N.J.
2. Marcovitch, S.: Volatile fluorine compounds for the control of insects, J. Econ. Entomol. 35:288, 1942.
3. Milby, T. H., Key, M. M., Gibson, R. L., and Stokinger, H. E.: Boron Compounds, in Gafafer, W. M. (ed.), Occupational Diseases—A Guide to Their Recognition, Publication No. 1097, U.S. Dept. of Health, Education, and Welfare, PHS, pp. 95–97, 1964.
4. NIOSH Criteria for a Recommended Stan-

dard . . . Occupational Exposure to Boron Trifluoride. U.S. Dept. of Health, Education, and Welfare, PHS, Center for Disease Control, Cincinnati, Ohio. DHEW (NIOSH) Publication No. 77-122, December, 1976.

5. Torkelson, T. R., et al.: The toxicity of boron trifluoride when inhaled by laboratory animals, Am. Ind. Hyg. Assoc. J. 22:263, 1961.

Carbon Monoxide
CO

During 1968–1975, CO was listed on death certificates as the underlying cause of 8764 deaths in the United States—5782 by motor vehicle exhaust, 1093 by incomplete combustion of domestic fuels and 1889 through occupational exposure at blast furnaces and kilns or to partially combusted industrial fuels. CO is an occupational hazard for workers involved with internal combustion engines, foundries, petroleum refineries, pulp mills and steel mills, among others.

Almost every industrial item manufactured today involves the use of heat, fire, combustion or oxidation at some point during its processing. For this reason, the possibilities of CO poisoning are ubiquitous. Such poisoning is thought to be the most common industrial poisoning, mainly because CO is odorless and tasteless, giving no warning of its presence under most circumstances, and because the early symptoms can resemble other diseases. Certain industries have been long recognized to be particularly hazardous in relation to CO exposures: iron and steel foundries, pulp paper mills, petroleum refineries, sintering mills and the manufacturers of formaldehyde and coke. Within these industries, the main sources of CO have been identified as emanating from the cupolas in the foundries, catalytic cracking units in petroleum refineries, lime kilns and the draft recovery furnaces in kraft paper mills, and the sintering of blast furnace feed. There are many other obvious but less-well-documented sources known to produce large quantities of CO, with the greatest hazards found in automotive and garage work, fork-lift truck operations, etc. Because the amounts of CO produced usually do not create problems, poisoning may occur with little warning if either the production of CO increases or ventilation is decreased, as may occur during cold weather.

See Chapter 3 for a discussion of the extremely important potential effects on intrauterine development and the newborn. Certain aspects of these effects concerning both sexes working with potential CO exposure must be reiterated. Carboxyhemoglobin is incapable of carrying oxygen. At any given level of CO in the air breathed, the rate at which blood becomes saturated with CO is directly proportional to cardiac output.

The dose-response relationship for CO is strongly time-dependent and reasonably well understood. Although CO levels of 200–400 ppm may cause headache and the levels of 800–1600 ppm produce unconsciousness, even 50 ppm for 120 minutes has been shown to reduce exercise tolerance in subjects with angina. The NIOSH-recommended standard for occupational exposure—35 ppm time-weighted average for a 40-hour workweek with 8 hours' exposure per day and a ceiling concentration of 200 ppm—is designed to avoid adverse cardiovascular effects.

With exposure to high concentrations such as 4000 ppm and above, transient weakness and dizziness may be the only premonitory warnings before coma; the most common early aftermath of severe intoxication is cerebral edema. Exposure to concentrations of 500–1000 ppm causes the development of headache, tachypnea, nausea, weakness, dizziness, mental confusion and, in some instances, hallucinations; the person may be cyanotic. Although an occasional individual will exhibit the unusual combination of hypoxia associated with a bright-red color of the fingernails, mucous membranes and skin, this "cherry-red" coloration usually is seen only at autopsy. Exposure to 50 ppm may cause aggravation of angina pectoris after 90 minutes; 50 ppm for 120 minutes may cause aggravation of intermittent claudication. Exposure to 50 ppm for 6–8 hours results in carboxyhemoglobin levels of 8–10%. Levels of carboxyhemoglobin over 60% usually are fatal; 50% is associated with collapse and syncope; above 25% there may be electrocardiographic evidence of a depression of the ST segment; between 15% and 25% there may be headache and nausea; with levels below 15% there may be headache and nausea; levels below 15% rarely produce symptoms. Reactions to given blood levels of carboxyhemoglobin are highly variable and some persons may be in a coma with a carboxyhemoglobin level of 38% whereas others may maintain an apparently clear sensorium with levels as high as 55%. Cigarette smokers reveal 2–10% blood carboxyhemoglobin and nonexposed persons have an average level of 1%. Several investigators have suggested that the results of behavioral tests such as time discrimination, visual vigilance, choice response tests, visual evoked responses and visual discrimination thresholds may be altered at levels of carboxyhemoglobin below 5%. Table 14–2 shows levels of carboxyhemoglobin concentrations.

TABLE 14–2.—CARBOXYHEMOGLOBIN CONCENTRATIONS*

CO, ppm	% COHb
0	0.36
5	1.1
8.7	1.7
10	1.9
15	2.6
20	3.4
30	4.7
40	6.1

*Carboxyhemoglobin concentrations after exposure to constant levels of CO, reaching equilibrium (at sea level).

Further research has shown that formation of carboxyhemoglobin is not the main mechanism of CO toxicity. In 1975, Goldbaum et al.[17] produced a definitive paper demonstrating that carboxyhemoglobinemia was of only minor or secondary importance in CO poisoning. In their experiments at the Armed Forces Institute of Pathology, 3 groups of 5 dogs each were used. Group I was given 13% by inhalation and Group II was bled to an anemic state, reducing the hemoglobin content of the blood by an average of 68%, and then had blood volumes restored to normal with saline and dextran. Group III was bled to the same anemic state as Group II but then transfused with packed red cells that contained 80% carboxyhemoglobin. All the dogs in Group I died within an hour with carboxyhemoglobin levels ranging between 54% and 90%. Group II dogs survived indefinitely. Most important was that Group III dogs survived indefinitely with determined carboxyhemoglobin levels of 60% (57–64%).

From the foregoing it is clear that even extensive combination of the hemoglobin with CO is not very dangerous. Other investigators have demonstrated that the true site of toxicity is the cytochrome a_3 oxidase in the mitochondria.[10, 13, 21] Therefore, the clinical condition of the patient is determined by the amount of cytochrome a_3 oxidase that is blocked. This is the same enzyme that is affected in cyanide poisoning and hydrogen sulfide poisoning. Fortunately, oxygen competes with CO for binding to cytochrome oxidase and, therefore, oxygen treatment is effective. Because it is not clinically possible to measure the level of impairment of the cytochrome system, our only laboratory index is the carboxyhemoglobin. It must be borne in mind that all of the published literature relates various degrees of incapacitation to the carboxyhemoglobin level. These must be interpreted as averages depending on whether the exposure is acute, chronic or prolonged. The actual clinical status of patients varies widely with any given level of carboxyhemoglobin.

When the tissues of the body become hypoxic due to cytochrome blockade, the heart must supply more blood by increasing both its rate and its output. Thus, the coronary arteries must supply more oxygen to the heart. The myocardium normally extracts 75% of the oxygen supplied to it via the coronary arteries, which is much more than the brain uses. Therefore, since anyone with coronary heart disease soon will suffer from hypoxia of the myocardium, the heart should be considered the first target organ in carbon monoxide poisoning because of the necessity for increased cardiac output. Normally, the myocardium extracts a pyruvate and lactate from the coronary circulation for oxidation. When the carboxyhemoglobin reaches a mean of 8.7%, the myocardium fails to extract either of these two substances and actually produces both.[9] Obviously, an 8.7% anemia is not the cause, but the mitochondrial cytochrome failure is the explanation.

The acute effects of CO on myocardial function in healthy adults, in patients with coronary artery disease and in patients with noncoronary heart disease have been amply described by investigators.[4,5,14,18] There is general agreement that the most vulnerable target organ for the low-level CO exposure is the heart. In 1949, Sjöstrand,[31] utilizing improved methods of measurements, demonstrated that the human body was a net producer of CO, identifying the source as the alphamethene bridge between the four porphyrin units in the heme molecule. During the "recycling" of the heme molecule reclaiming iron, four molecules of CO are released for every molecule of heme catabolized.[29] At this time, Sjöstrand also suggested a very practical means for estimating the body's level of carboxyhemoglobin through analysis of expired air.

Investigators have concluded that there are several ways in which CO at the most commonly found levels can clinically affect cardiac function or influence the occurrence and severity of coronary heart disease. These are: aggravation of angina pectoris, aggravation of intermittent claudication, alterations of electrocardiographic responses in normal subjects (these effects have been observed in certain occupations where exposure to CO is very high, as in firemen),[33,34] production or aggravation of atherosclerosis associated with the CO in smoking and, possibly, a decrement of survival in patients with acute myocardial infarctions. There is abundant documentation that an elevation of carboxyhemoglobin levels greater than 5% can affect adversely patients with angina pectoris and certain other cardiovascular diseases [2,3,7] and that exercise tolerance is decreased and anginal pains are of longer duration.

Not only should endogenous CO formation in the human body be considered but other external contaminants may further compound the problem. Most commonly encountered, especially in the smaller industrial establishments as well as in homes, is exposure to paint removers. These contain a variety of hydrocarbon ingredients, a major one being methylene chloride (dichloromethane, CH_2Cl_2), which has been shown to be metabolized rapidly to CO.[11] Under conditions of poor ventilation, such as insufficient air movement in a home garage, basement or small workplace, concentrations of methylene chloride vapors can accumulate quickly. Stewart and Hake[32] have shown that the use of such paint remover for a period of 3 hours easily can produce carboxyhemoglobin saturation of 5–10%. It is not possible to determine the extent of paint remover use in the U. S. private sector and perhaps equally difficult to determine occupational exposure to methylene chloride in the thousands of workplaces where solvents are in daily use. In terms of potential worker exposure, methylene chloride, although not the most hazardous chlorinated hydrocarbon, is somewhat unique in the context of CO sources. In addition to its common use as a paint or varnish remover, it is widely used in degreasing, as an aerosol propellent, as a solvent for paint, in plastic textile making, in producing photo films, in preparing certain oils and waxes and, at one time, as a general anesthetic. The NIOSH estimate of exposure in the United States is about 70,000 workers, but this estimate does not include home use.

The NIOSH recommends that employee exposure to carbon monoxide at the workplace be controlled to: (1) prevent acute CO poisoning, (2) protect the employee from deleterious myocardial alterations associated with levels of carboxyhemoglobin (COHb) in excess of 5% and (3) provide the employee protection from adverse behavioral manifestations resulting from exposure to low levels of CO. This recommended standard is designed to protect the safety and health of workers who are performing a normal 8-hour per day, 40-hour per week work assignment. It is not designed for the population at large and any extrapolation beyond the general worker population is unwarranted. Because of the well-defined relationship between smoking and the concomitant exposure to CO in inhaled smoke, the recommended standard may not provide the same degree of protection to those workers who smoke as it will to nonsmokers. Likewise, under conditions of reduced ambient oxygen concentration, such as would be encountered by workers at higher altitudes (e.g., 1500–2400 m above sea level), the permissible exposure stated in the recommended standard should be appropriately lowered to compensate for loss in the oxygen-carrying capacity of the blood. In addition, workers with physical impairments that interfere with normal oxygen delivery to the tissues (e.g., emphysema, anemia, coronary heart disease) will not be provided the same degree of protection as the healthy worker population. The document did not consider the fertile or pregnant woman.

Silk[30] pointed out the problems of *excursion values* making future epidemiologic studies extremely difficult from the standpoint of knowledge of the *continual levels* of true exposure to CO. The many difficult technical aspects of accurate assessment of CO content of the air in the workplace, particularly over long periods in blast furnace areas, were stressed by Silk.

Davies[15] discussed the problems of continual CO exposure in totally enclosed environments such as a nuclear submarine, with reference to nonsmokers and smokers and the effects on individual and over-all system performance and on health. Reference is made to his excellent presentation on the increasing number of workers "entrained" in sealed or "closed environments." There is concern for the health of these persons even though the majority are of the younger category of the work force. With the development of underwater activities, particularly for obtaining under-sea mineral and oil supplies, occupational-environmental factors will gain greater importance.

Davies states that the correlation of "smoking, COHb and cardiovascular disease is now well established, and there is probably no above-endogenous COHb level at which there is no increase in the risk of disease. A level perhaps could be found, however, from experimental and epidemiologic evidence, at which the increased risk is so low that it can be ignored." Wald et al.[38] showed that smokers with COHb levels greater than 5% were 21 times more likely to be affected by atherosclerotic disease than those whose level was less than 3%, and Astrup[8] quoted figures showing that nonatherosclerotic smokers generally had COHb levels less than 4.6% whereas atherosclerotics had levels of more than 6%. Knelson[24] demonstrated acute cardiodynamic changes in healthy persons and further electrocardiographic changes in persons with a prior abnormal ECG at COHb levels of 5% and above. Adams et al.[1] also demonstrated cardiodynamic changes in dogs at 4% COHb. Nevertheless, Eckhardt et al.[16] found no abnormal cardiac or brain pathologic changes in cynomolgus monkeys carrying COHb loads of 6–8% continually for 2 years. In humans, however, the evidence points to a substantial increase in disease risk associated with continual COHb loads above 3%. Therefore, allowing for the concurrent presence of other health hazards within a submarine atmosphere, for example, a maximal COHb burden of 2.5%, equivalent to an ambient carbon monoxide level of approximately 15 ppm, is recommended.

Jones and Sinclair[22] studied blast furnace workers at a large ironmaking plant, observing that these workers absorbed CO at work irrespective of their smoking habits. Studies in 1962 and 1974 showed similar results, with mean increases during working shifts of 2.0–2.6% carboxyhemoglobin. The prevalence of cardiovascular disease in this group and a matched control group showed no significant difference. The number of deaths of blast furnace workers from coronary thrombosis was not significantly higher than for other workers at the iron and steel works. On the evidence available to date, blast furnace workers are no more likely to develop arterial disease than are other steelworkers, despite showing increased carboxyhemoglobin levels of this order. On the evidence available to them at the time, Jones and Sinclair believed that the blast furnace workers were no more likely than other steelworkers to develop arterial disease. Not only does the occupational exposure of the blast furnace worker to CO vary from day to day but even from minute to minute throughout a working shift, and the physical levels of work or energy expenditure required can vary from mild to more than moderate levels. The increase in ventilatory minute volume may range from an average of 10 liters per minute to as high as 66 liters per minute.[22]

In determining significant levels of CO exposure in workers, the metabolic level of work has a great bearing on the intake of a potentially toxic (respirable) material into the human organ systems. Other concomitant stresses may be present, such as radiant-heat stress, higher humidity, psychic stress, dehydration and other potentially toxic substances, which cannot be ignored when making an occupational risk hazard evaluation.

In 1972–1975, almost every foundry in Finland was surveyed extensively for dust and other dangerous materials; at the same time, the health aspects of the foundry workers were also investigated.[19] Even though Finland has a population of about 4.5 million, close to that of Wisconsin, the scope of such an immense project, probably the first of its type, deserves praise and much of the results have a bearing on CO exposures applicable in other countries. Under the direction of The Institute of Occupational Health in Helsinki, a comprehensive plan was designed to survey the work environment in all Finnish foundries, although the practical problems of carrying out such a study were recognized. Various statistical sampling procedures would be used to concentrate on such typical hazards as silica dust, certain chemicals, metal fumes and carbon monoxide and their effects. In terms of manpower and funds, this project became the most extensive single research project ever carried out by that institute. This investigation involved about 25 research workers and assistants, 2 employer organizations, The Ministry of Commerce and Industry, The Ministry of Social Affairs and Health and The National Pensions Fund. It is worth noting that this project was not undertaken for scientific reasons alone but that labor organizations regarded it as equally important to determine hygienic data and instructions for the improvement of the individual foundries. The total number of workers in this project numbered slightly more than 4300 in 68 different foundries—iron, steel and nonferrous.

In 1976, Virtamo and Tossavainen[36] reported their results on carbon monoxide in foundry air, having measured the CO concentration in the air of 67 iron, steel or copper alloy foundries, making 1100 CO determinations. They measured blood carboxyhemoglobin levels of 145 workers from iron foundries, finding that the carboxyhemoglobin level of 6% was exceeded in 26% of the nonsmokers and in 71% of the smokers. As is typical in foundry work, CO concentrations exceeding the TLV were found around cupolas and in the casting areas, again demonstrating that a worker's exposure to CO depends on length of stay in these areas.

According to Koskela and coinvestigators,[25] when CO exposure is considered a causative factor for coronary disease, the failure to find excess mortality among those exposed may be due to too-small exposure differences between the "exposed" and the "nonexposed," i.e., the general population or other categories of foundry workers. First, all categories contain about the same proportion of smokers, and, therefore, the reference category is by no means "clean" with regard to CO exposure; second, CO exposure is intermittent in foundries and only part of the "exposed" workers actually have higher carboxyhemoglobin values than from smoking alone.[36] Health selection may have contributed also to the negative findings; its possible impact has been discussed elsewhere.[26] For these reasons, Koskela et al. concluded that their study must be regarded as rather noninformative with respect to a possible effect of CO exposure on coronary mortality.

In order to prevent the health hazard created by the presence of carbon monoxide in the air, factories should reduce the carbon monoxide concentrations in the air with engineering means and provide for the regular monitoring of both the carbon monoxide concentrations in the air and the carboxyhemoglobin levels of workers. Insulating furnaces against leaks and installing efficient local and general exhaust systems lower the carbon monoxide levels in the air of work sites. Also, foundries can reduce carbon monoxide concentrations in the casting areas by installing local exhaust systems, enclosing the conveyors and by blowing clean air into the work sites. A good ventilation system in the casting area is also important because other harmful gases, such as those formed from the pyrolysis of resin binders, can be present.[37]

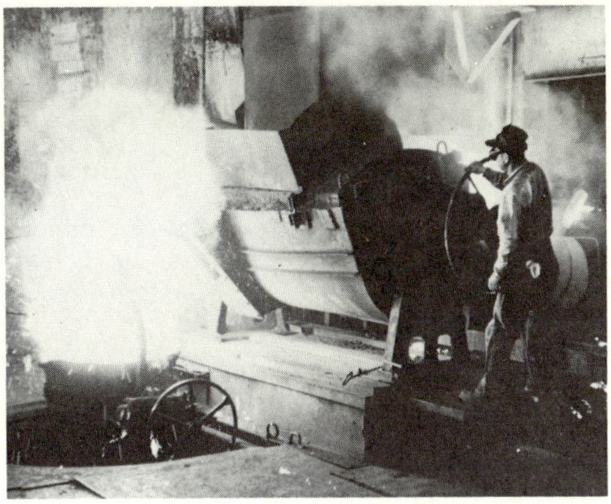

Fig 14–1.—At base of cupola area in an iron foundry.

While investigating workplace health hazards of fuelers of commercial jet aircraft at Kennedy International Airport, investigators from the NIOSH learned that in December, 1977, a 51-year-old fueler had been found dead in the cab of his fuel truck.[12] Since circumstances suggested the possibility of carbon monoxide poisoning, investigators examined the fuel trucks. It was noted that the exhaust pipe ran forward under the cab to a muffler mounted behind the front bumper. This configuration, apparently standard at airports, is intended to minimize the proximity of the exhaust system to the jet fuel in the truck and aircraft. CO levels were measured in the cabs of 3 airport fuel trucks in which the windows had been closed and the heaters turned on to simulate winter operating conditions. One of the 3 trucks had an average CO concentration of 180 ppm over a sampling period of 103 minutes. The other 2 had average levels less than 50 ppm. Fifteen other vehicles were examined; average CO levels in 7 exceeded 50 ppm; 1 of 7 exceeded 100 ppm and another, 300 ppm. Ambient CO levels in the test area were less than 1 ppm. It was not proved that CO contributed to the death of the fueler mentioned above, but the circumstances indicated the presence of a remediable health hazard.

The following recommendations were made to the employer: (1) minimize exposure time of the fuelers, (2) maximize fresh air ventilation in the trucks and (3) improve the maintenance of the vehicles.

Occupational exposure to carbon monoxide shall be controlled so that no worker shall be exposed at a concentration greater than 35 ppm determined as a time-weighted average (TWA) exposure for an 8-hour workday, as measured with a portable, direct reading, hopcalite-type carbon monoxide meter calibrated against known concentrations of CO, or with gas detector tube units certified under Title 42 of the Code of Federal Regulations, Part 84. No level of carbon monoxide to which workers are exposed shall exceed a ceiling concentration of 200 ppm.

Table 14–3 gives the standards or recommendations for occupational exposure to carbon monoxide. For procedures for calibration of equipment, sampling and analysis of CO samples, refer to the NIOSH Criteria Document.[28]

Treatment

1. Ensure that the airway is clear and give 100% oxygen by *tight-fitting* oronasal mask or endotracheal tube. The half-time for elimination of CO from hemoglobin is 5 hours and 20 minutes in normal fresh air. With a *tight-fitting* mask and 100% oxygen, this is lowered to 1 hour and 20 minutes. Hyperbaric oxygen (HBO) at 3 ATA lowers the elimination half-time to 23 minutes. The rate of elimination from cytochromes is not known but HBO appears to hasten the detachment of CO from the enzyme (competes with CO—law of mass action. For additional details, refer to Kindwall[23]).

2. Plastic disposable masks used in emergency rooms and nasal O_2 cannula are useless in CO poisoning (these do not deliver more than 35% oxygen).

3. *Correct acidosis if present*—very often pH is low and electrolyte determination on a severely poisoned patient is indicated. Correct with IV bicarbonate if the patient is well ventilated but be alert for hypokalemia.

4. The ECG is a good diagnostic indicator—sagging ST segments, especially in leads II, V_5 and V_6, are diagnostic of significant ischemia.

5. The preferred method for treatment in severe intoxication is by use of a hyperbaric chamber, if available, and is especially valuable if: *a)* The patient is unconscious or has a cloudy sensorium or any neurologic defect.

TABLE 14–3.—STANDARDS OR RECOMMENDATIONS FOR OCCUPATIONAL EXPOSURE TO CARBON MONOXIDE

15 ppm	National Aeronautics and Space Administration
18 ppm	Maximal Allowable Concentration, U.S.S.R.
25 ppm	ACGIH at altitudes of 1500 and 2500 meters
35 ppm	NIOSH, Sweden
50 ppm	Permissible-Exposure Limit, U.S.A. and West Germany
200 ppm	NIOSH ceiling
400 ppm	ACGIH Short-Term Exposure Limit

b) When the carboxyhemoglobin exceeds 25%.

c) ECG reveals ischemia.

Other General Control Recommendations

Because employees with overt cardiovascular disease may not be protected from an occupational exposure to 35 ppm of CO, a medical program should be instituted consisting of preplacement and periodic examinations with special attention to the cardiovascular system and to medical conditions that could be exacerbated by exposure to CO.

REFERENCES

Carbon Monoxide

1. Adams, J. D., Erickson, H. H., and Stone, H. L.: Myocardial metabolism during exposure to carbon monoxide in the conscious dog, J. Appl. Physiol. 34:238, 1973.
2. Anderson, E. W., et al.: Effect of low-level carbon monoxide exposure on onset and duration of angina pectoris, Ann. Intern. Med. 79:46, 1973.
3. Anderson, R. F., Allensworth, D. C., and DeGroot, W. J.: Myocardial toxicity from carbon monoxide poisoning, Ann. Intern. Med. 67:1172, 1967.
4. Aronow, W. S.: Effect of Carbon Monoxide on Angina, Intermittent Claudication, and Hemodynamics, in *Clinical Implications of Air Pollution Research* (Littleton, Mass.: Publishing Sciences Group, Inc., 1976), pp. 107–111.
5. Aronow, W. S.: Effect of cigarette smoking and of carbon monoxide on coronary heart disease, Chest 70:514, 1976.
6. Aronow, W. S., et al.: Effect of smoking cigarettes on cardiovascular hemodynamics, Arch. Environ. Health 28:330, 1974.
7. Aronow, W. S., and Isbell, M. W.: Carbon monoxide effect on exercise-induced angina pectoris, Ann. Intern. Med. 79:392, 1973.
8. Astrup, P.: Pathological effects of moderate carbon monoxide exposure, Staub 32:20, 1972.
9. Ayers, S. M., et al.: Systemic and myocardial hemodynamic responses to relatively small concentration of carboxyhemoglobin (COHb), Arch. Environ. Health 18:689, 1969.
10. Ball, E. G., Strittmalter, C. F., and Cooper, O.: The reaction of carbon monoxide, J. Biol. Chem. 193:635, 1951.
11. Benzon, H. T., et al.: Elevated carbon monoxide levels from exposures to methylene chloride, JAMA 239:2341, 1978.
12. Carbon Monoxide Exposure—N.Y.C. Morbidity and Mortality Weekly Report. U.S. Dept. of Health, Education, and Welfare, PHS, Center for Disease Control, HEW Publication No. (CDC) 79-8017, MMWR, Vol. 28, No. 22, pp. 254–255, June 8, 1979.
13. Chance, B., Erecinska, M., and Wagner, M.: Mitochondrial responses to CO toxicity, Ann. N. Y. Acad. Sci. 174:193, 1970.
14. Corya, B. C., Black, M. J., and McHenry, P. L.: Echocardiographic findings after acute carbon monoxide poisoning, Br. Heart J. 38:712, 1976.
15. Davies, D. M.: The application of threshold limit values for carbon monoxide under conditions of continuous exposure, Ann. Occup. Hyg. 18:21, 1975.
16. Eckhardt, R. E., MacFarland, H. N., Alarie, Y. C. E., and Busey, W. M.: The biologic effect for long-term exposure of primates to carbon monoxide, Arch. Environ. Health 25:381, 1972.
17. Goldbaum, L. R., Ramierez, R. G., and Absalon, K. B.: What is the mechanism of carbon monoxide toxicity?, Aviat. Space Environ. Med. 46:1289, 1975.
18. Goldsmith, J. R., and Aronow, W. S.: Carbon monoxide and coronary heart disease: A review, Environ. Res. 10:236, 1975.
19. Hernberg, S.: The Finnish foundry project. Background and general methodology, Scand. J. Work Environ. Health 2(Supp. 1):8, 1976.
20. Haag, W. M.: Methods to reduce carbon monoxide in the workplace, Prev. Med. 8:369, 1979.
21. Ingenito, A. J., Fiedler, P. C., and Procita, L.: Negative action of carbon monoxide on the isolated isovolumic heart with a hemoglobin-free perfusate, Fed. Proc. 33:503, 1974.
22. Jones, J. G., and Sinclair, A.: Arterial disease amongst blast furnace workers, Ann. Occup. Hyg. 18:15, 1975.
23. Kindwall, E. P.: Carbon Monoxide, in Zenz, C. (ed.), *Occupational Medicine: Principles and Practical Applications* (Chicago: Year Book Medical Publishers, 1975), pp. 605–612.

24. Knelson, J. H.: Luftsqualitatskriterien und immissionsgrenzwerte für kohlenmonoxid in den Vereinigten Staaten, Staub 32:180, 1972.
25. Koskela, R-S., et al.: A mortality study of foundry workers, Scand. J. Work Environ. Health 2(Supp. 1):73, 1976.
26. Koskela, R-S., Luoma, K., and Hernberg, S.: Turnover and health selection among foundry workers, Scand. J. Work Environ. Health 2(Supp. 1):90, 1976.
27. Micheal, L. W.: Compliance with the carbon monoxide standard in the workplace, Prev. Med. 8:289, 1979.
28. National Institute for Occupational Safety and Health, U. S. Dept. of Health, Education, and Welfare: Criteria for a Recommended Standard . . . Occupational Exposure to Carbon Monoxide. Center for Disease Control, National Institute for Occupational Safety and Health, Robert A. Taft Laboratories, 4676 Columbia Parkway, Cincinnati, Ohio 45226.
29. Ringold, W., et al.: Estimating recent carbon monoxide exposures: A rapid method, Arch. Environ. Health 5:308, 1962.
30. Silk, S. J.: The threshold limit value for carbon monoxide, Ann. Occup. Hyg. 18:29, 1975.
31. Sjöstrand, T.: Endogenous formation of carbon monoxide in man under normal and pathological conditions, Scand. J. Clin. Lab. Invest. 1:201, 1949.
32. Stewart, R. D., and Hake, C. L.: Paint-remover hazard, JAMA 235:398, 1976.
33. Stewart, R. D., et al.: Experimental human exposure to high concentrations of carbon monoxide, Arch. Environ. Health 26:1, 1973.
34. Stewart, R. D., Stewart, R. S., Stamm, W., and Seelen, R. P.: Rapid estimation of carboxyhemoglobin level in fire fighters, JAMA 235:390, 1976.
35. Vigilance performance (effects of CO). Effects of low level carbon monoxide on divided attention, pitch discrimination, and the auditory evoked potential. National Institute for Occupational Safety and Health, Cincinnati, Ohio, November, 1976.
36. Virtamo, M., and Tossavainen, A.: Carbon monoxide in foundry air, Scand. J. Work Environ. Health 2(Supp. 1):37, 1976.
37. Virtamo, M., and Tossavainen, A.: Gases formed from furan binding agents, Scand. J. Work Environ. Health 2(Supp. 1):50, 1976.
38. Wald, N., Howard, S., Smith, P. G., and Kjeldsen, K.: Association between atherosclerotic diseases and carboxyhaemoglobin levels in tobacco smokers, Br. Med. J. 1:761, 1973.
39. Zenz, C.: The epidemiology of carbon monoxide in cardiovascular disease in industrial environments. A review, Prev. Med. 8:279, 1979.

Chlorine

At workplace temperatures and pressures, chlorine is a yellowish green gas with a distinctive, irritating odor. Because of its reactivity, it is not found in the uncombined state in nature, but commonly as salt (NaCl). Chlorine is produced commercially by electrolysis of brine, electrolysis of fused sodium chloride or by oxidation of chlorides using chemical methods. By far the most important production method is the electrolysis of brine using diaphragm cells or mercury cells. U. S. chlorine production was estimated at 11,000,000 short tons in 1976. The pulp and paper industry uses chlorine primarily in the elemental form for bleaching pulp and paper; chlorine is used in the production of plastic and resins to make chlorinated solvents, to make ethylene glycol antifreeze and ethylene chloride (used in antiknock additives). Chlorine is also used in textile and household bleaches, refrigerants, pharmaceuticals, cosmetics, in the beneficiating of ores and in metal extraction. Exposure to chlorine can occur in any of these operations. In addition, exposure to chlorine can occur when hypochlorites are mixed with materials such as toilet bowl cleaners or vinegar and when chlorinated hydrocarbons are decomposed thermally or by actinic rays from welding.[6, 7] Some occupations with potential exposure to chlorine are aerosol propellent makers, alkali salt makers, aluminum purifiers, benzene hexachloride makers, bleachers, bleaching powder makers, bromine makers, broom makers, carpet makers, chemical synthesizers, calcium chloride makers, chlorinated solvent makers, chlorinated hydrocarbon insecticide makers, chlorine workers, color makers, disinfectant makers, dye makers, ethylene glycol makers, ethylene oxide makers, flour bleachers, fluorocarbon makers, gasoline additive workers, gold extractors, ink makers, iodine makers, iron detinners, iron dezincers, laundry workers, methyl chloride makers, paper bleachers, petroleum refinery workers, phosgene makers, photographic workers, pump bleachers, rayon makers, refrigerant makers, rubber makers, sewage treaters, silver extractors, sodium hydroxide makers, submarine workers, sugar refiners, sulfur chloride makers, swimming pool maintenance workers, tetraethyl lead makers, textile bleachers, tin recovery workers, vinyl chloride makers, vinylidene chloride makers, water treaters and zinc chloride makers. The NIOSH has estimated that 26,000 persons are employed in the chlor-alkali manufacturing industry, and about 15,000 workers have potential occupational exposure to chlorine.[5]

The main occupational exposure is by inhalation. Chlorine gas is a severe irritant of the eyes, mucous membranes, skin and respiratory system. Mild upper respiratory irritation may occur at 0.2–16 ppm; at 7–8 ppm, eye irritation; and cough at 30 ppm; 1000 ppm has proved fatal after a few breaths.[4] A major accidental exposure (community) to unmeasured but high concentrations for a brief period caused burning of the eyes with lacrimation, burning of the nose and mouth with rhinorrhea, cough, choking sensation and substernal pain.[1] These symptoms frequently were accompanied by nausea, vomiting, headache, dizziness and sometimes syncope. Of the 33 persons hospitalized, all suffered tracheobronchitis; 23 progressed to pulmonary edema and, of those, 14 developed pneumonitis. Respiratory distress and substernal pain generally subsided within the first 72 hours; cough increased in frequency and severity after 2–3 days and became productive of thick mucopurulent sputum; cough disappeared after 14 days. In another accidental exposure of 5 chlorine plant workers and 13 nonworkers, pulmonary function tests showed airway obstruction and hypoxemia; these cleared within 3 months except in 4 of the chlorine plant workers who still showed effects after 12–14 months.[2] In high concentrations, chlorine irritates the skin and causes sensations of burning and pricking, inflammation and vesicle formation. Liquid chlorine causes eye and skin burns on contact.

TREATMENT.—Immediate removal from exposure and hospitalization and observation for 3 days is advisable to guard against delayed pulmonary edema. Administer oxygen, provide clear airway by intubation and mechanical ventilation, if needed. Positive end-expiratory pressure breathing may be indicated and helpful. If the eyes are irritated, flush with water; if there is skin contact, lightly wash with mild soap and water.

The 1979 TLV: 1 ppm.

REFERENCES

Chlorine

1. Chasis, H., et al.: Chlorine accident in Brooklyn, Occup. Med. 4:152, 1947.
2. Kaufman, J., and Burkons, D.: Clinical, roentgenologic and physiologic effects of acute chlorine exposure, Arch. Environ. Health 23:29, 1971.
3. Manufacturing Chemists Association, Inc., Chemical Safety Data Sheet SD-80, Washington, D. C., pp. 23–26, 1970.
4. National Research Council, Committee on Medical and Biological Effects of Environmental Pollutants: Chlorine and Hydrogen Chloride, National Academy of Sciences, Washington, D. C., pp. 116–123, 1976.

5. NIOSH Criteria for a Recommended Standard . . . Occupational Exposure to Chlorine. U.S. Dept. of Health, Education, and Welfare, PHS, Center for Disease Control, HEW Publication No. (NIOSH) 76-170, Cincinnati, Ohio, May, 1976.
6. Rinzema, L. C.: Behavior of chlorohydrocarbon solvents in the welding environment, Int. Arch. Arbeitsmed. 28:151, 1971.
7. Rinzema, L. C., and Silverstein, L. G.: Hazards from chlorinated hydrocarbon decomposition during welding, Am. Ind. Hyg. Assoc. J. 33:35, 1972.

Chloroethanes

Chloroethanes are chlorinated organic compounds structurally related to ethane in which one or more of the hydrogen atoms have been replaced by a chlorine atom or atoms. Monochloroethane, for example, is shown to result from the replacement of one hydrogen atom in ethane by a chlorine atom.

At room temperature, monochloroethane is a gas, hexachloroethane is a solid and the eight other chloroethanes are liquids. Some of the chloroethanes are manufactured on a large scale and used extensively because of their low cost and excellent solvent properties.

Pentane (C_5H_{12}), hexane (C_6H_{14}), heptane (C_7H_{16}) and octane (C_8H_{18}) are members of a homologous series of aliphatic hydrocarbons with the empirical formula C(n)H(2n + 2). At room temperature, these four classes of alkanes are colorless, neutral liquids with a light petroleum odor. Pen-

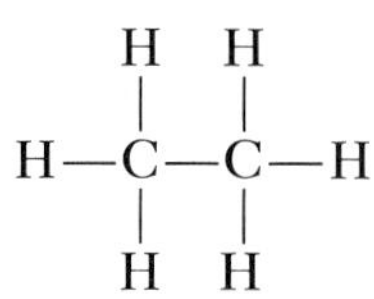

Ethane

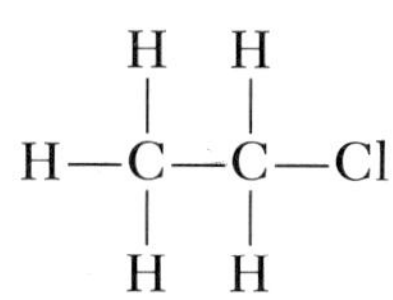

Monochloroethane

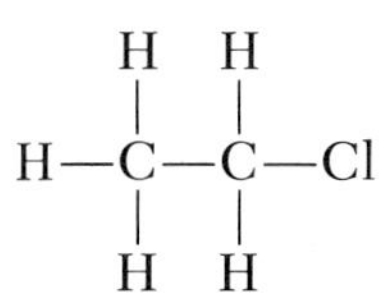

Chloroethane
(Ethyl Chloride)

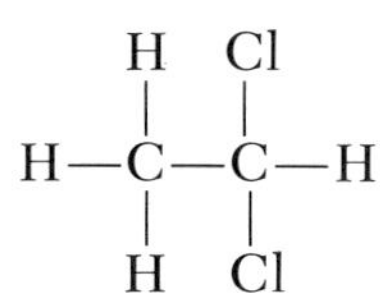

1,1-Dichloroethane

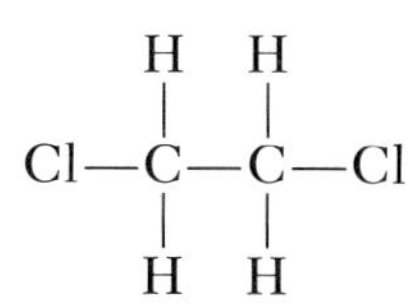

1,2-Dichloroethane
(Ethylene Dichloride)

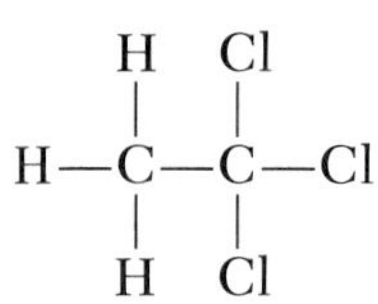

1,1,1-Trichloroethane
(Methyl Chloroform)

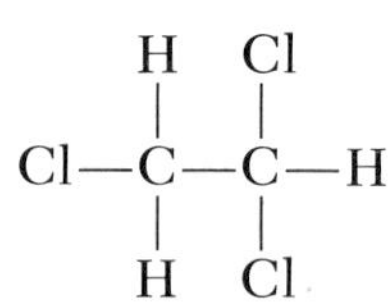

1,1,2-Trichloroethane

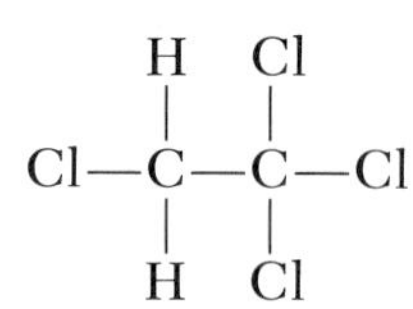

1,1,1,2-Tetrachloroethane

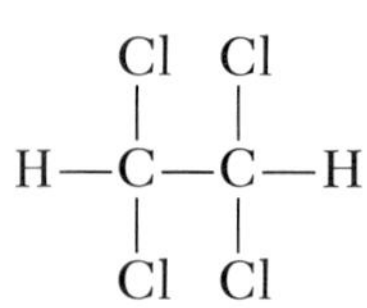

1,1,2,2-Tetrachloroethane

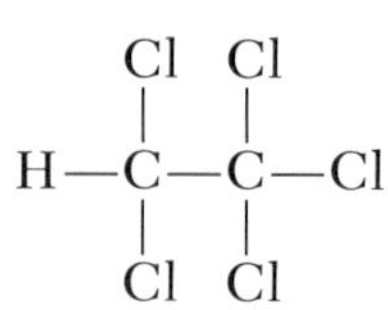

Pentachloroethane

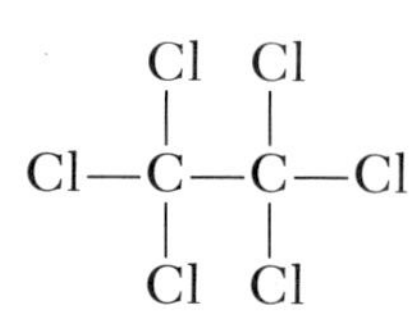

Hexachloroethane

tane, hexane, heptane and octane are produced almost exclusively from crude petroleum by catalytic cracking, thermal cracking, hydro-cracking and catalytic reforming. In the processes of catalytic and thermal cracking, high molecular weight hydrocarbons are broken down at high temperatures either with or without a catalyst into lower molecular weight mixtures. During the process of hydro-cracking, high molecular weight hydrocarbons are broken down with hydrogen at high pressures and temperatures without a catalyst. In catalytic re-forming, high molecular weight hydrocarbons are passed over a platinum catalyst at elevated temperatures in the presence of high-pressure hydrogen to produce lower molecular weight mixtures, which then are separated by distillation into high-purity fractions that include pentane, hexane, heptane and octane. One-third of the pentane produced in the United States comes from another source, fractional condensation of natural gas. Natural gas in the United States contains an average of 0.4% pentane by volume.

The estimated U. S. production of *n*-pentane and methylbutane (isopentane) in 1967 was 310,000 and 499,000 barrels per day, respectively. This is equivalent to approximately 48 million liters per day of *n*-pentane and 80 million liters per day of methylbutane. In 1974, the U. S. Tariff Commission reported an annual production of 280 million liters of hexane.

Alkanes are used in a variety of industrial applications and processes. A major use of pentane is in the formulation of gasoline. Hexane is used commercially as a solvent in glues, varnishes, cements and other products such as inks and also used in the seed oil industry to extract the natural oils from various seeds, including soybeans and cottonseed. Heptane and octane are used principally as solvents and to some extent in the formulation of gasoline.

Occupations with potential exposure to pentane, hexane, heptane and octane are adhesive workers, automobile fuel handlers, aviation fuel handlers, cabinet finishers, degreasing workers, farm fuel handlers, furniture makers, glue fabrication workers, gluing machine operators, laboratory workers (chemical), lacquerers, lacquer makers, laminators, leather cementers, metal degreasers, petrochemical process workers, petroleum distillation workers, petroleum extraction workers, petroleum refinery workers, plastics manufacturing workers, polyethylene laminating workers, printers, printing ink production workers, resin makers, rubber cement workers, shoe factory workers, spray painters and stainers, stain makers, synthetic chemical production workers, synthetic rubber workers, thermometer makers (low temperature), varnish makers, vegetable oil extraction workers and vinyl production workers. The NIOSH estimates that 10,000 workers in the United States are potentially exposed to pentane and heptane and 300,000 workers are potentially exposed to octane. It is not clear if these estimates take into account fuel handling operations. The NIOSH estimates that 2.5 million workers are potentially exposed to hexane.

Chloroethane production is estimated to be in excess of 4 billion kg in the United States. Although chloroethanes have been associated with cancer in laboratory animals, the NIOSH is unaware of any definitive evidence indicating that chloroethanes are carcinogenic in humans. The chloroethanes have long been known to be capable of producing harmful local and systemic effects. As summarized in Table 14–4, the chloroethanes may affect a variety of human organs and/or systems. The effects of chloroethane exposure vary from one compound to another, but most manifestations and laboratory findings associated with chloroethane toxicity are similar for the major routes of entry: inhalation, skin absorption and ingestion. Liver and/or kidney injury, pulmonary irritation and damage to the blood-forming system have been associated with inhalation of chloroethanes. Repeated or prolonged

TABLE 14–4.—ADVERSE EFFECTS OF CHLOROETHANE ON HUMAN ORGANS AND SYSTEMS [2, 8–11, 15]*

CHEMICAL	IMMUNOLOGIC-ALLERGIC	HEMATOLOGIC	CARDIOVASCULAR	PULMONARY	RENAL-UROLOGIC	GASTROINTESTINAL	HEPATIC-BILIARY	MUSCULOSKELETAL	NEUROLOGIC	DERMATOLOGIC	OPHTHALMOLOGIC	OTHER
monochloroethane	x		x	x		x			x	x	x	x
1,1-dichloroethane				x					x	x		
1,2-dichloroethane		x	x	x	x	x	x	x	x	x		x
1,1,1-trichloroethane		x	x			x	x		x	x	x	x
1,1,2,2-tetrachloroethane		x	x	x	x	x	x		x	x		x
hexachloroethane									x		x	

*Adverse human health effects have not been reported to the NIOSH for 1,1,2-trichloroethane, 1,1,2-tetrachloroethane and pentachloroethane.

skin exposure can defat the skin and cause dermatitis.

In addition to the toxic effects of chloroethanes and their metabolites, the oxidative decomposition of products produced in the presence of open flames, hot metals or lighted cigarettes should be taken into account. The chloroethane compounds may degrade to phosgene, hydrogen chloride and dichloracetylene. Phosgene is considered to be dangerous to life in 30–60 minutes at 12.5 ppm.[12]

LABORATORY ANIMAL STUDIES

Carcinogenicity

As of July, 1978, four of the eight chloroethanes selected by the NCI for testing have been shown to be carcinogenic in laboratory animals. Each compound was studied separately in male and female Osborne-Mendel rats and male and female $B_6C_3F_1$ mice. Each experiment consisted of a high-dose and a low-dose group of 50 animals each. Twenty animals of each species/sex combination served as untreated controls and 20 animals of each species/sex combination served as vehicle controls. The chloroethane compounds were administered to the test animals in a corn oil vehicle by gastric intubation (stomach tube) 5 days a week for 78 weeks. The vehicle controls were intubated with pure corn oil at the same rate as the high-dose animals.

The National Cancer Institute has concluded that under the conditions of the bioassay, 1,2-dichloroethane, 1,1,2-trichloroethane, 1,1,2,2-tetrachloroethane and hexachloroethane are carcinogenic in mice, inducing liver cancer in both sexes.[3-6] In addition, results of the NCI bioassay of 1,2-dichloroethane indicate that this compound also causes cancer in male and female rats. In mice, 1,1,2-trichloroethane was also associated with increased adrenal pheochromocytoma, a tumor that gives rise to high blood pressure and hyperglycemia. Toxic kidney damage was observed in all groups of both mice and rats treated with hexachloroethane.[4]

Although the occurrence of cancer in mice is highly significant, the results do not provide conclusive evidence that 1,1,2-trichloroethane, 1,1,2,2-tetrachloroethane or hexachloroethane causes cancer in rats. A statistically significant association between increased dosage and accelerated mortality was observed in rats treated with

TABLE 14–5.—CHLOROETHANE EXPOSURE STANDARDS

CHEMICAL	OSHA EXPOSURE STANDARD (ppm)	NIOSH RECOMMENDED EXPOSURE STANDARD (ppm)
monochloroethane	1000	none
1,1-dichloroethane	100	none
1,2-dichloroethane	50	5
1,1,1-trichloroethane	350	350
1,1,2-trichloroethane	10	none
1,1,1,2-tetrachloroethane	none	none
1,1,2,2-tetrachloroethane	5	1
pentachloroethane	none	
hexachloroethane	1	

hexachloroethane. The NCI has concluded that early mortality may have obscured a carcinogenic effect in these animals.

Other Adverse Effects in Animals

All of the chloroethane compounds are known to cause central nervous system depression in laboratory animals. This usually is expressed as abnormal weakness, intoxication, restlessness, irregular respiration, muscle incoordination and unconsciousness. Chloroethanes generally are irritating to the eyes and skin. Damage to the liver and/or kidneys has been demonstrated in various animal species following exposure to these compounds.[13]

It has been reported that some of the chloroethanes and their metabolites are mutagenic in bacterial systems.[1,6] Mutagenic activity, per se, should be considered a substantial liability. In addition, research suggests a correlation between mutagenicity in some bacterial strains and carcinogenicity in higher animals. Other adverse effects of the chloroethanes may vary from one compound to another.

Summaries of the current Department of Labor–Occupational Safety and Health Administration (OSHA) exposure standards[14] and the NIOSH recommended exposure standards for the chloroethane compounds are given in Table 14–5.

The OSHA exposure standards and the NIOSH recommended standards and control measures for the chloroethanes were developed before the carcinogenic potential of these compounds was recognized. Therefore, an assessment of the carcinogenicity of these compounds was not included. The levels currently recommended or adopted may not provide adequate protection from potential carcinogenic effects.

REFERENCES

Chloroethanes

1. Fishbein, L.: Industrial mutagens and potential mutagens I. Halogenated aliphatic derivatives, Mutat. Res. 32:267, 1976.
2. Gosselin, R. E., Hodge, H. C., Smith, S. P., and Gleason, M. N. (eds.): *Clinical Toxicology of Commercial Products: Acute Poisoning* (4th ed.; Baltimore: Williams & Wilkins, 1976).
3. National Cancer Institute. Bioassay of 1,2-Dichloroethane for Possible Carcinogenicity. U.S. Department of Health, Education, and Welfare, PHS, National Institute of Health, National Cancer Institute, Carcinogenesis Testing Program, DHEW Publication No. (NIH) 78-1305, January 10, 1978.
4. National Cancer Institute. Bioassay of Hexachloroethane for Possible Carcinogenicity. U.S. Dept. of Health, Education, and Welfare, PHS, National Institute of Health, National Cancer Institute, DHEW Publication No. (NIH) 78-1318, 1978.
5. National Cancer Institute. Bioassay of 1,1,2-Trichloroethane for Possible Carcinogenicity. U.S. Dept. of Health, Education, and Wel-

fare, PHS, National Institute of Health, National Cancer Institute, DHEW Publication No. (NIH) 78-1324, 1978,
6. National Cancer Institute. Bioassay of 1,1,2,2-Tetrachloroethane for Possible Carcinogenicity. U.S. Dept. of Health, Education, and Welfare, PHS, National Institute of Health, National Cancer Institute, DHEW Publication No. (NIH) 78-827, 1978.
7. National Cancer Institute. Chemicals Being Tested for Carcinogenicity by the Carcinogenesis Testing Program. Division of Cancer Cause and Prevention, National Cancer Institute, June 1, 1978.
8. National Institute for Occupational Safety and Health. Criteria for a Recommended Standard . . . Occupational Exposure to Ethylene Dichloride (1,2-Dichloroethane). U.S. Dept. of Health, Education, and Welfare, PHS, Center for Disease Control, National Institute for Occupational Safety and Health, DHEW (NIOSH) Publication No. 76-139, March, 1976.
9. National Institute for Occupational Safety and Health. Criteria for a Recommended Standard . . . Occupational Exposure to 1,1,1-Trichloroethane (Methyl Chloroform). U.S. Dept. of Health, Education, and Welfare, PHS, Center for Disease Control, National Institute for Occupational Safety and Health, DHEW (NIOSH) Publication No. 76-184, July, 1976.
10. National Institute for Occupational Safety and Health. Criteria for a Recommended Standard . . . Occupational Exposure to 1,1,2,2-Tetrachloroethane. U. S. Department of Health, Education, and Welfare, PHS, Center for Disease Control, National Institute for Occupational Safety and Health, DHEW (NIOSH) Publication No. 77-121, December, 1976.
11. National Institute for Occupational Safety and Health. NIOSH Current Intelligence Bulletin #25, Ethylene Dichloride. U.S. Dept. of Health, Education, and Welfare, PHS, Center for Disease Control, National Institute for Occupational Safety and Health, DHEW Publication No. (NIOSH) 74-149, April 19, 1978.
12. Patty, F. A., Fassett, D. W., and Irish, D. D. (eds.): *Industrial Hygiene and Toxicology* (2d ed.; New York: Interscience Publishers, 1963).
13. Sax, N. I.: *Dangerous Properties of Industrial Materials* (New York: Van Nostrand Reinhold Company, 1975).
14. United States Department of Labor, Occupational Safety and Health Administration. General Industry Standards (29 Code of Federal Regulations 1910), January, 1976.
15. U.S. International Trade Commission. Synthetic Organic Chemicals, United States Production and Sales, 1976. U.S. International Trade Commission, USITC Publication No. 833, 1976.

Cobalt Metal and Its Compounds

Occupational exposures and uses of cobalt metal are in alloying processes such as steel cutting, grinding, welding and melting, in ceramics, in glass as pigments, as a catalyst and in magnets (20% of all cobalt consumed). Exposures are through inhalation. Cobalt metal dust and fume cause chronic interstitial pneumonitis and skin sensitization. Rhabdomyosarcomata developed in rats injected intramuscularly with the powder of either pure cobalt metal or cobalt oxide.[10] Animals were exposed to the repeated inhalation of the cobalt metal blend used by the cemented carbide industry (see section on Tungsten, this chapter). A concentration of 20 mg/m^3 for 3 years produced hyperplasia of the bronchial epithelium and focal fibrotic lesions of the lungs, with developing granulomata. Daily inhalation of cobalt metal fume composed of approximately equal parts of cobalt, cobalt oxide and cobaltic-cobaltous oxide did not elicit these reactions. Guinea pigs developed acute pneumonitis, often rapidly fatal, from the intratracheal injection of cobalt metal or repeated inhalation of a mixture of 75% tungsten carbide and 25% cobalt.[7] Chronic interstitial pneumonitis has been reported in workers in the cemented carbide industry and cobalt has been conditionally implicated as the etiologic agent by a process of elimination of the other materials used in the industry. Symptoms range from shortness of breath, cough and dyspnea on exertion to permanent disability or death in some cases. Among 12 workers engaged in the manufacture of, or grinding with, tungsten carbide tools who developed interstitial lung disease there were 8 fatalities; serial chest roentgenograms over a period of 3–12 years revealed gradually progressive densities of a linear and nodular nature that gradually involved major portions of both lungs; cough, dyspnea on exertion and reduced pulmonary function occurred early in the course of the disease.[6] The disease has features of hypersensitivity; only a small percentage of people exposed are affected, and with little evidence of dose-response relationship. Cobalt and its compounds may produce an allergic dermatitis of an erythematous papular type, which usually occurs in skin areas subjected to friction, such as the ankles, elbow flexures and sides of the neck.[5]

Six groups of workers from the tungsten carbide industry with different degrees of exposure to cobalt have been studied by Alexandersson.[1] Nonexposed control groups from the same industries, matched with regard to sex, age and smoking, were compared. Respiratory tract irritative effects were reported with a higher frequency among exposed persons than among controls. It appeared that an average exposure to 0.06 mg Co/m^3 of air gives rise to respiratory tract reaction with changes mainly of an obstructive type. This reaction can be demonstrated over a working shift, decreasing when away from work (2 shifts), and even more over a weekend. However, regression was not complete, because there is a difference between the exposed persons and the matched controls of Monday morning before work. The same trend could be demonstrated in some of the other less-exposed groups. The reactions mentioned were most pronounced in smokers who also were exposed to cobalt.

Alexandersson and Hedenstierna[3] investigated exposure to cobalt dust and the effects on lung function in 155 employees and 74 matched control subjects. The cobalt-exposed subjects were divided into five groups: (A) low exposure to cobalt dust (avg. exposure 0.005mm<0.01 mg/m^3); (B) heavy exposure to cobalt dust (avg. exposure 0.06 mg/m^3); (C) dry polishing of sintered material (avg. exposure 0.01 mg/m^3); (D) wet polishing of sintered material (avg. exposure 0.008 mg/m^3); (E) inspectors (avg. exposure 0.002 mg/m^3). Pulmonary function was evaluated by means of spirometry and a single-breath nitrogen washout. Measurements were done (a) on Monday morning before work, (b) on Friday afternoon immediately after work and (c) after 4 weeks of holiday. Acute effects of cobalt exposure were tested by comparing the lung function values on Monday morning with those on Friday afternoon. Long-term effects were studied by comparing lung function in exposed persons and control subjects on Monday before work and by studying the effects on lung function after 4 weeks of holiday. Closing volume in relation to vital capacity (CV%) was increased in group B after exposure to cobalt during work. The less-exposed subjects in groups A, C and D tended to increase their CV% and indexes of intrapulmonary gas distribution during the week. Group E (the inspectors) showed no changes during the week. Thus, the findings indicated an impaired pulmonary function as a consequence of exposure to cobalt dust during the week in the moderately and highly exposed employees. A comparison with matched control subjects on Monday morning showed no differences except for those in group B. Thus, lung function returned to normal levels in groups A, C and D whereas the most heavily exposed employees in group B had a persisting reduction in lung function, which remained after 4 weeks of holiday. In conclusion, exposure to cobalt below the TLV (0.1 mg/m^3) at the time of their investigation (1977–1978) resulted in acute but, in general, subsiding pulmonary effects, interpreted as airway obstruction. For the most exposed subjects, a chronic reduction in lung function could not be excluded.

Alexandersson and Lidums[4] determined the normal range and lower limits of cobalt in blood and urine, noting cobalt content to be about 8.48 nmol/l in blood and 6.78 nmol/l in urine of a nonexposed group. After exposure, cobalt was rapidly excreted in urine. When the occupational exposure was relatively high there was rapid, continual decrease in excretion for about 24 hours and then a phase with slower excretion. When the exposure is low, the excretion in urine of cobalt is relatively constant, although it may be 4–10 times higher than in nonexposed persons. The slow excretion continues for a long time, sometimes at least 4 weeks after exposure. The variations in cobalt concentrations in blood are smaller but follow the exposure. When blood and urine concentrations of cobalt were compared on Friday afternoon, the correlation coefficient was 0.82. When the average exposure to cobalt for the whole week was compared with the cobalt concentration in urine, the correlation coefficient on Friday afternoon was 0.79 and on Monday morning 0.81. For blood, the correlation coefficient was 0.87 on Friday afternoon and 0.76 on Monday morning.

Work exposures in 8 cemented tungsten carbide plants in Sweden were evaluated by Alexandersson and Bergman.[2] Their findings revealed that exposure to cobalt varies a great deal from one category of production personnel to another. Some cobalt particles are small enough to penetrate the alveolar level and give rise to pulmonary reactions. The highest level of exposure to cobalt occurs among groups handling powder; declining levels occur among press operators, shapers, dry grinders, wet grinders, flat grinders and inspection personnel (in that order), the exposure levels of the two last-mentioned categories being very low, indeed. The concentration of airborne cobalt generally was below the Swedish TLV, 0.1 mg Co/m^3. For short periods, however, some of the workers handling powder may have exceeded the TLV, but, in these situations, the workers are instructed to use dust respirators.

REFERENCES

Cobalt Metal and Its Compounds

1. Alexandersson, R.: Undersökningar över effekter av exposition för kobolt. II. Reaktioner i andningsorganen vid olika grad av exposition i hårdmetallindustri, Arbete och Hälsa, Vetenskaplig Skriftserie, 2, 1979.
2. Alexandersson, R., and Bergman, K.: Undersökningar över effekter av exposition för kobolt. I. Undersögning över expositionsförhållandena i hårdmetallindustri, Arbete och Hälsa, Vetenskaplig Skriftserie, 20, 1978.
3. Alexandersson, R., and Hedenstierna, G.: Undersökningar över effekter av exposition för kobolt. III. Ventilationsformaga, distribution av inandningsgas och luftvägsavstängning under pågående arbete och efter expositionsuppehåll, Arbete och Hälsa, Vetenskaplig Skriftserie, 7, 1979.
4. Alexandersson, R., and Lidums, V.: Undersökningar över effekter av exposition för kobolt. IV. Koboltkoncentrationen i blod och urin som expositionsindikator, Arbete och Hälsa, Vetenskaplig Skriftserie, 8, 1979.
5. Browning, E.: *Toxicity of Industrial Metals* (2d. ed.; London: Butterworths, 1969), pp. 132–142.
6. Coates, E. O., and Watson, J. H. L.: Diffuse interstitial lung disease in tungsten carbide workers, Ann. Intern. Med. 75:709, 1971.
7. Delahant, A. B.: An experimental study of the effects of rare metals on animals' lungs, A.M.A. Arch. Ind. Hyg. 12:116, 1955.
8. Gilman, J. P. W., and Ruckerbauer, G. M.: Metal carcinogenesis. 1. Observations on the carcinogenicity of refinery dust, cobalt oxide, and colloidal thorium dioxide, Cancer Res. 22:152, 1962.
9. Hampel, C. A., and Hanley, C. G.: *The Encyclopedia of Chemistry* (3d ed.; New York: Van Nostrand Reinhold Co., 1973).
10. Heath, J. C.: The histogenesis of malignant tumours induced by cobalt in the rat, Br. J. Cancer 14:478, 1960.
11. Hygienic Guide Series: Cobalt (except the carbonyls), Am. Ind. Hyg. Assoc. J. 27:199, 1966.
12. Miller, C. W., et al.: Pneumoconiosis in the tungsten-carbide tool industry, A.M.A. Arch. Ind. Hyg. 8:453, 1953.

Cresols

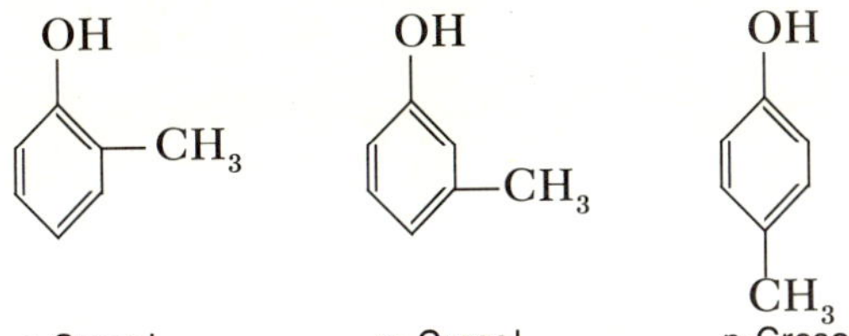

o-Cresol *m*-Cresol *p*-Cresol

The cresol isomers ($CH_3C_6H_4OH$) are monomethyl derivatives of phenol (or hydroxy derivatives of toluene) that have the methyl group ortho, meta or para to the hydroxyl group. The three isomers can occur alone or in various mixtures, either with one another or with other compounds. A mixture containing all three isomers often is referred to as tricresol and has a boiling range between 191° and 203° C. Commercial cresylic acids generally are defined as mixtures in which 50% of the material boils above 204° C. The cresol isomers usually are the major components of cresylic acids. Although some of these properties differ among the isomers, the oil/water partition coefficients suggest that their biologic distribution may be similar. Most nonsynthetic cresol used in industry is derived from petroleum or coal tar acids. Petroleum-based cresol is a by-product of the naphtha-cracking process and is present in the spent caustic liquor used to wash petroleum distillate. Coal tar acids are obtained from coke oven by-products, gas-retort oven tars and distilled tar by-products. The initial fractionation of petroleum or coal tar acids yields a phenolic mixture composed mainly of cresol, phenol and xylenols. Pure *o*-cresol can be obtained by further distillation of this mixture, but because of their similar boiling points, the meta and para isomers of cresol must be separated by other methods. Generally, these two isomers are used industrially as a mixture containing 40–65% *m*-cresol. Only small amounts of pure natural meta and para isomers are produced. There also are several methods of synthesizing the cresol isomers, particularly *p*-cresol. The catalyzed methylation of phenol is one of the methods used most often.

It is estimated that 70 million kg of cresol and cresylic acids were produced in the United States in 1975. The consumption of synthetic cresol varies to some extent from that of the natural products. Industry sources estimated that, in 1975, 28% of natural cresol was used for the production of wire enamel solvents, 20% for phosphate esters, 18% for phenolic resins, 6% for agricultural chemicals, 3% for disinfectants, 3% for ore flotation, 10% for miscellaneous purposes and 12% for export. In 1969, 29% of synthetic cresol was consumed for phenolic resins, 26% for tricresyl phosphate, 11% for disinfectants, 17% for antioxidants and automotive products, 7% for ore flotation and 10% for other purposes. A major use of *o*-cresol is in the manufacture of the herbicides dinitro-*o*-cresol (DNOC) and 2-methyl-4-chlorophenoxyacetic acid (MCPA). *p*-Cresol is used largely to produce the antioxidant 2,6-*ditert*-butyl-*p*-cresol (BHT), which is added to plastics and to food. Cresylic acids and *m*,*p*-cresol mixtures are used to make phenolic resins, tricresyl phosphate and cresyl diphenyl phosphate, the last two used mainly as plasticizers. Some minor uses of cresols are in the production of azo dyes and as perfume additives, nylon solvents, metal degreasing agents and synthetic tanning agents.

The NIOSH estimates that 11,000 people in the United States are occupationally exposed to cresol. This estimate is low, however, because it does not include workers who are intermittently exposed to a widely used commercial degreasing agent that contains cresol. Some representative occupations are: antioxidant producers, coal tar workers, cresol soap makers, cresol workers, cresylic acid makers, deodorant workers, disinfectant makers, disinfectors, DNOC producers, dye makers, enamel makers, flotation agent makers, flotation workers, foundry workers, glue workers, ink makers, ink remover makers, ink removers, insecticide workers, insulation enamal workers, oil additive makers, paint remover makers, paint removers, perfume makers, phenolic resin producers, phosphate ester producers, photographic developer workers, pitch workers, resin makers, roofers, rubber makers, scouring compound makers, stainers, stain makers, surfactant makers, tanning agent makers, tar distillery workers, textile sizers, varnish remover makers, varnish removers, veterinarians and wood scourers.

The ability of cresols to be absorbed through the skin and produce local and systemic effects has been demonstrated in humans.[5, 11–13, 16, 18, 24] The skin, considered to be the primary route of occupational exposure, is the site of most of the worker injuries reported from cresols. Skin contact with cresols has resulted in skin peeling on the hands,[16] facial peripheral neuritis,[16] severe facial burns[13] and damage to internal organs, including loss of kidney function[5] and necrosis of the liver and kidneys.[12] Cresols also have caused sensitization of the skin.[11, 24] Dermatitis developed on the fingers of workers who had been using a solution containing cresol and cresylic acid.[11] Of 30 workers in a synthetic plastics plant, 6 developed dermatitis on the hands and face resulting from exposure to cresol and phenol.[24] Although the information in these reports was insufficient to allow determination of dose-response relationships, industrial experience indicated that only small quantities of cresols were needed to produce chemical burns of the skin.

Animal studies also have indicated that cresols can cause local irritation and be absorbed after skin contact.[1, 4, 20] Discoloration of the skin, convulsions and death occurred in rats given dermal applications of 1 ml/kg of various coal tar-derived cresylic acids.[4] In rabbits that had any of the three cresol isomers applied dermally in doses of 1 ml/kg for 24 hours, severe edema, erythema or subdermal hemorrhaging developed.[1] Other effects included salivation, lacrimation, hypoactivity, tremors, convulsions, sedation and death.[1] Shelley[20] reported that repeated dermal application of 0.5% *p*-cresol caused depigmentation of the hair and epidermis and local corrosion of the skin in mice.

Appreciable concentrations of cresol vapors rarely are generated in industry because all three cresol isomers have low vapor pressures. However, a hazardous concentration of vapor may be generated at elevated temperatures, and there have been a few reports in the literature[6, 22] describing effects from inhalation of cresol vapor. Corcos[6] reported that 7 workers exposed to airborne cresol at an unspecified concentration developed headaches and nausea. Some workers also had hypertension, muscle irritability, convulsions and decreased kidney function.[6] Interviews with workers exposed to cresol and phenol at concentrations of 0.02–10 ppm (0.08–38 mg/m^3) in air did not delineate effects on the eyes, nose and throat.[8] The airborne concentration was reported as total phenols, so the actual exposure to cresol was not known. However, Uzhdavini et al.[22] found that 8 of 10 subjects experimentally exposed to *o*-cresol vapor at a concentration of 6 mg/m^3 complained of dryness of the throat and the sensation of an unspecified taste. Despite the lack of specific details regarding methodology, this is the only reference of human inhalation exposure to a pure cresol and should not be ignored. Although no reports of effects in humans from long-term exposure to cresols were found, toxic effects have been observed in animals repeatedly exposed by inhalation.[4,17,22] Campbell[4] reported irritation of the nose and eyes and some deaths in mice that inhaled coal tar- or petroleum-derived cresylic acid vapors at "saturated" air concentrations for 1 hour per day on 10 consecutive days. Uzhdavini et al.[22] observed some microscopic changes in mice exposed to *o*-cresol vapor aerosol at an average concentration of 50 mg/m^3 for 2 hours per day, 6 days per week for 1 month and in rats and guinea pigs exposed to *o*-cresol vapor at a concentration of 9 mg/m^3 for 6 hours per day, 5 days per week for 2 months and 4 hours per day, 5 days per week for another 2 months. These authors also reported irritation of the upper respiratory tract in humans exposed to airborne *o*-cresol at 6 mg/m^3 and in cats exposed at 5–9 mg/m^3. They did not comment on whether similar effects were found in rats and guinea pigs. Kurlyandskiy et al.[17] found that 0.05 mg/m^3 of tricresol vapor was the lowest concentration at which effects, including CNS excitability and protein denaturation, were noted in rats exposed for 3 months.

Several cases of cresol ingestion and its intravaginal applications have shown cresol to be corrosive to body tissues and to cause toxic effects on the vascular system, liver, kidneys and pancreas. Cresol introduced into the uteri of pregnant women has produced abortion,[19,23] extensive hemolysis,[19] erosion of blood vessels,[23] damage to the kidney tubules,[19] necrosis of the liver[19] and death.[19] Most cases of cresol ingestion have been the result of attempted[3,14,15] or successful[10,14] suicides. The smallest amount of cresol that produced death was 4 ml of a 25–50% cresol solution in an 11-month-old child.[14] Systemic effects observed after cresol ingestion reflected those observed after its use as an abortifacient and included elevated blood pressure,[15] damage to the vascular system[15] and kidneys[10,14,15] and acute pancreatitis.[10,15]

Although no data were found that compared the effects of *o*-, *m*- and *p*-cresol in humans, several animal studies[1,2,9,21] suggest that their biologic actions are similar. Mortality studies using dermal, oral, subcutaneous or intravenous administration generally have shown that *o*- and *p*-cresol are about equal in toxicity but that *m*-cresol is less toxic. The only inhalation study[1] that compared the three isomers showed no difference in effect between *m*- and *p*-cresol at identical concentrations; *o*-cresol was given at a somewhat higher concentration. The toxic effects other than mortality observed in these studies[1,9,21] were qualitatively similar for the three isomers and included skin irritation, CNS disturbances and liver and kidney damage. The urinary metabolites of the three isomers have also been found to be similar.[2] Compounds conjugated at the hydroxyl group accounted for the majority of the metabolites. In summary, the most frequently observed effects resulting from occupational exposure to cresols are burns of the skin and eyes. In addition to being strong tissue irritants, cresols may cause impairment of kidney and liver function and CNS and cardiovascular disturbances. The NIOSH recommends that an environmental limit for cresol of 10 mg/m^3 as a TWA concentration be established. It is believed that a TWA concentration of 10 mg/m^3 will protect the worker from the occupational health hazards associated with cresol, considering the limited information available, and, in addition, it will reduce the probability of cresol acting as a promoter. The workplace environmental limit recommended for cresol applies to the individual cresol isomers when they occur alone or to any mixture of the isomers.

REFERENCES

Cresols

1. Bio Fax Techniques—Methods Used in Determining Biological Activity of Chemicals. Northbrook, Ill., Industrial Bio-Test Laboratories, Inc., Vols, 3–5, 4–5, 5–5, 1969.

2. Bray, H. G., Thorpe, W. V., and White, K.: Metabolism of derivatives of toluene—4. Cresols, Biochem. J. 46:275, 1950.
3. Burg, K.: Double central pneumonia in a case of Lysol poisoning, Med. Klin. 23: 1134, 1929 (German).
4. Campbell, J.: Petroleum cresylic acids—a study of their toxicity and the toxicity of cresylic disinfectants, Soap Sanit. Chem. 17:103, 121, 1941.
5. Cason, J. S.: Report on three extensive industrial chemical burns, Br. Med. J. 1:827, 1959.
6. Corcos, A.:. Contribution to the study of occupational poisoning by cresols. Dissertation. Paris, Vigot Freres Editeurs, 62 pp., 1939 (French).
7. Criteria for a Recommended Standard . . . Occupational Exposure to Cresol. DHEW (NIOSH) Publication No. 78-133. Cincinnati, Ohio, U.S. Dept. of Health, Education, and Welfare, PHS, Center for Disease Control, National Institute for Occupational Safety and Health, 117 pp., 1978.
8. Cummins Northeastern Incorporated—Dedham, Massachusetts, Health Hazard Evaluation/Toxicity Determination Report No. 73-5-110. Cincinnati, Ohio, U.S. Dept. of Health, Education, and Welfare, PHS, Center for Disease Control, National Institute for Occupational Safety and Health, Hazard Evaluation Services Branch, 7 pp., 1974.
9. Deichmann, W. B., and Witherup, S.: Phenol studies—VI. The acute and comparative toxicity of phenol and *o*-, *m*- and *p*-cresols for experimental animals, J. Pharmacol. Exp. Ther. 80:233, 1944.
10. Dellal, V.: Acute pancreatitis following Lysol poisoning, Lancet 1:407, 1931.
11. Goodman, H.: Silk handler's disease of the skin. Dermatitis venenata due to isomers of cresol, Med. J. Rec. 138:349, 1933.
12. Green, M. A.: A household remedy misused. Fatal cresol poisoning following cutaneous absorption (a case report), Med. Sci. Law 15:65, 1975.
13. Herwick, R. P., and Treweek, D. N.: Burns from anesthesia mask sterilized in compound solution of cresol, JAMA 100:407, 1933.
14. Isaacs, R.: Phenol and cresol poisoning, Ohio State Med. J. 18:558, 1922.
15. Klimkiewicz, E., Klinger, M., Kurbiel, A., and Soltys, W.: A case of liquid phenol poisoning complicated by acute pancreatitis and acute renal failure, Wiad. Lek. 27:1211, 1974 (Polish).
16. Klinger, M. E., and Norton, J. F.: Toxicity of cresylic acid-containing solvent, U.S. Nav. Med. Bull. 3:438, 1945.
17. Kurlyandskiy, B. A., Partsef, D. P., and Chernomorskiy, A. R.: Methods for determination of mean daily MPC of tricresol in the atmosphere, Gig. Sanit. 5:85, 1975 (Russian).
18. Plant observation reports and evaluation. Menlo Park, Calif., Stanford Research Institute, 146 pp. (submitted to NIOSH under Contract No. CDC-99-74-31, October, 1977).
19. Presley, J. A., and Brown, W. E.: Lysol-induced criminal abortion, Obstet. Gynecol. 8:368, 1956.
20. Shelley, W. B.: *p*-Cresol. Cause of ink-induced hair depigmentation in mice, Br. J. Dermatol. 90:169, 1974.
21. Uzhdavini, E. R., Astafyeva, N. K., and Mamayeva, A. A.: The acute toxicity of lower phenols, Gig. Tr. Prof. Zabol. 18:58, 1974 (Russian).
22. Uzhdavini, E. R., Astafyeva, N. K., Mamayeva, A. A., and Bakhtizina, G. Z.: Inhalation toxicity of *o*-cresol, Tr. Ufim. Nauchno-Issled. Inst. Gig. Prof. Zabol. 7:115, 1972 (Russian).
23. Vance, B. M.: Intrauterine injection of Lysol as an abortifacient. Report of a fatal case complicated by oil embolism and Lysol poisoning, Arch. Pathol. 40:395, 1945.
24. Zalecki, M.: The results of examination of Cracow plant employees for detection of occupational skin diseases, Med. Pregl. 16:385, 1965 (Polish).

4,4′-Diaminodiphenylmethane (DDM)

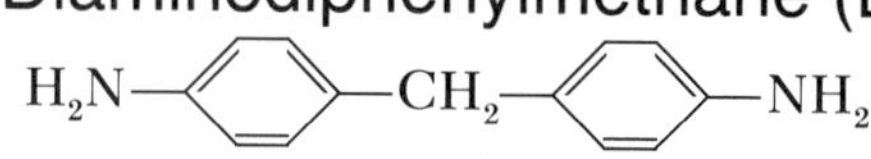

DDM, 4,4′-diaminodiphenylmethane, also known as *p,p*′-methylenedianiline (MDA), is an important chemical intermediate. More than 100 million kg per year of DDM are manufactured in the United States. DDM is produced by the condensation of aniline with formaldehyde in the presence of an acid catalyst. Approximately 99% of the DDM produced is consumed in its crude form (occasionally containing not more than 50% DDM and polyDDM) at its production site by reaction with phosgene in the preparation of isocyanates and polyisocyanates. These isocyanates and polyisocyanates are used in the manufacture of rigid polyurethane foams that find application as thermal insulation. Polyisocyanates are also used in the preparation of the semi-flexible polyurethane foams used for automotive safety cushioning. DDM is also used as an epoxy hardening agent, a raw material in the production of polyurethane elastomers, in the rubber industry as a curative for neoprene,[5] as an antifrosting agent (antioxidant), in footwear, a raw material in the production of Qiana Nylon and a raw material in the preparation of poly (amide-imide) resins (used in magnet wire enamels).

It is estimated that 2500 workers are exposed to DDM. Many of these exposures to DDM are in the preparation of isocyanates and polyisocyanates and on construction sites in the application of epoxy coatings. In 1965, the hepatotoxic effects of DDM in humans were first seen in the so-called Epping Jaundice outbreak in Great Britain. In this incident, 84 people who had eaten DDM-contaminated bread experienced hepatocellular damage evidenced by elevated SGOT and SGPT levels.[3,4] DDM also has been shown to produce liver lesions in a group of intragastrically fed rats[2] and has caused liver degeneration and spleen lesions in another group of DDM-fed rats.[8]

DDM in the occupational environment has been implicated in a number of cases of toxic hepatitis. During an 18-month period beginning April, 1972, 6 cases of hepatitis developed among about 300 men who used epoxy resins in the construction of a nuclear power plant in Alabama. Two chemicals, DDM and 2-nitropropane, were held suspect in this study.[11,12] In another study, 13 cases of hepatitis developed between 1966 and 1972 among workers who added DDM to a mixture to produce a hard plastic insulating material. All of these men became ill within a few days of working intensively with DDM.[6] One other case of hepatitis, possibly associated with DDM, was reported by a person who wrote to the Environmental Protection Agency describing an episode of acute hepatitis as well as CNS and pulmonary symptoms he experienced following exposure to a surfacing agent containing DDM.

The carcinogenic effects of DDM have also been studied. In one study, 16 rats were given 4 or 5 20-mg DDM doses by stomach tube over 8 months. A hepatoma and a hemangioma-like tumor of the kidney were found in one rat after 18 months and an adenocarcinoma of the uterus was found in another after 24 months.[9] In another report, of 48 rats given DDM intragastrically 5 times weekly, all developed liver cirrhosis, 4 developed hepatomas (2 benign) and others developed miscellaneous tumors.[7] In a third report, 50% of 50 DDM-injected rats developed tumors (4 hepatomas) compared wtih 26% of a control group.[10] There have been no reported human cancers associated with DDM.

If, as hypothesized in the Center for Disease Control study of nuclear power plant construction workers, not all workers are susceptible to liver injury after exposure to DDM, and if the 1–2% incidence of liver disease seen in this study were applied to all workers with possible exposure to DDM, we would expect to see 25–50 cases of DDM-associated toxic hepatitis a year.[1]

REFERENCES

4,4′- Diaminodiphenylmethane

1. DDM—Background Information on 4,4′-Diaminodiphenylmethane—Technical Evaluation and Review Branch Office of Extramural Coordination & Special Projects, National Institute for Occupational Safety and Health, Cincinnati, Ohio, January 30, 1976.

2. Gohlke, R., and Schmidt, P.: 4-4′-Diaminodiphenylmethane: Histological, enzyme, histochemical and autoradiographic investigations in acute and subacute experiments in rats with and without the additional stress of heat, Int. Arch. Arbeitsmed. 32:217, 1974.
3. Kopelman, H., Robertson, M. H., Sanders, P. G., and Ash, I.: The Epping Jaundice, Br. Med. J. 1:514, 1966.
4. Kopelman, H., Scheuer, P. J., and Williams, R.: The liver lesion of the Epping Jaundice, Q. J. Med. 35:553, 1966.
5. Lloyd, J. W., DeCoufle, P., and Moore, R. M., Jr.: Current intelligence—background information on chloroprene, J. Occup. Med. 17:263, 1975.
6. McGill, D. B., and Motto, J. D.: An industrial outbreak of toxic hepatitis due to methylenedianiline, N. Engl. J. Med. 291:278, 1974.
7. Munn, A.: Occupational Bladder Tumors and Carcinogens: Recent Developments in Britain, in Deichmann, W., and Lampe, K. F. (eds.), *Bladder Cancer. A Symposium* (Birmingham, Alabama: Aesculapius, 1974), p. 187.
8. Pludro, G., Karlowski, K., Mankowska, M., Woggon, H., and Udhe, W. J.: Toxicological and chemical studies of some epoxy resins and hardeners. I. Determination of acute and subacute toxicity of phthalic acid anhydride, 4-4′-diaminodiphenylmethane and of the epoxy resin Epilox EG-34, Acta Pol. Pharm. 26:352, 1969.
9. Schoental, R.: Carcinogenic and chronic effects of 4-4′-diaminodiphenylmethane, an epoxy resin hardener, Nature 219:1162, 1968.
10. Steinhoff, D., and Grundmann, E.: Zur Cancerogenen winkung von 4-4′-diaminodiphenylmethan und 2,4′-diaminodiphenylmethan, Naturwissenschaften 57:247, 1970.
11. Unpublished data, Center for Disease Control, 1974.
12. Williams, S. V., Bryan, J. A., and Wolf, F. S.: Toxic hepatitis and methylenedianiline, N. Engl. J. Med. 291:1256, 1974.

Disulfiram

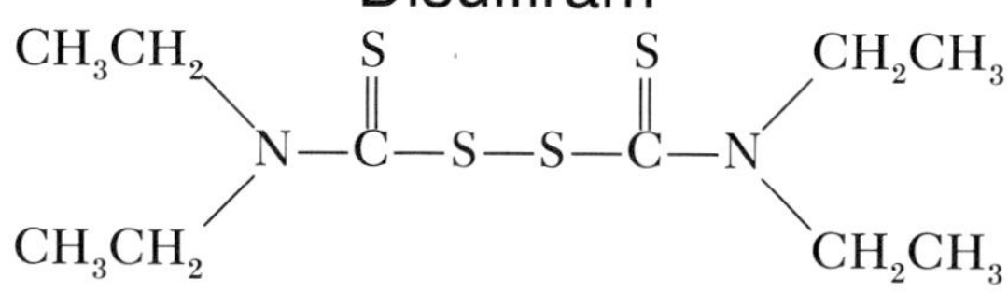

Disulfiram is a prescription drug used as an alcohol deterrent and *also is an accelerator used in the manufacture of rubber*. Disulfiram also may be used as a fungicide and insecticide. Disulfiram is widely used in alcoholism control programs under the trade names Antabuse and Ro-Sulfiram. The intake of even small quantities of ethanol (ethyl alcohol) while on disulfiram results in flushing, breathing difficulty, nausea, vomiting and low blood pressure. This violent and unpleasant reaction reinforces an individual's resolve to abstain from alcohol. The human therapeutic dose of disulfiram ranges from 125 to 500 mg per day; disulfiram therapy may continue for many months, even years.

Disulfiram was first noted for its effects on workers in a rubber plant, and its toxicity in the presence of ethyl alcohol was reported by Hald et al.[3] Disulfiram acts by inhibiting cytoplasmic and mitochondrial dehydrogenases in the liver, interfering with the ethanol-acetaldehyde-acetic acid pathway. The blocking action of disulfiram on aldehyde dehydrogenases led Plotnick[5] to investigate the effects of this on the detoxification or biotransformation of ethylene dibromide in the liver. Although the literature does not contain reports of carcinogenic effects of disulfiram in laboratory animals, the International Agency for Research in Cancer (IARC) has concluded that "the limited data available do not allow an evaluation of the carcinogenicity of disulfiram to be made."[4] The NIOSH estimates that approximately 70,000 workers have occupational exposure to disulfiram. This estimate is based on the

NIOSH National Occupational Hazard Survey that was conducted between 1972 and 1974 and included more than 500,000 employees at 4775 facilities. In addition, there may be as many as 100,000 people on disulfiram therapy for alcoholism.

LABORATORY ANIMAL STUDY OF TOXIC INTERACTION[2]

In the NIOSH-sponsored research, laboratory rats exposed to 20 ppm ethylene dibromide by inhalation (the current 8-hour TWA OSHA exposure standard) and also receiving a diet containing 0.05% disulfiram experienced exceedingly high mortality levels as well as a high incidence of tumors (including hemangiosarcomas of the liver, spleen and kidney). Even in those sites where tumors often occur spontaneously in rats, such as the mammary gland in females, the incidence of tumors appears to be increased and the tumors are occurring at an earlier than expected age. Although the clinical significance of the data has not yet been evaluated, great caution is indicated. The extent to which this toxic interaction is specific for ethylene dibromide and disulfiram is not known. Similar toxic interactions may occur between disulfiram, as well as chemicals structurally related to disulfiram, and other halogenated hydrocarbons.

NIOSH RECOMMENDATIONS

It is recommended, as an interim and prudent measure, that no worker be exposed to both ethylene dibromide and disulfiram. Workers should not be exposed to ethylene dibromide during the course of disulfiram therapy. Disulfiram (Antabuse, Ro-Sulfiram) should not be administered to workers having potential occupational exposure to ethylene dibromide except in those cases where, in the best judgment of the responsible physician, the benefit of disulfiram therapy strongly outweighs the risk to the particular patient. Whenever disulfiram [bis(diethylthiocarbamoyl) disulfide, tetraethylthiuram disulfide] is used in the workplace (e.g., as an accelerator in rubber production, as a fungicide or insecticide), precautions should be taken so that no worker is exposed to both ethylene dibromide and disulfiram.

REFERENCES

Disulfiram

1. Criteria for a Recommended Standard . . . Occupational Exposure to Ethylene Dibromide, U.S. Dept. of Health, Education, and Welfare, PHS, Center for Disease Control, National Institute for Occupational Safety and Health, Cincinnati, Ohio, August, 1977.
2. Current Intelligence Bulletin 23: Ethylene dibromide and disulfiram toxic interaction. National Institute for Occupational Safety and Health, Robert A. Taft Laboratories, 4676 Columbia Parkway, Cincinnati, Ohio, DHEW (NIOSH) Publication No. 78-145, April 11, 1978.
3. Hald, J., Jacobson, E., and Larsen, V.: The sensitizing effect of tetraethylthiuram disulphide (Antabuse) to ethyl alcohol, Acta Pharmacol. Toxicol. 4:285, 1948.
4. IARC Monographs on the Evaluation of Carcinogenic Risk of Chemicals in Man, 12:85, 1976.
5. Plotnick, H. B.: Carcinogenesis in rats of combined ethylene bromide and disulfiram, JAMA 239:1609, 1978.
6. Yodaiken, R. E.: Ethylene dibromide and disulfiram—a lethal combination (editorial), JAMA 239:2783, 1978.

Formaldehyde

This simple aldehyde, HCHO, is a colorless, irritating gas, soluble in water and used as an intermediate in the preparation of dyes, explosives, resins and synthetic lacquers. Large quantities are used to make melamine-formaldehyde, phenol-formaldehyde and urea-formaldehyde resins. Formaldehyde is used as a disinfectant and as a preservative in many products and processes and was one of the early pesticides. More recently, it is utilized to sterilize equipment and tubing prior to peritoneal dialysis, both in the home and in the hospital, where nearly 5 liters per patient per month is needed. Annual production as a 37–56% solution is estimated to be nearly 3 billion kg in the United States, approximately 30% being used for the production of urea-formaldehyde resins. According to the NIOSH, some 8000 workers are potentially exposed, but this estimate does not take into account hospital and other allied health workers.

Occupational exposure to formaldehyde may occur through ocular and dermal contact, most commonly by inhalation and rarely by ingestion.

On dermal contact, formaldehyde reacts with the active hydrogen in the protein molecules of the skin, resulting in cross-linking and precipitation of the proteins. Under chronic but mild exposure, an allergic skin rash can occur in sensitive persons. More severe exposures result in hardening and tanning of the skin due to coagulation necrosis. Most cases of dermatitis are caused by contact with aqueous formaldehyde solutions, although incidents have also been reported from respiratory exposures. Formaldehyde vapors and solutions cause severe eye burns. Prolonged exposure to low concentrations of the vapors can also result in irritation and inflammation of the eyelids.

At concentrations of 2–3 ppm, nearly all adults experience a mild burning sensation in the eyes, nose and throat. Few persons can tolerate these concentrations up to 8 hours without further discomfort, and most develop increasing upper respiratory irritation. At these levels, lacrimation occurs in most persons. Levels of 10 ppm may be tolerated for only minutes and marked tearing occurs in nearly all persons, even those supposedly inured. Solutions containing 25% formaldehyde, splashed in the eyes, have caused marked inflammation and corneal damage. Strong formaldehyde solutions on the skin and/or exposure to the vapor have caused primary skin irritation. Workers can develop eczematous skin reactions of the eyelids, face, neck, hands and flexor surfaces of the arms that can occur as little as only a few days after beginning work. Other eczematous reactions may not appear for months to years and are seen most commonly on the dorsum of the hands, fingers, wrists, forearms and other exposed portions of the body, especially those exposed to friction from clothing. Sensitization occurs in susceptible individuals (in some occupations up to 20–25% of the workers), and these sensitized individuals should not be exposed to any formaldehyde whatsoever. Breathing difficulties in the healthy adult worker occur at vapor concentrations between 10 and 20 ppm, and the intense sensation of burning of the eyes, nose and throat extends into the tracheal area, producing coughing. It is not certain at which levels severe bronchial and lower pulmonary tract inflammation might occur, but it is surmised that short exposures of 5–15 minutes at levels of 50–100 ppm can cause severe illness. Inhalation of high levels of formaldehyde vapor has caused pulmonary edema, pneumonitis and death.[4] Most persons can immediately perceive the presence of formaldehyde by odor at levels at or below 1 ppm.

Inhalation of formaldehyde vapors produces irritation and inflammation of the bronchi and lungs. In vitro studies of the action of aqueous formaldehyde on lung tissue showed that the tissue properties were altered, possibly by forming intermolecular cross-linkages. This mechanism probably also occurs in vivo, leading to lung damage. Once in the lungs, the formaldehyde vapors can be picked up by the bloodstream.

Of 25 workers using urea formaldehyde in a plastics factory, 4 were reported to have respiratory disease, according to Harris.[6] In a study of 63 production workers using a phenol-formaldehyde resin, Schoenberg and Mitchell[15] placed these workers into four exposure groups, based on years employed at their jobs, compared with a nonexposed group. By questionnaire, prevalence of symptoms of dyspnea, chest tightness and wheezing was noted in 45% of the exposed workers and in 7% of controls. Basic spirometric pulmonary tests revealed decreases in forced expiratory volume (FEV_1), and the ratio of FEV_1 to forced vital capacity significantly correlated with length of exposure, the highest reductions being in those workers exposed 5 or more years.

Ingestion of formaldehyde is followed immediately by inflammation of the mucosa of the mouth, throat and gastrointestinal tract. Absorption appears to occur in the intestines.[9] Once absorbed into the bloodstream, formaldehyde disappears rapidly. This rapid disappearance is due to condensation reactions with body tissue constituents such as proteins, with oxidation to formic acid. The main reaction appears to be initial oxidation to formic acid followed by further oxidation to CO_2 and H_2O. This pathway was shown to occur when rats were fed ^{14}C-labeled formaldehyde. In this study,[2] 40% of the ^{14}C was recovered as respiratory CO_2. The intraperitoneal application of ^{14}C-labeled formaldehyde to rats resulted in 82% of the dosages expired in the air as CO_2. Studies on the metabolism of methanol, for which formaldehyde is an intermediate, have shown the presence of several enzymes capable of catalyzing the oxidation of formaldehyde to formic acid. Westerfield[17] identified 6 different enzymes capable of catalyzing the conversion: aldehyde dehydrogenase, glyceraldehyde-3-phosphate dehydrogenase, aldehyde oxidase, xanthine oxidase, catalase and peroxidase. Strittmatter and Ball[16] isolated a formaldehyde-specific, NAD-dependent formaldehyde dehydrogenase from beef liver. This enzyme requires the presence of reduced glutathione. Similar formaldehyde dehydrogenase enzymes have been found in the liver of other mammals, including humans.

Mechanisms causing pulmonary disease from formaldehyde vapor have been suggested. Nicholls[13] has described in vitro histamine release from lung tissue with exposure to dimethylhydantoin-formaldehyde resin, an ingredient of many cosmetic hair lacquers. Technicians and staff members of a renal dialysis unit developed productive coughs and asthma. Bronchial provocation testing with formalin by Hendrick and Lane[7] was reported to have induced nonimmediate asthmatic reactions in 2 workers and prevented it in 1 person by beclomethasone inhalation. Humoral precipitating antibodies to aldehydes were found in 10 of 12 workers in an electronics plant by Oziganova et al.,[14] who also found that all these workers developed asthma when given inhalation challenge with formaldehyde-containing resin fume.

The cytotoxicity of formaldehyde was studied by using Ehrlich-Landschutz diploid (ELD) ascites tumor cells during short-time in vitro incubations. Holmberg and Malmfors[8] found that formaldehyde was highly toxic to ELD cells at a concentration of 100 ppm after a 1-hour incubation and with 50 ppm after a 2-hour incubation. The frequency of irreversibly injured cells at the end of 5 hours of incubation did not increase remarkably compared to the frequency at the 1- and 2-hour incubations.

The liver and the erythrocytes appear to be the sites for the rapid oxidation of formaldehyde to formic acid. Malorny et al.[9] showed that human blood rapidly oxidized formaldehyde to formic acid after absorption of erythrocytes in vitro. Matthies[10-12] found that aldehyde dehydrogenase present in the erythrocytes was responsible for catalyzing this reaction. In vivo studies in dogs and cats also showed a rapid appearance of formic acid in the plasma. Once formed, formic acid can undergo any one of three reactions to final detoxification: (1) oxidation to CO_2 and H_2O and exhalation of the CO_2 from the lungs, (2) elimination in the urine as sodium salt or (3) entry into the one-carbon pool. This pathway is capable of handling minor quantities with relatively little difficulty. However, large doses overload

TABLE 14–6.—FORMALDEHYDE

A. Occupational Standards (8-hour workday)	
OSHA	3 ppm
ACGIH	2 ppm
NIOSH	1 ppm
Sweden	1 ppm
B. National Academy of Science recommendations for spacecraft	
60-minute exposure	1 ppm
90-day exposure	0.1 ppm
6-month exposure	0.1 ppm
C. Residential Standards (24 hours per day)	
ASHRAE	0.2 ppm
West Germany	0.1 ppm
Denmark	0.12 ppm (established in law 1979)
Sweden	0.1–0.4 ppm (established in law 1978)*
Netherlands	0.1 ppm (established in law 1977)

*0.1 to 0.2 proposed, 1979

the detoxification mechanism, resulting in acidosis and tissue damage from protein cross-linkages.[9]

Complaints of irritation and disturbed sleep after exposures to formaldehyde at 1–2 ppm form the basis for recommending a ceiling concentration limit of 1 ppm (1.2 mg/m^3) in workplaces where exposure to formaldehyde can occur, and the NIOSH recommends respiratory protection. A preplacement medical examination is recommended, as well as other clinical studies; if judged necessary by the responsible physician and as indicated by circumstances of exposure, for all employees subject to occupational exposure to formaldehyde, which has been established by the NIOSH as "exposures to formaldehyde at concentrations exceeding 0.5 ppm (0.6 mg/m^3) based on a 30-minute sampling period."

REFERENCES

Formaldehyde

1. American Conference of Governmental Industrial Hygienists: Formaldehyde. Documentation of the TLVs for Substances in Workroom Air, 3d ed., pp. 118–119, Cincinnati, Ohio, 1976.
2. Buss, J., Kuschinsky, K., Kewitz, H., and Koransky, W.: Enterale Resorption von Formaldehyde, Arch. Exp. Path. Pharmakol. 247:380, 1964.
3. Fisher, A. A.: *Contact Dermatitis* (2d ed.; Philadelphia: Lea & Febiger, 1973), pp. 47–48.
4. Formaldehyde, A Recommended Standard for Occupational Exposure to . . . ., NIOSH, U.S. Dept. of Health, Education, and Welfare, PHS, Center for Disease Control, 4676 Columbus Parkway, Cincinnati, Ohio 45226, December, 1976.
5. Formaldehyde—Investigation of Selected Potential Environmental Contaminants—Atlantic Research Corp., U.S. Dept. of Commerce. National Technical Information Service, PB-256 839, August, 1976.
6. Harris, D. K.: Health problems in the manufacture and use of plastics, Br. J. Ind. Med. 10:255, 1953.
7. Hendrick, D. J., and Lane, D. J.: Occupational formalin asthma, Br. J. Ind. Med. 34:11, 1977
8. Holmberg, B., and Malmfors, T.: The cytotoxicity of some organic solvents, Environ. Res. 7:183, 1974.
9. Malorny, G., Rietbrock, N., and Schneider, M.: Die Oxydation des Formaldehyds zu Ameiscansaure in blat. Ein Breitrag Zum Stoffwechsel des Formaldehyds, Arch. Exp. Path. Pharmakol. 250:419, 1965.
10. Matthies, H.: Die wirkung von aldehyden aud die methämoglob intruckbildung in eythrocyten, Biochem. Z. 329:341, 1957.
11. Matthies, H.: Die wirkung von aldehyden aud die methämoglob intruckbildung in

eythrocyten, Biochem. Z. 329:421, 1957.
12. Matthies, H.: Vergleichende Untersuchungen über die aldehydedehydrogenase kernloser erythrocyten, Biochem. Z. 330:169, 1958.
13. Nicholls, P. J.: Release of histamine from lung tissue in vitro by dimethylhydantoin-formaldehyde resin and polyvinylpyrrolidone, Br. J. Ind. Med. 33:127, 1975.
14. Oziganova, V. N., Ivanova, I. S., and Deuva, L. A.: Bronchial asthma in radio equipment assemblers, Sov. Med. 8:139, 1977.
15. Schoenberg, J. B., and Mitchell, C. A.: Airway disease caused by phenolic (phenol-formaldehyde) resin exposure, Arch. Environ. Health 30:574, 1975.
16. Strittmatter, P., and Ball, E. G.: Formaldehyde dehydrogenase, a glutathione-dependent enzyme system, J. Biol. Chem. 213:445, 1955.
17. Westerfield, W. W.: The metabolism of alcohol, Tex. Rep. Biol. Med. 13:559, 1955.
18. Woodbury, M. A., and Zenz, C.: Formaldehyde in Homes. A report to the U.S. Dept. of Health, Education, and Welfare, Washington, D.C., October 24, 1978.

Hydrazines

The biologic effects of hydrazines on humans and on animals described here include those of 5 compounds: hydrazine (H_2NNH_2), methylhydrazine (CH_3NHNH_2), 1,1-dimethylhydrazine ($(CH_3)_2NNH_2$), 1,2-dimethylhydrazine ($CH_3NHNHCH_3$) and phenylhydrazine ($C_6H_5NHNH_2$). All these hydrazines are at least slightly basic and polar, and they are strong reducing agents. The hydrazine bases are used in the production of salts and hydrazones that are used in surfactants, detergents, plasticizers, pharmaceuticals, insecticides and herbicides. Three of the hydrazines (hydrazine, methylhydrazine and 1,1-dimethylhydrazine) have been used as rocket propellants. Hydrazines are very reactive and have wide use, and they are capable of causing a variety of biologic effects. There has been great interest in the toxicologic implications of the hydrazines, and there have been many animal studies conducted on the 3 hydrazines used as rocket fuels. Comprehensive reviews have been prepared by various groups, including the U. S. Air Force[1,2,9] and the International Agency for Research on Cancer (IARC).[10] The Committee on Toxicology of the National Academy of Sciences[6] also provided documentation on establishing guidelines for short-term community air exposures. The NIOSH has expressed concern about the possible tumorigenicity of a number of chemicals, including several hydrazines. In the 1976 edition of the *NIOSH's Registry of Toxic Effects of Chemical Substances*,[3] several hydrazines were listed as animal carcinogens, based primarily on the 1974 report of studies by the IARC. Little information is available on the decomposition of the hydrazines in air and water. Hydrazine is thermodynamically unstable and may decompose into hydrogen, ammonia and nitrogen. The reaction rate reportedly is slow at room temperatures but increases at elevated temperatures, particularly in the presence of metals such as copper.

Hydrazine, methylhydrazine, 1,1-dimethylhydrazine and 1,2-dimethylhydrazine are characterized by a fishy, ammonia-like odor. These 4 compounds are clear, colorless, flammable or combustible, hygroscopic liquids that are soluble in water, ethanol and other polar solvents. Phenylhydrazine has a faint aromatic odor and occurs as yellow monoclinic crystals or oil. It is miscible with alcohol, ether, chloroform and benzene but only sparingly soluble in water. Occupations with potential exposure to hydrazines are agricultural chemical workers, analytical chemists, anticorrosion additive workers, boiler operators, catalyst reclaimers, chlorine scavenger makers, drug makers, dye makers, explosives makers, foamed plastic makers, fuel cell makers, herbicide makers, hydraulic fluid workers, hydrazine and hydrazine-derivative makers, insecticide makers, jet fuel handlers, jet fuel makers, nitron makers, organic chemical synthesizers, oxygen scavenger makers, photographic developer makers, rocket fuel handlers, rocket fuel makers, rubber workers, silverplating workers, solder flux makers, solderers, textile dyers (acrylic and vinyl), vat dye makers and water treaters.

The potential for worker exposure to the hydrazines is primarily through two routes of exposure—inhalation and contact with skin or eyes. Hydrazine, methylhydrazine and 1,1-dimethylhydrazine were readily absorbed through the shaved skin of dogs. Each compound was detectable in the blood in 30 seconds, and signs of acute toxicity ensued. Two drops of anhydrous hydrazine applied to the shaved skin of rats, as well as 3 ml applied to rabbits, were lethal, suggesting that even a small spill on the skin of workers could be toxic. In general, the compound with the highest vapor pressure, 1,1-dimethylhydrazine, should be the least toxic by skin absorption because of rapid evaporation. Since 1,1-dimethylhydrazine is toxic by this route, other hydrazines are likely to have a similar effect. In regard to eye damage, as little as 2 drops of a 25% solution of hydrazine applied to the eyes of animals caused permanent damage.[11] Methylhydrazine, 1,1-dimethylhydrazine and 1,2-dimethylhydrazine, however, produced only temporary mild effects. These effects probably are pH dependent, since alkaline compounds would be expected to cause more damage to eye surfaces; thus, the eye damage expected for phenylhydrazine and the salts of hydrazines may be similarly related to pH. The salts would be at least as water soluble, if not more so, than the free bases, and many are acidic, suggesting that they would be more readily removed by tear formation or induced flushing.

Hydrazine as the vapor or liquid is a severe skin and mucous membrane irritant, a convulsant, a hepatotoxin and a carcinogen in animals. In animals, hydrazine is absorbed through the skin as well as by inhalation and orally; systemic effects include weight loss, weakness, vomiting, excited behavior and convulsions; the chief histologic findings are fatty degeneration of the liver and nephritis. In dogs, hemolysis occurs after intravenous injection but not from inhalation of the vapor. Inhalation by animals results in bronchitis, pulmonary edema and damage to the liver and kidneys. In humans, the vapor is immediately irritating to the nose and throat and causes dizziness and nausea; itching, burning and swelling of the eyes develop over a period of several hours. Severe exposure of the eyes to the vapor causes temporary blindness lasting for about 24 hours. The liquid in the eyes or on the skin causes severe burns. Recurrent exposure to hydrazine hydrate has been reported to cause contact dermatitis of the hands without systemic intoxication. Hydrazine or hydrazine salts are carcinogenic in mice after oral administration (pulmonary adenocarcinoma; hepatocarcinoma) or intraperitoneal injection (pulmonary carcinoma) and in rats after oral administration (pulmonary adenocarcinoma). There are no special tests.

The worker must be protected to minimize the risks of systemic toxicity, eye damage and sensitization, which can result from contact with the hydrazines and their salts, and of cancer, which is predicted to be a possible result of contact with or inhalation of these hydrazines. For these reasons, occupational exposure to hydrazines is defined as work in any area where one or more of the hydrazines is stored, produced, processed, transported, handled or otherwise used and present in such a manner that vapors or aerosols may be released into workroom air or that the hydrazines may spill or splash onto the skin or into the eyes. Because even small spills of hydrazines on the skin can result in severe systemic toxicity, all employees assigned to such a work area, even temporarily, for any purpose, including maintenance or repair, should be regarded as occupationally exposed. Workers in areas where hydrazines are used, in either open or closed systems, should be considered to be occupationally exposed, since there is no effective way to demonstrate that a closed system remains completely free from leaks. Conversely, workers assigned only to control rooms in which no air from other hydrazine-containing areas is present should not be considered occupationally exposed.

REFERENCES

Hydrazines

1. Back, K. C., Carter, V. L., Jr., and Thomas, A. A.: Occupational Hazards of Missile Operations with Special Regard to the Hydrazine Propellants, in JANNAF Working Group on Safety and Environmental Protection—Minutes of April 10-77 Meeting—John F. Kennedy Space Center, Florida. Laurel, Maryland. Johns Hopkins University, Chemical Propulsion Information Agency, Applied Physics Laboratory, pp. 25–47, 1977.
2. Clark, D. A., et al.: Pharmacology and toxicology of propellant hydrazines in Aeromedical Reviews, review 11-68. Springfield, Virginia, U.S. Dept. of Commerce, National Technical Information Service (NTIS AD 688 500), 126 pp. 1968.
3. Christensen, H. E., Fairchild, E. J., Carroll, B. S., and Lewis, R. J., Sr.: Registry of Toxic Effects of Chemical Substances, 1976 ed., DHEW Publication No. (NIOSH) 76-191. Rockville, Maryland, U.S. Dept. of Health, Education, and Welfare, PHS, Center for Disease Control, National Institute for Occupational Safety and Health, pp.594–598, 1976.
4. Criteria for a Recommended Standard . . . Occupational Exposure to Hydrazines. U.S. Department of Health, Education, and Welfare, PHS, Center for Disease Control, DHEW (NIOSH) Publication No. 78-172, Cincinnati, Ohio, National Institute for Occupational Safety and Health, June, 1978.
5. Evaluation of Atmospheric Concentrations of Hydrazine and Unsymmetrical Dimethylhydrazine in and around the Rocky Mountain Arsenal. Hydrazine Facility, Industrial Hygiene Special Study No. 35-0101-77. Aberdeen Proving Ground, Aberdeen, Maryland, U.S. Dept. of the Army, U.S. Army Environmental Hygiene Agency, 21 pp., 1977.
6. Guides for Short-Term Exposures of the Public to Air Pollutants. V. Guide for Hydrazine, Monomethylhydrazine, and 1,1-Dimethylhydrazine. Springfield, Virginia, U.S. Dept. of Commerce, National Technical Information Service (NTIS PB 224 337), 57 pp., 1974.
7. Haun, C. C., and Kinkead, E. R.: Chronic Inhalation Toxicity of Hydrazine, in Proceedings of the 4th Annual Conference on Environmental Toxicology. Springfield, Virginia, U.S. Dept. of Commerce, National Technical Information Service (NTIS AD 781 031), pp. 351–363, 1973.
8. Haun, C. C., MacEwen, J. D., Vernot, E. H., and Egan, G. F.: The Acute Inhalation Toxicity of Monomethylhydrazine Vapor, Report No. AMRL-TR-68-169. Wright-Patterson Air Force Base, Ohio, U.S. Air Force, Air Force Systems Command, Aerospace Medical Division, Aerospace Medical Research Laboratories, Toxic Hazards Division, Toxicology Branch, 48 pp., 1969.
9. Melvin, W. W., and Johnson, W. S.: Survey of Information Relevant to Occupational Health Standards for Hydrazines. Springfield, Virginia, U.S. Dept. of Commerce, National Technical Information Service (NTIS AD AO22 851), 75 pp., 1976.
10. Some Aromatic Amines, Hydrazine and Related Substances, *n*-Nitroso Compounds and Miscellaneous Alkylating Agents. IARC Monographs on the Evaluation of Carcinogenic Risk of Chemicals to Man. Lyon, France, International Agency for Research on Cancer, Vol. 4, pp. 127–172, 1974.
11. Thienes, C. H., et al.: Final Report on Acute and Chronic Toxicity of Hydrazine. Los Angeles, University Park, University of Southern California School of Medicine, Dept. of Pharmacology and Toxicology, 51 pp., 1948.
12. Toth, B., and Wilson, R. B.: Blood vessel tumorigenesis by 1,2-dimethylhydrazine dihydrochloride (symmetrical). Gross, light and electron microscopic descriptions, I. Am. J. Pathol. 64:585, 1971.
13. Toxic Hazards Research Unit Annual Tech-

nical Report—1975. Springfield, Virginia, U. S. Dept. of Commerce, National Technical Information Service (NTIS AD AO19 546 LLC), pp. 101–111, 1975.
14. Wattenburg, L. W.: Inhibition of dimethylhydrazine-induced neoplasia of the large intestine by disulfiram, J. Natl. Cancer Inst. 54:1005, 1975.
15. Wilson, R. B.: Species variation in response to dimethylhydrazine, Toxicol. Appl. Pharmacol. 38:647, 1976.

Hydrogen Cyanide and Cyanide Salts

Synonyms for hydrogen cyanide (HCN) are hydrocyanic acid, prussic acid and formonitrile. For the purpose of this document, cyanide salts are defined as sodium cyanide (NaCN), potassium cyanide (KCN) and calcium cyanide ($Ca(CN)_2$). The word cyanide or the symbol CN is used to designate salts as well as hydrogen cyanide.

HCN is used primarily in the production of chemical intermediates and in fumigation. It can be produced in electroplating, metallurgy, photographic development and various other occupations. The estimated United States consumption of HCN for 1973 was approximately 310,000 short tons. The number of workers with potential exposure to HCN has been estimated by the NIOSH to be approximately 1000.

Sodium cyanide and potassium cyanide are used primarily in the extraction of ores, electroplating, metal treatment and various manufacturing processes. The number of workers with potential exposure to NaCN has been estimated by the NIOSH to be 20,000. The number of workers potentially exposed to KCN and $Ca(CN)_2$ has not been estimated. Hydrogen cyanide and its sodium, potassium and calcium salts manifest their toxicity by way of a common mechanism, namely, inhibition of the respiratory enzyme cytochrome oxidase. This inhibition causes cellular anoxia and, if a large enough dose is received, results in death. Skin contact with a solution of cyanide salts can cause itching, discoloration or corrosion, which most likely is due to the alkalinity of the solution. Cyanide salt aerosols can cause upper respiratory irritation. Enlargement of the thyroid glands and changes in the chemical and cellular composition of the blood of employees exposed to cyanide have also been reported. An increased occurrence of the subjective symptoms of headache, weakness, changes in taste and smell, irritation of the throat, vomiting, effort dyspnea, lacrimation, abdominal colic, precordial pain and nervous instability has been noted among workers having long-term occupational exposure to low concentrations of HCN. The NIOSH recommends that workers occupationally exposed to cyanide have comprehensive preplacement and annual medical examinations. Engineering controls should be used wherever feasible to maintain cyanide concentrations at or below the prescribed limits and respirators should be used only in certain nonroutine or emergency situations.

Medical surveillance shall be made available as specified below for all workers occupationally exposed to HCN or cyanide salts.

A. Preplacement and annual medical examinations shall include:

1. An initial or interim work and medical history with special attention to skin disorders and those nonspecific symptoms, such as headache, nausea, vomiting, dizziness or weakness, that may be associated with chronic exposure.

2. A physical examination giving particular attention to skin, thyroid and the cardiovascular and upper respiratory systems.

3. An evaluation of the advisability of the worker's use of negative- or positive-pressure respirators.

B. Initial medical examinations shall be made available to presently employed workers within 6 months of the promulgation of a standard.

C. The responsible physician and the employer shall be aware of substances used in the workplace and shall ensure that employees trained in first-aid measures are on duty whenever there is potential occupational exposure to HCN or a cyanide salt.

D. Two physicians' treatment kits shall be immediately available to trained medical personnel at each plant where there is a potential for the release of, accidental or otherwise, or for contact with, hydrogen cyanide or cyanide salts. One kit should be portable in order that it may be carried by medical personnel while accompanying a patient to the hospital. The other kit should be kept under lock and key to ensure that it is intact and available when and if needed. The key should be readily available at all times to the work supervisor on duty, and the storage place should be of such construction as to allow accessibility in the event of loss of the key.

E. First-aid kits shall be immediately available if there is a potential for exposure to cyanide salts. This kit shall contain as a minimum 2 boxes of ampules (2 dozen), each containing 0.3 ml of amyl nitrite. Ampules shall be replaced biannually or sooner if needed to ensure their potency. The amyl nitrite ampules should be protected from high temperatures. In all cases, the contents of the medical and first-aid kits shall be replaced before the manufacturer's assigned expiration dates.

In case of contact, immediately flush skin or eyes with plenty of water for at least 15 minutes; get medical attention. Remove contaminated clothing and wash before reuse.

Carry patient to fresh air.

Have patient lie down.

Remove contaminated clothing but keep patient warm.

Start artificial respiration if breathing stops.

Administer antidote (amyl nitrite ampule).

Transport patient to the nearest medical treatment facility. Hyperbaric oxygen therapy has proved helpful (see section on Carbon Monoxide, this chapter).

TEMPORARY ANTIDOTE

If cyanide gas is inhaled: Break an amyl nitrite ampule in a cloth and hold lightly under nose for 15 seconds. Repeat at about 15-second intervals.

If cyanide is swallowed: Break an amyl nitrite ampule in a cloth and hold lightly under nose for 15 seconds. Repeat inhalation of amyl nitrite 5 times at about 15-second intervals. If patient is conscious or when consciousness returns, give emetic (1 tablespoonful of salt to each glass of warm water) and repeat until vomit fluid is clear. Do not give an emetic to an unconscious or barely conscious person.

More recently, physicians have used 100% oxygen together with hydroxocobalamin given intravenously. Hydroxocobalamin combines with cyanide to form cyanocobalamin (vitamin B_{12}). Graham et al.[1] have reported their results with this newer form of treatment in acute cases.

The following warning sign shall be affixed in a readily visible location at or near entrances to areas containing HCN and where there is reasonable potential for emergencies:

DANGER
CYANIDE HAZARD AREA
UNAUTHORIZED PERSONS KEEP OUT
DO NOT WORK ALONE IN THIS AREA
IN EMERGENCY: (Here include, as applicable,

1. Location of gas masks and other emergency equipment.
2. Instructions for sounding emergency alarm.
3. Location of first-aid equipment and supplies.
4. Instructions for summoning medical aid.)

The sign shall be printed both in English and in the predominant language of non-English-reading workers. All workers shall receive training and information on the hazards and safe work practices in handling HCN and cyanide salts and on first-aid procedures in poisoning by these compounds.

The NIOSH recommends the promulgation of new federal standards so that employee exposure to hydrogen cyanide and the cyanide salts does not exceed 5 mg/m^3 of air (expressed as CN), determined as a ceiling concentration based on a 10-minute sampling period. Because of the ready hydrolysis of calcium cyanide in humid air, it is required that whenever the air is analyzed for cyanide salts, a concurrent analysis be made for HCN. Neither respective ceiling value may be exceeded nor may the combined values exceed 5 mg/m^3 measured as CN during a 10-minute sampling period.

REFERENCES

Hydrogen Cyanide and Cyanide Salts

1. Graham, D. L., Laman, D., Theodore, J., and Robin, E. D.: Acute cyanide poisoning complicated by lactic acidosis and pulmonary edema, Arch. Intern. Med. 137:1051, 1977.
2. National Institute for Occupational Safety and Health. A Recommended Standard for Occupational Exposure to . . . Hydrogen Cyanide and Cyanide Salts. U.S. Dept. of Health, Education, and Welfare, PHS, Center for Disease Control, NIOSH, 1975.

Hydrogen Fluoride (HF)

Anhydrous hydrogen fluoride is a colorless liquid or gas that fumes in moist air and has a pungent, irritating odor. Its aqueous solutions also are colorless and fume above a concentration of 40–48%. It is manufactured by allowing sulfuric acid to react with acid-grade fluorspar (97% calcium fluoride) in heated rotary or stationary kilns. Hydrogen fluoride is evolved as a gas, purified and then condensed as liquid anhydrous hydrogen fluoride. Between 1876 and 1931, considerable quantities of aqueous hydrofluoric acid were produced and used for cleaning sand from castings and for etching glass. In 1931, anhydrous hydrogen fluoride was first produced commercially and use of anhydrous hydrogen fluoride as a catalyst in alkylation processes for making high-octane fuel blends began in 1942. Prior to 1954, the steel industry was the largest consumer of fluorspar, from which hydrogen fluoride is generated. Since then, the quantity of fluorspar used for the manufacture of hydrogen fluoride has surpassed that used in the steel industry. In 1958 and 1971, approximately 52% of all fluorspar consumed in the United States was used for making hydrogen fluoride. In 1974, production reached 375,000 tons. Currently, the major uses of hydrogen fluoride are in the production of cryolite for the aluminum industry, in the manufacture of fluorocarbon compounds, as a catalyst in alkylation processes, in steel pickling, uranium processing, enamel stripping, glass and quartz etching and polishing, and in various electroplating operations. Hydrogen fluoride often is produced by other industrial processes using fluorides, e.g., welding and aluminum production. Some occupations with potential exposure to hydrogen fluoride: aircraft workers, alkylation plant workers, alloy steel cleaners, alloy steel makers, aluminum fluoride makers, aluminum workers, ammonium fluoride makers, bleachers, brass cleaners, brewers, brick cleaners, casting cleaners, ceramic workers, chemists, copper cleaners, cryolite makers, crystal glass polishers, dye makers, electric arc welders, electroplaters, enamel etchers, fermentation workers, fertilizer makers, filter paper makers, fluoborate makers, fluoride makers, fluorine makers, fluocarbon makers, fluorochemical makers, fluosilicate makers, freon makers, genetron makers, glass etchers, graphite purifiers, hydrogen fluoride workers, incandescent lamp frosters, isotron makers, laundry workers, metal cleaners, metal polishers, neon sign makers, oil well acidizers, ore dissolvers, petroleum refinery workers, phosphate rock workers, phosphoric acid makers, plastic makers, polish workers, quartz crystal makers, rocket fuel handlers, rocket fuel makers, stainless steel cleaners, stainless steel makers, steel casting picklers, stone cleaners, uranium refiners and yeast makers.

Occupational exposure main routes of entry are by inhalation and skin contact. Hydrogen fluoride as a gas is a severe respiratory irritant, and in solution causes severe and painful burns of the skin. Animals repeatedly exposed to 17 ppm showed damage to the lungs, liver and kidneys, but at 8.6 ppm there was only occasional lung injury.[1] Fatalities occurred in 3 of 6 workers exposed to spills of 70% solutions on the skin and inhalation of the vapor; despite prompt showering with water for skin burns, death from pulmonary edema occurs 2 hours after exposure.[7] A chemist exposed to hydrogen fluoride splashed on the face and upper extremities developed pulmonary edema 3 hours after exposure and died 10 hours later.[5] In human subjects, 120 ppm was the highest concentration that could be tolerated for 1 minute due to onset of conjunctival and respiratory irritation with stinging of the skin. Repeated experimental human exposures to concentrations of 2 ppm for 6 hours daily caused a slight stinging of the eyes and skin of the face, with nasal irritation.[6] Repeated exposures to low concentrations at work may produce chronic irritation of the nose, throat and bronchi. Hydrogen fluoride solutions in contact with skin, if untreated, result in marked tissue destruction; the fluoride ion readily penetrates skin and deep tissue, causing necrosis of soft tissues and decalcification of bone.[2] When skin contact is with solutions of less than 20% hydrogen fluoride, the burns do not become manifest for several hours; burns from solutions greater than 20% generally are felt in a matter of minutes, and severe eye injuries from splashes may occur.[3] In one case of eye burns from a fine spray of hydrofluoric acid in the face, considerable loss of corneal epithelium occurred despite immediate and copious flushing with water and irritation for 3 hours with a 0.5% solution of benzethonium chloride; within 19 days there was recovery of normal vision.[4]

The determination of fluoride concentration in the urine may be utilized to gauge the degree of absorption of hydrogen fluoride following suspected overexposure.

TREATMENT.—Persons who have had contact with hydrofluoric acid should be subjected immediately to a drenching shower of water. Contaminated clothing should be removed as rapidly as possible, even while the person is under the shower. The high risk of either immediate or delayed onset of pulmonary edema following inhalation of the gas requires that oxygen be administered under pressure immediately after a severe exposure and continued as long as necessary; close observation should be continued for 24–48 hours. It is essential that the exposed area be washed with copious quantities of water for a sufficient period of time to remove all hydrofluoric acid from the skin or eyes. Skin burns have been treated with immediate application of iced hyamine chloride or Zephiran solution and continued application for 1–4 hours; severe deep or especially painful burns have been treated by local infiltration with 10% calcium gluconate following block anesthesia of the affected part.[2, 9] The 1979 TLV:3 ppm.

REFERENCES

Hydrogen Fluoride

1. ACGIH Hydrogen Fluoride as HF, Documentation of TLVs for Substances in Workroom Air (3d ed., 2d printing), Cincinnati, Ohio, p. 131, 1974.
2. Dibbell, D. G., et al.: Hydrofluoric acid burns of the hand, J. Bone Joint Surg. (Am.) 52:931, 1970.
3. Fleming, A. J. et al., *Modern Occupational*

Medicine (2d ed.; Philadelphia: Lea & Febiger, 1960), pp. 392–393, 403–405.
4. Grant, W. M.: *Toxicology of the Eye* (2d ed.; Springfield, Ill.: Charles C Thomas, Publisher, 1974), pp. 557–559.
5. Kleinfeld, M.: Acute pulmonary edema of chemical origin, Arch. Environ. Health 10:942, 1965.
6. Largent, E. J.: The metabolism of fluorides in man, A.M.A. Arch. Ind. Hyg. 21:318, 1960.
7. Mayer, L., and Guelich, J.: Hydrogen fluoride (HF) inhalation and burns, Arch. Environ. Health 7:445, 1963.
8. NIOSH Criteria for a Recommended Standard . . . Occupational Exposure to Hydrogen Fluoride. U.S. Dept. of Health, Education, and Welfare, PHS, Center for Disease Control, HEW Publication No. (NIOSH) 76-143, March, 1976.
9. Reinhardt, C. F., et al.: Hydrofluoric acid burn treatment, Am. Ind. Hyg. Assoc. J. 27:166, 1966.

Hydrogen Sulfide

H_2S

Hydrogen sulfide is a ubiquitous, acute-acting toxic substance and a leading cause of sudden death in the workplace. Brief exposures to hydrogen sulfide at high concentrations have caused conjunctivitis and keratitis, and exposures at very high concentrations have caused unconsciousness, respiratory paralysis and death. Eye irritation, cough, sore throat, vague gastrointestinal symptoms and photophobia may occur with low-level exposures; with overwhelming exposures, collapse and respiratory arrest can develop within minutes.

Hydrogen sulfide is used as a common reagent in chemical laboratories in the preparation of sulfide and organic sulfur compounds such as sulfuric acid and 1-dodecanethiol. The potential for release of high concentrations of hydrogen sulfide in work areas where the gas occurs as a by-product (e.g., petroleum wellheads, petroleum refineries, tanneries and sulfur products processing) has been a major cause of concern for worker safety. Hydrogen sulfide occurs naturally in most petroleum and natural gas deposits and as a bacterial decomposition product of protein. The NIOSH estimates that 125,000 workers in the United States are exposed or potentially exposed to hydrogen sulfide.

To provide a sufficient margin of safety in protecting against the immediate acute effects (and possible chronic effects) of hydrogen sulfide, a ceiling concentration of 15 mg/m^3 is recommended as an occupational exposure limit. Due to the rapid, often lethal effects of exposure to a high concentration of hydrogen sulfide, a work practice requirement for continual monitoring is recommended in situations in which there is potential exposure to a concentration of 70 mg/m^3 hydrogen sulfide or greater.

Hydrogen sulfide is especially dangerous when it occurs in low-lying areas or confined work spaces or when it exists in high concentrations under pressure. As a result, work practices, such as continual monitoring and the use of specified respiratory protective equipment in certain work situations, are of great importance.

Liquid manure systems in the United States are increasing as farms modernize and become more concerned with the efficient recycling of energy-rich waste. Numerous deaths in swine, beef and dairy animals have been associated with these systems. Furthermore, several farm workers have died after entering recently emptied liquid manure tanks or have drowned after falling into full tanks.[5]

CASE REPORT: A 16-year-old farm worker collapsed and died on December 8, 1977 while steam cleaning gutters inside a calf barn in Eau Claire, Wisconsin. The apparent cause of his death was the inhalation of toxic gases, with hydrogen sulfide (H_2S) the probable active agent.

The source of the gases was decomposing liquid manure that had been agitating for 30–60 minutes in a 50,000-liter tank beneath the barn. The boy had been working inside the barn approximately 30 feet from the tank for about 10 minutes when he was overcome by gases. While trying to rescue him, 2 other workers experienced syncopal episodes but recovered. No animals died during the incident; however, no calves were in the affected area of the barn at the time of exposure.

The farm worker had been in good health. He had no chronic illnesses, took no medication and had no history of drug abuse. Autopsy findings were consistent with inhalation of a toxic gas resulting in emesis and aspiration. H_2S was implicated as the causative agent by air tests done under similar conditions 2 days after the incident. The tests showed that H_2S concentrations at the site of death after 8 minutes of manure agitation were 70 ppm. (By comparison, the NIOSH recommends a maximal exposure concentration of no more than 10 ppm over a 10-minute period; when concentrations reach 50 ppm, evacuation is recommended.) Other gases, such as nitric oxide, nitrogen dioxide and sulfur dioxide, which have been associated with deaths in silos, were not detected. Carbon monoxide was ruled out at autopsy by blood tests, methane was thought not to have been present, since two open-flame heaters were in use, and ammonia was considered unlikely to have existed in high concentrations because its odor and irritation properties act as excellent warning signals.

Several factors appear to have contributed to the hazardous conditions present at the time of the incident. For example, the manure tank was full and the contents had been agitating longer than usual before pumping began. The barn was inadequately ventilated that day (outside temperature was -16^0 C. Only 1 of its 5 fans was in use, and then only intermittently, and a westerly wind blew through the only open door. In addition, the calves' high protein diet made the formation of H_2S more likely.

A number of toxic gases are released from decomposing manure, but H_2S, carbon dioxide, methane and ammonia are of principal concern. Several preventive measures may be taken to reduce farm workers' risk of toxic gas exposure from liquid manure systems. These steps include improving ventilation and developing contingency plans for evacuating animals and workers from enclosed farm buildings while the manure is agitating. In addition, agricultural authorities have recommended that workers who must enter a closed space containing a manure tank should wear self-contained air packs and safety harnesses, and that reserve workers should be stationed outside.[3,5]

Slowly decaying fish may deplete a ship's hold of oxygen and lead to the production of toxic quantities of hydrogen sulfide (H_2S), ammonia (NH_3) and carbon dioxide (CO_2). From 1966 to 1971, reports of 3 deaths and 4 cases of unconsciousness from asphyxia among Danish commercial fishermen led to a survey of the air content in the holds of 13 large industrial fishing cutters.[1] In 7 of these ships, the oxygen concentration was found to be dangerously low (7 vol. %, range 3–20). There were concentrations of CO_2 greater than 20 vol. % (range 0–40) and NH_3 (200 ppm) in 9 vessels. These high concentrations are sufficient to cause immediate toxicity or asphyxia in man, and the median levels are above the threshold limit values recommended for occupational exposure in industrial workplaces. Whereas most large fishing craft have equipment to ventilate the holds of ships before crewmen enter, small vessels do not. The toxicity of air in the holds of small vessels has not previously been viewed as a potential hazard.

Sodium bisulfate and sodium metabisulfite have been used in a $1^1/_4$% solution since 1956 as a dip for the preservation of fresh shrimp. The white powder emits a pungent odor of sulfur dioxide, particularly when it is not kept cool, and this odor may be enhanced when mixed with warm salt water. The finding of measurable levels of sulfhemoglobin in the blood of the crewmen in the absence of methemoglobin suggests that their sulfur exposure may have been due in part to the inhalation of a high concentration of sulfur dioxide gas.

During July, 1978, 2 crewmen of a shrimp fishing vessel died and the captain was hospitalized following toxic exposure to the atmosphere of the ship's hold. The hold was refrigerated with ice and contained approximately 4000 pounds of shrimp caught in the preceding 11 days at sea. Both crewmen previously had been involved in dipping the shrimp into a sodium bisulfite solution used routinely to control "black-spot," a discoloration associated with decay. When the first crewman descended into the hold to pack the freshly caught shrimp on ice, he collapsed immediately into coma. The captain went into the hold to resuscitate the first crewman and also fell unconscious. The second crewman followed the first 2 men into the hold and also collapsed. The captain regained consciousness long enough to climb out of the hold and notify the Coast Guard; shortly thereafter he was evacuated by helicopter and brought to the hospital.

At autopsy of the crewmen who died, no specific gross pathologic changes were noted. The bodies and blood samples smelled distinctly of sulfur. Sulfhemoglobin determinations performed on frozen blood specimens showed levels of 6% and 12% (normal level is zero); neither carboxyhemoglobin nor methemoglobin was present. Inquiries by the Coast Guard and the Louisiana Department of Health and Human Resources have identified 4 similar episodes since 1970 that resulted in 9 deaths and 2 hospitalizations. Two of these episodes involved shrimpers exposed to the sodium bisulfite dip. Four other deaths in ships' holds occurred in 2 separate incidents involving government inspectors.

TREATMENT.—Immediate removal from exposure and ensure that the airway is clear. Give 100% oxygen by tight-fitting oronasal mask or endotracheal tube. Hyperbaric oxygen at 3 atmospheres has been successful (see the section on Carbon Monoxide for details).

Because of the acute toxicity of hydrogen sulfide, any person who might be exposed to sudden high concentrations of the gas or is controlling the handling of the gas should not be subject to episodes of fainting, epileptic seizures or other conditions that might alter his state of consciousness and endanger himself or others. A person with chronic conjunctivitis, asthma or other chronic respiratory diseases may be more sensitive to the effects of H_2S exposure, and the physician should consider those potential effects in determining whether individuals with such histories should be subject to exposure, even at low levels.

REFERENCES

Hydrogen Sulfide

1. Dalgaard, J. B., et al.: Fatal poisoning and other health hazards connected with industrial fishing, Br. J. Ind. Med. 29:307, 1972.
2. Donham, K. J., Rubino, M., Thedell, T. D., and Kammermeyer, J.: Potential health hazards to agricultural workers in swine confinement buildings, J. Occup. Med. 10:383, 1977.
3. Fletcher, W. J.: Safety hazards associated with livestock waste. Presented at the winter meeting of the American Society of Agricultural Engineers, Chicago, December, 1971.
4. Idyll, P. P.: How to use sodium bisulfite to control "black-spot" on shrimp. Florida State Board of Conservation and the Marine Laboratory, University of Miami, Coral Gables, Florida, Special Services Bulletin No. 12, August, 1956.
5. Midwest Plan Service: Livestock Waste Facilities Handbook. Ames, Iowa, Iowa State University, 1975.
6. Morbidity and Mortality Weekly Report: Deaths from asphyxia in fishermen. Center for Disease Control, Vol. 27, No. 34, pp. 309–315, August 25, 1978.
7. Muehling, A. J.: Swine housing and waste management: A research review. Urbana, Ill., Cooperative Extension Service, University of Illinois, pp. 65–78, 1969.
8. National Institute for Occupational Safety and Health: Criteria for a Recommended Standard . . . Occupational Exposure to Hydrogen Sulfide. (DHEW [NIOSH] Publication No. 77–158), Cincinnati, Ohio, NIOSH, pp. 1–149, 1977.

Iron Oxide and Hematite

Hematite, a major source of iron, is found in two forms—red hematite (red iron ore), consisting of about 70% iron (Fe_2O_3), and brown hematite, a hydrated sesquioxide of iron, with 42% iron content. Of importance is that most ores mined may contain between 10% and 12% free silica.

Occupational exposures may occur to dust and fumes of iron oxide in mining, both underground or open-pit, to chippers and grinders, arc welders, in various metal processing in foundries and in silver polishing (using fine iron oxide as a polishing rouge).

Inhalation of iron oxide fume or dust may cause a clinical entity known as "benign pneumoconiosis," often labeled "siderosis," based on x-ray findings and work history. Iron oxide alone does not cause fibrosis in the lungs of animals, and it is probable that the same applies in humans.[6] Heavy exposures of 6–10 years usually are required before changes recognizable by x-ray can occur; the retained dust gives x-ray shadows that may be indistinguishable from fibrotic pneumoconiosis.[4,9] Eight of 25 welders exposed chiefly to iron oxide for an average of 18.7 (range 3–32) years had reticulonodular shadows on chest x-rays consistent with siderosis but no reduction in pulmonary function; exposure levels[4,8] ranged from 0.65 to 47 mg/m^3. In another study, 16 welders with an average exposure of 17.1 (range 7–30) years also had x-rays suggesting siderosis and spirograms that were normal; however, the static and functional compliance of the lungs was reduced; some of the welders were smokers.[10] The welders with the lowest compliance complained of dyspnea. Signs of "benign pneumoconiosis" with x-ray shadows that may be indistinguishable from fibrotic pneumoconiosis are found. It should be noted that in industrial situations, iron oxide fumes usually exist with other metallic fumes, and the effects of the combined substances should be considered.

Axelson and Sjöberg[1] studied a working population with high exposure to iron oxides who were engaged in sulfuric acid production from pyrite ore (FeS_2). Some 500 workers had been annually occupied in a factory founded in 1905 with particularly heavy iron oxide exposure throughout the years up to the mid-1950s. The production process, based on oxidation of pyrite ore to produce sulfur dioxide, further oxidized to sulfur trioxide, was used. The remaining content of the pyrite is iron oxides, almost exclusively hematite, Fe_2O_3, with 1–2% of copper and small amounts of arsenic, nickel and cobalt metals found as impurities along with the iron oxides. The arsenic content (as iron arsenate, $FeAsO_4$) was estimated at about 0.01–0.1% (based on arsenic weight) whereas most of the copper was extracted. It was estimated that the iron oxide content of the factory air might have been in the order of 50–100 mg/m^3 for many of the workers through a considerable time of the shift. It was well known that a heavy, dark "mist" of iron oxide was characteristic in several workplaces in this factory. The particle size was estimated to have been less than 10μ for 25% of the dust, with 5–10% less than 5μ. Axelson and Sjöberg added that, despite the very heavy exposures, no cases of siderosis were found in this plant. In this case-referent study, Axelson and Sjöberg found no excess cancer in the respiratory system or other sites. It was suggested that earlier reports of respiratory cancers thought to be associated with iron oxides might be due to other and concomitant risk factors.

Judging from experiences in Sweden,[2] the increased lung cancer mortality among various mining populations was explained to be most likely due to exposure to radon and radon daughters rather than to iron oxides, along with a possible relationship to diesel exhaust gases.[7] Hernberg[5] summarized the evidences for and against the carcinogenic properties of iron ore dust and concluded that the carcinogenic effect for humans still is an open question.

An epidemiologic survey of welders was conducted in the Caterpillar Tractor Company plants in Peoria, Illinois, by Emmett et al.[3] in 1976. Comparison groups consisted of 77 white males who had been welders at this plant for a total of longer than 10 years, 75 white males who were not welders but had been employed in other crafts in the vicinity of welding operations at this plant for more than 8 years and 58 white male parts and tool employees who had neither worked as welders or in the vicinity of welding operations but had been employed at this plant for more than 10 years. The investigators reported a statistically significant increase in the prevalence of cough in the morning and at other times during the day in the welders. Those in the welding and exposed groups reported significantly more phlegm at times other than the morning compared with the control group. There was no significant difference in the prevalence of other chest symptoms, of major respiratory illness, of abnormalities on physical examination of the respiratory system or of abnormalities detectable on posteroanterior chest x-ray among the groups. The observed/expected FEV_1 and observed/expected MMF were significantly reduced in smokers contrasted with nonsmokers. There was a significant reduction in the observed/expected FEV_1 and observed/expected FVC in both the welding and exposed groups compared with the controls. There were indications that smoking and occupation might interact in producing decrements in observed/expected FVC, observed/expected FEV_1 and observed/expected MMF. The decrements in pulmonary function compared to the control group were similar in both the welding and exposed groups, suggesting that other factors rather than the ambient workplace atmospheres might be responsible.

The 1979 TLV for iron oxide fumes: 5 mg/m^3. Methods of control are seen in Figures 14–2 and 14–3.

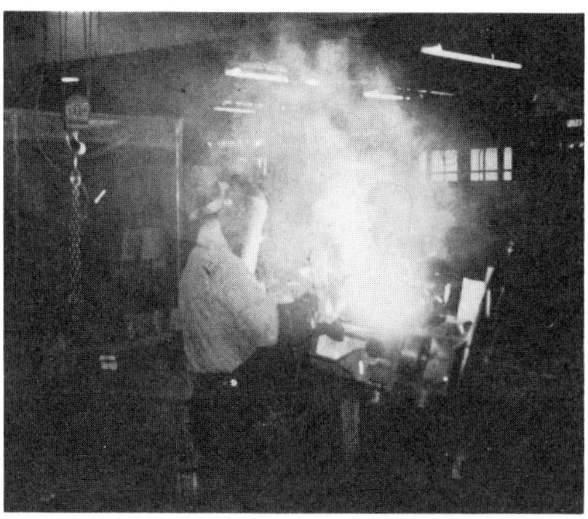

Fig 14–2.—Production welding before exhaust system was installed. Note dense fumes, which are mainly iron oxide.

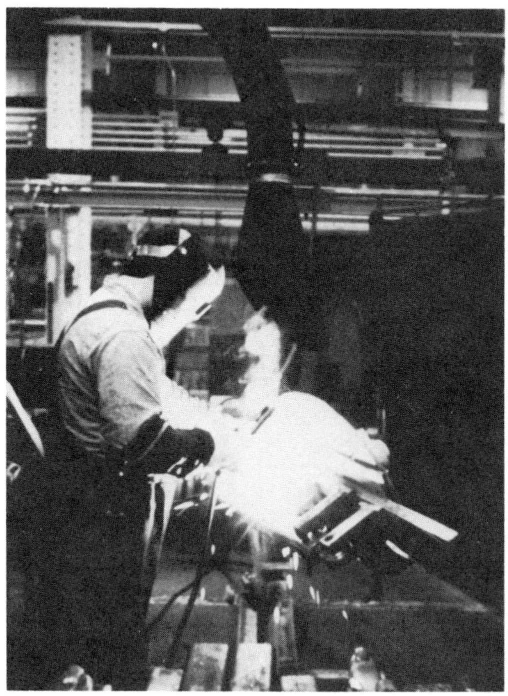

Fig 14–3.—Welding fumes effectively captured by local exhaust. The materials in the air are collected on a special filter, similar to that of a vacuum cleaner.

REFERENCES

Iron Oxide and Hematite

1. Axelson, O., and Sjöberg, A.: A case-referent study on cancer incidence and exposure to iron oxide dust, J. Occup. Med. 21:419, 1979.
2. Axelson, O., and Sundell, L.: Mining, lung cancer and smoking, Scand. J. Work Environ. Health 4:46, 1978.
3. Emmett, E., Buncher, C., and Suskind, R.: An epidemiologic survey of welders, Department of Environmental Health, College of Medicine, University of Cincinnati, Cincinnati, Ohio, 1976.
4. Harding, H. E., et al.: Clinical, radiographic, and pathological studies of the lungs of electric-arc and oxyacetylene welders, Lancet 2:394, 1958.
5. Hernberg, S.: Incidence of cancer in populations with exceptional exposure to metals, in *Origins of Human Cancer,* Cold Spring Harbor Laboratory, 1977.
6. Jones, G., and Warner, C.: Chronic exposure to iron oxide, chromium oxide, and nickel oxide fumes of metal dressers in a steelworks, Br. J. Ind. Med. 29:169, 1972.
7. Jorgensen, H.: A study of mortality from lung cancer among miners in Kiruna, 1950–1970, Work Environ, Health 10:127, 1973.
8. Kleinfeld, M., et al.: Welders' siderosis, Arch. Environ. Health 19:70, 1969.
9. Sentz, F., and Rakow, A.: Exposure to iron oxide fume at arcair and powder-burning operations, Am. Ind. Hyg. Assoc. J. 30:143, 1969.
10. Stanexcu, D., et al.: Aspects of pulmonary mechanics in arc welders' siderosis, Br. J. Ind. Med. 24:143, 1967.

Isocyanates

The diisocyanates and polyisocyanates may be considered together, since they have similar commercial applications and present similar toxicologic problems.

Isocyanates react with a wide variety of compounds containing active hydrogen atoms to produce such products as rigid or flexible foams, surface coatings, adhesives, rubbers and fibers. Wide application of the products ranges from packaging, insulation materials, upholstery in automobiles, furniture and shoe soles. Most of the flexible foams are produced in large-scale operations in the form of slabs, blocks or sheets, which, after curing, should contain no free isocyanates. Such operations generally are quite amenable to engineering controls. A significant proportion of the rigid polyurethane foams, however, is generated with portable equipment, or virtually no equipment at all, by mixing the polymerizing ingredients, resins, polyols, polyethers, emulsifiers, catalysts, water and sometimes "frothing" or "blowing" agents on site and pouring them into the mold or structural cavity that is to be filled with the rigid foam. Another method of application of rigid foam is by spraying the polymerizing ingredients immediately after mixing onto a surface that is to be coated with a layer of foam. In such situations, the problems of limiting concentration in the breathing zone are difficult. Occupations with potential exposures are: abrasion resistant rubber makers, adhesive workers, aircraft builders, insulation workers, lacquer workers, mine tunnel coaters, organic chemical synthesizers, plastic foam makers, plasticizer workers, polyurethane sprayers, polyurethane foam makers, ship burners, ship welders, spray painters, textile processors, upholstery makers and wire coating workers. The NIOSH has estimated the number of workers with potential exposure to be approximately 40,000. Vapor pressures have a particular importance in the assessment of the relative toxicity of different isocyanates, since the principal industrial hazard is a respiratory hazard arising from the inhalation of atmospheric isocyanate.

In addition, it should be borne in mind that isocyanates may enter the respiratory tract not only in the vapor phase but also as airborne dusts and aerosols.

TDI (TOLUENE DIISOCYANATE)

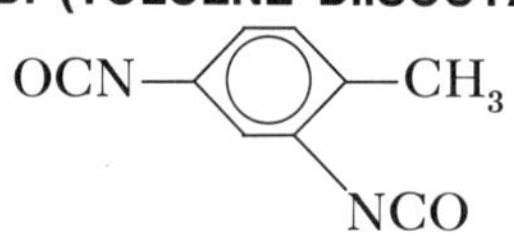

TDI is manufactured from toluene diamine by reaction with carbonyl chloride (phosgene). Isocyanates are chemical compounds containing the N=C=O group. The two isomers most commonly used are 2,4-toluene diisocyanate and 2,6-toluene diisocyanate; commercially available are three isomer ratios: (1) 100% 2,4; (2) 80% 2,4:20%2,6; and (3) 65% 2,4:35% 2,6.

TDI is the most widely used isocyanate, being utilized in almost all the applications in which isocyanates are used, as precursors in the production of polyurethanes, polyureas, polyamides, allophanates and simple polymers of the isocyanates themselves. All these compounds are collectively referred to as "polyurethanes" or "polyurethane plastics."

The vapor is a strong irritant to the eyes, mucous membranes and skin and is a potent sensitizer of the respiratory tract. Exposed human subjects experienced irritation of the eyes, nose and throat, a choking sensation and a productive cough of a paroxysmal type, often with retrosternal soreness and chest pain. Higher concentrations produce a sensation of oppression or constriction of the chest; there may be bronchitis and severe bronchospasm; pulmonary edema may occur also. Nausea, vomiting and abdominal pain may complicate the presenting symptoms. Although the acute effects may be severe, their importance is overshadowed by respiratory sensitization in susceptible individuals after repeated exposure to levels of TDI of 0.02 ppm and below. The onset of symptoms of sensitization may be insidious, becoming progressively more pronounced with continued exposure over a period of days to months; initial symptoms may be nocturnal dyspnea and/or nocturnal cough with progression to asthmatic bronchitis. Often when the respiratory illness has become incapacitating and the worker has been hospitalized or otherwise removed from the worksite, a return to work causes an acute and severe asthmatic attack almost immediately or within a few hours. In another pattern, if a worker has had only minimal upper respiratory symptoms or no apparent acute asthmatic reaction to the same or slightly higher level, the asthmatic reaction may be severe, sometimes resulting in status asthmaticus, which may be fatal. It is not known whether all persons or only those with a history of atopy are potentially susceptible to sensitization to TDI. A third type of respiratory response to inhaled TDI is a small decrease in FEV_1 in most or all workers exposed to concentrations as low as 0.002 ppm in the absence, in many cases, of overt symptoms of respiratory irritation. Splashes of TDI liquid in the eye will cause severe conjunctival irritation and lacrimation. On the skin, the liquid produced a marked inflammatory reaction; sensitization of the skin occurs but is uncommon due to proper work practices; there seems to be little relation between skin sensitivity and respiratory sensitivity to TDI.[8] If exposure occurs, promptly flush the eyes with water and wash the skin with soap or mild detergent and water. Consideration should be given to hospitalization and observation for the possible delayed onset of pulmonary edema or status asthmaticus. Exposure to TDI shall be controlled so that no worker shall be exposed to a TWA of more than 0.005 ppm (0.036 mg/m^3) for any 8-hour workday or for any 20-minute period to more than 0.02 ppm (0.14 mg/m^3).

HDI (HEXAMETHYLENE DIISOCYANATE)

HDI is a volatile liquid isocyanate. It has been used in the treatment of leather, the preparation of surface coatings and the production of solid elastomers. It is a powerful skin and respiratory irritant and is known to have caused respiratory sensitization.

NDI (NAPHTHALENE DIISOCYANATE)

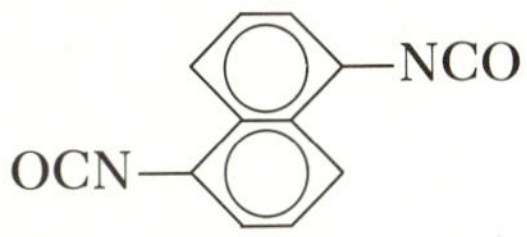

NDI is a solid isocyanate at room temperature that is used in the manufacture of urethane elastomers. It is relatively nonirritating to the skin in crystalline form. Having a low volatility, it is unlikely to present a vapor hazard unless heated, but at the elevated temperatures required for processing, the vapor pressure is such that a number of cases of respiratory sensitization due to contact with the heated material have been recorded.

MDI (DIPHENYLMETHANE DIISOCYANATE)

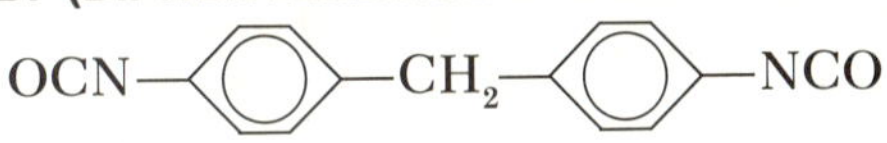

MDI is an isocyanate that may vary in physical form, being produced either as a viscous liquid or as a solid material. It is extensively and increasingly used in the manufacture of polyurethane foams, adhesives and solid urethane elastomers. It is also suitable for use in certain spray applications. Having a low volatility, it constitutes much less of a practical hazard than TDI and at room temperature can be handled without fear of a vapor hazard. When airborne spray droplets are inhaled, respiratory irritation and sensitization may result. The main toxic effect of MDI is the development of respiratory sensitization, leading to asthma and allergic bronchitis. The asthmatic response may be delayed several hours after the last exposure and a reduction in the FVC and FEV_1 may occur. At high levels, irritation to the nose and throat, chest tightness and pain may occur. Sensitive individuals may also develop dermatitis. There are no specific diagnostic tests, although some physicians find hematocrit and WBC count, with differential cell count to determine eosinophils, to be useful to rule out infection, other allergies, etc. The demonstration of isocyanate-specific antibodies in sera has been investigated as a possible biologic test of sensitization, but this test has not become standardized for routine use. There is no specific treatment.

METHYL ISOCYANATE

The vapor is an irritant to the eyes, mucous membranes and skin and it can cause pulmonary irritation and sensitization. Exposure of humans to high concentrations can cause cough, dyspnea, increased pulmonary mucous secretions and chest pains. Isocyanates cause pulmonary sensitization in susceptible individuals; should this occur, further exposure must be avoided, since extremely low levels of exposure may trigger an asthmatic episode. Cross sensitization to unrelated materials probably does not occur. Experimental exposure of 4 human subjects for 1–5 minutes caused the following effects: 0.4 ppm, no effects; 2 ppm, lacrimation, irritation of the nose and throat; 4 ppm, symptoms of irritation more marked; 21 ppm, unbearable irritation of eyes, nose and throat.[5] A cotton plug saturated with the liquid was applied to the ear of a rabbit for 30 minutes and caused erythema, edema, necrosis and perforation; a few drops of the liquid on the ear of a rabbit caused destruction of tissue. The liquid in contact with the eye may cause permanent damage. The TLV for methyl isocyanate is fixed at 0.02 ppm (ceiling value).

DADI (DISANISDINE DIISOCYANATE)

This isocyanate is a gray-brown crystalline solid that is used in the manufacture of some elastomers and adhesives. Its vapor pressure up to 150° C is negligible, so vapor inhalation hazards are greatly reduced. Nevertheless, care must be taken to avoid breathing dust arising from the material.

TRIPHENYLMETHANE TRIISOCYANATE

This isocyanate, which usually is in liquid form as a 20% solution in methylene chloride, is used chiefly in bonding applications.

In general, its toxicity is comparable to that of MDI, but it is a more potent skin irritant because of the solvent. It usually contains a trace of free phenyl monoisocyanate, which may contribute to its irritant properties and frequently it is used in combination with other diisocyanates. It may constitute a respiratory hazard (as in the case of MDI) when used in spray applications.

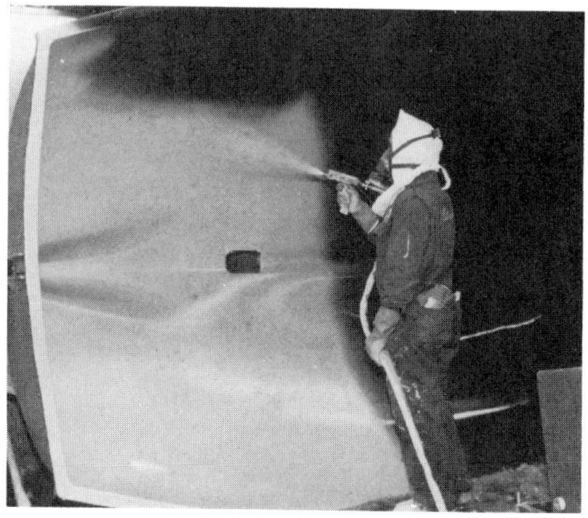

Fig 14–4.—Spray application of special coating. Worker has proper clothing and suitable respiratory protective equipment.

POLYMETHYLENE POLYPHENYLISOCYANATE

This high molecular weight, low volatile polyisocyanate is a viscous liquid used chiefly in the manufacture of surface coatings, adhesives and polyurethane foams. Polymethylene polyphenylisocyanate has a low order of hazard, since, in normal conditions of industrial use, vapor concentrations are unlikely to approach the TLV of 0.02 ppm. During spray operations, however, great care will be required to ensure protection against inhalation of airborne droplets. It does not appear to have any significant irritant properties in contact with the skin.

Polyurethane paints are those in which an organic isocyanate is used as a constituent. The most likely source of free isocyanate is the two-pack paint system, which separates the active isocyanate-containing catalyst from the inert base material. Respiratory problems have been reported from the use of single-pack moisture-cured surface coatings. Toluene diisocyanate, hexamethylene diisocyanate, diphenyl methane diisocyanate and isophorone diisocyanate may be incorporated in polyurethane paint systems. The volatile isocyanates usually are modified to reduce their vapor pressure but always will contain a small percentage of residual free volatile parent isocyanate (this usually is less than 0.7% residual isocyanate related to 100% of the polyisocyanate used as a catalyst in the paint system). A health hazard may arise from the inhalation of free volatile parent isocyanate when the paint is applied by brush at room temperature. A greater hazard, however, arises when the paint is spray-applied, for, in addition to the free parent isocyanate, the paint also contains a high proportion of nonvolatile isocyanate groups, which, although chemically combined in the paint, will cause respiratory problems if the paint spray is inhaled. An oronasal mask fitted with cartridges effective against dust and 1% organic vapors is satisfactory if the paint is applied by brush. A compressed-air-fed respirator should be worn if the polyurethane paint is spray-applied (Fig. 14–4.)

POLYURETHANE PREPOLYMERS

Prepolymers are manufactured by reacting a polyol with a molar excess of diisocyanate in the absence of water. The prepolymer itself, therefore, is a large molecule of very low volatility with reactive isocyanate groups at its ends. The commercial prepolymer, however, will contain traces of the diisocyanate used to make it, and this will be far more volatile. Prepolymers are used in the manufacture of semirigid and rigid foams, surface coatings and elastomers. They are also used as binding agents in the manufacture of reconstituted polyether foam. Surface coatings with nonyellowing characteristics can be produced only from prepolymers based on aliphatic or alicyclic diisocyanates (methylene bis-4 cyclohexylene isocyanate, isophorone diisocyanate or hexamethylene diisocyanate, etc.). It is possible to mask the isocyanate groups of diisocyanates or prepolymers by reacting them reversibly with other chemicals, e.g., phenolic compounds, tertiary alcohols, etc. In this way, the free isocyanate is safely held in chemical combination until the masking is unblocked by heating or chemical displacement of the blocking agent with compounds containing more highly reactive hydrogen atoms. *Isocyanate prepolymers and marked isocyanates always should be handled with the same precautions as the isocyanate itself.*

The British Rubber Manufacturers' Association[5] has prepared detailed processing precautions and medical recommendations for processes involving the handling and use of isocyanates. They urge that use should not be undertaken without a proper understanding of the potential hazards involved and the provision of adequate supervision of, and safeguards for, personnel. Such supervision should include:

1. Pre-employment screening and selection.
2. Periodic health checks.
3. Health checks on return to work after absence due to illness.
4. First-aid instruction and facilities.

REFERENCES

Isocyanates

1. American Conference of Governmental Industrial Hygienists: Toluene-2,3-Diisocyanate (TDI). Documentation of the Threshold Limit Values for Substances in Workroom Air, 3d ed., Cincinnati, Ohio. pp. 167, 260–261, 1974.
2. Criteria for a Recommended Standard . . . Occupational Exposure to Diisocyanates DHEW (NIOSH) HSM 78-215, Cincinnati, Ohio, U.S. Dept. of Health, Education, and Welfare, PHS, Center for Disease Control, National Institute for Occupational Safety and Health, 1978.
3. Criteria Document: Recommendations for Occupational Exposure Standard for Toluene Diisocyanate, HSM 73-1102, U.S. Dept. of Health, Education, and Welfare, National Institute for Occupational Safety and Health, 1974.
4. Hygienic Guide Series: Toluene diisocyanate, Am. Ind. Hyg. Assoc. J. 28:90, 1967.
5. Isocyanates in Industry, Operating and Medical Codes of Practice. British Rubber Manufacturers' Association, Ltd. BR. M. A. Scala House, Birmingham, Rev. ed., 1977.
6. Manufacturing Chemists Association, Inc.: Chemical Safety Data Sheet SD-73, Toluene Diisocyanate. Washington, D.C., pp. 6, 16–19, 1971.
7. Rye, W. A.: Human responses to isocyanate exposure, J. Occup. Med. 14:306, 1973.
8. Wegman, D. S., et al.: A dose-response relationship in TDI workers, J. Occup. Med. 16:258, 1974.

4,4′-Methylenebis(2-Chloroaniline)

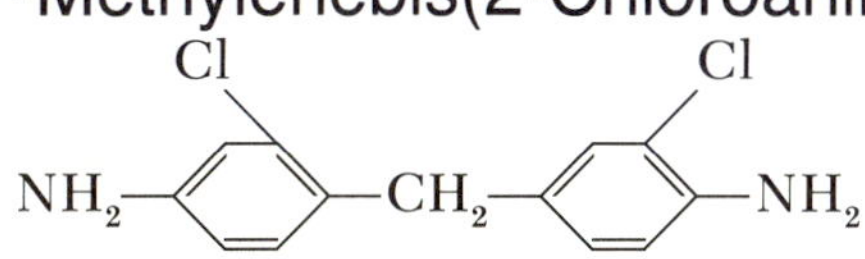

4,4′-Methylenebis(2-chloroaniline), more commonly referred to as MOCA, a registered trade name of the Du Pont Company, has the formula $C_{13}H_{12}C_{12}N_2$. Common or trade names include: 4,4′-methylenebis(2-chloroaniline), DACPM, MBOCA,MOCA, Curaline M, Curene 442 and Cyanaset. It is commercially important as a curing agent for diisocyanate-based polymers (polyurethanes) and epoxy resin systems used in the manufacture of certain products, particularly integral-skin polyurethane semirigid foam as used for crash padding, and solid urethane rubber moldings, such as gear blanks and industrial tires. This compound is used to vary the hardness, flexibility and impact strength of these products. During the melting of the solid, when temperatures of about 200° C are used, the release of irritant and toxic vapors (primarily ortho-chloroaniline) may occur. The NIOSH estimated through a national survey that in the early 1970s approximately 55,000 U. S. workers were potentially exposed to 4,4′-methylenebis(2-chloroaniline). The majority of these workers were employed in small to medium-sized establishments. Based on information presented by the NIOSH (Appendix I), 4,4′-methylenebis(2-chloroaniline) was one of 14 substances for which the Occupational Safety and Health Administration (OSHA) promulgated an emergency temporary standard on May 3, 1973. Even though not enforceable as a federal standard, several states, including California, continued to enforce the standard under state law. In 1972, the American Conference of Governmental Industrial Hygienists (ACGIH) included 4,4′-methylenebis(2-chloroanaline) as an experimental carcinogen in Appendix A of its Threshold Limit Values booklet[1] without a recommended environmental limit. The experimental carcinogen designation was applied by the ACGIH to industrial substances found to be of high potency for inducing tumors under experimental conditions in animals. In 1975, the ACGIH revised their designation for experimental carcinogens to be "Occupational Substances Suspected of Oncogenic Potential for Workers" and assigned 4,4′-methylenebis(2-chloroaniline) a threshold limit value of 0.02 ppm with a skin notation. The documentation for this TLV apparently was not based on a consideration of the carcinogenic potential of this chemical but was established with the belief that this limit was "sufficiently low as to prevent systemic poisoning, provided skin contact is avoided."[2] The documentation included a warning that worker exposure by all routes should be reduced to a minimum in light of the warning of the potency for the chemical to induce tumors in animals.[3]

4,4′-methylenebis(2-chloroaniline) possesses the general toxicity characteristics of aromatic amines and may, if introduced into the human body, produce cyanosis from methemoglobin formation.[9] From an occupational health standpoint, there is greater concern for 4,4′-methylenebis(2-chloroaniline)'s carcinogenic potential, evidence for which comes primarily from animal bioassays as well as in vitro mutagenicity studies. Results reported by 5 independent groups of investigators clearly demonstrate 4,4′-methylenebis(2-chloroaniline) to be oncogenic in the rat, mouse and dog. Ingestion of daily doses of 4,4′-methylenebis(2-chloroaniline) by mice and rats has resulted in the appearance of cancers of the liver, kidneys, lungs, skin and mammary glands. Urinary bladder cancer was produced in female beagle dogs fed doses of 4,4′-methylenebis(2-chloroaniline) that varied from 8 to 15 mg/kg body weight per day for up to 9 years.[10] Based on positive oncogenic results in 3 animal test species, the NIOSH recommends that 4,4 -methylenebis(2-chloroaniline) be treated as a potential occupational carcinogen. Because a significant route of entry into the body is by skin absorption,[3,5,6] efforts must be made to prevent skin contact with 4,4′-methylenebis(2-chloroaniline), whenever possible. The use of protective clothing made of butyl rubber, neoprene or spunbonded olefin has been shown to assist in the reduction of worker exposure through skin contact.[4,8]

Although research information is not yet available to demonstrate a quantitative relationship between skin absorption of 4,4′-methylenebis(2-chloroaniline) and urinary levels in workers, occupational experience indicates that urinary monitoring is necessary as an adjunct to the monitoring of airborne 4,4′-methylenebis(2-chloroaniline) in the skin.[6] The finding of 3,3′-methylenebis(2-chloroaniline) in the urine demonstrates that exposure has occurred and can indicate work situations that need additional control efforts. Likewise, monitoring of workplace surfaces can identify where contamination problems exist and where the potential for workplace exposure is greatest. Detailed procedures for monitoring work surfaces for 4,4′-methylenebis(2-chloroaniline) contamination are presented in the NIOSH Criteria Document.[7]

CONTROL GUIDELINES

The National Institute for Occupational Safety and Health recommends that employee exposure to 4,4′-methylenebis(2-chloroaniline) (MOCA) in the workplace be controlled so that no worker will be exposed to concentrations in excess of 3 mg/m^3 of (breathing zone) air, determined as a time-weighted average (TWA) concentration for up to a 10-hour workshift, 40-hour workweek over a working lifetime. The recommended exposure level of 3 μg/m^3 is the lowest level at which 4,4′-methylenebis(2-chloroaniline) can be reliably measured at this time. The control guidelines contain recommendations for medical surveillance, informing employees of hazards, sanitation, work practices, labeling and posting, personal protective clothing and equipment, monitoring and record keeping.

Although compliance with these recommendations should materially reduce the risk of developing cancer from 4,4′-methylenebis(2-chloroaniline), no absolutely safe concentration can be established for a carcinogen at this time. The employer should regard the recommended permissible exposure level as the upper boundary of exposure and make every effort to keep exposure by all routes as low as possible.

In approximately 22 years of industrial experience with the manufacture of 4,4′-methylenebis(2-chloroaniline), Du Pont has found no evidence of a carcinogenic effect in its workers.[4]

REFERENCES

4,4′-Methylenebis(2-Chloroaniline)

1. American Conference of Governmental Industrial Hygienists, Committee on Threshhold Limits: Threshold Limit Values for Chemical Substances and Physical Agents in Workroom Environment with Intended Changes for 1972. Cincinnati, Ohio, ACGIH, p. 39, 1972.
2. American Conference of Governmental Industrial Hygienists, Committee on Threshold Limits: Threshold Limit Values for Chemical Substances and Physical Agents in the Workroom Environment with Intended Changes for 1975. Cincinnati, Ohio, ACGIH, p. 42, 1975.
3. American Conference of Governmental Industrial Hygienists: Documentation of the Threshold Limit Values for Substances in Workroom Air and Supplements for Those Substances Added or Changed Since 1971, 3d ed. Cincinnati, Ohio, ACGIH, p. 337, 1974.
4. Du Pont Company Adiprene . . . "MOCA" and LD-813. Du Pont Product Bulletin Ap-710-1, E. I. du Pont de Nemours & Company, Elastomer Chemicals Department, Wilmington, Delaware, 1977.
5. International Agency for Research on Cancer (IARC) Monograph on the Evaluation of Carcinogenic Risk of Chemicals to Man. Some aromatic amines, hydrazine and related substances, *N*-nitroso compounds and miscellaneous alkylating agents, Vol. 4, World Health Organization, Lyon, France, pp. 65–71, 1974.
6. Linch, A. L., O'Connor, G. B., Barnes, J. R., Killian, A. S., Jr., and Neeld, W. E., Jr.: Methylene-bis-ortho-chloroaniline (MOCA). Evaluation of hazards and exposure control, Am. Ind. Hyg. Assoc. J. 32:802, 1971.
7. NIOSH Special Hazard Review with Control Recommendations for 4,4′-Methylenebis

(2-chloroaniline), U.S. Dept. of Health, Education, and Welfare, PHS, Center for Disease Control, (NIOSH) DHEW Publication No. 78-188, Cincinnati, Ohio, 1978.

8. Personal communication from W. J. Touhey, Jr., E. I. Du Pont de Nemours & Company, Wilmington, Delaware, to J. L. Haln, State of California Dept. of Health, Proposed Standard — 4,4′Methylenebis(2-chloroaniline), June 26, 1978.
9. Ryan, J. D.: MOCA (TM). A Diamine Curing Agent for Isocyanate-containing Polymers. Du Pont Product Bulletin, E. I. du Pont de Nemours & Company, Elastomer Chemicals Department, Wilmington, Delaware, 1971.
10. Stula, E. F., Barnes, J. R., Sherman, H., Reinhardt, D. F., and Zapp, J. A., Jr.: Urinary bladder tumors in dogs from 4,4′-methylenebis(2-chloroaniline) (MOCA), J. Environ, Pathol. Toxicol. 1:31, 1977.

Nitric Acid

Nitric acid (HNO_3) is a powerful oxidizing agent, reacting with most metals, and is used in enormous quantities to produce fertilizer, dyes and plastics. The well-known "Ostwald process" produces ammonia (NH_3) from atmospheric nitrogen, which is oxidized to nitrogen dioxide. Nitric acid is unstable, decomposing on contact with heat and exposure to light, water, nitrogen dioxide and oxygen.

Occupational exposures may occur by inhalation and/or skin contact. Nitric acid vapor or mist is a severe irritant to the eyes, mucous membranes and skin. When nitric acid is exposed to air or comes into contact with organic matter, it decomposes to yield a mixture of oxides of nitrogen, including nitric oxide and nitrogen dioxide, both equally or more hazardous than nitric acid. Exposure to high concentrations of nitric acid vapor or mist causes pneumonitis and pulmonary edema, which may be fatal; onset of symptoms may be delayed for 4–30 hours. In contact with the eyes, the liquid produces severe burns, which may result in permanent damage and visual impairment. On the skin, the liquid in concentrated solutions may cause deep ulcers and stain the skin a bright yellow or yellowish brown color. The vapor and mist may erode teeth. Ingestion of the liquid will cause immediate pain and burns of the gastrointestinal tract.

TREATMENT.—Prompt removal from exposure and immediate flushing with water. Consider hospitalization for observation for the possible delayed onset of pulmonary edema.

The TLV of 2 ppm was set mainly to prevent irritation and erosion of teeth.[1]

REFERENCES

Nitric Acid

1. American Conference of Governmental Industrial Hygienists: "Nitric Acid," Documentation of the Threshold Limit Values for Substances in Workroom Air, 3d ed., Cincinnati, Ohio, pp.181–182, 1976.
2. Hygienic Guide Series: Nitric acid, Am. Ind. Hyg. Assoc. J. 25:426, 1964.
3. Manufacturing Chemists Association, Inc.: Chemical Safety Data Sheet, DS-5, Nitric Acid, Washington, D.C., pp.15–17, 1961.
4. National Institute for Occupational Safety and Health, U.S. Dept. of Health, Education, and Welfare: Criteria for a Recommended Standard . . . Occupational Exposure to Nitric Acid. NIOSH Publication No. 76-141 (HEW), Cincinnati, Ohio, 1976.

2-Nitropropane

$CH_3CHNO_2CH_3$

A recently completed inhalation study indicates that 2-nitropropane, a widely used solvent in industrial coatings and printing inks, causes liver cancer in rats. In this study, sponsored by the National Institute for Occupational Safety and Health (NIOSH), all laboratory rats exposed to 207 ppm 2-nitropropane over a 6-month period developed hepatocellular carcinoma or hepatic adenoma. Although this study suggests that 2-nitropropane is carcinogenic, its carcinogenic potential in man has not yet been researched.[1] Solvent systems containing 2-nitropropane are used in coatings (e.g., vinyl, epoxy, nitrocellulose and chlorinated rubber), printing inks and adhesives. Occupational exposure to these products may occur in various industries, including industrial construction and maintenance, printing (rotogravure and flexographic inks), highway maintenance (traffic markings), shipbuilding and maintenance (marine coatings), furniture, food packaging and plastic products. The NIOSH estimates that 100,000 workers are potentially exposed to 2-nitropropane in these and other industries.

Synonyms for 2-nitropropane include dimethylnitromethane, isonitropropane, nitroisopropane and 2-NP. Trade names under which 2-nitropropane is marketed include NiPar S-20th (commercial grade 2-nitropropane) and NiPar S-30th (mixtures of 1- and 2-nitropropane). 2-Nitropropane (in concentrations ranging from approximately 5% to 25%) is used in a number of solvent systems to contribute desirable properties such as improved drying time, more complete solvent release, better flow and film integrity, retardation of blushing, greater wetting ability, improved electrostatic spraying and increased pigment dispersion. Of the estimated 15 million kg of 2-nitropropane produced annually in the United States, 6 million kg are sold domestically; the remainder is either used internally by the companies producing it, or exported.

In an inhalation study conducted by Huntingdon Research Center under a NIOSH contract (HEW/NIOSH Project No 210-75-0039), Sprague-Dawley male rats and New Zealand White male rabbits were exposed to commercial grade 2-nitropropane for 7 hours per day, 5 days per week. One group of 50 rats and 15 rabbits was exposed to 207 ppm 2-nitropropane, a second group of the same size was exposed to 27 ppm and a third group was maintained as a control. Ten rats from each group were killed after exposure periods of 2 days, 10 days, 1 month, 3 months and 6 months. Liver neoplasms, described as hepatocellular carcinoma or hepatic adenoma, were observed in all 10 rats killed after 6 months of exposure to 207 ppm 2-nitropropane. No tumors were observed in any other animals in this study, including controls. However, hepatocellular hypertrophy, hyperplasia and necrosis were reported in rats exposed to 207 ppm 2-nitropropane for 3 months. In addition, elevated liver weights were found in rats exposed to 207 ppm 2-nitropropane for 1, 3 and 6 months. Liver histopathology, as well as the liver weights, of rats exposed to 27 ppm 2-nitropropane did not differ from controls. Although certain shortcomings do exist in the conduct of this study,* the experiment is sufficient to merit the concern of the occupational health community.

The effects of 2-nitropropane inhalation in laboratory animals have also been studied by Treon and Dutra.[2] Five species of laboratory animals (2 animals of each species per exposure level) were exposed to various concentrations of 2-nitropropane. Acute exposures ranged up to 9000 ppm for short time periods (as low as 1 hour) whereas chronic exposure levels ranged down to 83 ppm 2-nitropropane for as long as 26 weeks. Treon and Dutra reported no histologic changes in the monkeys, rabbits, guinea pigs and rats exposed to 328 ppm or less, regardless of exposure time. However, both cats died within 17 days of exposure to 328

*The 50 rats exposed to 207 ppm 2-nitropropane were weanling rats (younger and smaller than the other exposed rats and the control group) that were introduced to replace rats experiencing excess mortality during the first few days of exposure to 400 ppm 2-nitropropane. In addition, throughout the entire study, exposure to 2-nitropropane was conducted while food and water were present, thus introducing the potential for exposure by the oral route.

ppm and had severe liver damage and slight to moderate damage to the kidney and heart. There are a number of published reports concerning acute health effects of occupational exposure to 2-nitropropane.[1] One report of 2 workers attributed the death of one and liver damage in both workers to high-level exposure to 2-nitropropane while painting the inside of a tank. Another paper relates that continual exposure to concentrations of 20–45 ppm 2-nitropropane caused workers in one plant to experience nausea, vomiting, diarrhea, anorexia and severe headaches. A third report indicates that workers exposed to from 165 to 445 ppm mixed 1- and 2-nitropropane also experienced nausea, dizziness, headaches and diarrhea. In addition, Williams et al.[3] reported an excess of toxic hepatitis among construction workers applying epoxy resins to the walls of a nuclear power plant. Although the hepatitis in this case was attributed to exposure to a known hepatotoxin, *p,p'*-methylenedianiline(4,4'-diaminodiphenylmethane), these men were also observed to have used 2-nitropropane to remove the hardened resin from their skin.

The current Occupational Safety and Health Administration (OSHA) standard for occupational exposure to 2-nitropropane is 25 ppm. However, in light of the new information generated by the Huntingdon study, and while the carcinogenic potential of 2-nitropropane is being evaluated further, the NIOSH believes that it would be prudent to handle 2-nitropropane in the workplace as if it were a human carcinogen.

REFERENCES

2-Nitropropane

1. Current Intelligence Bulletin No. 17: 2-Nitropropane. U.S. Dept. of Health, Education, and Welfare, PHS, Center for Disease Control, National Institute for Occupational Safety and Health, Cincinnati, Ohio, April, 1977.
2. Treon, J. F., and Dutra, F. R.: Physiological response of experimental animals to the vapor of 2-nitropropane, Arch. Ind. Hyg. Occup. Med. 5:52, 1952.
3. Williams, S. V., et al.: Toxic hepatitis and methylenedianiline (letter to editor), N. Engl. J. Med. 291:1256, 1974.

Nitrosamines

Although *N*-nitrosamines are thought to be an important group of human carcinogens, their role as an increased occupational risk factor has not been established. The formation of diethanolnitrosamine in cutting fluids was first postulated and reported from Sweden by Zingmark and Rappe,[6] who measured diethanolnitrosamine in a specifically formulated "grinding fluid" containing nitrite and triethanolamine.

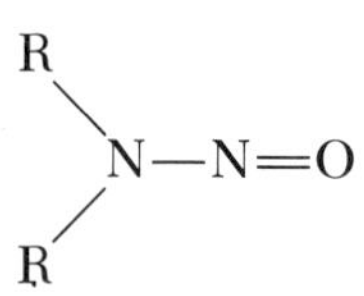

They surmised that the potential hazard of working with these types of products should not be underestimated. Four hundred to more than 1000 ppm diethanolnitrosamine in 8 commercial cutting fluids produced by different manufacturers has been found.[1] Studies conducted during an actual machining operation showing the presence of 1000 ppm diethanolnitrosamine in the diluted cutting fluid prior to use and 384 ppm after use strongly suggest that machine operators may be continually exposed to nitrosamines.

In 1977, Zingmark and Rappe[6] presented further evidence of formation of *N*-nitrosamines from secondary and tertiary amines with nitrite in acidic solution, noting that the acid catalyzes the reaction by forming nitrous acid, which then participates in the *N*-nitrosation. The reaction proceeds very slowly under alkaline conditions because of the low concentration of nitrous acid. Nevertheless, analyses of grinding fluid concentrates containing triethanolamine, nitrite and water show that small amounts of *N*-nitrosodiethanolamine are formed during storage even though the pH values of the fluids are between 10.2 and 11.4. The fluids Zingmark and Rappe tested had been stored for 5–7 months and showed an *N*-nitrosamine concentration ranging from 400 to 800 ppm. These analyses clearly show that the mixing of nitrite and an amine in a technical product always should be regarded with some suspicion as to *N*-nitrosamine formation, especially if the product is stored. *N*-nitrosodiethanolamine has been shown to induce cancer in rats, although high doses are required.[3]

Occupational exposure to cutting fluids, primarily among machine operators, has been studied for possible health effects. A recent published account by Decoufle[2] relates that a slight excess mortality *(not statistically significant)* from respiratory and digestive cancers was observed among male workers exposed to cutting fluids in metal machining jobs. Nomenclature for cutting fluid is not standardized. The term generally applies to substances used in drilling, gear cutting, grinding, milling and other machining operations for the purpose of cooling, lubricating and removing metal or plastic chips, filings and cuttings from the contact area. These substances are variously referred to as cutting, cooling, grinding, industrial, lubricating and synthetic oils or fluids.[5]

Commercial cutting fluids can be divided into four categories:

Cutting Oils or Straight Oils—contain mineral oil, fat and additives. These oils are water insoluble.

Soluble Cutting Oils—contain mineral oil, fat, emulsifiers (may include amines), additives (rarely nitrite*) and water.

Semisynthetic Cutting Oils—contain mineral oil, water, fat, a soluble base (usually including amines), emulsifiers (may include amines) and additives (usually including nitrite).

Synthetic Cutting Fluids—a soluble base (usually including amines), additives (usually including nitrite) and water.

Various proprietary cutting fluids are produced by more than 1000 companies in the United States. The NIOSH estimates that 780,000 persons are occupationally exposed in the manufacture and use of cutting fluids. Synthetic cutting fluids, semisynthetic cutting oils and soluble cutting oils may contain nitrosamines and are found either as contaminants in amines or as products from the reaction of amines (e.g., triethanolamine) with nitrite. Straight oils do not contain nitrites or amines but may contain polynuclear aromatic compounds.

Practical industrial hygiene practices that can minimize dermal and respiratory exposures to cutting fluids are as follows:

1. *Engineering controls*.—The most effective control of any contaminant is control at the source of generation. Effective engineering measures include the use of local exhaust ventilation, with a suitable collector.

2. *Substitution*.—The substitution of a cutting fluid that does not contain either nitrosamine amines or the necessary ingredients (amines and nitrites) for nitrosamine formation is another possible control measure. Since many of the proprietary ingredients of cutting fluids have not undergone complete toxicologic evaluation, caution should be used when contemplating any change from one cutting fluid formulation to another, giving full consideration to the potential hazards of the substitute.

3. *Respirators*.—Personal respiratory protective devices should be used only as an interim measure while engineering controls are being installed, for nonroutine use and during emergencies. Considering the carcinogenic potential and the lack of a standard for nitrosamines as a group, the only available personal respiratory protective measure is the use of a positive-pressure-supplied air respirator or a positive-pressure self-contained breathing apparatus (see section on Respiratory Protection, this chapter).

4. *Protective clothing*.—Impervious clothing should be provided and should be replaced and properly maintained. Nonimpervious clothing is not suggested, but, if used, it should be re-

*Some consumers may incorporate additives containing nitrite into the soluble cutting oil while preparing it for use.

moved and laundered frequently to remove all traces of cutting fluids before being reworn. (Laundry personnel should be made aware of the potential hazard from handling contaminated clothing.)

5. *Personal cleanliness*.—All exposed areas of the body and any area that becomes wet with cutting fluids should be washed with soap or mild detergent. Frequent showering is recommended, and these facilities should be made available in the workplace.

6. *Isolation*.—Where possible, any operations involved with cutting fluids should be placed in an isolated area to reduce exposure to employees not directly concerned with the operations.

7. *"Barrier creams."*—Barrier creams may provide limited protection against dermal irritation and skin absorption; however, the barrier cream should not contain secondary or tertiary amines (which may react to form nitrosamines in the presence of nitrites). Reliance must not be placed solely on such preparations for hygienic controls.

REFERENCES

Nitrosamines

1. Current Intelligence Bulletin: Nitrosamines in cutting fluids. U. S. Dept. of Health, Education, and Welfare, PHS, Center for Disease Control, National Institute for Occupational Safety and Health, Cincinnati, Ohio, October, 1976.
2. Decoufle, P.: Cancer mortality among workers exposed to cutting-oil mist, Ann. N.Y. Acad. Sci. 271:94, 1976.
3. Fan, T. Y., et al.:*N*-nitrosodiethanolamine in synthetic cutting fluids: A part-per-hundred impurity, Science 196:70, 1977.
4. Lijinsky, W.: Health problems associated with nitrites and nitrosamines. AMBIO, Royal Swedish Academy of Sciences/ Universtetsforlaget (Sweden), Vol. 5, pp. 67–72, 1976.
5. Pittelkow, R.: Occupational Dermatoses, in Zenz, C. (ed.), *Occupational Medicine: Principles and Practical Applications* (Chicago: Year Book Medical Publishers, 1975), pp. 191–230.
6. Zingmark, P-A., and Rappe, C.: On the formation of *N*-nitrosodiethanolamine from a grinding fluid under simulated gastric conditions. AMBIO, Royal Swedish Academy of Sciences/Universitetsforlaget (Sweden), Vol. 5, pp. 237–238, 1977.

Organotins

Organotins are defined as compounds having at least one covalent carbon-tin bond. The organotins are divided into 4 major groups, mono-, di-, tri- and tetraorganotins. Organotins, as a class, show widely varying chemical and physical properties. The chemical names for the organotin compounds often are long and cumbersome. Common names are available for only a few compounds and abbreviations for chemical names have been used in the NIOSH criteria document to refer to organotin compounds.[1] Since isomers differ in their toxicity, different isomeric forms of the compounds have also been identified by specific abbreviations. A few of the abbreviations are shown here; a more detailed list is found in the criteria document: MBTA (mono-*n*-butyltin acid), DBDA (dibutyltin diacetate), DBDC (dibutyltin dichloride), DMDC (dimethyltin dichloride), DOTO (di-*n*-octyltin oxide), TBTA (tribultyltin acetate), TBTB (tributyltin bromide), TBTL (tributyltin laurate), TETB (triethyltin bromide), TMTC (trimethyltin chloride), TPTF (triphenyltin fluoride), TeAT (tetraamyltin) and TeMT (tetramethyltin).

Commercially, organotin compounds are used in three major types of applications: as stabilizers in polymers, as biocides and as catalysts. As stabilizers, organotin compounds, particularly the dialkyltins, prevent degradation of halogen-containing polymers and polyamides and of such nonhalogenated products as lubricating oils, hydrogen peroxide and polyolefins and other plastics. The largest use of organotin stabilizers is in polyvinyl chloride (PVC), where the dibutyltin and dioctyltin derivatives are the most important. Diorganotin derivatives are used as heat stabilizers for plastics, as catalysts in the production of polyurethane foams and in the cold curing of silicone rubber, whereas triorganotin derivatives are used mainly in biocidal applications. As corrosion inhibitors in chlorinated heat-exchange fluids and as heat stabilizers in polyvinyl chloride, diorganotin additives act by binding hydrochloric acid formed by thermal decomposition. Diorganotins containing mercaptide ligands stabilize polymers by reacting with organic radicals formed during decomposition. Other diorganotins combine with labile chloro-groups and reactive double bonds, which increases the stabilities of polymeric chains. Trialkyltin derivatives are used as preservatives of polymeric chains. Trialkyltin derivatives are used as preservatives for wood, textile, paper, leather and glass and both trialkyl- and triaryltins are used as rodent repellents, molluscicides, fungicides and insecticides. In general, the triorganotins show greater toxicity than the diorganotins.

World production of organotin compounds has shown a sustained increase since the 1940s—in 1976, more than 25 million kg. Workers in manufacturing operations involving the various organotin formulations or as paint sprayers or PVC compounders represent occupational groups with the greatest potential for exposure; the NIOSH estimates that 30,000 employees in the United States may be exposed to organotin compounds.

The main route of entry is by inhalation and skin absorption. The *organic compounds of tin,* chiefly solids and liquids, cause irritation of the eyes, throat and skin; some produce cerebral edema whereas others cause hepatic necrosis. Oral administration of a preparation of organic tin containing diethyltin di-iodide and up to 10% triethyltin for treatment of human furunculosis resulted in 217 cases of poisoning, of which 100 were fatal. After a latent period of 4 days there was severe, persistent headache followed by vertigo, visual disturbances, including photophobia, abdominal pain, vomiting and urinary retention; the more severe cases showed transient or permanent paralysis and psychic disturbances. Residual symptoms in those who recovered included persistent headache, diminished visual acuity, partial paresis, focal anesthesia and, in 4 severe cases, flaccid paraplegia with incontinence. The most significant lesion found at autopsy was cerebral edema. Repeated oral administration to rats of 50 mg/kg of dibutyltin chloride resulted in inflammation of bile ducts and hepatic necrosis; repeated skin applications of 10 mg/kg caused severe local skin injury and bile duct damage. Triethyltin sulfate administered repeatedly to rats at 10 mg/kg caused tremors and paresis, which in some animals progressed to complete paralysis and death; it was equally toxic by mouth and by injection. In mice, tributyltin chloride had a marked hemolytic action whereas dibutyl and tributyl and tetrabutyl tin were less markedly hemolytic. Workers exposed to the vapor or fumes of butyltin compounds developed sore throat and cough several hours after exposure. Chemical burns from organic tin compounds may result from only brief contact with the skin; pain usually is moderate and itching is the chief symptom; healing usually is complete within 7–10 days. When a worker was splashed in the face with a tributyltin compound, lacrimation and severe conjunctivitis appeared within minutes, despite immediate lavage, and persisted for 4 days; at the end of 7 days, the eyes appeared normal.

Skin contact is to be prevented by work practices, engineering design and controls and the use of personal protective equipment.

There are no biologic tests to monitor human exposures.

TREATMENT.—Immediate removal from exposure; flush the eyes with water; wash the skin with soap or mild detergent and water. Recovery usually is complete. TLV:0.1 mg/m^3, measured as tin.

REFERENCE

Organotins

1. National Institute for Occupational Safety and Health, Criteria for a Recommended Standard . . . Occupational Exposure to Organotin Compounds. U.S. Dept. of Health, Education, and Welfare, PHS, Center for Disease Control, DHEW (NIOSH) Publication No. 77-115, Cincinnati, Ohio, November, 1976.

Oxides of Nitrogen (Nitrogen Dioxide and Nitric Oxide)

Nitrogen dioxide (NO_2) is one of several oxides of nitrogen. It is a reddish brown or dark orange gas; its dimer, nitrogen tetroxide (N_2O_4), is colorless. At temperatures between $-9.3°C$ and 135°C, nitrogen dioxide and nitrogen tetroxide coexist as a mixture of gases. Below $-9.3°C$, a colorless solid consisting of nitrogen tetroxide is formed whereas above 135°C, the gas consists mostly of nitrogen dioxide. In evaluations of occupational exposures to the mixtures of these two compounds, however, the results customarily are expressed in terms of nitrogen dioxide. The conversion of molecular nitrogen into nitrogenous compounds is known as fixation of nitrogen. In the upper atmosphere, this is brought about through photochemical processes in which nitrogen and oxygen atoms from dissociated molecules combine to form nitric oxide. At ground level, the combination of nitrogen and oxygen takes place thermally in flames, explosions and electric discharges.

Ultraviolet energy or sufficiently high temperatures to accomplish this in the occupational environment are encountered in electric or gas welding, in the combustion of fuels, for example, in furnaces or internal combustion engines, and in the detonation of explosives. Nitric oxide is also produced when nitrogen dioxide is dissolved in warm water. Both nitric oxide and nitrogen dioxide are formed when nitric acid reacts with reducing agents. For dilute nitric acid, the resultant mixture contains predominantly NO whereas for concentrated nitric acid more NO_2 is produced. However, nitric oxide and nitrogen dioxide rarely exist independently in the occupational environment.

Elkins[7] calculated that with a nitric oxide concentration of 200 ppm, nitrogen dioxide would be formed at a rate of about 11 ppm/minute. If the nitric oxide concentration were 100 ppm, the oxidation rate could drop to 2.8 ppm/minute whereas with 25 ppm of nitric oxide, it would take more than 5 minutes of 1 ppm of nitrogen dioxide to be formed. For this reason, both nitric oxide and nitrogen dioxide should be sampled simultaneously. The presence of other factors, such as moisture, metal fumes or ultraviolet radiation, may either accelerate or slow down the actual rate of oxidation of nitric oxide in air.[17] As a result, it is not practicable to estimate the concentration of one of the nitrogen oxides solely on the basis of a measurement of the other. Mixtures of the oxides of nitrogen are also produced in other ways, such as from the combustion of nitrogen-containing materials or from reactions of nitric acid with metals or organic matter. At the time of release, these mixtures may contain substantial percentages of nitrogen dioxide. Somewhat more nitrogen dioxide is to be expected where nitrogen-containing compounds are decomposed. Where nitric acid is a reactant in acid dipping, nitrogen dioxide will be the predominant oxide released.

SOURCES OF EXPOSURE.—Although nitric oxide is the oxide of nitrogen initially produced in the welding arc or flame, its con-

TABLE 14-7.—APPROXIMATE DISTRIBUTION OF NITROGEN OXIDES GENERATED FROM VARIOUS OPERATIONS*

SOURCE	NO_2 %	NO %
Carbon arc	9	91
Oxyacetylene torch	8	92
Cellulose nitrate combustion	19	81
Diesel exhaust	35	65
Dynamite blast	52	48
Acid dipping	78	22

*From NIOSH Criteria Document.[4]

centration in such operations is only rarely reported. In many field studies and controlled laboratory experiments, concentrations of nitric oxide have been reported as "nitrous gases" or "nitrogen oxides" whereas other field investigations and controlled studies have expressed concentrations of nitric oxide as "nitrogen dioxide." Differences in describing environmental levels, coupled with the variety of sampling and analytic methods used to assess the environments, virtually preclude direct comparison and interpretation between these studies. In a simulation of cutting torch operations causing toxicity, Norwood et al.[16] reported separate figures for concentrations of nitric oxide and nitrogen dioxide in 2 of 10 samples. This study showed nitrogen dioxide to be 13% of the total oxides found 15 minutes after cutting began. The nitrogen dioxide increased to 33% after an additional 25 minutes. Nitrogen dioxide is dissociated by ultraviolet radiation, producing nitric oxide plus oxygen atoms. The oxygen atoms, in turn, react with nitrogen dioxide at a very rapid rate, producing nitric oxide and oxygen molecules.[10] Thus, according to Silverman and Husain,[17] ultraviolet rays emitted in arc welding would counteract the oxidation of nitric oxide to nitrogen dioxide. On the other hand, ozone produced in the arc could oxidize nitric oxide to nitrogen dioxide or to even higher oxides, such as nitrogen pentoxide. They also pointed out that iron and moisture present could have a converse influence, reducing nitrogen dioxide to nitric oxide and possibly to ammonia or nitrogen. In addition, freshly formed iron fumes may react with nitrogen oxides to produce particulate nitrites and nitrates, with a consequent reduction in the amount of gaseous oxides present.[17] In their own welding experiments, conducted in a test chamber, Silverman and Husain[17] found that approximately equal concentrations of nitric oxide and nitrogen dioxide totaling approximately 30 ppm showed no appreciable changes in the ratio of the gases after a period of 2–3 hours.

In general, it has been found that hot metals decompose nitric oxide, forming the metal oxide and nitrogen.[17] This may explain the higher rate of formation of oxides of nitrogen when an oxyacetylene flame does not touch metal.[16, 18] Norwood et al.[16] found that as much as 250 ppm of nitrogen oxides were formed where the flame was not in contact with metal and only 47 and 71 ppm in tests where stainless steel was being melted. Similarly, Steel and Sanderson[18] reported that the concentrations of nitrogen dioxide produced by flame alone were several times greater than the concentrations observed when metals were being flame-cut. Another example[1] of occupational hazard concerns exposure to exhaust gases from ice-resurfacing machines in ice arenas. Such exposures made the machine operators, as well as arena patrons, ill on a number of occasions. Investigations of 45 ice arenas in Minnesota showed nitrogen oxides concentrations (reported as nitrogen dioxide) as high as 40 ppm. However, concentrations of carbon monoxide were elevated, suggesting that nitrogen oxides were not the only cause of adverse effects. Since the form of nitrogen emitted from internal combustion engines exists largely as nitric oxide at the time of discharge, workers employed in automobile parking or repair garages may have occupational exposures. The production of nitric oxide by the catalytic oxidation of ammonia is the first step in the manufacture of nitric acid. Kennedy[12] reported that underground blasting operations with both nitroexplosives and gunpowder produce levels of the oxides of nitrogen up to 88 ppm after normal firing of a commonly used blasting explosive and up to 167 ppm after "misfires" (incomplete detonation). Conventional powder shots may cause momentary concentrations of up to 56 ppm and concentrations as high as 150 ppm after multiple firings. Commins et al.[3] noted that concentrations of nitric oxide and nitrogen dioxide reaching several hundred ppm were produced in a freshly filled agricultural silo during various stages of the decomposition process. The maximal concentrations of nitric oxide and nitrogen dioxide were found on the fifth day after loading the silo. At that time, a distinct layer of brown gas was observed at the center of the silo. In general, concentrations decreased with increased height above the surface of the silage. Measurements were also made before and after operation of the silo-filling blower. Use of the blower did reduce the levels of nitric oxide and nitrogen dioxide; however, high concentrations of these gases still remained near the surface of the silage. It is difficult to estimate how many people are exposed to oxides of nitrogen, since hazardous occupations also involve all workers located in the vicinity of operations or processes having conditions conducive to the generation of nitrogen oxidation, i.e., furnaces, boilers, welding, internal combustion engines and nitrogen oxides produced from numerous chemical processes. The difficulty in delineating the incidence of exposure has been shown by Storlazzi[19] in a study of welding and burning operations in U.S. naval shipyards. Although only 6000 workers were directly engaged in such activities, approximately 60,000 workers were indirectly exposed to the by-products of these operations. The NIOSH estimates that 1,500,000 workers are potentially exposed to the oxides of nitrogen. In view of the factors mentioned, this figure is low.[4] An estimated[15] 300,000 tons of nitrogen oxides are produced annually from industrial processes and 10 million tons result from fuel combustion. These are rough estimates at best and do not distinguish between the various nitrogen oxides. From the many cases found in the medical literature, it is known that serious, even lethal, concentrations of nitrogen oxides may be encountered. Similar serious consequences have been reported from chemical processes.[2, 5, 6, 11, 20]

Cases of marked illness from NO_2 have been from accidental exposures to arc or gas welding (in confined spaces), in unventilated farm silos, following explosions, using nitrogen-containing explosives and with the use of nitric acid. Nitrogen dioxide gas is a respiratory irritant; it causes pulmonary edema and rarely, among survivors, bronchiolitis obliterans. Brief exposure of humans to concentrations of about 250 ppm causes cough, production of mucoid or frothy sputum and increasing dyspnea. Within 1–2 hours, the person may develop pulmonary edema with tachypnea, cyanosis, fine crackles and wheezes throughout the lungs and tachycardia. Alternatively, there may be only increasing dyspnea and cough for several hours; the symptoms then gradually subside over a 2–3-week period. The condition then may enter a second stage of abruptly increasing severity; fever and chills precede a relapse, with increasing dyspnea, cyanosis and recurring pulmonary edema. Death may occur in either the initial or second stage of the disease; a severe second stage may follow a relatively mild initial stage. The subject who survives the second stage usually recovers over 2–3 weeks; however, some do not return to normal but experience varying degrees of impaired pulmonary function. The radiographic features in the acute initial stage vary from normal to those of typical pulmonary edema; most reports mention a pattern of nodular shadows on the chest film at the outset. The roentgenogram then may clear, only to show miliary mottling as the second stage commences, progressing to the development of a confluent pattern. Results of pulmonary function tests in the acute stage show reduction in lung volume and diffusing capacity; similar findings are recorded in the volume and diffusing capacity. The same findings are recorded in the second stage. Pathologic examination of the acute lesion shows extensive mucosal edema and inflammatory cell exudation. The delayed lesion shows the histologic appearance of bronchiolitis obliterans; small bronchi and bronchioles contain an inflammatory exudate that tends to undergo fibrinous organization, finally obliterating the lumen.[4, 13] The effects expected in humans from exposure to nitrogen dioxide for 60 minutes are: 100 ppm, pulmonary edema and death; 50 ppm, pulmonary edema with possible subacute or chronic lesions in the lungs; 25 ppm, respiratory irritation and chest pain. A concentration of 50 ppm is moderately irritating to the eyes and nose; 25 ppm is irritating to some persons.

Exposure causes cough, mucoid or frothy sputum production, increasing dyspnea, chest pain, signs and symptoms of pulmonary edema with cyanosis, tachypnea, tachycardia and eye irritation. Consideration should be given to hospitalization and observation for the possible delayed onset of pulmonary edema and to treatment with corticosteroids if pulmonary edema occurs.

Occupational exposure to nitrogen dioxide (NO_2) shall be controlled so that workers are not exposed to nitrogen dioxide at greater than a ceiling concentration of 1 ppm by volume (1.8 mg/m^3) as determined by a sampling time of 15 minutes. Nitric oxide (NO) causes narcosis in animals. Exposure of mice to 2500 ppm for 6 or 7 minutes caused narcosis, and death occurred within 12 minutes. Some early reports attributed the toxicity of nitric oxide to the formation of methemoglobin; however, more recent studies indicate that nitric oxide reacts in vitro with normal (ferrous) hemoglobin but, in exposed animals, this interaction does not occur and no methemoglobin is formed. Nitric oxide is converted spontaneously in air to nitrogen dioxide; hence, some of the latter gas invariably is present whenever nitric oxide is found in the air. At concentrations below 50 ppm, however, this reaction is slow, and frequently substantial concentrations of nitric oxide may occur with negligible quantities of nitrogen dioxide. Nitrogen dioxide causes delayed pulmonary edema.

REFERENCES

Oxides of Nitrogen

1. Anderson, D. E.: Problems created for ice arenas by engine exhaust, Am. Ind. Hyg. Assoc. J. 32:790, 1971.
2. Charleroy, D. K.: Nitrous and nitric gas casualties, U.S. Naval Med. Bull. 44:435, 1945.
3. Commins, B. T., Raveney, F. J., and Jesson, M. W.: Toxic gases in tower silos, Ann. Occup. Hyg. 14:275, 1971.
4. Criteria for a Recommended Standard . . . . Occupational Exposure to Oxides of Nitrogen (Nitrogen Dioxide and Nitric Oxide). U.S. Dept. of Health, Education, and Welfare, PHS, Center for Disease Control, National Institute for Occupational Safety and Health, HEW (NIOSH) Publication No. 76-149, Cincinnati, Ohio, March, 1976.
5. Darke, C. S., and Warrack, A. J. N.: Bronchiolitis from nitrous fumes, Thorax 13:327, 1958.
6. Desgranges, J. B.: Observation and comments on a sudden death caused by nitrous gas, J. Med. Chir. Pharm. 8:487, 1804 (French).
7. Elkins, H. B.: Nitrogen dioxide. Rate of oxidation of nitric oxide and its bearing on the nitrogen dioxide content of electric arc fumes, J. Ind. Hyg. Toxicol. 28:37, 1946.
8. Gleason, M. N., et al.: *Clinical Toxicology of Commercial Products* (4th ed.; Baltimore: Williams & Wilkins, 1976), Section III, pp. 175–180.

9. Gray, E. L.: Oxides of nitrogen: Their occurrence, toxicity hazard, A.M.A. Arch. Ind. Hyg. 19:479, 1959.
10. Harris, L., and Siegel, B. M.: Reactions of nitrogen dioxide with other gases, J. Am. Chem. Soc. 63:2520, 1941.
11. Hortsch, W.: Nitric oxide poisoning with motor hemiparalysis, Arch. Gewerbepathol. Gewerbehyg. 11:402, 1942 (German).
12. Kennedy, M. C. S.: Nitrous fumes and coalminers with emphysema, Ann. Occup. Hyg. 15:285, 1972.
13. Levy, S. A.: Occupational Pulmonary Diseases, in Zenz, C. (ed.), *Occupational Medicine: Principles and Practical Applications* (Chicago: Year Book Medical Publishers, Inc., 1975), pp. 117–155.
14. Miles, F. D.: *Nitric Acid Manufacture and Uses* (London: Oxford University Press, 1961), pp. 1–8.
15. Nationwide Inventory of Air Pollutant Emissions 1978, NAPCA Publication No. AP-73. Raleigh, N.C., National Air Pollution Control Administration, pp. 14–16, 1970.
16. Norwood, W. D., et al.: Nitrogen dioxide poisoning due to metal-cutting with oxyacetylene torch, J. Occup. Med. 8:301, 1966.
17. Silverman, L., and Husain, S. I.: A study of nitrogen oxide concentrations during arc, Arch. Ind. Hyg. Occup. Med. 3:135, 1951.
18. Steel, J., and Sanderson, J. T.: The thermal degradation of protective coating. A basic study. Part I. Zinc-rich epoxy primers, Am. Ind. Hyg. Assoc. J. 26:449, 1965.
19. Storlazzi, I. D.: Hygiene of welding in U.S. naval shipyards, Arch. Ind. Health 19:307, 1959.
20. Zadek, J.: Mass poisoning by the inhalation of nitrous fumes (nitrite intoxications), Berl. Klin. Wochenschr. 53:246, 1916 (German).

Ozone

O_3

This highly reactive gas can form during inert gas-shielded arc welding; it is formed in and around electrical equipment at high voltages, especially during pulse testing of motors, generators and other devices (usually above 600 volts); it is found in air- and water-purifying devices and infrequently with certain copy and reproductive devices using powerful ultraviolet light sources.

Airline flight attendants on trans-Pacific flights reported an increased incidence of respiratory symptoms, attributed to high-altitude ozone exposure. An epidemiologic survey of flight attendants on 3 airlines with differing potential for ozone exposure was evaluated by Ostrov.[5] They were (1) an international carrier ("high exposure"), (2) a mixed domestic/foreign carrier ("intermediate exposure") and (3) a domestic carrier ("low exposure"). Respiratory questionnaires and flight diaries were completed by 1330 flight attendants on the 3 airlines. For symptoms that had been preclassified as ozone-related—chest pain, dyspnea, persistent cough, sore throat and nosebleeds—a gradient in age-adjusted incidence with that airline was noted. A gradient was not evident for 12 nonspecific symptoms considered unrelated to ozone. Flight diaries for 5008 flight days showed that the incidence of ozone-related symptoms increased with duration and altitude of flights, two indirect measures of ozone exposure. Although lacking environmental ozone data, these results suggest that ozone exposure is an occupational hazard for flight attendants and that more efficient in-flight air-treatment systems must be installed on high-altitude aircraft.

Typically irritated are mucous membranes, especially the eyes, nose and throat and the lungs. The characteristic odor is readily detectable at low concentrations (0.01–0.05 ppm). Ozone produces local irritation of the eyes and mucous membranes. At low levels, a disagreeable irritation and dryness of the eyes, mouth and throat occurs at concentrations of 0.05–0.1 ppm for 10–30 minutes. At high levels, marked eye irritation, cough, a choking sensation with substernal pain and dyspnea develop. Pulmonary edema can occur and, within several hours, signs of bronchopneumonia. Lung function can be impaired up to 24 hours following exposure to 0.6–0.8 ppm for 2 hours.[2,4] If substantial exposure has occurred or is suspected, hospitalization is advisable because of delayed-onset pulmonary edema.

The 1979 TLV: 0.1 ppm, a level thought to prevent radiomimetic effects.[1]

REFERENCES

Ozone

1. American Conference of Governmental Industrial Hygienists: Documentation of the TLVs for Substances in Workroom Air, 3d ed., pp. 194–195, Cincinnati, Ohio, 1976.
2. Committee on Medical and Biologic Effects of Environmental Pollutants: Ozone and other photochemical oxidants, pp. 402–415, Washington, D.C., National Academy of Sciences, 1977.
3. Jaffe, L. S.: Photochemical air pollutants and their effects on men and animals. II. Adverse effects, Arch. Environ. Health 16:241, 1968.
4. Nasr, A. N. M.: Ozone poisoning in man: Clinical manifestations and differential diagnosis—a review, Clin. Toxicol. 4:461, 1971.
5. Ostrov, P.: Ozone exposure in airline flight attendants, Epidemiology and Intelligence Service Bulletin, C.D.C., Atlanta, Georgia, 1979.
6. Tabershaw, I. R., Ottoboni, F., and Cooper, W. C.: Oxidants: Air quality criteria based on health effects, J. Occup. Med. 10:464, 1968.

Selected Petroleum-Derived Solvents

Almost all occupational health specialists have been confronted with workers who have had some contact or exposure to Stoddard solvent, mineral spirits, petroleum ether, kerosene, rubber solvent, varnish makers' and painters' naphtha and benzene. These chemicals are used in enormous quantities in virtually all industries.

Occupations with potential exposure to these refined petroleum solvents are adhesive makers, ammonia synthesis workers, asphalt coating workers, ceramic production workers, degreasers (metal), detergent makers, dry cleaners, enamel makers (synthetic), farmers, fat and oil processors, fungicide handlers, garage workers, heating fuel handlers, herbicide handlers, hydrogen manufacturing workers, ink production workers, insecticide handlers, jet fuel handlers and makers, kerosene handlers, laboratory workers (chemical), lacquerers, leather japanners, metal cleaners, naphtha workers, oil processors, painters, paint makers, perfume extraction workers, petrochemical workers, petroleum refinery workers, photographic chemical makers, printers, resin makers, rocket fuel handlers and makers, rubber coaters and makers, stainers, stain makers, typesetters, varnish makers, wax makers, wood preservation makers and wool process workers.

Eyes, nose and throat irritation, dermatitis and effects on the nervous system have been found in workers exposed to some refined petroleum solvents.

BENZENE

Benzene is derived primarily through the refinement and fractionation of crude petroleum, has a boiling point of 80.1° C (176° F) at 760 mm Hg and may be a contaminant of some refined petroleum solvents, especially if the solvent has a boiling range near or encompassing the boiling point of benzene. The extent of this contamination will also vary, depending on the inherent chemical composition of the crude oil and the method of distillation in the refinery. It has been shown that the vapor pressure of benzene in mixtures deviates from Raoult's law and, therefore, the benzene vapor concentration resulting from handling such mixtures frequently will be higher than would be expected from the composition of the solvent. If the benzene content of a solvent ranged from 1% to 4% in volume, ordinary use of the solvent would not produce benzene vapor hazards, but if the concentration of benzene were greater than 5%, the possibility of "substantial" exposure to benzene vapors resulting from "free" use of the solvent must be considered.

Benzene has been recognized as causing serious deleterious effects such as blood dyscrasias in humans and experimental animals, and, in 1974, the NIOSH issued criteria and recommendations for occupational exposure to this compound. Acute poisoning by benzene results primarily from its narcotic action. The inhalation of a high concentration of benzene (i.e., 3000 ppm for 0.1–1 hour) may cause a state of excitation and euphoria (benzol jag), followed by drowsiness, fatigue, vertigo, nausea and vomiting. With higher concentrations (i.e., 7500 ppm for 0.5–1 hour) or longer exposure times, convulsions followed by paralysis, loss of consciousness and death from respiratory failure may result. The inhalation of small amounts of benzene over long periods has caused blood dyscrasias, including aplastic anemia, leukopenia and thrombocytopenia. Additional signs and symptoms of chronic toxicity may include headache, dizziness, fatigue, loss of appetite, irritability, nervousness and nosebleed and other hemorrhagic manifestations. In 1976, the NIOSH issued an *Update Criteria and Recommendations for a Revised Benzene Standard* and recognized that there now was sufficient evidence to conclude that benzene is leukemogenic. Since benzene causes progressive, malignant diseases of the hematopoietic system, the NIOSH recommended that, for regulatory purposes, benzene should be considered carcinogenic in man and also recommended that the use of benzene as a solvent or diluent in open operations should be prohibited. The NIOSH recommended that occupational exposure be controlled so that no worker will be exposed to benzene in excess of 3.2 mg/m^3 (1 ppm) in air as determined by an air sample collected at 1 liter/minute for 2 hours.

As a consequence of the toxicity and carcinogenic potential of benzene, the benzene content of a solvent should be determined, and, if it is found to be present, air monitoring should be instituted to ensure compliance with the federal standard.[52]

STODDARD SOLVENT

Stoddard solvent is a mixture of hydrocarbons, predominantly C9 to C11, that has a boiling range between 160° and 210° C (320–410° F). Chemically, Stoddard solvent is a mixture of 30–50% straight and branched chain paraffins, 30–40% naphthenes and 10–20% aromatic hydrocarbons. Although Stoddard solvent and mineral spirits are not always considered the same petroleum products and are used differently for different purposes in industry, their boiling ranges (Stoddard solvent, 160–210° C; mineral spirits, 150–200° C) are almost identical and, therefore, their chemical compositions are similar. In fact, many investigators use the terms mineral spirits and Stoddard solvent interchangeably, and some consider Stoddard solvent to be a specific type of mineral spirits. Currently there are four classes of Stoddard solvent: regular Stoddard solvent, 140 flash solvent, odorless solvent and low end point solvent. Stoddard solvent, used primarily as a dry cleaning agent, can be produced from a straight-run distillate of paraffinic or mixed base crude. It was reported in 1964 that U.S. industry used 700 million liters of Stoddard solvent. Four liters of Stoddard solvent will clean about 12–16 kg of clothes. It was estimated in 1964 that 55% of the volume of dry cleaning in the United States is carried out in Stoddard solvent. The NIOSH estimates that 75,000 workers in the United States are potentially exposed to Stoddard solvent.

Braunstein[3] reported follicular dermatitis on the hands and arms of a worker after 2 weeks of dermal exposure to liquid Stoddard solvent. This worker also complained of nausea when initially inhaling the solvent. Eventually, he developed obstructive jaundice and subacute yellow atrophy of the liver.

Scott et al.[41] observed 4 cases and Prager and Peters[37] 1 case of aplastic anemia after dermal exposure to liquid Stoddard solvent.

In 1974, Markel and Shmunes[30] cited the results of a Stoddard solvent hazard evaluation of a greeting card company. Workers were exposed to Stoddard solvent at 99–1906 mg/m^3 (average 438 mg/m^3) in their working environment and the authors concluded that, under the conditions found at the time of the survey, Stoddard solvent was not toxic and did not constitute a hazard to health.

In 1974, Larsen and Shmunes[25] found that Stoddard solvent used to clean polishing machines probably was the cause of dermatitis in several industrial workers. These workers also complained of headache and eye and nose irritation. Although Stoddard solvent concentrations of less than 20 ppm (115 mg/m^3) were detected, the authors believed that higher concentrations could have occurred immediately after the polishing machines were cleaned with Stoddard solvent and could have been the cause of the headache and eye and throat irritation.

Carpenter et al.[5] determined both the odor and the sensory thresholds for Stoddard solvent. The odor threshold was found to be between 0.5 and 5 mg/m^3 (0.09 and 0.9 ppm). The sensory threshold was found to be between 850 and 2700 mg/m^3 (150 and 470 ppm) for a 15-minute exposure. No irritation was noted at 140 mg/m^3 (24 ppm) whereas slight, transient eye irritation occurred in 1 volunteer at 850 mg/m^3 and in all at 2700 mg/m^3, some with tearing. Slight dizziness also was reported at 2700 mg/m^3 by some of the subjects. The volunteers experienced olfactory fatigue at all of the concentrations tested, but recovered fully within 10 minutes after exposure ended.

Nelson et al.[34] similarly observed that volunteers exposed to Stoddard solvent for 3–5 minutes at air concentrations in excess of 400 ppm (2290 mg/m^3) suffered irritation of the eyes, nose and throat.

Carpenter et al.[7] described odor threshold sensory irritation in humans exposed to 140 flash aliphatic solvent. The odor threshold was about 4 mg/m^3 (0.6 ppm). Minor eye irritation was the only discomfort noted by subjects exposed to 140 flash aliphatic solvent at either 110 or 310 mg/m^3 (17 or 47 ppm) for 15 minutes. This response was expressed by the same subjects during each inhalation period and did not persist after exposure. All subjects reported olfactory fatigue at both concentrations. The subjects believed that 310 mg/m^3 (49 ppm) could be an acceptable concentration for an 8-hour day.

As mentioned below in the discussion of mineral spirits, dermal exposure to Stoddard solvent has been associated with several cases of aplastic anemia[37, 41] but, from present knowledge concerning benzene-free solvents, this seems unlikely to occur. But the benzene content of Stoddard solvents should be evaluated to ensure that the federal exposure limit for benzene is not exceeded.

MINERAL SPIRITS

Mineral spirits are a mixture of hydrocarbons that have a boiling range of 150–200° C (302–392° F). These compounds have also been termed white spirits, petroleum spirits and light petrol. As mentioned above, Stoddard solvent is considered by some investigators to be synonymous with mineral spirits. Mineral spirits are clear, colorless liquids with a "pleasant sweetish odor" and contain about 30–65% paraffins, 15–55% naphthenes and 10–30% aromatic hydrocarbons. Mineral spirits are used as a general-purpose thinner, a solvent for paint and varnish industries and a dry cleaning agent. The NIOSH estimates that 61,000 workers in the United States are potentially exposed to mineral spirits.

In 1975, Åstrand et al.[2] reported on the effects of white spirits (mineral spirits) on human alveolar air and blood solvent concentrations during rest and exercise. The white spirits used in the study consisted of 83% aliphatic and 17% aromatic compounds. In the initial trials, men were exposed at 2500 or 5000 mg/m^3 for an unspecified period. Nausea and vertigo were apparent at both concentrations. No differences were noted in heart rate, alveolar ventilation or oxygen uptake either at rest or during exercise at an intensity of 50 watts during exposure at 1250 and 2500 mg/m^3 of white spirits. In addition, their studies[2] indicated that more solvent reaches the blood during exercise than during rest. This finding, in the absence of changes in alveolar ventilation, suggests changes in the respiratory transport.

In 1975, Gamberale et al.[14] reported the effects of exposure to white spirits (mineral spirits) on humans. Performance tests were conducted in perceptual speed, reaction time, short-term memory, numerical ability and manual dexterity. Men exposed to white spirits at 625, 1250, 1875 and 2500 mg/m^3 for 4 continuous 30-minute periods showed no impairment in the 5 performance tests. Exposure to 4000 mg/m^3 of white spirits for 50 minutes had no effect on perceptual speed, numerical ability and manual dexterity. There was, however, a definite prolongation of reaction time and a possible impairment of short-term memory as a result of exposure at 4000 mg/m^3. The authors concluded that there was a risk of subjective distress and adverse effects on psychomotor and intellectual functions in a worker exposed at 2500 mg/m^3 who is doing light industrial work, since the alveolar air concentrations of white spirits in workers at rest exposed at 4000 mg/m^3 were similar to the white spirits alveolar air concentrations of workers exposed at 2500 mg/m^3 engaged in light physical activity.[2,14]

Since the composition of mineral spirits and Stoddard solvents is similar, it is recommended that dermal exposure to mineral spirits be avoided. The benzene content of mineral spirits should be evaluated to ensure that the federal exposure limit for benzene is not exceeded.

PETROLEUM ETHER

Petroleum ether is a mixture of volatile aliphatic hydrocarbons with a boiling range of about 30–60° C (86–104° F). Petroleum ether sometimes is referred to as benzin, benzine, petroleum benzin, canadol, light ligroin and "Skellysolve." Reference sometimes is made to high-boiling petroleum ether; this terminology is essentially synonymous with ligroin or varnish makers' and painters' naphtha.

Physically, petroleum ether is a clear, colorless, nonfluorescent, volatile liquid. It has a characteristic odor and is highly flammable. Chemically, petroleum ether consists primarily of pentane and isohexane. It typically contains no aromatics. It is a low-boiling fraction obtained from the fractional distillation of petroleum. Petroleum ether is used as a solvent for oils, fats and waxes; a detergent; a fuel; in paints and varnishes; an insecticide; and in photography.

In 1970, Spruit et al.[42] reported that dermal exposure to petroleum ether caused disruption of the horny layer of the skin in humans. The average time of exposure before the appearance of irritation was about 20 minutes. No other reports have been found concerning the dermal toxicity of petroleum ether, but Oettel[36] conducted a study using pentane and hexane, the major constituents of petroleum ether, to evaluate the toxicity of these compounds and reported in 1936 that dermal exposure to pentane or hexane for up to 1 hour resulted in the development of irritation in humans characterized by erythema, hyperemia, swelling and pigmentation. After 5 hours of exposure, these alkanes produced skin blisters.

Several studies have related industrial exposure to hexane with the development of polyneuropathy.[20, 45, 50, 51] In 1969, Yamamura[51] reported the effects on workers after exposure to hexane, a constituent of the glue used in the production of sandals. The concentration of hexane in the air ranged from 1759 to 8793 mg/m^3. The initial symptoms included sensory impairment in the distal portion of the extremities. Inoue et al.,[22] in a follow-up study on the sandal workers, indicated that polyneuropathy could have developed as a result of exposure at concentrations of *n*-hexane below 1759 mg/m^3. In 1971, Herskowitz et al.[20] examined employees working in a furniture factory who were exposed to *n*-hexane. Air samples of hexane were found to average 2286 mg/m^3 and peaked at 4573 mg/m^3. The patients complained of one or more of the following symptoms: abdominal cramps, burning sensations, numbness and weakness of the distal extremities and paresthesia. In 1972, Yamada[50] investigated 17 workers reporting symptoms of intoxication from exposure to hexane vapor. Six were employed by a pharmaceutical company and used a 95% hexane solution to remove oil from the surface of tablets. The airborne hexane concentration in the center of the workroom was 1759 mg/m^3, but, in the immediate work area, the concentration was 3517 mg/m^3. The initial worker complaints were fatigue and loss of appetite, followed by paresthesia in distal parts of the extremities and difficulty in walking. In 1975, Takeuchi et al.[45] reported on 4 persons exposed to petroleum benzine who worked in a brocade sash cleaning shop in a poorly ventilated workroom. In general, within 1–9 months, the workers experienced fatigue, loss of appetite, difficulties in walking, muscle weakness, paresthesia, irritability, insomnia and weight loss. Although determination of the air concentrations of petroleum benzine was not made at the time the workers developed their illness, analysis of the concentrations of petroleum benzine and its major constituents in the workroom air was made subsequently. The concentration of petroleum benzine and *n*-hexane did not exceed 4400 and 844 mg/m^3, respectively. The authors indicated that if the concentration of petroleum benzine rose higher than 4400 mg/m^3, irritation of mucous membranes would have become unbearable and a narcotic effect would have occurred. The effects of dermal exposure were not measured, but such a route could not be disregarded as a potential mode of intoxication. In all the above cases, the authors[20, 22, 40, 50, 51] concluded that the workers had signs and symptoms of polyneuropathy. Gaultier et al.[15] stated that alkanes other than *n*-hexane may also cause polyneuropathy.

In 1967, Miyagaki[32] reported the neurotoxic effects of *n*-hexane exposure in mice. The animals exposed at *n*-hexane concentrations greater than 879 mg/m^3 for 24 hours per day, 6 days per week for 1 year developed signs of neurotoxicity whereas mice similarly exposed at 352 mg/m^3 of hexane showed no abnormalities.

Truhaut et al.[47] exposed rats to a technical grade of hexane at a concentration of 2000 ppm, 5 hours per day, 5 days per week for 1–6 months. The hexane contained 0.3% *n*-pentane, 25.1% 2-methylpentane plus cyclopentane, 18.4% 3-methylpentane, 48.8% *n*-hexane, 8% methylcyclopentane, 1.2% methylhexane and 1.2% benzene. Studies on the sciatic and saphenous nerves indicated that this solvent caused a decrease in the conduction rate, an increase in the refractory period and a decrease in the excitability of the nerves.

The TWA concentration limit for all C5–C8 alkanes recommended by the NIOSH is 350 mg/m^3; the NIOSH also recommends that a TWA concentration for petroleum ether, a mixture of 80% *n*-pentane and 20% isohexane, be set at 350 mg/m^3.

This recommended standard assumes additive toxic effects between hexane and pentane, which is a premise consistent with data and analysis presented in the NIOSH criteria document on alkanes.[11]

KEROSENE

Kerosene is a mixture of petroleum hydrocarbons, with carbon chain lengths that range from C9 to C16 carbon atoms per molecule, and distills between 175° and 325° C (347–617° F). Synonyms for kerosene include astral oil, coal oil and No. 1 fuel oil. Physically, kerosene usually is a pale yellow or water-white, mobile, low volatile, oily liquid that has a flashpoint (closed cup) of about 38–74° C (100–165° F) and therefore is considered a combustible compound. The composition of kerosene varies depending on the source of crude oil and the method of refining. Kerosene is a complex mixture of aliphatic, naphthenic and alkylated aromatic hydrocarbons. A typical analysis of kerosene indicates that there are about 25% normal paraffins, 12% branched paraffins, 30% monocycloparaffins, 12% dicycloparaffins, 1% tricycloparaffins, 16% mononuclear aromatics and 5% dinuclear aromatics. The aromatic content of kerosene ranges from 5% to 20%. The predominant aromatic molecular types include indenes, diphenyls, methylnaphthalenes and tetralins. Additional chemical and physical properties of kerosene are given in the NIOSH criteria document.[12]

Kerosene can be produced in a refinery using a straight-run-treated distillate from paraffinic or mixed crude, a solvent-treated distillate from paraffinic or mixed crude or a solvent-treated distillate from aromatic crude. Deodorized kerosene (washed with fuming sulfuric acid, followed by a sodium plumbite solution and sulfur) is a highly refined product of low aromatic content, often used in insect sprays.

Kerosene is used as a fuel, as a carrier for pesticides, as a weed-killer, as a mold-release agent in the ceramic and pottery industry, as a cleaning solvent and in asphalt coatings, enamels, paints, thinners and varnishes. In 1975, the United States produced 55,673,000 barrels of kerosene. The NIOSH estimates that 310,000 workers in the United States are potentially exposed to kerosene.

Several investigators have shown that kerosene can cause dermatitis.[13, 40, 44] In addition, several studies have examined the mechanism of action of the kerosene-induced skin irritation.[26, 28, 29]

In 1955, Johnson[23] investigated a presumable sensitivity of a person to kerosene. The patient developed hypoplastic anemia with a deficiency of all cell elements and hypoplastic marrow after recurrent exposure to kerosene for a 3-year period. The author suggested, however, that aromatic hydrocarbons of the benzol series present in kerosene may have been responsible for the myelotoxicity in this individual.

Hiebel et al.[21] observed bone marrow depression after dermal exposure to kerosene in 1 patient and by a combination of dermal and oral routes in 2 patients.

In 1946, Carpenter and Smyth[9] related that the application of 0.5 ml of deodorized kerosene into the eye of rabbits produced no adverse effects. However, Volkova et al.[48] found that animals exposed to unpurified kerosene in an aerosol developed conjunctivitis.

In 1969, Volkova et al.[48] noted that aerosols of purified kerosene were less toxic than aerosols of unpurified kerosene. Exposure to unpurified kerosene at 500 mg/m^3 caused respiratory irritation and leukocytosis.

In 1976, Carpenter et al.[8] determined the odor and sensory thresholds for deodorized kerosene determined in a group of volunteers. The odor threshold was approximately 0.6 mg/m^3 (0.09 ppm). Fifteen-minute exposures to kerosene at a mean measured vapor concentration of 140 mg/m^3 (20 ppm) were easily tolerated without sensory irritation. A slight decrease in olfactory acuity, but not total fatigue, was noted in 2 subjects. The 140 mg/m^3 concentration of deodorized kerosene was deemed by the subjects to be acceptable for an 8-hour workday, based on the 15-minute exposure.

Light petroleum hydrocarbons, such as kerosene, have a low toxicity when ingested and retained in the stomach, but if the solvent is aspirated directly into the lungs, extensive lung damage and death can occur.[18] Several investigators[17, 18, 40, 43] have reported that 0.1–0.2 ml of kerosene administered into the trachea can cause death. In addition, there are numerous cases of kerosene poisoning in humans by aspiration or ingestion of the liquid.[31, 35, 36] There is no present reason for suggesting that these solvents, if they are free from carcinogenic aromatics such as benzene, would cause cancer, birth defects or germinal mutations.

Kerosene has been shown to cause skin irritation[8, 13, 24, 29, 44] and possibly bone marrow depression,[10, 21, 23] probably from benzene absorption,[10, 23] after dermal exposure. Therefore, when this substance is used, care must be taken to prevent dermal exposure. Thirty minutes of dermal kerosene exposure has caused changes in skin structure.[29] The skin has developed a burning sensation during the first hour of kerosene exposure, erythema by the second hour and blister formation by the twelfth hour.[27] A solution of 40% kerosene has been shown to be innocuous to the human skin, but 55%, 70% and 85% kerosene solutions caused dermatitis in 24%, 85% and 100% of volunteers, respectively.[44] Naphthenic-type kerosene has a greater skin-irritating potential than paraffinic-type kerosene.[24] Kerosene has also been shown to augment the toxicity of a skin-sensitizing agent.[38] Thus, it is possible that other sensitizing agents that may come into contact with the worker's skin may heighten the response to dermal kerosene exposure. Kerosene never should be ingested, since, in addition to its oral toxicity,[33] aspiration can occur and result in pneumonitis and possibly death.[1, 16, 17, 19, 46, 49] The benzene content of the kerosene also should be evaluated to ensure that federal exposure limits are not exceeded.

VARNISH MAKERS' AND PAINTERS' NAPHTHA

Varnish makers' and painters' (VM and P) naphtha is a mixture of hydrocarbons that has a boiling range of approximately 95–160° C (203–320° F). Sometimes it is known as benzine, Naphtha 76, ligroin or high-boiling petroleum ether. Physically, VM and P naphtha is a colorless to yellow liquid that has an aromatic odor and it is composed of about 45–60% paraffins, 30–45% naphthenes and 5–13% aromatics. A sample of VM and P naphtha showed 55% paraffins, 30% monocycloparaffins, 2% dicycloparaffins and 12% alkylbenzenes. It is used as a quick-evaporating paint thinner of moderate solvent power. The NIOSH estimates that about 600,000 workers in the United States are potentially exposed to all "specialized" naphthas.

Carpenter et al.[4] reported the effects of exposure to VM and P naphtha on human odor and sensory responses. The authors concluded that the odor threshold was about 5 mg/m^3 (0.86 ppm). In assessing the sensory responses to VM and P naphtha, Carpenter et al. subjected volunteers to 15-minute exposures to the naphtha at concentrations ranging from 660 to 4100 mg/m^3 (140–880 ppm). Olfactory fatigue was noted at all concentrations. Solvent concentrations up to 2100 mg/m^3 (450 ppm) caused only slight or transitory eye and throat irritation in 2 of 7 subjects, which the authors considered "sporadic sensory responses." At the highest concentration tested, 4100 mg/m^3 (880 ppm), definite throat and eye irritation was produced.

Since C5–C8 alkanes, Stoddard solvent and mineral spirits are primary irritants,[3, 11, 25] VM and P naphtha, whose boiling range overlaps the ranges of these solvents, has solvent properties similar to these other solvents. VM and P naphtha is, accordingly, also considered to be a dermal irritant. Thus, contact of the skin as well as the eyes should be avoided. The benzene content of VM and P naphtha should be evaluated to ensure that federal exposure limits are not exceeded.

RUBBER SOLVENT

Rubber solvent is a mixture of hydrocarbons that boils in the range of 45–125° C (113–257° F). This solvent sometimes is referred to as benzine and lacquer diluent.

Physically, rubber solvent usually is a clear, colorless liquid and is less volatile than petroleum ether. Rubber solvent is primarily a mixture of paraffins (chiefly C5–C8) and aromatics. The actual composition will vary depending on the boiling range, the refinery stocks from which the solvent is produced and the method of preparation. In general, rubber solvent has 70–90% paraffins, 11–22% naphthenes and 9–22% aromatics. Rubber solvent can be produced from a straight-run petroleum distillate of paraffin base crude. It is used as a rubber cement diluent and as an agent in rubber dope mixing and rubber spreading. In 1965, the United States produced 28,857,000 barrels (1 barrel = 159 liters or 42 gallons) of what was described as special naphthas (including rubber solvent and varnish makers' and painters' naphtha), which represented 0.7% of the total production of petroleum products and, in 1975, 27,325,000 barrels of naphthas.

The NIOSH estimates that about 600,000 workers in the United States are potentially exposed to all "specialized" naphthas.

Carpenter et al.[6] exposed volunteers for about 10 seconds to rubber solvent vapor to determine its odor threshold. The authors concluded that the most probable threshold concentration was about 40 mg/m^3 (10 ppm) given the determined range of 6.4–64 mg/m^3 (1.6–16 ppm). Volunteers were also exposed to rubber solvent vapor at one of a series of concentrations from 1700 to 8100 mg/m^3 (430–2000 ppm) for one 15-minute period per day. Slight transitory eye, nose and throat irritation responses were noted at concentrations of 3100 mg/m^3 (780 ppm) and above, as well as 4 cases of light-headedness and 1 of headache at the 8100 mg/m^3 concentration, both of which were reported to have subsided within 10 minutes after exposure. At the 3100 mg/m^3 concentration, 1 volunteer reported eye irritation and 2 others throat irritation. One of 6 exposed to rubber solvent at 8100 mg/m^3 reported eye and throat irritation.

The authors[6] also reported the toxic effects of rubber solvent inhalation in animal toxicity studies. Groups of rats were exposed at 11,000, 21,000, 39,000 or 96,000 mg/m^3 (2800, 5300, 9800 or 24,200 ppm) for a single 4-hour period. Impairment of coordination and eye irritation were observed at concentrations greater than 11,000 mg/m^3. Convulsions and death occurred at 96,000 mg/m^3. The calculated 4-hour LC_{50} was reported to be 61,000 mg/m^3 (15,000 ppm). Female beagles were exposed to rubber solvent vapors at concentrations of 5900, 12,000 or 25,000 mg/m^3 (1500, 3300 or 6300 ppm) for a single 4-hour period. Loss of coordination was observed at concentrations of 13,000 and 25,000 mg/m^3. No observable effects occurred at 5900 mg/m^3.

The acute CNS effects of a 4-hour exposure to rubber solvent vapors at 49,000 mg/m^3 (12,400 ppm) were examined in male cats.[6] A time-related and sequential pattern of events occurred that included ataxia, loss of proprioception, salivation, relaxation of the nictitating membrane, unconsciousness, tremors and convulsions. Gross and microscopic examination of tissues showed no lesions related to solvent exposure.

Male rats and beagles were exposed to either 0, 1900, 3700 or 7900 mg/m^3 (0, 480, 930 or 2000 ppm) of rubber solvent 6 hours per day, 5 days per week for up to 62–63 days.[6] There were no animal deaths attributed to rubber solvent. There were no changes in body weight gain, blood chemistry or hematology that resulted from exposure to the solvent. Serum alkaline phosphatase was higher after 62 days in all rats exposed to rubber solvent, but the authors suggested that this finding was an artifact that resulted from very low control alkaline phosphatase levels. Microscopic examination of various organ sections showed no tissue damage that could be attributed to the solvent vapors. There was a significant increase in the specific gravity of the urine of dogs exposed at 7900 mg/m^3 for 62 days. The significance was not reported by the investigators.

Although no specific data on the dermal effects of rubber solvent have been found, alkanes and solvents that boil below 232° C (450° F) are known to be primary irritants[11,21] and, therefore, rubber solvent should be considered to be a dermal irritant. Dermal exposure to this solvent, therefore, should be minimized. The benzene content of rubber solvent should be evaluated to ensure that the federal exposure limit for benzene is not exceeded.

GENERAL CONTROL MEASURES

It is recommended that 350 mg/m^3 be adopted as a TWA concentration limit for up to a 10-hour work shift in a 40-hour workweek for petroleum ether, rubber solvent, varnish makers' and painters' naphtha, mineral spirits and Stoddard solvent. On a volume/volume basis, these concentrations are equal to about 114 ppm for petroleum ether, 88 ppm for rubber solvent, 75 ppm for varnish makers' and painters' naphtha, 55 ppm for mineral spirits and 59 ppm for Stoddard solvent. The recommended TWA concentration limit for kerosenes is 100 mg/m^3 (about 14 ppm). In addition, a ceiling concentration limit of 1800 mg/m^3 (about 590 ppm of petroleum ether, 454 ppm of rubber solvent, 386 ppm of varnish makers' and painters' naphtha, 282 ppm of mineral spirits and 306 ppm of Stoddard solvent), based on a sample collection period of 15 minutes, is recommended to protect workers from short-term exposures that might cause effects, such as vertigo or other adverse reactions, that could result in accidents. No ceiling limit is believed needed for kerosene.

It is recognized that many workers handle small amounts of petroleum ether, rubber solvent, varnish makers' and painters' naphtha, Stoddard solvent, mineral spirits and kerosene or work in situations where, regardless of the amount used, there is only negligible contact with these substances. Under these conditions, it should not be necessary to comply with many of the provisions of these recommended standards, which have been prepared primarily to protect workers' health under more hazardous circumstances. Concern for the workers' health requires that protective measures be instituted below the enforceable limit to ensure that exposures stay below that limit. For these reasons, an action level for petroleum ether, rubber solvent and varnish makers' and painters' naphtha has been defined as 200 mg/m^3 (about 66 ppm for petroleum ether, 50 ppm for rubber solvent and 43 ppm for varnish makers' and painters' naphtha), thereby delineating those work situations that do not require the expenditure of health resources for environmental and medical monitoring and associated record keeping. The action levels for Stoddard solvent, mineral spirits and kerosene are identical to the TWA concentration for these solvents because of the lower volatility of these solvents and the lower likelihood of developing toxicity. The action levels have been chosen on the basis of professional judgment rather than on quantitative data that delineate nonhazardous areas from areas in which a hazard may exist. Because of nonrespiratory hazards such as those resulting from skin or eye contact or from ingestion of petroleum ether, rubber solvent, varnish makers' and painters' naphtha, mineral spirits, Stoddard solvent and kerosene, it is recommended that appropriate work practices and protective measures be required regardless of the air concentration.

REFERENCES

Petroleum-Derived Solvents

1. Albert, W. C., and Inkley, S. R.: The efficacy of steroid therapy in the treatment of experimental kerosene pneumonitis, Am. Rev. Respir. Dis. 98:888, 1968.
2. Åstrand, I., Kilbom, A., and Övrum, P.: Exposure to white spirit. I. Concentration in alveolar air and blood during rest and exercise, Scand. J. Work Environ. Health 1:15, 1976.
3. Braunstein, L. E.: Subacute yellow atrophy of the liver due to solvent, JAMA 114:136, 1940.
4. Carpenter, C. P., et al.: Petroleum hydrocarbon toxicity studies. II. Animal and human response to vapors of varnish makers' and painters' naphtha, Toxicol. Appl. Pharmacol. 32:263, 1975.
5. Carpenter, C. P., et al.: Petroleum hydrocarbon toxicity studies. III. Animal and human response to vapors of Stoddard solvent, Toxicol. Appl. Pharmacol. 32:282, 1975.
6. Carpenter, C. P., et al.: Petroleum hydrocarbon toxicity studies. IV. Animal and human response to vapors of rubber solvent, Toxicol. Appl. Pharmacol. 33:526, 1975.
7. Carpenter, C. P., et al.: Petroleum hydrocarbon toxicity studies. VIII. Animal and human response to vapors of 140 flash aliphatic solvent, Toxicol. Appl. Pharmacol. 34:413, 1975.
8. Carpenter, C. P., et al.: Petroleum hydrocarbon toxicity studies. XI. Animal and human response to vapors of deodorized kerosene, Toxicol. Appl. Pharmacol. 36:443, 1976.
9. Carpenter, C. P., and Smyth, H. F.: Chemical burns of the rabbit cornea, Am. J. Ophthalmol. 29:1363, 1946.
10. Cavanagh, J. R., and Wilner, P. R.: Aplastic anemia due to kerosene, M. Ann. D.C. 8:140, 1939.
11. Criteria for a Recommended Standard . . . Occupational Exposure to Alkanes (C5–C8). U.S. Dept. of Health, Education, and Welfare, PHS, Center for Disease Control, National Institute for Occupational Safety and Health, 1978.
12. Criteria for a Recommended Standard . . . Occupational Exposure to Refined Petroleum Solvents, U.S. Dept. of Health, Education, and Welfare, Cincinnati, Ohio, DHEW (NIOSH) Publication No. 77-192, PHS, Center for Disease Control, National Institute for Occupational Safety and Health, 247, 1977.
13. Deichmann, W. B., Kitzmiller, K. V., Witherup, S., and Johansmann, R.: Kerosene intoxication, Ann. Intern. Med. 21:803, 1944.
14. Gamberale, F., Annwall, G., and Hultengren, M.: Exposure to white spirit. II. Psychological functions, Scand. J. Work Environ. Health 1:31, 1976.
15. Gaultier, M., Rancurel, G., Piva, C., and Efthymioc, M. L.: Polyneuritis and aliphatic hydrocarbons, J. Eur. Toxicol. 6:294, 1973 (French).
16. Gerarde, H. W.: Kerosine. Experimental and clinical toxicology, Occup. Health Rev. 16:17, 1964.
17. Gerarde, H. W.: Toxicological studies on hydrocarbons. IX. The aspiration hazard and toxicity of hydrocarbons and hydrocarbon mixtures, Arch. Environ. Health 6:329, 1963.
18. Gerarde, H. W., and Eckardt, R. E.: Aspiration hazards of petroleum products, in XIVth International Congress of Occupational Health, Madrid, Spain, Sept. 16–21, 1963. International Congress Series No. 62. New York, Excerpta Medica Foundation, Vol. II, pp. 723–727, 1964.
19. Gross, P., McNerney, J. M., and Babyak, M. A.: Kerosene pneumonitis. An experimental study with small doses, Am. Rev. Respir. Dis. 88:656, 1963.
20. Herskowitz, A., Ishii, N., and Schaumburg, H.: *N*-hexane neuropathy. A syndrome occurring as a result of industrial exposure, N. Engl. J. Med. 285:82, 1971.
21. Hiebel, J., Gant, H. L., Schwartz, S. O., and Friedman, I. A.: Bone marrow depression following exposure to kerosene. A report of 3 cases, Am. J. Med. Sci. 246:91, 1963.
22. Inoue, T., et al.: Industrial health survey of high incidence of *n*-hexane intoxication among vinyl sandal manufacturers, Jpn. J. Ind. Health 12:73, 1970 (Japanese).
23. Johnson, D. E.: Hypoplastic anemia following chronic exposure to kerosene, J. Am. Med. Wom. Assoc. 10:421, 1955.
24. Klauder, J. V., and Brill, F. A.: Correlation of boiling ranges of some petroleum solvents with irritant action on skin, Arch. Dermatol. Syphilol. 56:197, 1947.
25. Larsen, L. B., and Shmunes, E.: Occupational health case report, No. 6—Stoddard solvent, J. Occup. Med. 16:276, 1974.
26. Lupulescu, A. P., and Birmingham, D. J.: Effect of lipid solvents on protein, DNA, and collagen synthesis in human skin. An electron microscopic autoradiographic study, J. Invest. Dermatol. 65:419, 1975.
27. Lupulescu, A. P., and Birmingham, D. J.: Effect of protective agent against lipid-solvent-induced damages. Ultrastructural

and scanning electron microscopical study of human epidermis, Arch. Environ. Health 31:33, 1976.
28. Lupulescu, A., Birmingham, D., Habowski, J., and Pinkus, H.: Electron microscopic autoradiography of 3H-kerosene in human epidermis, J. Cell Biol. 59:204A, 1973.
29. Lupulescu, A. P., Birmingham, D. J., and Pinkus, H.: An electron microscopic study of human epidermis after acetone and kerosene administration, J. Invest. Dermatol. 60:33, 1973.
30. Markel, H. L., and Shmunes, E.: Health Hazard Evaluation, Report No. 72-33-129 (Barker Greeting Card Co.). Cincinnati, Ohio, U.S. Dept. of Health, Education, and Welfare, National Institute for Occupational Safety and Health, Hazard Evaluation Services Branch, 15 pp., 1974.
31. McNally, W. D.: Kerosene poisoning in children. A study of 204 cases, J. Pediatr. 48:296, 1956.
32. Miyagaki, H.: Electrophysiological studies of the peripheral neurotoxicity of *n*-hexane, Jpn. J. Ind. Health 9:660, 1967 (Japanese).
33. Narasimhan, M. J., Jr., and Ganla, V. G.: Experimental studies on kerosene poisoning, Acta Pharmacol. Toxicol. 25:214, 1967.
34. Nelson, K. W., et al.: Sensory response to certain industrial solvent vapors, J. Ind. Hyg. Toxicol. 25:282, 1943.
35. Nunn, J. A., and Martin, F. M.: Gasoline and kerosene poisoning in children, JAMA 103:472, 1934.
36. Oettel, H.: Effect of organic liquids on the skin, Arch. Exp. Pathol. Pharmakol. 83:641, 649, 693, 1936 (German).
37. Prager, D., and Peters, C.: Development of aplastic anemia and the exposure to Stoddard solvent, Blood 35:286, 1970.
38. Rebello, J. A., and Suskind, R. R.: The effect of common contactants of cutaneous reactivity to sensitizers, J. Invest. Dermatol. 41:67, 1963.
39. Rector, D. E., Steadman, B. L., Jones, R. A., and Siegel, J.: Effects on experimental animals of long-term inhalation exposure to mineral spirits, Toxicol. Appl. Pharmacol. 9:257, 1966.
40. Schwartz, S. I., Breslau, R. C., Kutner, F., and Smith, D.: Effects of drugs and hyperbaric oxygen environment on experimental kerosene pneumonitis, Dis. Chest 47:353, 1965.
41. Scott, J. L., Cartwright, G. E., and Wintrobe, M. M.: Acquired aplastic anemia. An analysis of thirty-nine cases and review of the pertinent literature, Medicine 38:119, 1959.
42. Spruit, D., Malten, K. E., and Lipmann, E. W. R. M.: Horny layer injury by solvents. II. Can the irritancy of petroleum ether be diminished by pretreatment?, Berufs-Dermatosen 18:269, 1970.
43. Steele, R. W., Conklin, R. H., and Mark, H. M.: Corticosteroids and antibiotics for the treatment of fulminant hydrocarbon aspiration, JAMA 219:1434, 1972.
44. Tagami, H., and Ogino, A.: Kerosene dermatitis, Dermatologica 146:123, 1973.
45. Takeuchi, Y., Mabuchi, C., and Takagi, S.: Polyneuropathy caused by petroleum benzine, Int. Arch. Arbeitsmed. 34:185, 1975.
46. Truffa, O., and Montalenti, P.: Acute pneumopathy and icterus from accidental ingestion of kerosene, Minerva Med. 60:1403, 1969 (Italian).
47. Truhaut, R., et al.: Preliminary electrophysiologic results following experimental poisoning with technical hexane and heptane in white rats, Arch. Mal. Prof. 34:417, 1973 (French).
48. Volkova, A. P., Tsetlin, V. M., Zhuk, E. B., and Iizotova, E. P.: Toxicity of kerosene as a solvent used in aerosol cylinders, Gig. Sanit. 34:24, 1969 (Russian).
49. Wolfsdorf, J., and Kundig, H.: Kerosene poisoning in primates, S. Afr. Med. J. 46:619, 1972.
50. Yamada, S.: Polyneuritis in workers exposed to *n*-hexane, its cause and symptoms, Jpn. J. Ind. Health 9:651, 1972 (Japanese).
51. Yamamura, Y.: *N*-hexane polyneuropathy, Folia Psychiatr. Neurol. Jpn. 23:45, 1969.
52. Zenz, C.: Benzene—attempts to establish a lower exposure standard in the United States. A review, Scand. J. Work Environ. Health 4:103, 1978.

Phosgene

$COCl_2$

This highly toxic substance can be found as gaseous or liquefied phosgene, with inhalation as the main route of exposure; it also is highly irritating to skin. Synonyms for phosgene include carbonyl chloride, carbon oxychloride, chloroformyl chloride and CG (designation used by military agencies).

Phosgene, originally known as a war gas during World War I, today is used primarily as a chemical intermediate in the manufacture of isocyanates. In the United States, more than 300 million kg are produced, with approximately 85% of this used in isocyanate manufacture, most isocyanate manufacturers producing phosgene for their own use. The NIOSH estimated that 10,000 workers have potential occupational exposure to phosgene during its manufacture and use. Also, phosgene can be formed by the decomposition of chlorinated hydrocarbons when these compounds are exposed to heat or ultraviolet radiation.

Phosgene gas is a severe respiratory irritant, and skin contact with the liquid may cause severe burns. In concentrations of 1–2 ppm, phosgene causes eye discomfort, and at higher concentrations, lacrimation and conjunctivitis can produce severe eye irritation. Three ppm is thought to be the least concentration capable of causing immediate irritation to the human throat; 4 ppm causes immediate irritation of the eyes; 4.8 ppm causes cough, and even brief exposure to 50 ppm may prove rapidly fatal. With moderate exposure, the presenting symptoms often are a dryness or a burning sensation in the throat, vomiting, pain in the chest and dyspnea. The onset of symptoms of severe respiratory distress may be delayed for up to 72 hours, the latent interval depending on the concentration and duration of exposure. Delayed onset of pulmonary edema is characterized by cough, abundant "foamy" sputum, progressive dyspnea and severe cyanosis. Pulmonary edema may progress to pneumonia, and cardiac failure may intervene.

Because of the often-delayed onset of symptoms following potentially lethal exposures to phosgene, education of employees and medical observation following suspected overexposures are extremely important. Medical examinations, including pulmonary function tests, are necessary to evaluate recovery from overexposure and to detect chronic lung changes.

In case of known or suspected overexposure to phosgene, first-aid measures must be taken immediately, followed by prompt medical evaluation and care. Overexposed persons should not be permitted unnecessary physical exertion and should be carried to a vehicle to receive medical assistance. Pressurized oxygen and attendants trained in its use shall be available in the event that they are needed for persons in respiratory distress. In case of skin or eye contact with liquid phosgene, contaminated clothing must be removed quickly and the exposed body areas flushed with copious amounts of water. Because of the often-delayed onset of symptoms following overexposure to phosgene, surveillance or monitoring of the patient by a physician or by trained paramedical personnel is required for the 24-hour period following overexposure. A posteroanterior chest film should be taken in each instance of known or suspected overexposure to phosgene for comparison with preplacement chest films. Pulmonary function tests may be useful during convalescence.

Occupational exposure to phosgene shall be controlled so that no worker is exposed to phosgene at a concentration greater than one-tenth part phosgene per million parts of air (0.1 ppm) determined as a TWA concentration for up to a 10-hour workday, 40-hour workweek, or to more than two-tenths part phosgene per million parts of air (0.2 ppm) as a ceiling concentration for any 15-minute period.

REFERENCE

Phosgene

1. NIOSH, A Recommended Standard for Occupational Exposure to Phosgene. U.S. Dept. of Health, Education, and Welfare, PHS, Center for Disease Control, National Institute for Occupational Safety and Health, Robert A. Taft Laboratories, 4676 Columbia Parkway, Cincinnati, Ohio 45226, 1976.

Polybrominated Biphenyls (PBBs)

These highly brominated compounds have been used as flame retardants, mainly in plastics requiring high heat resistance, such as for electronic insulating materials, TV and other electric cabinets and housings and in auto and truck plastics, where the PBB is added as a fine powder to the plastics. The PBBs have been used on synthetic fibers as well. (PBBs no longer are manufactured in the United States.)

The general formula is:

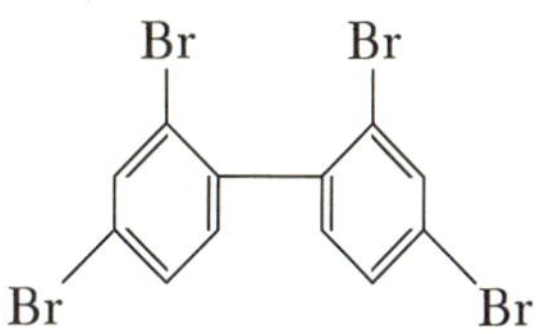

About 1 million kg were produced annually in the United States, but there are no reports of adverse human reactions in the manufacturing and subsequent use. When the PBBs are added to the mixing process to make various plastics (i.e., acrylonitrile-butadiene-styrene ["ABS"]), along with other materials such as pigments, the subsequent reactions yielding finished products result in plastic that has durable qualities, so that none of the ingredients originally used, and potentially hazardous, poses any problem to persons handling, fabricating and assembling such PBB-containing products. Only very high heat may release decomposition products, which may be entirely different compounds.

In mid-1973, one of these PBB compounds was accidentally mixed into an animal feedstock, resulting in widespread distribution involving thousands of animals, including cattle, chickens, sheep and swine. This product had an average bromine content of 6 bromine atoms per biphenyl molecule, also containing traces of tetra-, penta- and heptabromobiphenyls, brominated benzenes and traces of hexa- and pentabromonaphthalene. Embryotoxicity, teratogenicity and various degrees of neurologic dysfunctions were reported in animals and in livestock fed contaminated feed-stock. The PBBs were detected in the food chain, and a study by the Michigan Department of Public Health revealed that nearly 2000 farm families had eaten their own contaminated meats. The range of contamination was several thousand parts per million in the meat of dairy cows to less than one part per billion in milk sold in supermarkets. Extensive studies were made of those persons involved, but no significant differences in the incidence of symptoms between the group of "heavily exposed" farmers and controls was found.

This inadvertent contamination serves to point out how potentially hazardous materials may be accidentally dissipated into the community environment, involving the population at large (see Chapter 3 for further discussion). Again, such examples illustrate the importance of physicians and others concerned with occupational health and safety having some familiarity with the materials and processes in their communities (see Chapter 13 regarding material safety data sheets—"MSDS").

No adverse occupational exposures have been reported and TLVs for the polybrominated biphenyl compounds have not been established.

REFERENCES

Polybrominated Biphenyls

1. Lillis, R., et al.: Comparison of findings among residents on Michigan dairy farms and consumers of produce from these farms, Environ. Health Perspect. 23:105, 1978.
2. Tilson, H. A., et al.: Some neurotoxic effects of polybrominated biphenyl (PBB) compounds in rodents, Environ. Health Perspect. 20:244, 1977.

3. Valciukas, J. A., et al.: Comparative neurobehavioral study of a polybrominated biphenyl-exposed population in Michigan and a nonexposed group in Wisconsin, Environ. Health Perspect. 23:199, 1978.

Radon and Its Daughters

Synonyms for radon daughters are radon progeny, radon decay products, radium A, radium B, radium C, radium C′, radium D, radium E, radium F and radium G. The short half-life daughters (radium A, B, C and C′), which are associated with radon in air, commonly are referred to as "radon daughters" collectively and are also known as ^{218}Po, ^{214}Pb, ^{214}Bi and ^{214}Po. Radium D–G are also technically radon daughters, but radium D has a half-life of 22 years, so it often becomes dissociated from radon and produces its own decay products (daughters).

OCCUPATIONAL EXPOSURES

Radon and its daughters are found in most underground mines, in uranium mills, in chemical plants that handle radium and in medical installations that use "radon seeds" for radiotherapy. Encapsulated radium retains all the generated radon. However, the "needles" and capsules sometimes develop minute holes that permit escape of radon.

Radon is a noble gas and a decay product of radium, which, in turn, is a decay product of uranium. Whenever radium-containing material is open to air, radon tends to diffuse out into the air. While in the air, it decays, creating its daughters, which are metals. Since they are solids, they attach themselves to the nearest solid object, which usually is a dust particle. Radon and its short half-life daughters emit a wide spectrum of alpha, beta and gamma radiation. Suspended ions created by radon decay and dust suspended in air become quite radioactive. Unattached ions and ions attached to dust have different deposition sites when included. The average half-life of the short half-life daughters is collectively about $^1/_2$ hour, which means that radiation stops soon after a worker leaves a contaminated area. Radon and its daughters have no odor, cannot be seen and radiation from them cannot be felt.

The principal hazard from radon and its daughters is from ionizing radiation. Radioactive particles in the air (either free or attached to dust) are inhaled and are deposited within the tracheobronchial tree. The radiation dose contribution from the beta and gamma rays is so small compared to the contribution from alpha particles that it generally is disregarded. When radon is at or near equilibrium with its daughters, approximately 95% of the radiation dose to the tracheobronchial epithelium is delivered by radon daughters and 5% is delivered by radon alpha emission.

The ionizing radiation induces metaplasia and atypical cell growth in the tracheobronchial epithelium, which frequently develops into bronchial carcinoma. Radiation of terminal airways may lead to emphysema and pulmonary fibrosis. The frequency of carcinoma is greatly increased and the latent period is decreased when exposed persons smoke cigarettes, a synergistic effect. The resultant risk of cancer in the exposed population is dependent on the amount of cumulative radon daughter exposure, age distribution of the population, time since beginning of exposure, amount of cigarette smoking and chest size. Individuals who smoke heavily and who have had high cumulative radon daughter exposures have an extremely high risk of respiratory cancer.

Although there is some radiation exposure to skin, eyes, gut, nasopharynx, bone and kidneys from exposure to radon daughters in air, no excess malignancy of these organs has been observed in studies of uranium miners who have had high radon daughter exposures.

RECOMMENDED CONTROLS

Control of radon and its daughters generally is accomplished by ventilation. Sufficient air changes per hour must be made to prevent the build-up of radon by emanation from mine walls (or from water seepage) and to prevent the build-up of the daughters toward an equilibrium condition. In some situations, simple ventilation provides inadequate control and must be supplemented by methods of reducing emanation of radon into workplaces (pressurizing mines, closing off of unused workings or covering mine walls with a sealant that is impervious to radon) or by local removal of particles from the air (filters, electrostatic precipitators, etc.)

Many respirators are quite effective in removing radon daughters from air, but they do not remove radon. Even the disposable nuisance dust type of respirators remove a substantial fraction of radon daughters. However, respirators generally are uncomfortable and their use is resisted by workers, so their use generally should be limited to exposures of short duration when it is not feasible to control radon daughter levels by ventilation.

If the inhalation hazard is controlled, there is no hazard to eyes, skin or gut. There are no other known hazards from radon and its daughters.

CLINICAL MONITORING

No clinical or biologic monitoring methods are recommended for routine use, but several have been investigated and may be feasible under some circumstances. These consist of periodic examination of sputum by the Papanicolaou technique, whole-body gamma counting and determination of lead-210 in urine, blood or hair.

TABLE 14–8.—WORKDAY AIR EXPOSURE CONCENTRATIONS

AUTHORITY	YEAR	WORKING LEVEL* MONTHS/YEAR	SHORT-TERM AIR EXPOSURE CONCENTRATIONS	
			^{222}RADON (uc/ml)	CONCENTRATIONS (WORKING LEVELS)
Nuclear Regulatory Commission (10 CFR Part 20 as amended)	1975	4.0	3×10^{8}	0.33

*A "Working Level" (WL) is defined as any combination of short-lived ^{222}Rn daughters (^{218}Po, ^{214}Pb, ^{214}Bi and ^{214}Po) in 1 liter of air, without regard to the degree of equilibrium, that will result in the ultimate emission of 1.3×10^5 MeV of alpha particle energy. Exposure at 1 WL for 170 hours (usual working time per month) results in one Working Level Month (WLM). Conversion of WLM to rads is uncertain due to many poorly known variables, but usually is considered to be between 1 and 3 rads per 1 WLM.

REFERENCES

Radon and Its Daughters

1. Andrew, H. L.: *Radiation Biophysics* (2d ed.; Englewood Cliffs, N.J.: Prentice-Hall, Inc., 1974).
2. Christensen, H. E., and Zenz, C.: Compounds Associated with Carcinogenesis, in Zenz, C. (ed.), *Occupational Medicine: Principles and Practical Applications* (Chicago: Year Book Medical Publishers, 1975), pp. 843–868.
3. Voelz, G. L.: Radiologic Health in Occupational Medicine Practice, in Zenz, C. (ed.), *Occupational Medicine: Principles and Practical Applications* (Chicago: Year Book Medical Publishers, 1975), pp. 499–551.

Sodium Hydroxide

Sodium hydroxide, also called caustic soda, soda lye or white caustic, is produced commercially by electrolysis of a sodium chloride solution or from lime and soda ash. Total *United States production* of sodium hydroxide in 1974 was *10 billion kg*, attesting to the enormous use of this substance in only one industrialized country! The NIOSH estimates that 150,000 U.S. workers are potentially exposed to the alkali. It is used in the manufacture of rayon, mercerized cotton, soap, paper, aluminum, petroleum, chemicals and dyestuffs. It is also used for metal cleaning, electrolytic extraction of zinc, tin plating, oxide coating, laundering and bleaching.

Major hazards are by inhalation and skin contact (often concomitantly). Sodium hydroxide is a strong alkali; the mist, dust and solutions cause severe injury to the eyes, mucous membranes and skin. Although inhalation usually is of secondary importance in occupational exposures, the effects from the dust or mist will vary from mild irritation of the nose at 2 mg/m^3 to severe pneumonitis, depending on the severity of exposure. The greatest industrial hazard is rapid tissue destruction of eyes or skin on contact with either the solid or the concentrated solutions. Contact with the eyes causes disintegration and sloughing of conjunctival and corneal epithelium, corneal opacification, marked edema and ulceration; after 7–13 days, either gradual recovery begins or there is progression of ulceration and corneal opacification. Complications of severe eye burns are symblepharon with overgrowth of the cornea by a vascularized membrane, progressive or recurrent corneal ulceration and permanent corneal opacification. On the skin, solutions of 25–50% cause the sensation of irritation within about 3 minutes; with solutions of 4%, this does not occur until after several hours. If not removed from the skin, severe burns with deep ulceration will occur; exposure to the dust or mist may cause multiple small burns, with temporary loss of hair. Ingestion produces severe pain in the esophagus and stomach, corrosion of the lips, mouth, tongue and pharynx and the vomiting of large pieces of mucosa; cases of squamous cell carcinoma of the esophagus have occurred with patent periods of 12–42 years after ingestion; these cancers undoubtedly were sequelae of tissue destruction and possibly scar formation rather than from a direct carcinogenic action of sodium hydroxide itself.

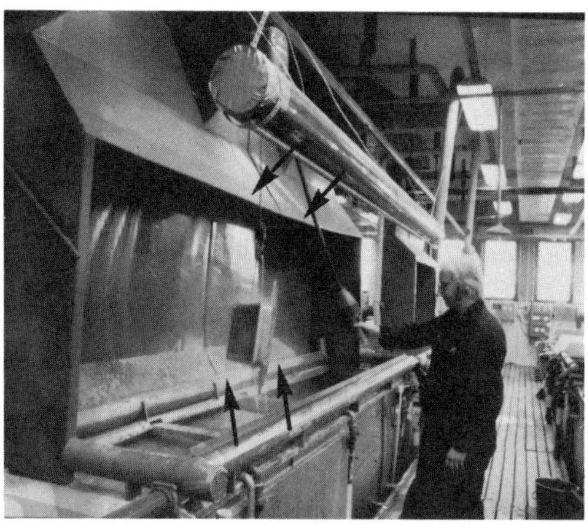

Fig 14–5.—Alkaline pickling. In order to avoid mists of sodium hydroxide in the breathing zone, yet be able to operate the lift over the bath, additional air inlets *(arrows)* were designed, constructed and placed so that the air would blow away from the worker's face. (Courtesy of Eric Ortman, M.D., LM Ericsson Co., Mölndal, Sweden.)

TREATMENT.—Remove from exposure. Immediately flush the eyes and skin with water. If swallowed and the person is conscious, immediately administer water orally. Consideration should be given to hospitalization and observation for the onset of pneumonitis.

The NIOSH recommends a ceiling concentration of 2.0 mg sodium hydroxide/m^3 as determined by a sampling period of 15 minutes. The present federal standard is 2.0 mg sodium hydroxide/m^3 as an 8-hour time-weighted average consideration. Samples representative of the exposure in the breathing zones of at least 25% of the employees in each operation or process shall be collected. Every employee shall be included in the sampling at least once every 2 years.

The NIOSH recommends that workers subject to sodium hydroxide exposure have comprehensive preplacement medical examinations. Medical examinations shall be made available promptly to all workers with signs or symptoms of skin, eye or upper respiratory tract irritation resulting from exposure to sodium hydroxide. Containers of sodium hydroxide shall be labeled to warn of the severe burns and blindness that may result, and personal protective equipment must be made available to protect eyes, face and skin from contact with sodium hydroxide. Engineering controls shall be used wherever feasible to maintain airborne sodium hydroxide at concentrations below the prescribed limit, and respirators may be used only in certain nonroutine or emergency situations.

REFERENCES

Sodium Hydroxide

1. American Conference of Governmental Industrial Hygienists: "Sodium Hydroxide," Documentation of the Threshold Limit Values for Substances in Workroom Air, 3d ed., Cincinnati, Ohio, p. 345, 1974.
2. Manufacturing Chemists Association, Inc.: Chemical Safety Data Sheet DS-9, Caustic Soda, Washington, D.C., pp. 16–17, 1968.
3. National Institute for Occupational Safety and Health, U.S. Dept. of Health, Education, and Welfare: Criteria for a Recommended Standard . . . Occupational Exposure to Sodium Hydroxide, No. (NIOSH) 76:105, Cincinnati, Ohio, 1975.

Styrene

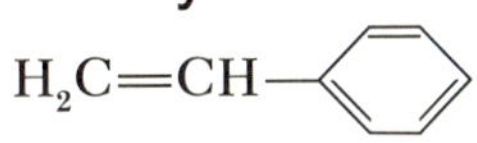

Styrene, or vinyl benzene, is one of the most widely used chemicals, with a world-wide production of about 7 million tons in 1977. This vast production is the greatest single use of benzene (50% of world capacity) and the third greatest use of ethylene next to polyethylene and polyvinyl chloride production. Styrene-butadiene rubber and tire production accounts for 10% of styrene use, the remainder for plastics, coatings and resins. "ABS" (acrylonitrile-butadiene-styrene) resin enjoys vast use for cars, trucks, sheets, pipes and similar products, much of the "ABS" plastics being used in making television cabinets and in other electrical manufacturing. It is estimated that more than 1 million workers, world-wide, are exposed to detectable styrene concentrations.

Considerable quantities of styrene are used in spraying and hand rolling of styrene-modified polyester plastics with fiberglass reinforcement in manufacturing boats of all sizes, swimming pools and various containers of large and small size. Much of the manufacturing goes on in small factories, especially in the numerous shops for the boat-building industry, often employing many women in these semiskilled activities (Figs 14–6 and 14–7).

Axelson[1] described in detail toxicity, metabolism, excretion and medical and hygienic controls. At the International Symposium on Styrene[8] Härkönen[4] reported on experimental and clinical toxicology of styrene, including mutagenic effects and certain neurophysiologic findings.

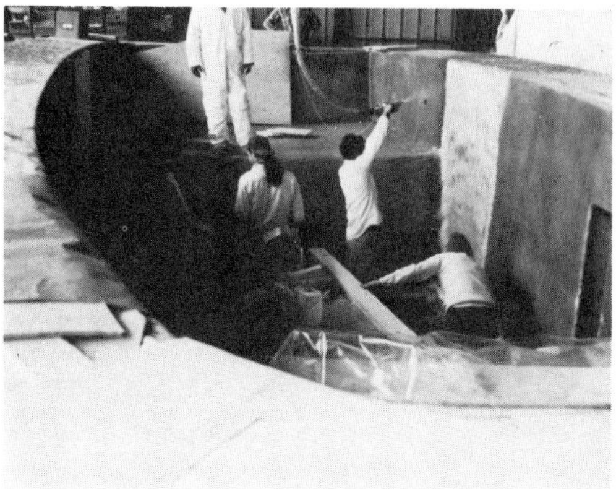

Fig 14–6.—Young men and women building a large boat hull, using fiberglass polyester resins. Boat builders use from 41% to 44% styrene in these laminating stages, which, for the most part, are hand applied. Exhaust ventilation and respiratory protective equipment are absent.

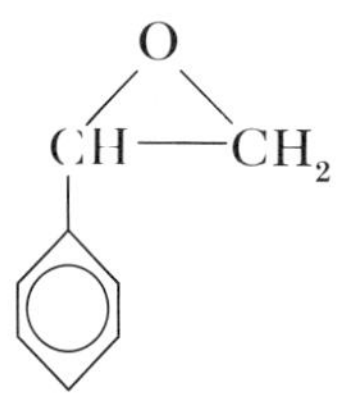

Styrene oxide

Styrene is converted by liver microsomes to its epoxide, styrene oxide, which is further metabolized by epoxide hydratase to styrene glycol. Because of its structural similarity to vinyl chloride, styrene has been tested for mutagenicity and other biotoxic effects.[8,9] Vainio et al.,[13] based on their studies, suggested that more detailed investigations on the mutagenic and carcinogenic potential of styrene and styrene oxide are warranted, pointing out the need for an epidemiologic study on workers in industry.

The neurotoxic effects of styrene have been known for some time, both in animals and in humans. Roth and Klimkova-Deutschova[11] reported that styrene in occupational exposure induces electroencephalographic abnormalities more often than several other chemicals. Seppäläinen and Härkönen[12] described neurophysiologic findings among 96 men (no women were included) occupationally exposed to styrene. They concluded that the EEG examination is useful in the study of the neurotoxic effects of styrene.

Holmberg[6] reported on his findings of an investigation begun in June, 1976, in Finland, concerning the possibility of mothers of children with central nervous defects having been exposed during pregnancy to noxious influences at work. This investigation was designed as a semiprospective case referent study to cover 12 months and comprised a series of mothers of all children with central nervous defects reported to the Finnish Register of Congenital Malformations, where notification to this Register is compulsory. In addition to the information obtained through this Register, information on work exposure to noxious influences was obtained. Holmberg reported central nervous defects in 2 children of mothers exposed to chemicals in the reinforced plastic industry. With the use of a specially designed questionnaire, with emphasis on occupational exposure to chemical agents at work, information was gained by personal interview with 2 mothers who had been employed in the reinforced plastic industry and had been exposed at work to a combination of styrene, polyester resin, organic peroxides and acetone during their pregnancy. When the number of fertile women in this

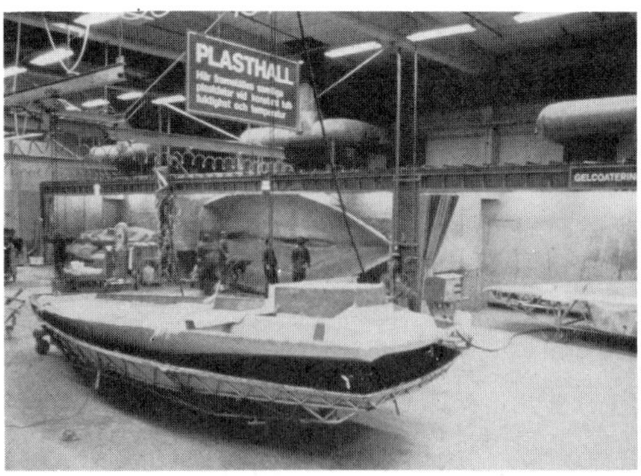

Fig 14–7.—A modern plastic boat-building factory. Note extensive exhaust system (Courtesy of Mr. Håkan Widman, Mölnycke Marin, Mariestad, Sweden.)

industry is considered (some 250), along with the low rate of anencephaly and hydrocephalus in the general population—diagnoses made of the children of these case mothers (0.5/1000 live births in Finland)—this occupational group seems overrepresented. Holmberg clearly indicated that in man, as far as is known, no teratogenic activity has been reported for styrene or its metabolites, but emphasized that the majority of malformations in human subjects remain without a causal explanation, and that every lead toward their clarification seems worth reporting.

Engström et al.[3] determined the uptake, distribution and elimination of styrene in male subjects, with special reference to storage in cutaneous adipose tissue, exposing 7 men to styrene vapor concentrations of 210 mg/m^3 (50 ppm) in inspired air, using a bicycle ergometer to simulate work intensities of 50, 100 and 150 watts. (Exposures were 30 minutes at rest and three 30-minute periods at work.) Styrene was found to be highly soluble in blood and tissues, and the equilibrium between concentrations in arterial blood and alveolar air was not achieved during short-term exposure. The mean uptake was 490 mg, corresponding to 63% of the amount inspired. Respiratory elimination of styrene 19 hours after exposure revealed that about 3% of the styrene was retained in the body during exposure. Needle biopsies of subcutaneous adipose tissue were made before exposure and ½, 2, 4 and 20–24 hours after exposure in all subjects. In 4 of the subjects, biopsies were obtained 1–2 weeks after exposure to styrene. The concentrations of styrene in adipose tissue were determined by gas chromatography after evaporation into nitrogen at a high temperature. Twenty-four hours after exposure ceased, the mean concentration of styrene in adipose tissue was at about the same level as 2–4 hours after exposure, i.e., about 3.5 mg/kg. Of considerable interest was that the retention of styrene in adipose tissue was found as late as 13 days after this short experimental exposure at a concentration in inspired air closely corresponding to the Swedish TLV (40 ppm). Engström and coworkers estimated the half-life of the concentration of styrene in adipose tissue to be about 2–4 days, despite the rapid metabolism of styrene, and they considered occupational exposure to be accompanied by a risk of accumulation of styrene in adipose tissue because of the slow elimination. Clearly, the results of these investigations focus on a reorientation of the concepts of the absorption, metabolism and excretion of styrene and other similar substances with lipid affinity. Parallels can be drawn between styrene and other commonly used solvents, in the past thought to be relatively "safe" in terms of acute and chronic exposures. This means that the traditional concepts of "metabolism" of many substances must be reconsidered in the light that immediate metabolism may not occur, but that a "storage" or "retention" may occur, an added factor for concern because of lipid affinity for many substances and potential effects on the nervous system. Metabolism and elimination following the ordinary work shift of 8 hours, along with weekends, may prove to be insufficient time for long-term work under existing limit values for many substances, especially when work effort is at an energy level far above a "sedentary," "sitting" or "resting" level. This storage or retention of styrene was further demonstrated in workers fabricating polyester storage tanks. Engström et al.[2] studied 3 male employes during a workweek, monitoring from Tuesday to Friday the concentration of styrene in the ambient air continually in the breathing zone. The uptake was estimated as the product of the time-weighted average concentration in inspiratory air, the mean 8-hour pulmonary ventilation and the percentage uptake in the lungs measuring pulmonary ventilation with a respirometer. The percentage styrene uptake was estimated on the basis of the concentrations in inspiratory and alveolar air and the amount of body fat was estimated by an anthropometric method. Concentrations of styrene in subcutaneous adipose tissue were determined by gas chromatography after needle biopsy before and after the work shift of Monday, Wednesday and Friday. They found that the time-weighted average concentration of styrene in inspiratory air during the workweek was 32–85 mg/m^3, i.e., below half of the Swedish TLV (210 mg/m^3), and the mean daily uptake was 193–558 mg. On Monday morning, the concentration of styrene in adipose tissue was 2.8–8.1 mg/kg and on Friday afternoon 4.7–11.6 mg/kg. The concentrations were higher in the 2 subjects with a higher exposure, of longer duration, as compared to the concentrations in a recently employed worker, who was exposed to lower concentrations in inspiratory air. Both of the 2 former workers had a large estimated amount of body fat (27 and 41 kg). The calculated half-life of the concentration of styrene in adipose tissue after the end of exposure was 5.2 and 2.8 days in these 2 men and an elimination time of about 5 weeks in the subject with the slowest elimination, before the limit of detection (0.1 mg/kg) was reached. Increased cardiorespiratory and vascular demands during pregnancy, described in other sections in this chapter, imply that the transport and potential storage in fetal tissues to a variety of chemicals must be viewed in the light of these recent investigations by Engström et al., who distinctly revealed a "half-life" of styrene in male workers after exposure ceased to be in excess of 5 days.

REFERENCES

Styrene

1. Axelson, O.: Styrene, in Zenz, C. (ed.), *Occupational Medicine: Principles and Practical Applications* (Chicago: Year Book Medical Publishers, 1975), pp. 816–820.
2. Engström, J., Åstrand, I., and Wigaeus, E.: Exposure to styrene in a polymerization plant: Uptake in the organism and concentration in subcutaneous adipose tissue, Scand. J. Work Environ. Health 4:324, 1978.
3. Engström, J., Bjurström, R., Åstrand, I., and Övrum, P.: Uptake, distribution and elimination of styrene in man: Concentration in subcutaneous adipose tissue, Scand. J. Work Environ. Health 4:315, 1978.
4. Härkönen, H.: Styrene, its experimental and clinical toxicology: A review, Scand. J. Work Environ. Health 4(Suppl. 2):104, 1978.
5. Heinonen, O. P., Slone, D., and Shapiro, S.: *Birth Defects and Drugs in Pregnancy* (Littleton, Mass.: Publishing Sciences Group, Inc., 1977).
6. Holmberg, P. C.: Central nervous defects in two children of mothers exposed to chemicals in the reinforced plastics industry. Chance or causal relationship?, Scand. J. Work Environ. Health 3:212, 1977.
7. Hygieniska Gränsvärden, Directives concerning limit values for air contaminants at places of work. National Board of Occupational Safety and Health, Stockholm, Sweden, May, 1978.
8. International Symposium on Styrene. Proceedings of the Occupational and Toxicological Aspects, Helsinki, April 17–19, 1978, Scand. J. Work Environ. Health 4(Suppl. 2):264, 1978.
9. Loprieno, N., et al.: A. Mutagenicity of industrial compounds: Styrene and its possible metabolite styrene oxide, Mutat. Res. 40:317, 1976.
10. Roberfroid, M., et al.: Acute biotoxic effect of styrene on rat liver: Correlation with enzyme-mediated mutagenicity of benzpyrene and acrylonitrile, Scand. J. Work Environ. Health 4(Suppl. 2):163, 1978.
11. Roth, B., and Klimkova-Deutschova, E.: The effect of the chronic action of industrial poisons on the electroencephalogram of man, Rev. Czech. Med. 9:217, 1963.
12. Seppäläinen, A. M., and Härkönen, H.: Neurophysiological findings among workers occupationally exposed to styrene, Scand. J. Work Environ. Health 3:140, 1976.
13. Vainio, H., et al.: A study of the mutagenic activity of styrene and styrene oxide, Scand. J. Work Environ. Health 3:147, 1976.

Sulfur Dioxide

SO_2

Sulfur dioxide is a colorless gaseous by-product of processes such as smelting of sulfide ores, combustion of coal or fuel oils containing sulfur as an impurity, paper manufacturing and petroleum refining. Industrially, sulfur dioxide is used in the manufacture of sodium sulfite and as an intermediate in the manufacture of sulfuric acid. It is also used in refrigeration, bleaching, fumigating and preserving operations and as an antioxidant in the melting, pouring and heat treatment of magnesium. The NIOSH estimates that 500,000 workers have potential exposure to sulfur dioxide. Occupational exposure to sulfur dioxide may occur in many industries, including petroleum refining, smelting, preserving industries, utility companies and paper making.

Sulfur dioxide gas is a severe irritant to the eyes, mucous membranes and skin. Its irritant properties are due to the rapidity with which it forms sulfurous acid on contact with moist membranes. Approximately 90% of all sulfur dioxide inhaled is absorbed in the upper respiratory passages, where most effects occur; however, it may produce respiratory paralysis and may also cause pulmonary edema. Exposure to concentrations of 10–50 ppm for 5–15 minutes causes irritation of the eyes, nose and throat, rhinorrhea, choking, cough and, in some instances, reflex bronchoconstriction with increased pulmonary resistance. Some 10–20% of the healthy young adult population are estimated to be hypersusceptible to the effects of sulfur dioxide whereas the phenomenon of adaptation to irritating concentrations is a recognized occurrence in some workers. Workers repeatedly exposed to 10 ppm experienced upper respiratory irritation and some nosebleeds, but the symptoms did not occur at 5 ppm. In another study, initial cough and irritation did occur at 5 ppm and 13 ppm, but subsided after 5 minutes of exposure.[1,4] In a human experimental study with the subjects breathing through the mouth, brief exposure to 13 ppm caused a 73% increase in pulmonary flow resistance; 5 ppm resulted in a 40% increase; 1 ppm produced no effects.[5] Exposure of the eyes to liquid sulfur dioxide from pressurized containers causes corneal burns and opacification, resulting in a loss of vision. Liquefied SO_2 on the skin produces skin burns from the freezing effect of rapid evaporation.

The TLV of 5 ppm was set to prevent respiratory irritation.

TREATMENT.—Remove from exposure. Immediately flush the eyes with water and wash the skin with soap or mild detergent and water. Hospitalization is recommended for observation for possible delayed pulmonary edema.

REFERENCES

Sulfur Dioxide

1. American Conference of Governmental Industrial Hygienists: Sulfur Dioxide. Documentation of the Threshold Limit Values for Substances in Workroom Air, pp. 238–239, Cincinnati, Ohio, 1974.
2. Hygienic Guide Series: Sulfur dioxide, Am. Ind. Hyg. Assoc. Q. 16:332, 1955.
3. National Institute for Occupational Safety and Health, U.S. Dept. of Health, Education, and Welfare: Criteria for a Recommended Standard . . . Occupational Exposure to Sulfur Dioxide, U.S. Government Printing Office, Washington, D.C., 1974.
4. Occupational Exposure to Sulfur Dioxide, Federal Register, 40:54520-54534, November 24, 1975.
5. Whittenberger, J. L., and Frank, R. N.: Human exposure to sulfur dioxide, Arch. Environ. Health 7:244, 1963.

Sulfuric Acid

The NIOSH estimates that 200,000 workers are potentially exposed to sulfuric acid in such industries as the manufacture of phosphate fertilizers, storage batteries, household detergents, the pickling of steel and alkylation operations in petroleum and petrochemical manufacture. Occupational exposures are by inhalation and skin contact.

Sulfuric acid mist is a severe irritant to the eyes, respiratory tract and skin. Concentrated sulfuric acid destroys tissue due to its severe dehydrating action whereas the dilute form acts as a milder irritant due to acid properties. The LC_{50} of mist of 1 micron particle size for an 8-hour exposure was 50 mg/m^3 for adult guinea pigs and 18 mg/m^3 for young animals. Continual exposure of guinea pigs to 2 mg/m^3 for 5 days caused pulmonary edema and thickening of the alveolar walls; exposure of guinea pigs to 2 mg/m^3 for 1 hour caused an increase in pulmonary airway resistance from reflex bronchoconstriction. A worker sprayed in the face with liquid fuming sulfuric acid suffered skin burns of the face and body as well as pulmonary edema from inhalation. Sequelae were pulmonary fibrosis, residual bronchitis and pulmonary emphysema; in addition, necrosis of the skin resulted in marked scarring. In human subjects, concentrations of about 5 mg/m^3 were objectionable, usually causing cough, with an increase in respiratory rate and impairment of ventilatory capacity. Workers exposed to concentrations of 12.6–35 mg/m^3 had a markedly higher incidence of erosion and discoloration of teeth than was noted in unexposed individuals. Splashed in the eyes, the concentrated acid causes extremely severe damage, often leading to blindness, whereas dilute acid produces more transient effects from which recovery may be complete. Repeated exposure of workers to the mist causes chronic conjunctivitis, tracheobronchitis, stomatitis and dermatitis. Although ingestion of the liquid is unlikely in ordinary industrial use, the highly corrosive nature of the substance may be expected to produce serious mucous membrane burns of the mouth and esophagus.

Common symptoms and signs are: eye, nose and throat irritation, bronchitis and pulmonary edema. Prolonged exposure may cause conjunctivitis, stomatitis, dental erosion, tracheobronchitis and dermatitis; skin and eye burns result from splashes. Urinary sulfates may go up 10 times after very high levels of exposures, although urinary levels vary greatly.

TREATMENT.—Remove from exposure and immediately flush the eyes and skin with water. Consideration should be given to hospitalization and observation for the delayed onset of pulmonary edema.

The NIOSH has concluded that adherence to the present federal standard of 1 mg/m^3 (in air), in conjunction with a strong program of good work practices, will protect workers from sulfuric acid exposure for up to a 10-hour workday, 40-hour workweek over a "working lifetime."

REFERENCES

Sulfuric Acid

1. Amdur, M. O., et al.: Toxicity of sulfuric acid mist to guinea pigs, A.M.A. Arch. Ind. Hyg. 5:318, 1952.
2. American Conference of Governmental Industrial Hygienists: Sulfuric Acid. Documentation of the Threshold Limit Values for Substances in Workroom Air, 3d ed., Cincinnati, Ohio, pp. 239–240, 1974.
3. Grant, W. M.: *Toxicology of the Eye* (2d ed.; Springfield, Ill.: Charles C Thomas, Publisher, 1974), pp. 959–960.
4. National Institute for Occupational Safety and

Health, U.S. Department of Health, Education, and Welfare: Criteria for a Recommended Standard . . . Occupational Exposure to Sulfuric Acid. HEW Publication No. (NIOSH) 74-128, U.S. Government Printing Office, Washington, D.C., 1974.

o-Tolidine

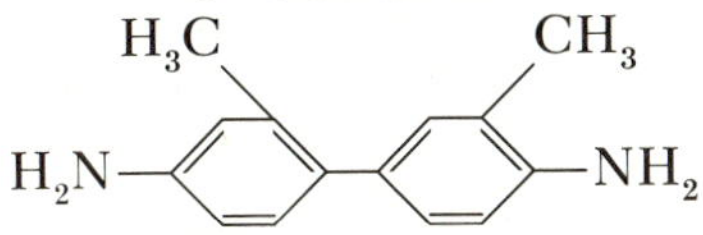

o-Tolidine (3,3′-dimethyl, 4,4′-diamino diphenyl) is a crystalline solid. *o*-Tolidine is used both as a dye and as an intermediate in the production of other dyes. It is widely used in small quantities as a laboratory analytic reagent and is a moiety of the commonly used biologic stain trypan blue. *o*-Tolidine is used in small quantities in chlorine test kits by water companies and swimming pool owners and in test tapes in clinical laboratories. Although other chemicals are preferred, *o*-tolidine has been used as a curing agent for urethane resins, in part because some of the other curing agents, e.g., 4,4′-methylene bis (2-chloraniline) (MOCA), were proposed for stringent regulation as carcinogens.

The major U.S. manufacturer of *o*-tolidine makes an average of 100,000 kg of *o*-tolidine salts, e.g., hydrochloride, each year. Smaller quantities are produced by other companies. U.S. production data on *o*-tolidine base are not available. Many chemical companies buy *o*-tolidine in bulk from other, principally foreign, manufacturers, repackage it and sell it in smaller units; sometimes they refine it. About 150,000 kg of *o*-tolidine base and 100,000 kg of *o*-tolidine salts are imported annually.

Workers potentially exposed to *o*-tolidine are: analytical chemistry workers, artists, chemical distributors, dye makers, forest service chemists, glucose diagnostic tape makers, leather dye workers, medical laboratory workers, organic chemists, *o*-tolidine makers, sanitarians, sewage treatment plant workers, swimming pool test kit makers, swimming pool service personnel, textile dryers, toluene diisocyanate makers, urethane curers and waterworks attendants. Workers exposed to the greatest amounts of *o*-tolidine probably are dye makers, toluene diisocyanate makers, clinical or analytical chemistry laboratory workers and repackagers. Workers in a variety of occupations may be exposed to small quantities of *o*-tolidine for analytic purposes, among them water and sewage plant attendants, sanitarians, forest service chemists, swimming pool service representatives and chemical test tape or kit makers. It is estimated that less than 100 employees are exposed to large quantities of *o*-tolidine in the United States, but as many as 200,000 may be exposed to small quantities.

Inhalation and skin absorption are main routes of entry. *o*-Tolidine absorption, whether from inhalation of the vapor or by skin absorption of the liquid, causes anoxia due to the formation of methemoglobin and hematuria. The earliest manifestations of poisoning in humans are headache and cyanosis of the lips, mucous membranes, the fingernail beds and the tongue. As the lack of oxygen increases there is growing weakness, dizziness and drowsiness, leading to stupor, unconsciousness and even death if treatment is not prompt. Transient microscopic hematuria has been observed in *o*-tolidine workers, presumably of renal origin, since no alterations in the bladder mucosa were observed by cystoscopy. In the eye of a rabbit, the liquid caused a severe burn. Excessive drying of the skin may result from repeated or prolonged contact.

TREATMENT.—Any *o*-tolidine on the body must be removed, including immediate removal of contaminated clothing, including shoes, washing of the entire body with plenty of soap or mild detergent and water. Shampoo the hair and scalp, clean fingernails and toenails, clean nostrils and ear canals. Give oxygen. Hospitalization is recommended. Determine methemoglobin in blood and repeat every 3–6 hours for 18–24 hours. Repeat shower and skin cleansing if methemoglobin appears to rise after 3–4 hours. Consideration may be given to the intravenous administration of methylene blue at high levels of methemoglobin in an attempt to accelerate the conversion of methemoglobin; however, the use of this agent is controversial because of its toxic effects.

REFERENCES

o-*Tolidine*

1. American Conference of Governmental Industrial Hygienists: "*o*-Tolidine." Documentation of the Threshold Limit Values for Substances in Workroom Air, 3d ed., Cincinnati, Ohio, pp. 261–262, 1974.
2. Mangelsdorff, A. F.: Treatment of methemoglobinemia, A.M.A. Arch. Ind. Hyg. 14:148, 1956.
3. Manufacturing Chemists Association, Inc.: Chemical Safety Data Sheet DS-82, *o*-Tolidine, Washington, D.C., pp. 13–14, 1961.
4. National Institute for Occupational Safety and Health: Criteria for a Recommended Standard . . . Occupational Exposure to *o*-Tolidine. U.S. Dept. of Health, Education, and Welfare, PHS, Center for Disease Control, NIOSH, 1978.

Trimellitic Anhydride (TMA)

TMA is used as a curing agent for epoxy and other resins, in vinyl plasticizers, paints and coatings, polymers, polyesters, agricultural chemicals, dyes and pigments, pharmaceuticals, surface-active agents, modifiers, intermediates and specialty chemicals. The NIOSH estimates that approximately 20,000 American workers currently are at risk of exposure to TMA in its various applications. The sole domestic producer of TMA is Amoco Chemicals Corporation, which has a 50-million-pound-per-year plant at Joliet, Illinois.

The National Institute for Occupational Safety and Health (NIOSH) recommends that TMA be handled as an extremely toxic agent in the workplace. Exposure to this compound may result in noncardiac pulmonary edema (apparently without benefit of a pulmonary irritation warning), immunologic sensitization and irritation of the pulmonary tract, eyes, nose and skin. There is no current Occupational Safety and Health Administration (OSHA) exposure standard for TMA. The Amoco Chemicals Corporation, the producer, suggests a limit of "0.05 mg/m^3 or less for susceptible individuals."[1]

HUMAN TOXICITY

The ability of TMA to cause pulmonary edema (lungs) has been reported by Rice et al.[5] Two workers who had been employed by the same company for only a short period (3 and 6 weeks) received multiple inhalation exposures to an epoxy resin containing TMA when it was sprayed on heated pipes. The levels of TMA were not available to the authors. No mention was made of severe irritation of the upper respiratory tract while the workers were receiving their exposures, suggesting little or no warning of subsequent damage to the lungs. The possibility that the pulmonary edema was the result of a hypersensitivity reaction therefore must be considered. Resins can be sensitizers (e.g., toluene diisocyanate or TDI), although most of the reported effects have been those of direct irritation.[4]

Sensitization to TMA was noted by Zeiss

et al.[6] Respiratory symptoms were observed in 14 workers employed in the synthesis of TMA. The authors suggest three distinct syndromes induced by inhalation of TMA. The first, rhinitis and/or asthma, developed over an industrial exposure period of weeks to years. After this period, the sensitized worker exhibited symptoms immediately following exposure to TMA dust or fumes, which abated after the work exposure had stopped. The second syndrome, termed "TMA flu" by the workers, also required a sensitization period of exposure and was characterized by delayed onset, cough, wheezing and labored breathing starting 4–8 hours after a work shift and peaking at night. These respiratory symptoms usually were accompanied by malaise, chills, fever, muscle and joint aches and appeared to be associated with relatively high exposures to TMA during particular work shifts. The third syndrome, which followed initial high exposure to TMA, was primarily an irritant effect. It was characterized by a "running" nose without itching or sneezing, occasional nosebleed, cough, labored breathing and occasional wheezing. Symptoms usually abated after 8 hours and rarely lasted into the night.

The above studies suggest harmful respiratory effects of TMA at relatively high concentrations, but even at lower concentrations, some workers may develop an immunologic sensitization over a period of time.

Fawcett et al.[2] also observed sensitization in a worker exposed to TMA in the production of tubular steel shop fittings coated with an epoxy resin. The chemical agent responsible for asthma symptoms of 6 workers was identified by careful inhalation challenge testing simulating work exposure. Typical attacks that began 1 year after onset of TMA exposure consisted of cough and breathlessness, lasting for 30 minutes, which subsided, only to be followed the same evening by sneezing, which persisted for about 24 hours. Subsequent attacks were prevented by avoiding exposure.

Data on occupational exposures to TMA were also obtained during a NIOSH Health Hazard Evaluation of a paint and varnish company during the manufacture of an epoxy paint.[3] The Health Hazard Evaluation was conducted at the request of employees who were concerned about possible harmful effects of TMA exposure during processing and decontamination operations. The occupational airborne exposure levels averaged 1.5 mg/m^3 TMA (with a range from "none detected" to 4.0 mg/m^3) during processing operations and 2.8 mg/m^3 TMA (ranging from "none detected" to 7.5 mg/m^3) during decontamination operations. A total of 13 employees (5 present and 8 former employees) were interviewed and examined briefly. Employees' symptoms and compaints were: eye irritation, nasal irritation, shortness of breath, wheezing, cough, heartburn, nausea, headache, skin irritation and throat irritation. Three of the former workers stated that they had left that department for health reasons. Complaints subsided when non-TMA-containing products were being formulated.

The Occupational Health and Safety Division, Department of Labor, Alberta, Canada, has reported to the NIOSH that they are aware of employee reactions in two plants using TMA-epoxy powder pipe coatings. One plant, started in 1971, had a number of employees with an immediate reaction. After instituting engineering and administrative controls there has been no further incidence. In the second plant, begun in 1974, the first adverse reaction occurred in 1975. There have been 9 cases of adverse reactions reported to date. Most of these employees were kept in intensive care while they recuperated and were advised by their physicians to seek new jobs. However, some returned to their previous jobs and became ill again. Due to the unavailability of a good analytic method for TMA, occupational levels could not be documented until November, 1977. The TMA concentrations found ranged from 0.11 mg/m^3 to 0.27 mg/m^3.

The NIOSH recommends that TMA be handled in the workplace as an extremely toxic substance because it can cause noncardiac pulmonary edema, immunologic sensitization and severe respiratory irritation. Exposure to TMA should be limited to as few employees as possible while minimizing workplace exposure levels. The area in which it is used should be restricted to those employees necessary to the process or operation. Furthermore, consideration should be given to isolating the TMA exposure area so that adjacent workers are not also exposed.

REFERENCES

Trimellitic Anhydride

1. Amoco-Industrial Hygiene Toxicology and Safety Data Sheet, Environmental Health Services, Medical and Health Services Department, July 8, 1976.
2. Fawcett, I. W., Taylor, A. J., and Pepys, J.: Asthma due to inhaled chemical agents-epoxy resin systems containing phthalic acid anhydride, trimellitic acid anhydride and triethylene tetramine, Clin. Allergy 7:1, 1977.
3. National Institute for Occupational Safety and Health, Health Hazard Evaluation Determination, Report No. 74-111-283.
4. Patty, F. A. (ed.): *Industrial Hygiene and Toxicology*, 2d ed. rev., Vol. II (New York: John Wiley & Sons, Inc., Interscience, 1963).
5. Rice, D. L., Jenkins, D. E., Gray, J. M., and Greenberg, S. D.: Chemical pneumonitis secondary to inhalation of epoxy pipe coating, Arch. Environ. Health 32:183, 1977.
6. Zeiss, C. R., Patterson, R., Pruzansky, J. J., Miller, M. M., Rosenberg, M., and Levitz, D.: Trimellitic anhydride-induced airway syndromes: Chemical and immunologic studies, J. Allergy Clin. Immunol. 60:96, 1977.

Tungsten

Tungsten (atomic number 74) is listed in the periodic table under period 6 of the transition elements, along with chromium and molybdenum. Tungsten closely resembles molybdenum in all of its physical and chemical properties. In the pure metallic state, tungsten is gray and has a luster somewhat like that of steel. The commercial tungstate minerals are wolframite ($(Fe,Mn)WO_4$), scheelite ($CaWO_4$), ferberite ($FeWO_4$) and hubnerite ($MnWO_4$). Worldwide, wolframite is the most important ore containing tungsten whereas scheelite is the principal domestic ore. Most tungsten deposits are low grade and are upgraded by concentration techniques. The tungsten concentrates produced contain at least 60% tungstic oxide. The total U.S. consumption of tungsten concentrate in 1975 was 7 million kg, of which 2.5 million kg were domestically produced, 3 million kg were imported primarily from Canada, Thailand, Peru, the People's Republic of China and Portugal and the remainder was released from government stockpiles. In 1975, the United States produced 6 million kg of tungsten products and consumed 6 million kg, including 72.5% in alloys for cutting and wear-resistant materials, 11.5% in mill products from metal powder, 9.2% in steel, 2.9% in superalloys, 2.4% in chemicals and ceramics, 0.03% in cast iron and 1.47% in miscellaneous products.

The principal health hazards from tungsten and its compounds may arise from inhalation of aerosols during mining and milling operations. Compounds of tungsten to which workers are exposed are ammonium-*p*-tungstate, oxides of tungsten (WO_3, W_2O_5, WO_2), metallic tungsten and tungsten carbide. In the production and use of tungsten carbide tools for machining, exposure to the cobalt used as a binder or cementing substance[8, 10] may be the most important hazard to the health of the employees (see Cobalt, this chapter). Since the cemented tungsten carbide industry uses such other metals as tantalum, titanium, niobium, nickel, chromium and vanadium in the manufacturing process, the occupational exposures generally are to mixed dusts. Potential occupational exposures to sodium tungstate are found in the textile industry, where the compound is used as a mordant and fireproofing agent, and in the production of tungsten from some of its ores, where sodium tungstate is an intermediate product. Potential exposures to tungsten and its compounds are also found in the ceramics, lubricants, plastics, printing inks, paint and photographic industries. Some of the occupations with potential exposures to tungsten and its compounds are: alloy makers, carbonyl workers, ceramic workers, cemented tungsten carbide workers, cement makers, dye makers, dyers, flameproofers, high-speed tool steelworkers, incandescent-lamp makers, industrial chemical synthesizers, ink makers, lamp-filament makers, lubricant makers, melting-pouring-casting workers, metal sprayers, ore-refining and foundry workers, pigment makers, papermakers, penpoint makers, petroleum refinery workers, photographic developers, spark plug makers, textile dryers, tool grinders, tungsten and molybdenum miners, waterproofing makers and welders. The NIOSH estimates that at least 30,000 employees in the United States are potentially exposed to tungsten and its compounds, based on actual observations in the National Occupational Hazards Survey.

EFFECTS ON MAN.—Occupational exposures to tungsten and its compounds have been reported to have primary effects on the respiratory system. In the cemented tungsten carbide (hard-metal) industry, exposure to a combination of cobalt and tungsten sometimes has resulted in "hard-metal disease." The pulmonary involvement presented in a number of reports was characterized clinically by upper respiratory tract irritation, coughing, exertional dyspnea and weight loss. As the condition of the workers worsened with prolonged exposure in this environment, extrinsic asthma, diffuse interstitial pneumonitis, fibrosis, pneumoconiosis or combinations of these were evident. Actually, these findings represent two forms of respiratory disease; the first is a type of bronchial asthma and the second a disabling and progressive interstitial fibrosis.[2]

The chief component in the tungsten carbide mixture responsible for cases of respiratory disease is thought to be cobalt, a binder used with the tungsten carbide in the process of its fabrication by power metallurgy. Animal experiments by Harding,[4] Delahant[3] and Schepers[9] indicate that cobalt is the hazardous material. Kerfoot[5] designed an animal inhalation study simulating conditions to which workers in the tungsten carbide industry are exposed in an attempt to define permissible limits of exposure to cobalt metal powder.

Two groups of miniature swine were exposed to an inhalation of pure cobalt metal powder at levels of 0.1 mg/m^3 (present Threshold Limit Value for workers) and 1.0 mg/m^3. Both exposures were carried out for 3 months at 6 hours per day and 5 days per week. Since the pulmonary reactions to cobalt are thought to be mediated through a hypersensitivity mechanism,[1] the animals were first exposed to a sensitization week of cobalt at the exposure level for each group. A 10-day lapse period followed this initial exposure to develop possible sensitized animals, which then were exposed for 3 months. Some of the animals were held in clean air after the exposure period to determine whether any symptoms cleared on removal from the cobalt. These cobalt animals were compared to a control group throughout the study.

A definite increase in collagen was laid down by resident fibroblasts in the central areas of the alveolar septa. The exposure of blood vessels to the alveolar space and thus the oxygen exchange membrane appears relatively free from collagenization. Such focal changes probably have had a beginning functional effect on the lung, especially with respect to compliance, which were manifested in the pulmonary function testing. Therefore, the marked abnormalities in compliance evidenced in the respiratory tests correlate with the findings of the electron microscopic change of increased septal collagen. Kerfoot concluded from this study that the present (1979, dust and fumes as Co) TLV of 0.1 mg/m^3 for cobalt seems to be inadequate.

REFERENCES

Tungsten

1. Bruckner, H. C.: Extrinsic asthma in a tungsten carbide worker, J. Occup. Med. 9:518, 1966.
2. Coates, E. O., and Watson, J. H. L.: Diffuse interstitial lung disease in tungsten carbide workers, Ann. Intern. Med. 75:709, 1971.
3. Delahant, A. B.: An experimental study of the effects of rare metals on animal lungs, A.M.A. Arch. Ind. Hyg. 12:116, 1955.
4. Harding, H. E.: Notes on the toxicology of cobalt metal, Br. J. Ind. Med. 7:76, 1950.
5. Kerfoot, E. J.: Chronic animal inhalation toxicity to cobalt. NIOSH, U.S. Dept. of Health, Education, and Welfare, PHS, Center for Disease Control, Cincinnati, Ohio, Contract No. HSM 099-71-19, 1973.
6. Materials Survey—Tungsten. Springfield, Va., U.S. Dept. of Commerce, National Technical Information Service, 126 pp. (NTIS PB 242 220), 1956.
7. NIOSH Criteria for a Recommended Standard . . . Occupational Exposure to Tungsten and Cemented Tungsten Carbide. U.S. Dept. of Health, Education, and Welfare, PHS, Center for Disease Control, DHEW (NIOSH) Publication No. 77-127, September, 1977.
8. Plant observation reports and evaluation. Menlo Park, Calif., SRI International, 150 pp. (submitted to NIOSH under contract No. CDC-99-75-31), March, 1977.
9. Schepers, G. W. H.: The biological action of particulate cobalt metal, tantalum oxide, cobalt oxide, tungsten metal, tungsten carbide, and carbon tungsten carbide and cobalt, A.M.A. Arch. Ind. Hyg. 12:121, 1955.
10. Tungsten, in Fairhall, L. T.: *Industrial Toxicology* (Baltimore: Williams & Wilkins, 1957), pp. 128–129.

Vinyl Acetate

Vinyl acetate, $CH_3COOCH{=}CH_2$, is a colorless, flammable liquid at room temperature with a vapor pressure of 100 mm Hg at 21.5° C. Initially, its odor is pleasant but quickly becomes sharp and irritating; the threshold of odor detection has been reported to be as low as 1 mg/m^3 (0.284 ppm), but olfactory fatigue has been reported at 19.5 ppm (68.3 mg/m^3). Vinyl acetate is produced by a vapor-phase reaction between ethylene and acetic acid in the presence of a palladium catalyst or between acetylene and acetic acid in the presence of a zinc acetate catalyst. In the United States, 800 million kg of vinyl acetate were produced in 1977. Vinyl acetate is used primarily in polymerization processes to produce polyvinyl acetate, polyvinyl alcohol and vinyl chloride-vinyl acetate copolymer. These polymers, usually made as emulsions, suspensions, solutions or resins, are used to prepare adhesives, paints, paper coatings and textile finishes and low molecular weight polyvinyl acetate is used as a chewing gum base. Vinyl acetate is extremely flammable and forms explosive mixtures at from 2.6% to 13.4% by volume in air. Occupational exposure to vinyl acetate may occur in any work involving the production, storage, transport or use. Occupations with potential exposure to vinyl acetate are: chemical synthesis workers, equipment cleaners, equipment repairers, maintenance workers, monomer-containing-aerosol producers, monomer loaders and unloaders, monomer production workers, monomer samplers and gagers, monomer transport workers, polymer compounders, polymer fabricators, polymer loaders and unloaders, polymer packagers, polymer processors, polymer production workers, polymer transport workers, quality-control laboratory workers and warehouse workers. The NIOSH estimates that approximately 70,000 workers work with vinyl acetate in the United States.

Exposure to vinyl acetate occurs primarily via inhalation of the vapor and contact of the liquid or vapor with the skin and eyes. In humans, exposure to vinyl acetate vapor at lower concentrations (68.3–75.6 mg/m^3) has resulted in reversible eye and upper respiratory irritation.[7, 12] Dermal exposure to the liquid may result in irritation of the skin.[7, 13] Vinyl acetate was lethal[13] to all (presumably 6) rats exposed for 2 hours at 28,000 mg/m^3, and 4-hour LC_{50}s for exposed rats, guinea pigs, mice and rabbits[5, 12] ranged from 5411 to 21,753 mg/m^3. No pathologic data were reported for the animals that died from these exposures.[5, 12, 13] The one beagle exposed[12] to vinyl acetate at 13,388 mg/m^3 and all of the rats exposed[13] at 3500 mg/m^3 survived. Upper respiratory difficulty, eye and nose irritation and increased macrophages in the lungs were noted in rats exposed at 7000 mg/m^3 periodically for 3 weeks.[8] Deese and Joyner[7] found that each of 3 persons exposed to vinyl acetate at 75.6 mg/m^3 experienced hoarseness or coughing and eye irritation; 1 person became hoarse when exposed at about 15 mg/m^3. Ocular effects have also been reported from contact with airborne vinyl acetate. Exposure to vinyl acetate at 840 mg/m^3 caused some eye blinking and reddening of the sclerae in a dog,[12] 651 mg/m^3 caused eye irritation and tearing in dogs[11] and 0.5 ml of vinyl acetate caused severe irritation or mild burns when applied to a rabbit's eye.[13] The lowest concentration that caused eye irritation in humans[7] (1 of 3 subjects) was 20.0 mg/m^3. Two reports[7, 13] suggested that skin irritation can result in humans after dermal contact with (presumably liquid) vinyl acetate. One report[13] noted that this irritation might result in blisters. Deese and Joyner[7] reported that skin irritation or rash was noted by 3 of 31 vinyl acetate workers. Union Carbide investigators[13] reported that the dermal LC_{50} in rabbits was greater than 5 ml/kg in a 24-hour covered-skin contact test with liquid vinyl acetate, but they also stated that undiluted vinyl acetate on the skin of the shaved abdomen of a rabbit caused no reaction. Evidence of possible adverse effects of vinyl acetate on the human nervous system is meager. Gofmekler[10] found that 0.32 mg/m^3 was the minimal concentration of vinyl acetate capable of inducing EEG desynchronization as a conditioned response; 0.21 mg/m^3 did not produce this effect. Goeva[9] found that rats given vinyl acetate in oral doses of 0.1 mg/kg for 7 months exhibited fewer positive responses to a conditioned stimulus and took longer to develop conditioned reflexes than either controls or rats fed 0.01 mg/kg of vinyl acetate. It is questionable whether these particular studies[9, 10] demonstrated adverse changes, so it does not now seem appropriate to conclude that vinyl acetate exposure in the work environment at these concentrations will induce biologically significant effects on the nervous system. The readily identifiable odor of vinyl acetate appears to be one means by which workers are warned of its presence in the work environment. Determinations of the threshold of odor detection have given varying results. For example, Deese and Joyner[7] reported that all of 3 subjects detected a marked odor of vinyl acetate at 75.6 mg/m^3; a "slight" odor was reported by 3 of 4 exposed at 14.7 and 1.4 mg/m^3. In an experimental study,[12] all of 9 volunteers detected the odor of vinyl acetate at 4.6 mg/m^3 but, with one questionable exception, they did not detect its odor at 2.1 mg/m^3. Minimal perceptible (threshold) and maximal imperceptible concentrations for odor detection were determined by Gofmekler[10] to be 1.0 and 0.7 mg/m^3, respectively. These findings indicate that the odor threshold of vinyl acetate probably ranges from 1.0 to 3.3 mg/m^3; their variability probably reflects differences in methods of determination and possibly in the development by the test subjects of adaptation to the odor. Although a noticeable odor of vinyl acetate may indicate a potential hazard, it is not quantitatively reliable. Olfactory fatique has also been observed during exposure to vinyl acetate. Vinyl acetate at 68.3–250.3 mg/m^3 produced olfactory fatigue in all exposed volunteers.[12] Olfactory fatigue was complete in all of 3 persons exposed at 68.3 mg/m^3 and in 1 of 3 at 119.7 mg/m^3 after 3–116 minutes; 2 of 3 subjects at the latter concentration and all of 4 at 250.3 mg/m^3 experienced partial olfactory fatigue.

A Threshold Limit Value (TLV) of 10 ppm or 30 mg/m^3 was recommended by the Threshold Limits Committee of the American Conference of Governmental Industrial Hygienists (ACGIH)[3] in 1969 and adopted[4] in 1971. A Short-Term Exposure Limit (STEL) of 20 ppm or 60 mg/m^3 was recommended[2] in 1976. The Documentation of Threshold Limit Values[1] noted 4-hour LC_{50} values in rats, mice and rabbits of 4000, 1550 and 2500 ppm, respectively. No evidence of circulatory abnormalities or evidence of altered metabolism was noted in dogs exposed 6 hours per day to vinyl acetate for about 11 weeks at average concentrations of from 91 to 186 ppm. The documentation stated that Gage[8] had found rats unaffected by repeated exposures at 100 ppm and had recommended 50 ppm as a working standard. The documentation also noted a report of 15 years' industrial experience with 21 vinyl acetate chemical operators in whom hoarseness and coughing ("slight irritation") were observed at around 22 ppm. The medical records and multiphasic examinations were stated to have revealed no evidence of chronic effects from concentrations of 5–10 ppm. The Threshold Limits Committee recommended a TLV of 10 ppm, citing the evidence that irritation may be experienced at around 20 ppm but not at 10 ppm and in the light of evidence that neither acute nor chronic effects occur from repeated daily exposure for many years.[2] Australia, Belgium, Finland, the Netherlands, Sweden and Switzerland have maximal allowable concentrations (MACs) for vinyl acetate of 10 ppm, or 30 mg/m^3. The MAC for vinyl acetate in the USSR, Poland and Yugoslavia is 10 mg/m^3 (2.8 ppm). The Rumanian limits consist of average and maximal vinyl acetate concentrations of 50 and 100 mg/m^3 (14 and 28 ppm), respectively. The ILO report noted that MACs or ceiling values are used because time-weighted averages (TWAs) should not be applied to fast-acting substances, e.g., irritants and narcotics, or to substances that are particularly toxic. There is no current U.S. federal occupational standard for vinyl acetate.

REFERENCES

Vinyl Acetate

1. American Conference of Governmental Industrial Hygienists, Committee on Threshold Limit Values: Documentation of Threshold Limit Values for Substances in Workroom Air, 3d ed., 1971. Cincinnati, Ohio, ACGIH, 2d printing, pp. 276–277, 1974.
2. American Conference of Governmental Industrial Hygienists: TLVs—Threshold Limit Values for Chemical Substances in Workroom Air Adopted by ACGIH for 1976. Cincinnati, Ohio, ACGIH, p. 30, 1976.
3. American Conference of Governmental Industrial Hygienists: Threshold Limit Values of Airborne Contaminants and Intended Changes Adopted by ACGIH for 1969. Cincinnati, Ohio, ACGIH, p.18, 1969.
4. American Conference of Governmental Industrial Hygienists: Threshold Limit Values of Airborne Contaminants and Physical Agents with Intended Changes Adopted by ACGIH for 1971. Cincinnati, Ohio, ACGIH, p.27, 1971.
5. Carpenter, C. P., Smyth, H. F., Jr., and Pozzani, U. D.: The assay of acute vapor toxicity, and the grading and interpretation of results on 96 chemical compounds, J. Ind. Hyg. Toxicol. 31:343, 1949.
6. Criteria for a Recommended Standard . . .

Occupational Exposure to Vinyl Acetate, DHEW (NIOSH) Publication No. 78-205. Cincinnati, Ohio, U.S. Dept. of Health, Education, and Welfare, PHS, Center for Disease Control, National Institute for Occupational Safety and Health, 78 pp., 1978.

7. Deese, D. E., and Joyner, R. E.: Vinyl acetate. A study of chronic human exposure, Am. Ind. Hyg. Assoc. J. 30:449, 1969.
8. Gage, J. C.: The subacute inhalation toxicity of 109 industrial chemicals, Br. J. Ind. Med. 27:1, 1970.
9. Goeva, O. E.: Maximum permissible concentration of vinyl acetate in water basins, Hyg. Sanit.(USSR) 31:209, 1966.
10. Gofmekler, V. A.: Maximum admissible concentration of acetates in the atmosphere, Gig. Sanit. 25:9, 1960 (Russian).
11. Report of Toxicity of Vinyl Acetate. Unpublished report submitted to American Conference of Governmental Industrial Hygienists by E. I. du Pont de Nemours & Co., Inc., Central Research and Development Dept., Haskell Laboratory for Toxicology and Industrial Medicine, 7 pp., January, 1967.
12. Summary of Responses of Animals and Humans to the Vapors of Vinyl Acetate. Unpublished report submitted to American Conference of Governmental Industrial Hygienists by Carnegie-Mellon University, Mellon Institute, Pittsburgh, Pa., 3 pp., October, 1968.
13. Toxicology Studies—Vinyl Acetate HQ. New York, Union Carbide Corporation, Industrial Medicine and Toxicology Dept., 2 pp., 1958.

Welding and Metal Fumes

Metal fumes are formed by condensation, evaporation and oxidation of metals in air, emanating from high-temperature processes such as brazing, soldering, oxyacetylene cutting, welding (electric and gas), heat treating, metallizing and making iron and steel refining metals from ores and scraps in foundries, especially during the melting and pouring. Potential exposures range from soldering on electronic assembly lines to that of furnace tenders, foundry workers, including molders, crane operators, laborers and others assigned to work in the immediate work areas. Scrap workers are particularly prone to exposure, as the emission of metal fumes (and smoke) depends on the quality of the scrap that is handled. During cutting and welding, lead and zinc fumes are unexpectedly encountered from galvanized and painted scrap metal, with pyrolysis of grease, oil, plastics and rubber contributing to workplace contamination and occupational exposures (Fig 14–8). Decomposition of the organic ingredients in foundry molds and cores (cereal binders, coal and various other materials) produces complex organic compounds, including polyaromatic hydrocarbons. Fumes, as well as gases produced by welding and gas (torch) cutting, must be controlled to prevent health risks to workers. Depending on the metals, rods, fluxes and their alloying constituents, contaminants may be carbon monoxide, carbon dioxide, fluorides, phosgene, phosphine, oxides of nitrogen and ozone. It must be recognized that not all of these substances are present simultaneously. The metal oxides formed, often as fumes, can be aluminum, beryllium, cadmium, chromium, cobalt, copper, fluorides, iron, lead, manganese,

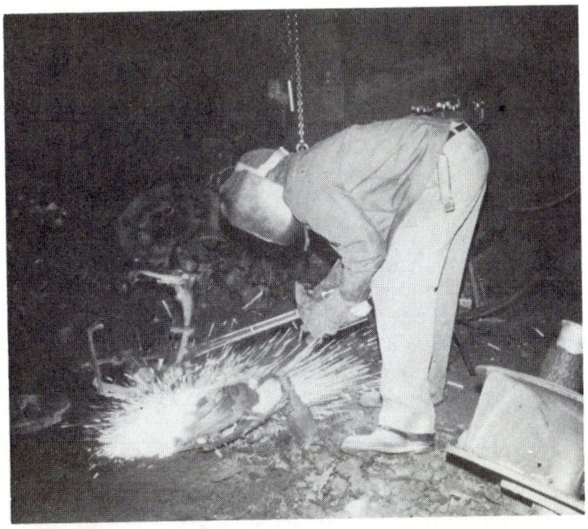

Fig 14–8.—Oxyacetylene torch cutting in a foundry.

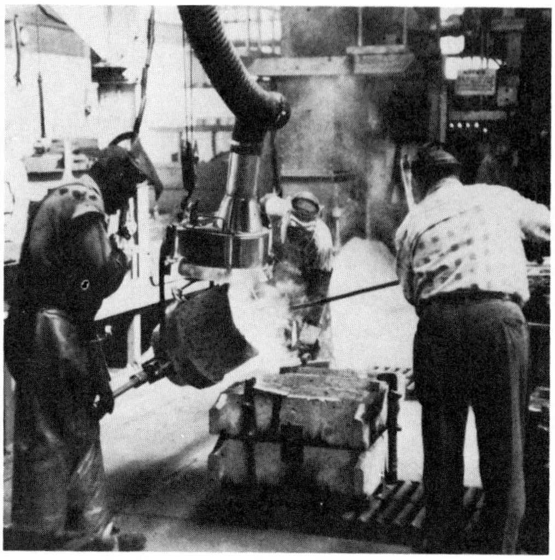

Fig 14–9.—Exhaust hood and flexible duct over ladle of molten metal (nonferrous alloy) effectively capturing fumes.

magnesium, molybdenum, nickel, titanium, tungsten, vanadium, zinc, zirconium and others.

Tossavainen[2] analyzed airborne metal fumes in 36 Finnish foundries (10 steel, 15 iron and 11 copper alloy), finding that airborne concentrations of lead, copper and zinc during metal and casting could present a health hazard when iron or steel scrap is melted in induction or electric (arc) furnaces and when copper alloy castings are melted, poured or ground. Enclosing furnaces, removing fumes during pouring and casting with local exhaust (Fig 14–9) and good general ventilation can reduce or prevent exposures.[1] See sections on Cobalt, Iron Oxide and Hematite, this chapter, for clinical factors related to potential occupational exposures.

REFERENCES

Welding and Metal Fumes

1. Berg, B. A., and Zenz, C.: Clinical and environmental control of lead in nonferrous foundries, J. Am. Ind. Hyg. Assoc. 28:175, 1967.
2. Tossavainen, A.: Metal fumes in foundries, Scand. J. Work Environ. Health 2(Suppl. 1):42, 1976.
3. Virtamo, M., and Tossavainen, A.: Gases formed from furan binding agents, Scand. J. Work Environ. Health 2(Suppl. 1):50, 1976.

General Principles of Treatment

A. For gases such as ammonia, chlorine, hydrofluoric acid, hydrogen sulfide, nitric acid, oxides of nitrogen and sulfur dioxide.

1. The presence of the agent when it is inhaled usually is evanescent and, therefore, cannot be washed away or otherwise removed, i.e., when only the skin is involved.

2. When the patient arrives for treatment, one is faced mainly with the problems caused by the presence of the agent.

3. Arterial blood gases are of primary importance to aid in determination of the extent of damage. Never discharge a patient significantly exposed to irritant gas without obtaining an arterial blood sample.

4. Supportive measures include suctioning (intubation may be required), volume cycle ventilator support (positive and expiratory pressure [PEEP]), steroids and antibiotics, after a culture has been taken. If the eyes are involved, an ophthalmologic consultation is recommended.

B. For gases with delayed action on the lungs.

1. Phosgene may cause severe pulmonary edema, often seen several hours after exposure. Treatment is similar to that for irritant gases described above except that PEEP may be most useful. A unique property of hydrogen sulfide is that it can kill by directly paralyzing the respiratory center within seconds of heavy exposure. Remember that hydrogen sulfide often produces olfactory fatigue, making its presence undetectable to those who have been previously exposed to lesser amounts. Delayed pulmo-

nary edema can occur. Hyperbaric oxygen has proved to be valuable in treatment of hydrogen sulfide poisoning (Kindwall, E. P., St. Luke's Hospital, Milwaukee, Wisconsin, unpublished).

2. Oxides of nitrogen (nitrogen dioxide and nitrogen tetroxide) have a delayed action on the lungs. A worker may be exposed for 8 hours during the day with no ill effects and later, while at home, may lapse into pulmonary edema, which can be fatal. Treatment is as noted above.

Elements of Respiratory Protection (A Summary)

IRWIN MARGOLIS, M.D., JULIAN B. OLISHIFSKI, P.E., and CARL ZENZ, M.D.

Many types of respirators are used for protection against a variety of conditions that may be encountered in different work activities. Each has a particular field of application and limitations from the viewpoint of protection, as well as advantages and disadvantages from the viewpoint of operational procedures and maintenance. Ordinarily, "respirators" are not intended to constitute "first-line defense" against hazardous materials but rather to offer a worker temporary protection. The most effective control measures must be built on engineering principles, described previously and shown in the figures throughout this chapter.

The conditions to be protected against range from those that are mainly a nuisance, as odor or mild "irritation," to those that are immediately dangerous to life. The hazard may be due to one or more toxic contaminants or to an atmosphere deficient in oxygen. The contaminants may be in the gaseous or particulate state or in combination. Protection may be needed for only minutes, as in rescue operations, or for several hours, i.e., for "sand blasting" (Fig 14–10) or paint spraying.

Respirators generally fall in the following classifications: (a) atmosphere-supplying respirators, (b) air-purifying respirators (gas and vapor [gas mask and chemical cartridge], particulate [dust, fog, fumes, mist, smoke and sprays] and combination gas, vapor and particulate) and (c) combination atmosphere-supplying and air-purifying respirators (Figs 14–11 through 14–13).

It is the responsibility of the employer to provide a respiratory protection program meeting established requirements. The employer must provide respirators, ensure that employees use the respirators in a proper manner when wearing of respirators is required and must ensure that employees are properly instructed in the use of respirators assigned to their use and to test for leakage, proper fit and proper operation. The employer must provide a program of cleaning, sanitizing, inspecting, maintaining, repairing and storing of respirators to ensure that employees are provided with clean respirators in good operating condition.

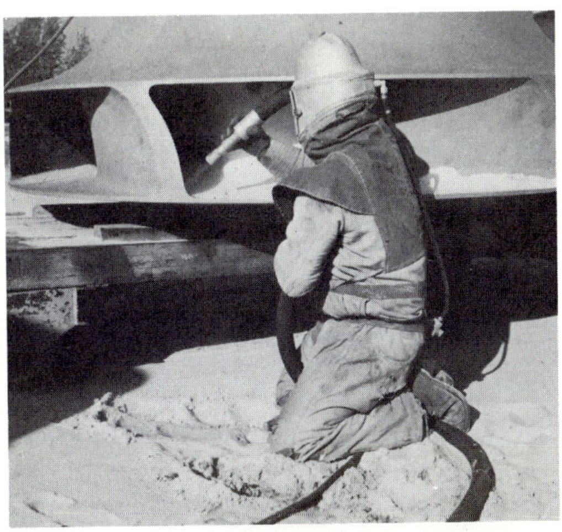

Fig 14–10.—Sandblasting an impeller. Note large amount of silica (sand) used.

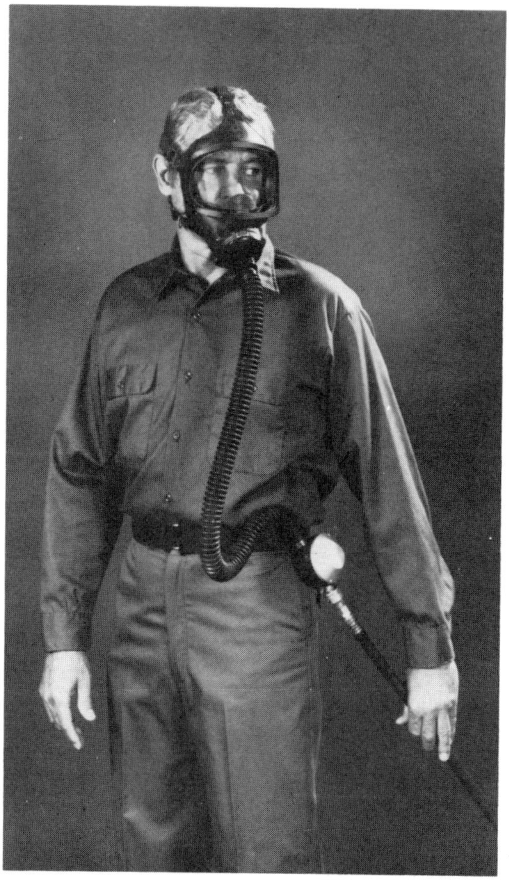

Fig 14–11.—A demand-flow airline respirator with belt-mounted regulator, used with hose to an approved respirable compressed air source, up to 100 meters. (Courtesy of Mine Safety Appliance Co.)

Requirements for approval of many types of respirators have been established by the Secretary of the Interior and the Secretary of Health, Education, and Welfare and are published as Title 30, Code of Federal Regulations, Part II (30 CFR 11).[13]

An air-purifying respirator for protection against particulates is equipped with a mechanical filter designed to remove particulate matter from the inspired air by capture on the filter, usually a fibrous pad (Fig 14–14). These respirators consist of a soft, resilient, full, half or quarter mask facepiece to which is attached one or two filters through which the inspired air is drawn. Check valves, present in most mechanical-filter respirators, prevent exhaled breath from passing through the filters and allow it to be forced out through an exhalation valve in the facepiece to the surrounding atmosphere. The facepiece is held securely to the wearer's face by the head harness or headband.

The useful life of the mechanical filters is limited by the build-up of resistance to inhalation as the contaminant is removed by the filter. The higher the concentration of contaminant in the air drawn into the filter, and the greater the wearer's requirement for ventilation when using a nonpowered respirator, the more rapidly the resistance to inhalation increases. The requirement for ventilation depends on several variables. The most obvious is the amount of energy a worker is expending. This is a function of the task performed, the position in which it is performed and other external stresses, such as heat and humidity, that the worker

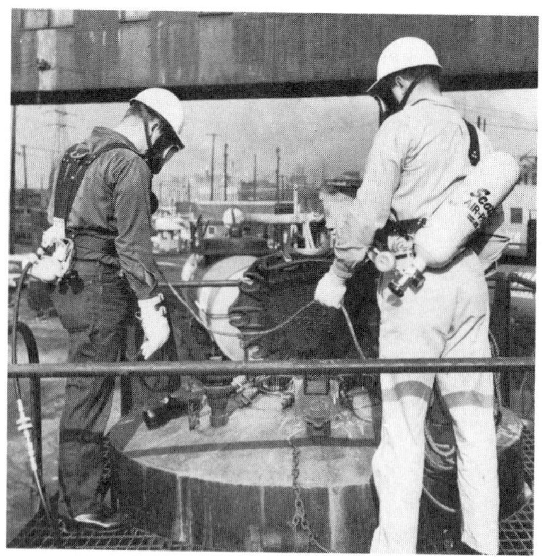

Fig 14–12.—Examples of emergency respirators. The airline respirator has an auxiliary air supply to allow escape in case the line should break.

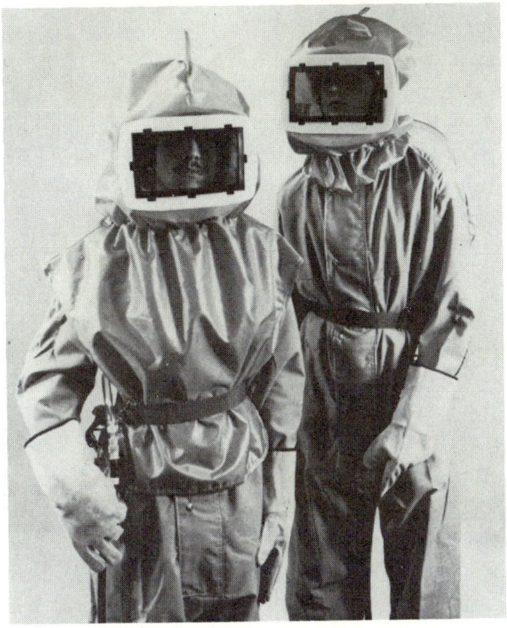

Fig 14–13.—Continuous supplied-air respirators affording full face, head and neck protection. Useful during paint spraying, chemical handling, bagging, buffing, grinding, sandblasting, pesticide applying, etc. (Courtesy of E. D. Bullard Co.)

is subjected to during the performance of the task.[10] The resting respiratory ventilation of a worker depends on body size. It has been thought that women have a lower tidal volume and minute volume ventilation on the basis of sex. This, however, does not seem to be true. Differences in ventilation are related to body size and conditioning rather than to sex. Resting and exercise ventilation studies on normal young women show ventilation to be equivalent to that of males of equal body size. For exposures within threshold limit values, men and women must be considered equally in terms of potential respirable exposures.[5]

A powered air-purifying positive-pressure respirator contains a motor-blower that draws the contaminated air of the workplace through a mechanical filter and discharges it into a facepiece, hood or helmet. The device can be designed to ensure a positive pressure in the facepiece, so that high protection can be achieved. Since leakage through the facepiece seal is reduced and inhalation resistance is eliminated, lower facepiece sealing forces can be used. In addition, the air sweeping through the mask may provide some facial cooling, reducing moisture build-up in the mask. Acceptance of this device by the worker should be higher than that of the conventional air-purifying respirators.

The air supply system for the powered air-purifying respirator may be designed to be worn by a worker or separately mounted with an airline connection to the worker, but this additional weight and bulk may be uncomfortable to some workers. As with the nonpowered air-purifying respiratory devices, the filter service life will depend on the concentration of air contaminant.

The positive-pressure-supplied air respirator is an airline respirator consisting of a half mask or full facepiece to which respirable air is supplied through a small-diameter hose. The airline respirator is the most com-

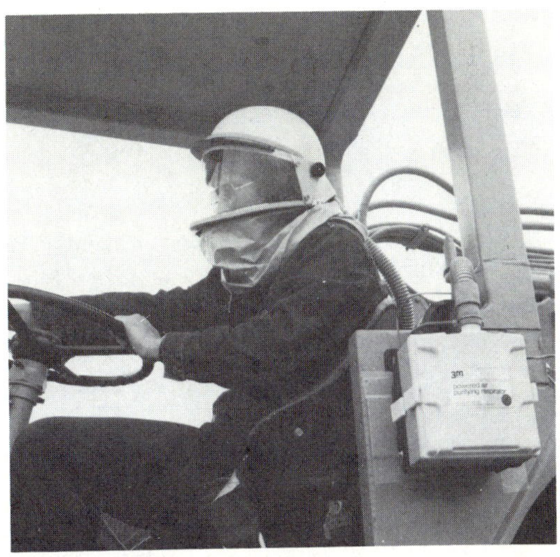

Fig 14–14.—A powered air-purifying helmet, useful in certain jobs, such as pesticide applications in agriculture, forestry and construction work. (Courtesy of 3M Co.)

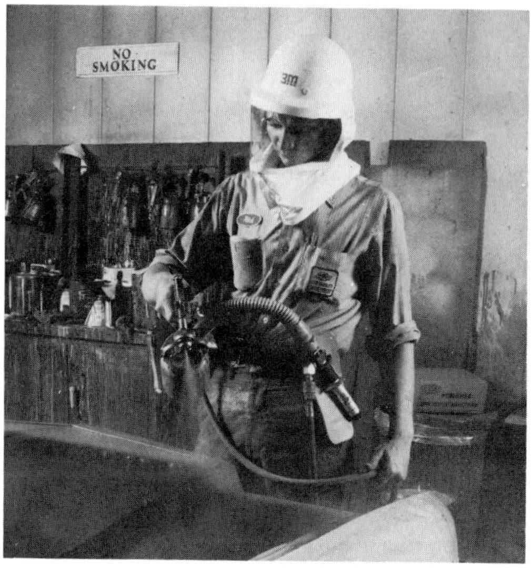

Fig 14–15.—A lightweight air-supplied hood for respiratory protection, useful in many occupations. (Courtesy of 3M Co.)

fortable to wear for prolonged periods, offers little or no resistance to inhalation and the flow of air usually provides a cooling and refreshing effect. The worker supports little weight other than the facepiece and a short connecting hose. A limitation is the necessity for trailing the small-diameter hose connecting the facepiece to the air source, which limits the range of travel (Fig 14–15).

Problems and Precautions

Providing adequately fitting respirators is complicated by the wide range of facial sizes and shapes that must be accommodated because of factors such as age, sex and race. Women have need for smaller-sized face-fitted equipment, as pointed out in Chapter 6. Facial hair, such as beards or sideburns, *makes it difficult to achieve an airtight seal* between the facepiece and the face, particularly with the half-mask type of respirator. Hair stubble resulting from failure to shave daily can cause inward leakage of contaminated air. Therefore, workers who must wear respirators with half or full facepiece should be instructed about the need for regular shaving habits. Even in cool environments, there is a build-up of moisture between the skin and the seal, which may compensate for small amounts of hair growth, and the rubber or plastic seal between the mask and face also improves with time because of gradual conformation of the skin to the edge of the mask.

Most respirators affect workers' visual capabilities. The half mask and the attached elements can appreciably restrict normal downward vision. Diminished vision in the full-face mask may be caused not only by the facepiece but also by the design and placement of the eyepieces. Respiratory protection for individuals wearing safety or corrective glasses may pose certain drawbacks, since the device often rests high on the face, making wearing of glasses uncomfortable. For a full-face mask, a proper face seal may not be established if the temple bars of the eyeglasses extend through the sealing edge. Some full-facepiece designs provide for the mounting of special corrective lenses within the facepiece. Although more expensive, these types are preferred for regular use by workers with need for visual correction.

Speech transmission through a respirator is decreased, annoying and fatiguing to workers. Movements of the jaws in speaking may cause leakage between the facepiece and face, especially with the commonly used half-mask respirator. The worker's comfort and acceptance of the distress caused by wearing a respirator are no less important than the device's effectiveness. These factors, such as improperly fitted respirators and uncomfortable resistance to breathing as a result of increased physical effort on the job (the energy requirements of some heavier jobs result in *respiratory air movement up to 50–60 liters per minute*, which can severely impede air flow), are the major drawbacks to respirator use in the absence of suitable exhaust systems.

Whole-body protective suits (Fig 14–16) significantly increase respiratory work loads,

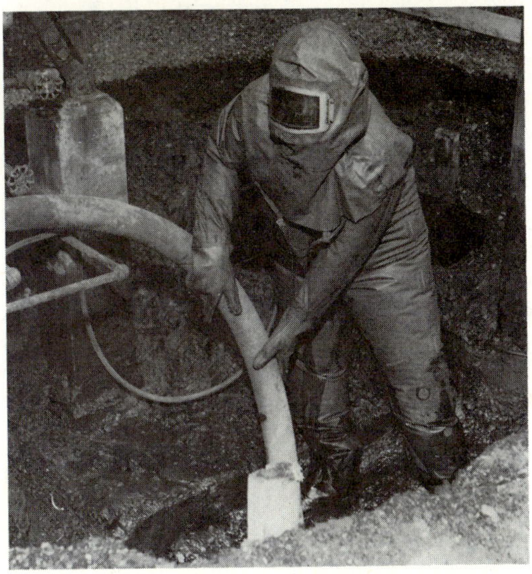

Fig 14–16.—The worker is encased from the neck down in a one-piece suit with integral boots and gloves. His head and shoulders are covered with an airline-fed hood. Fabric is butyl-covered cotton.

altering cardiorespiratory and thermoregulatory responses, resulting in early onset of fatigue. When occupational hazards exist, demanding use of such suits or a self-contained breathing apparatus (which can weigh 15 kg or more), submaximal and maximal work performance is greatly reduced and rest pauses are required. Limitations of air supply pose serious risks, especially in firemen and other emergency or rescue workers who must use self-contained breathing devices. These factors were reported by Levy et al.[4] in 1975 and by Raven et al.[10, 11] in 1977 and 1979.

Pulmonary Function Testing in the Conduct of Occupational Health Controls

A most useful technique for the detection of early lung function changes and for assessment of pulmonary function is that procedure termed "spirometry," capable of discerning early changes and identifying obstructive and, to some extent, restrictive lung diseases. Spirometric methodology now has reached a stage where it is practical and efficient for the assessment of subtle and early changes in respiratory function.

The most commonly used test of pulmonary function utilizes the spirogram. This is a volume versus time tracing of a maximal expiratory effort (Fig 14–17). The FEV_1, both as a percentage of predicted and a percentage of the forced vital capacity, is valuable in determining the presence or absence of airway obstruction. Although Congress passed a Medical Device Act in 1976 and, as mentioned earlier in this chapter, a great number of regulatory standards require or recommend "pulmonary function testing," technical concerns such as accuracy and reproducibility, as well as standardization of procedures, are vital if meaningful data are to be obtained. Many types of spirometric devices have been developed, marketed and, indeed, proliferated to measure several parameters of pulmonary function, such as volume versus flow or volume versus time. These devices can vary in ease of use, accuracy, reproducibility, to say nothing of cost. As a minimum, to produce acceptable spirometric results, a mechanical spirometer must be able to measure a volume of at least 7 liters (which can measure approximately 97% of the normal adult population) and be accurate within ±3% (within the physiologic range of variability of subjects who have taken the multiple spirometric test).

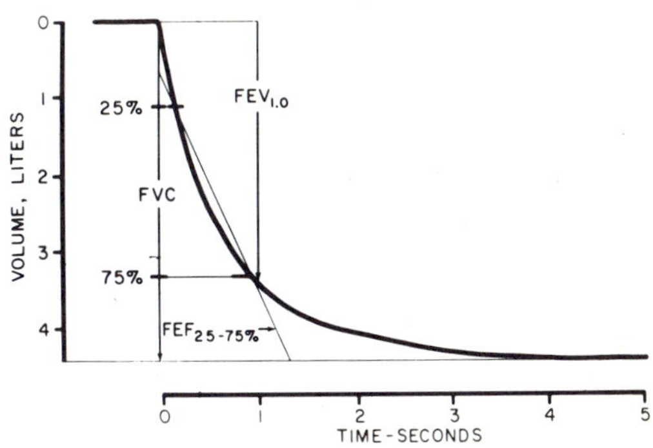

Fig 14–17.—Schematic representation of the basic pulmonary spirogram. (See text for explanation.)

Another important feature of a spirometer is that it must be capable of accepting flow rates of 0–12 liters per second and be able to record data directly for a period of at least 10 seconds. Ease of calibration, stability of calibration, with a minimum of technical failure are necessary. Equally important along with equipment are the skills of the personnel who administer and may interpret test results. Although seemingly simple, the spirogram is effort-dependent (the test subject and, to a limited extent, the technician as well) and requires an experienced technician to ensure a valid and reproducible result. Studies have shown significant improvement in the percentage of satisfactory tests obtained with the number of repetitions of each study done on a subject from 2 to 5 times. The spirogram is only one of many pulmonary function tests and must be interpreted ultimately in light of clinical findings and with the awareness that the interpreter is dealing with a screening situation in most industrial settings.

One can assume that if a worker has only mild airway obstruction, defined as FEV_1/FVC greater than 60%, the worker should have minimal, if any, difficulty in using nondisposable dust, mist, fume and chemical cartridge respirators.

When making recommendations concerning workers' use of positive-pressure respirators, the clinical entities, which may cause problems, include severe or uncontrolled asthma, emphysema (bullous or otherwise) and a history of recurrent pneumothorax. Workers with any of these findings may have a higher risk than expected for barotrauma when using positive-pressure respirators.

In summary, prevention of occupational pulmonary diseases is dependent on recognition of potential hazards in the workplace, minimizing, reducing and eliminating the hazard(s), protecting the worker by engineering controls and other methods, described and illustrated in this and other chapters, medical awareness and assistance in worker selection, education, training and safe placement. Physical examinations, including chest x-rays and pulmonary function tests, must not be relied on to ensure long-term good health of workers but may be used to preselect workers who may be inadvertently exposed to potentially hazardous substances.

Appreciation is given to Ernest M. Dixon, M.D., Lawrence Birkner, M.S., and Frank A. Ubel, M.D., for their assistance.

REFERENCES

Respiratory Protection

1. American Conference of Governmental Industrial Hygienists: *Industrial Ventilation* (14th ed.; Lansing, Mich.: American Conference of Governmental Industrial Hygienists, 1976), pp. 5–1 to 5–116.
2. American National Standards Institution, Inc.: American National Standard Practices for Respiratory Protection, ANSI Z88. 2-1969, New York, 1969.
3. Environmental Monitoring, National Academy of Sciences, Washington, D.C., 1977.
4. Levy, S. A., Margolis, I., and Zenz, C.: Ergonomics study shows effect of full-body suit on energy use, Occup. Health Saf. 45:12, 1976.
5. Margolis, I.: Personal communication. St. Luke's Hospital, Milwaukee, Wisconsin, December, 1978.
6. NIOSH Certified Equipment List: National Institute for Occupational Safety and Health, 4676 Columbia Parkway, Cincinnati, Ohio, July 1, 1978.
7. NIOSH Research Report—Evaluation of two-way valves for respiratory testing. National Institute for Occupational Safety and Health, 4676 Columbia Parkway, Cincinnati, Ohio, December, 1974.
8. NIOSH Research Report—Ventilation requirements for grinding, butting and polishing operations, No. 75-107. National Institute for Occupational Safety and Health, 1974.

9. Olishifski, J. B. (ed).: *Fundamentals of Industrial Hygiene* (2d ed; Chicago: National Safety Council, 1979).
10. Raven, P. B., Dodson, A., and Davis, T. O.: Stresses involved in wearing PVC supplied-air suits: A review, Am. Ind. Hyg. Assoc. J. 40:592, 1979.
11. Raven, P. B., et al.: Maximal stress test performance while wearing a self-contained breathing apparatus, J. Occup. Med. 19:802, 1977.
12. Ulfvarson, U.: Statistical evaluation of the results of measurements of occupational exposure to air contaminants: A suggested method of dealing with short-period samples taken during one whole shift when noncompliance with occupational health standards is being determined, Scand. J. Work Environ. Health 3:109, 1977.
13. U.S. Department of Labor, Occupational Safety and Health Administration, Occupational Safety and Health Standards: General Industry Safety and Health Regulations, Part 1910, June 27, 1974.
14. White, T., Schultz, A., and Lundgren, K-M.: Effects of a welding helmet and dust respirators on respiration at rest and during exercise, Scand. J. Work Environ. Health 1:249, 1975.

APPENDIX

A Summary of NIOSH Recommendations for Occupational Health Standards

SUBSTANCE, AGENT OR ENVIRONMENTAL FACTORS	MAIN USES, SOURCES AND POTENTIAL OCCUPATIONAL EXPOSURES, I.E., INHALATION (I), SKIN CONTACT (S), SKIN ABSORPTION (SA), ORAL (O)	NIOSH CHIEF HEALTH EFFECTS CONSIDERED
Acetylene $HC=CH$	Oxyacetylene welding, cutting and soldering; has been used as illuminating gas; the manufacture of acetaldehyde, acetic acid and as a fuel additive for certain engines (I)	Indirect asphyxia
Acrylamide $CH_2=CHCONH_2$	Used in making polymers and in papermaking flocculating processes; soil stabilizer; waterproofing (I), (S)	Skin, eye and nervous system effects
Acrylonitrile $CH_2=CHCN$	Chemical intermediate to make organic products such as certain pesticides; as fumigants; making acrylic fibers (I)	Lung and bowel cancer
Aldrin/dieldrin	Insecticide (I), (SA), (O)	Cancer (in animals)
Alkanes $C_5=C_8$	In petroleum products and certain solvents (I), (S), (SA)	Skin and nervous system effects
Allyl chloride $CH_2=CHCH_2Cl$	Used for synthesis of allyl compounds (I), (SA)	Liver, kidney and lung effects
Ammonia NH_3	To make fertilizer, nitric acid; manufacturing explosives; plastics; many chemicals; used as a refrigerant; found in petroleum refining (I), (S)	Airway irritation
Antimony	Compounds such as sulfides used in making rubber and pyrotechnics; an alloying agent with other metals such as lead, copper or tin; chlorides used as coloring agents and catalysts; fluorides used in organic synthesis and pottery manufacture (I), (O)	Skin irritation; lung effects

N.B.: NIOSH TWA recommendations based on up to a 10-hour exposure unless otherwise indicated.

CURRENT OSHA OCCUPATIONAL ENVIRONMENTAL STANDARD	NIOSH RECOMMENDATION FOR OCCUPATIONAL ENVIRONMENTAL EXPOSURE LIMIT	SPECIAL COMMENTS; CLINICAL TESTS, IF AVAILABLE
2500 ppm (10% of lower explosive limit)	No exposure in excess of 2500 ppm (2662 mg/m^3)	Employers to check for and inform employees of contaminants such as arsine and phosphine
0.3 mg/m^3, 8-hr TWA (skin)	0.3 mg/m^3 TWA	Skin and eye contact to be prevented
2 ppm, 8-hr TWA, 10 ppm ceiling (15-minute) (skin)	Not greater than 4 ppm (8.7 mg/m^3) by recommended method	Chest x-ray required. First-aid and medical kits to be available during use. Hazardous liquid, skin. Federal standard promulgated October 3, 1978 (See Chapter 14)
0.25 mg/m^3, 8-hr TWA (skin)	Lowest reliably detectable level; 0.15 mg/m^3 TWA by NIOSH validated method. Skin contact to be prevented	
1000 ppm, 8-hr TWA, pentane; 500 ppm, 8-hr TWA *n*-hexane	350 mg/m^3 TWA (approx. 120 ppm pentane; 100 ppm hexane; 85 ppm heptane; 75 ppm octane. Mixtures to be not greater than 350 mg/m^3 TWA; 1800 mg/m^3 ceiling singly or mixtures (15-minute)	Action level defined as 200 mg/m^3 for these substances
1 ppm, 8-hr TWA	1 ppm TWA (3.1 mg/m^3); 3 ppm ceiling (9.3 mg/m^3) (15-minute)	Urine, blood and pulmonary function testing required
50 ppm, 8-hr TWA	50 ppm ceiling (34.8 mg/m^3) (5-minute)	Hazardous liquid; eye damage
0.5 mg/m^3, 8-hr TWA	0.5 mg/m^3 TWA	Chest x-ray, pulmonary function testing and electrocardiogram required

SUBSTANCE, AGENT OR ENVIRONMENTAL FACTORS	MAIN USES, SOURCES AND POTENTIAL OCCUPATIONAL EXPOSURES, I.E., INHALATION (I), SKIN CONTACT (S), SKIN ABSORPTION (SA), ORAL (O)	NIOSH CHIEF HEALTH EFFECTS CONSIDERED
Arsenic, inorganic As	As fungicides and insecticides; commonly a by-product in copper smelting ores, in certain alloys such as copper and lead and in pigment production; as a rodenticide (I), (SA), (O)	Dermatitis; lung and lymphatic cancer
Benzoyl peroxide $(C_6H_5CO)_2O_2$	Used in curing plastics, bleaching flour and in certain oils (I)	Airway and eye irritation; skin effects
Benzyl chloride $C_6H_5CH_2Cl$	Making benzyl compounds, dyes, resins and perfumes (I), (S)	Irritation; skin and eye effects
Beryllium Be	Alloying in certain electrical products; nonsparking tools (I), (S)	Lung cancer
Boron trifluoride BF_3	As a catalyst; flux for soldering magnesium and as a fumigant (I)	Respiratory system effects
Cadmium Cd	Electroplating; certain engraving processes; batteries; aluminum soldering; an alloying agent in some bearings; deoxidizer in nickel plating (I)	Lung and kidney effects
Carbaryl	Insecticide (I), (SA), (O)	Nervous and reproductive system effects

CURRENT OSHA OCCUPATIONAL ENVIRONMENTAL STANDARD	NIOSH RECOMMENDATION FOR OCCUPATIONAL ENVIRONMENTAL EXPOSURE LIMIT	SPECIAL COMMENTS; CLINICAL TESTS, IF AVAILABLE
10 μg/m³, 8-hr TWA	2 μg As/m³ ceiling (15-minute)	Chest x-rays required. Federal standard promulgated May 5, 1978. Determination may be done on urine (100 ml) or gastric secretion (50 ml) or hair or nails (at least 0.5 gm). Urine may be an indication of recent exposure; hair may be used for past exposure; a first urine sample in the morning may be used for chronic exposure Normal ranges: Urine—0–10 μg/liter 10–100 μg/liter minimal elevation 100–1000 μg/liter chronic elevation 1000 μg/liter acute poisoning Hair—upper limit of 30 μg/100 gm
5 mg/m³, 8-hr TWA	5 mg/m³ TWA	
1 ppm (5 mg/m³), 8-hr TWA	5 mg/m³ ceiling (15-minute)	Chest x-ray and pulmonary function testing required
3 μg/m³, 8-hr TWA; 5 μg/m³ acceptable ceiling; 25 μg/m³ maximal ceiling (30 minutes)	0.5 μg/m³ (130 minutes)	Pulmonary function, chest x-ray and sputum cytology required
1 ppm ceiling	None recommended	Adequate procedures for sampling and analysis not available; pulmonary function testing required
0.1 mg/m³, 8-hr TWA: 0.3 mg/m³ ceiling (fume); 0.2 mg/m³, 8-hr TWA; 0.6 mg/m³ ceiling (dust)	40 μg Cd/m³ TWA; 200 μg Cd/m³ ceiling (15-minute)	Urine and pulmonary function testing required. 50 ml urine or 3 ml whole blood preserved with heparin or EDTA Normal ranges: Urine—0.5–11 μg/liter Blood—0–10 μg/liter normal 10–100 μg/liter—chronic exposure
5 mg/m³, 8-hr TWA	5 mg/m³ TWA	Medical warnings of possible effects on reproductive system and minimal exposure during pregnancy required; skin and eye contact to be prevented (see Chapters 3 and 13)

SUBSTANCE, AGENT OR ENVIRONMENTAL FACTORS	MAIN USES, SOURCES AND POTENTIAL OCCUPATIONAL EXPOSURES, I.E., INHALATION (I), SKIN CONTACT (S), SKIN ABSORPTION (SA), ORAL (O)	NIOSH CHIEF HEALTH EFFECTS CONSIDERED
Carbon black	Pigment in plastics, rubber and other materials; making inks and certain electrical apparatus; as a decolorizing agent (I)	Lung, heart and skin effects
Carbon dioxide CO_2	A by-product of many chemical reactions such as ammonia production, limekiln operations and in fermenting processes (I)	Respiratory effects
Carbon disulfide CS_2	Widely used solvent for oils, resins and waxes; solvent for certain lipids, sulfur, rubber, phosphorus; as an insecticide and used to make rayon fibers (I), (SA)	Heart, nervous and reproductive system effects
Carbon monoxide CO	Common by-product of combustion and in engine exhaust (I)	Heart effects
Carbon tetrachloride CCl_4	Solvent used for fats, oils, lacquers, varnishes; in rubber making and resin production. Has been used as a degreasing and cleaning agent in fire extinguishers (now forbidden) (I), (SA)	Liver cancer in animals
Chlorine Cl	Bleaching agent and synthetic chemical making; sterilization of water supplies and swimming pools; in detinning and dezincing iron; metal fluxing (I)	Eye and airway irritation
Chloroform $CHCl_3$	Aerosol propellents; purifying and extracting antibiotics and other pharmaceuticals; making of fluorocarbons for refrigerants; plastics; solvent uses (I)	Liver or kidney and central nervous system effects
Chloroprene $CH_2{=}CClCH{=}CH_2$	Synthetic rubber manufacturing	Reproductive effects; potential for cancer
Chromic acid CrO_3	Compounds used in electroplating, leather tanning and to make certain colored glass (I), (S)	Nasal ulceration
Chromium (VI)	Steel alloys, especially stainless and heat-resisting steels; as a pigment in paints, plastics and as a corrosion inhibitor (I)	Lung cancer; skin ulcers; lung irritation
Chrysene	Dye making (I), (S), (SA)	Cancer

CURRENT OSHA OCCUPATIONAL ENVIRONMENTAL STANDARD	NIOSH RECOMMENDATION FOR OCCUPATIONAL ENVIRONMENTAL EXPOSURE LIMIT	SPECIAL COMMENTS; CLINICAL TESTS, IF AVAILABLE
3.5 mg/m^3, 8-hr TWA	3.5 mg/m^3 TWA; 0.1 mg/m^3 TWA in presence of polycyclic aromatic hydrocarbons	Chest x-rays, pulmonary function testing, sputum cytology recommended
5000 ppm, 8-hr TWA	10,000 ppm TWA (18,000 mg/m^3); 30,000 ppm ceiling (54,000 mg/m^3) (10-minute)	
20 ppm, 8-hr TWA	1 ppm TWA (3 mg/m^3); 10 ppm ceiling (30 mg/m^3) (15-minute)	Employees to be advised of potential effects on reproductive system
50 ppm, 8-hr TWA	35 ppm TWA (40 mg/m^3); 200 ppm ceiling (229 mg/m^3)	Preserved whole blood is necessary; at least 2 ml is required. Container should be tightly capped
10 ppm, 8-hr TWA; 25 ppm acceptable ceiling; 200 ppm maximal ceiling (5 minutes in 4 hours)	2 ppm ceiling (12.6 mg/m^3) (60-minute)	
1 ppm ceiling	0.5 ppm ceiling (1.45 mg/m^3) (15-minute)	Chest x-rays required
50 ppm ceiling	2 ppm ceiling (9.78 mg/m^3) (60-minute)	Current federal standard should be TWA
25 ppm, 8-hr TWA	1 ppm ceiling (3.6 mg/m^3) (15-minute)	Chest x-ray and pulmonary function testing required; medical warnings to workers concerning reproductive effects in animals; pregnant workers to be counseled about continuing work with chloroprene (see Chapter 3)
0.1 mg/m^3 ceiling	0.05 mg Cr 03/m^3 TWA; 0.1 mg Cr 03/m^3 ceiling (15-minute)	
110 μg/m^3 ceiling	1 μg/m^3 for carcinogenic Cr (VI); 25 μg/m^3 TWA for other Cr (VI); 50 μg/m^3 ceiling (15-minute)	Employer must demonstrate absence of carcinogenic Cr (VI); x-ray required
None	To be controlled as an occupational carcinogen	Control recommendations also included for polycyclic aromatic hydrocarbons

SUBSTANCE, AGENT OR ENVIRONMENTAL FACTORS	MAIN USES, SOURCES AND POTENTIAL OCCUPATIONAL EXPOSURES, I.E., INHALATION (I), SKIN CONTACT (S), SKIN ABSORPTION (SA), ORAL (O)	NIOSH CHIEF HEALTH EFFECTS CONSIDERED
Coal gasification plants	Various gases, tars, solvents, fumes, dusts, heat, noise, vibrations (I), (S), (SA)	Various effects, depending on substances present; carcinogenic potential
Coal tar products	From using coal tar pitches as a binding agent; in carbon electrodes and in pitch-melting operations (I), (S)	Lung and skin cancer
Coke oven emissions	Main source is from coke ovens used to manufacture coke and in steel making (I)	Lung cancer
Cotton dust	Cotton processing (I)	Pulmonary disease (byssinosis)
Cresols $CH_3C_6H_4CH$	Making antiseptics, disinfectants, insecticides, plasticizers and resins (I), (SA)	Skin, liver, kidney and pancreas effects
Cyanide, hydrogen and cyanide salts	Heat treating of metals such as iron and steel; electroplating; making mirrors; as a fumigant (calcium cyanide); in photographic processing; in extraction of gold and silver (I), (SA), (O)	Thyroid, blood and respiratory system effects
DDT	Insecticide (I), (SA), (O)	Cancer in animals
Decomposition products of fluorocarbons	Formed at high temperatures during certain cutting, fabricating, machining, grinding of fluorocarbon plastics (about 500° C and higher, depending on type of polymer)	Lung effects; polymer fume fever
Dibromochloropropane $CH_2BrCHBrCH_2Cl$	Nematocide (I), (SA)	Male sterility; renal and liver effects

CURRENT OSHA OCCUPATIONAL ENVIRONMENTAL STANDARD	NIOSH RECOMMENDATION FOR OCCUPATIONAL ENVIRONMENTAL EXPOSURE LIMIT	SPECIAL COMMENTS; CLINICAL TESTS, IF AVAILABLE
	Existing federal occupational exposure limits or NIOSH	Extensive work practice and control procedures recommended. Document limited to those technologies most likely to be operational in the U.S.
None	0.1 mg/m^3 TWA (cyclohexane-extractable fraction)	Includes coal tar, creosote and coal tar pitch. Pulmonary function testing, chest x-rays and sputum cytology required
150 μg/m^3, 8-hr TWA	Work practices to minimize exposure to emissions	Sputum cytology and chest x-ray required. Federal standard promulgated October 22, 1976
200 μg/m^3, 8 hr TWA (yarn manufacturing); 750 μg/m^3, 8-hr TWA (slashing and weaving operations); 500 μg/m^3, 8-hr TWA (all other operations)	200 μg/m^3 lint-free cotton dust	Pulmonary function testing required. Federal standard promulgated June 23, 1978
22 mg/m^3, 8-hr TWA (skin)	10 mg/m^3 TWA	Applies to mixtures of cresols and cresylic acid. Hazardous substance, skin and eyes. Possible delayed effects (See Chapter 14)
10 ppm, 8-hr TWA (alkali cyanides)	5 mg CN/m^3 ceiling (4.7 ppm) (10-minute)	Concurrent measurement required for HCN when measuring for cyanide salt. Trained first-aid personnel and first-aid kits to be available during use. Hazardous liquids, skin and eyes (See Chapter 14)
1 mg/m^3, 8-hr TWA (skin)	Lowest reliably detectable level; 0.5 mg/m^3 TWA by NIOSH validated method. Skin contact to be avoided	(See Chapters 3 and 13)
None	None recommended	Workroom air to be monitored for inorganic fluorides and hydrogen fluoride
1 ppb, 8-hr TWA; eye and skin contact to be avoided	10 ppb ceiling (0.1 mg/m^3) (30-minute)	Medical warnings to workers of reproductive system abnormalities, including sterility and notice of findings of cancer in animals following direct gastric application. Federal standard promulgated March 17, 1978 (see Chapter 3)

SUBSTANCE, AGENT OR ENVIRONMENTAL FACTORS	MAIN USES, SOURCES AND POTENTIAL OCCUPATIONAL EXPOSURES, I.E., INHALATION (I), SKIN CONTACT (S), SKIN ABSORPTION (SA), ORAL (O)	NIOSH CHIEF HEALTH EFFECTS CONSIDERED
Diisocyanates	Plastics production (I), (S)	Respiratory effects and sensitization; irritation
Dinitro-ortho-cresol $CH_3C_6H_2OH(NO_2)_2$	In making certain pesticides, herbicides and insecticides; as a fungicide (I), (SA)	Central nervous system and metabolic effects
Dioxane $C_4H_8O_2$	Solvent for many organic materials (I), (SA)	Liver and kidney effects; cancer
Epichlorohydrin C_3H_5OCl	Making synthetic glycerin, epoxy resins, pharmaceuticals, insecticides, agricultural and textile chemicals, adhesives, coatings, plasticizers (I), (SA)	Skin, kidney, liver and respiratory effects
Ethylene dibromide CH_2BrCH_2Br	A fumigant; found in certain gasolines and solvent for fats, oils and waxes (I), (SA)	Damage to skin, eyes, heart, liver, spleen, respiratory and central nervous systems; potential for cancer and mutagenesis
Ethylene dichloride	Vinyl chloride making; fumigant; insecticide; in degreasing compounds; as an antiknock agent in fuels; in rubber cements (I), (SA), (O)	Cancer; nervous system, respiratory, heart and liver effects
Ethylene oxide C_2H_4O	Sterilizing agent; fumigant; fungicide; in organic chemical synthesis (I)	Mutagenesis; cancer
Ethylene thiourea	Accelerator in rubber and plastic making; a contaminant in certain fungicides (I), (SA)	Carcinogenesis and teratogenesis
Fibrous glass	Insulation and reinforced plastics (I), (S)	Eye, skin and airway effects

CURRENT OSHA OCCUPATIONAL ENVIRONMENTAL STANDARD	NIOSH RECOMMENDATION FOR OCCUPATIONAL ENVIRONMENTAL EXPOSURE LIMIT	SPECIAL COMMENTS; CLINICAL TESTS, IF AVAILABLE
0.02 ppm (0.14 mg/m^3) ceiling (TDI); 0.02 ppm (0.2 mg/m^3) ceiling (MDI)	All values are in μg/m^3; toluene diisocyanate (TDI): 35 TWA, 140 ceiling; diphenylmethane diisocyanate (MDI): 50 TWA, 200 ceiling; hexamethylene diisocyanate (HDI): 35 TWA, 140 ceiling; naphthalene diisocyanate (DNI): 40 TWA, 170 ceiling; isophorene diisocyanate (IPDI): 45 TWA, 180 ceiling; dicyclohexylmethane (hydrogenated MDI): 55 TWA, 210 ceiling; other diisocyanates to be controlled to 20 ppb ceiling and 5 ppb TWA	Chest x-ray and pulmonary function testing required (See Chapter 14)
0.1 mg/m^3, 8-hr TWA (skin)	0.2 mg/m^3 TWA	Blood and urine monitoring required. Hazardous substance, skin and eyes; possible delayed effects
100 ppm, 8-hr TWA (skin)	1 ppm ceiling (3.6 mg/m^3) (30-minute)	Blood and urine testing required; hazardous liquid, skin
5 ppm, 8-hr TWA (20 mg/m^3)	20 mg/m^3 TWA; 19 mg/m^3 ceiling (15-minute)	Medical warning of infertility effects required; hazardous liquid, skin (see Chapter 3)
20 ppm, 8-hr TWA; 30 ppm acceptable	1 mg/m^3 ceiling (0.13 ppm) (15-minute)	Medical warnings to workers of potential reproductive abnormalities and cancer following direct administration in animals; hazardous liquid; contact to be prevented (see Chapter 3)
50 ppm, 8-hr TWA; 100 ppm acceptable ceiling; 200 ppm maximal ceiling (5 minutes in 3 hours)	1 ppm TWA (4 mg/m^3); 2 ppm ceiling (2 mg/m^3) (15-minute)	Nursing infants at risk (See Chapter 3)
90 mg/m^3 (50 ppm), 8-hr TWA	90 mg/m^3 (50 ppm) TWA; 135 mg/m^3 (75 ppm) ceiling (15-minute)	Recommendations for blood monitoring and medical counseling concerning mutations (see Chapter 3)
None	Use of encapsulated form in industry; worker exposure to be minimized	Workers to be informed of carcinogenic and teratogenic hazards. Special attention to be given to thyroid function tests (see Chapter 3)
15 mg/m^3 total dust; 5 mg/m^3 respirable fraction (nuisance dust)	3,000,000 fibers/m^3 TWA (fibers of 3.5 microns diameter and 10 microns length); 5 mg/m^3 TWA (total fibrous glass)	NIOSH recommends that this limit also apply to other man-made fibers

SUBSTANCE, AGENT OR ENVIRONMENTAL FACTORS	MAIN USES, SOURCES AND POTENTIAL OCCUPATIONAL EXPOSURES, I.E., INHALATION (I), SKIN CONTACT (S), SKIN ABSORPTION (SA), ORAL (O)	NIOSH CHIEF HEALTH EFFECTS CONSIDERED
Fluorides, inorganic	Aluminum reduction and in certain steel making, fluoride acts as a flux in melts, in kiln firing of bricks or ceramics, glass making sources or in calcining of fluoride-containing minerals and in drying and grinding ores (I), (O)	Kidney and bone effects
Formaldehyde HCHO	In formic esters; leather making, plastics and resins, rubber and as a disinfectant; urea formaldehyde resins in plywood and foam insulation "particle" or "chip" board (I), (S)	Irritation; lung effects
Glycidyl ethers	Reactive diluents in epoxy resin systems (I), (SA)	Skin and mucous membrane effects; sensitization potential; tumorigenesis and mutagenesis
Hydrazines NH_2NH_2	Making organic hydrazine compounds; reducing agent and in rocket fuels (I), (SA)	Liver, blood, eye and skin effects; cancer
Hydrogen fluoride HF	Etching glass; as a catalyst in high octane gasoline production (I), (S)	Skin, eye and airway irritation; bone effects
Hydrogen sulfide H_2S	Common by-product in many industrial processes, especially around oil wells and in petroleum processing plants; in agricultural wastes; fishing vessel holds; sewage plants (I)	Irritation; severe, acute effects on nervous and respiratory systems
Hydroquinone $C_6H_4(OH)_2$	In photographic developers and reducers; widely used as an antioxidant in plastics and rubber (I), (O—rare)	Eye and skin effects
Isopropyl alcohol $CH_3CHOHCH_3$	Making acetone; as a solvent in cosmetics, skin lotions and making pharmaceuticals (I), (SA)	Mucous membrane irritation; possible cancer threat in manufacturing process
Kepone	Pesticide, in production and use (I), (SA)	Nervous system effects; liver cancer

CURRENT OSHA OCCUPATIONAL ENVIRONMENTAL STANDARD	NIOSH RECOMMENDATION FOR OCCUPATIONAL ENVIRONMENTAL EXPOSURE LIMIT	SPECIAL COMMENTS; CLINICAL TESTS, IF AVAILABLE
2.5 mg/m³, 8-hr TWA	2.5 mg F/m³ TWA	Urine monitoring required. At least 3 ml of serum should be submitted. Avoid tubes that may have contained an anticoagulant such as sodium fluoride to obviate the possibility of contamination. Normal range: less than 50 μg/100 ml
3 ppm, 8-hr TWA; 5 ppm acceptable ceiling; 10 ppm maximal ceiling (30-minute)	1.2 mg/m³ ceiling (1 ppm) (30-minute)	Hazardous liquid, skin
45 mg/m³ ceiling (allylglycidyl ether); 270 mg/m³, 8-hr TWA (*n*-butyl glycidyl ether); 2.8 mg/m³, 8-hr TWA (di-2,3-epoxypropyl ether); 240 mg/m³, 8-hr TWA (isopropyl glycidyl ether); 60 mg/m³, 8-hr TWA (phenyl glycidyl ether)	45 mg/m³ (AGE); 30 mg/m³ (BGE); 1 mg/m³ (DGE); 240 mg/m³ (IGE); all ceiling values (15-minute)	Possible additive effects with mixture
1.0 mg/m³ (1.1-dimethyl hydrazine); 22 mg/m³ (phenyl-hydrazine) as 8-hr TWA values; 0.35 mg/m³ ceiling (methyl-hydrazine)	0.4 mg/m³ (hydrazine); 0.15 mg/m³ (1.1-dimethyl-hydrazine); 0.6 mg/m³ (hydrazine); 0.08 mg/m³ (methyl-hydrazine); all as ceiling values (120-minute)	Blood and urine monitoring, chest x-ray required; bowel examination required for some workers
3 ppm, 8-hr TWA	2.5 mg F/m³ TWA (approx. 6 ppm); 5.0 mg/m³ ceiling (approx. 12 ppm) (15-minute, fluoride ion)	Pelvic x-ray (male) and urine testing required
20 ppm acceptable ceiling; 50 ppm maximal ceiling (10-minute)	15 mg/m³ ceiling (approx. 10 ppm) (10-minute)	Continual monitoring required if potential exists for exposure to 70 mg/m³ or greater; evacuation required at this level
2 mg/m³, 8-hr TWA	2 mg/m³ ceiling (15-minute)	Special provisions for darkroom use
400 ppm, 8-hr, TWA	400 ppm TWA (984 mg/m³); 800 ppm ceiling (1968 mg/m³) (15-minute)	More stringent work practices and medical surveillance for manufacturing workers
None	1 μg/m³ ceiling (15-minute)	Liver function testing required (see Chapter 3)

SUBSTANCE, AGENT OR ENVIRONMENTAL FACTORS	MAIN USES, SOURCES AND POTENTIAL OCCUPATIONAL EXPOSURES, I.E., INHALATION (I), SKIN CONTACT (S), SKIN ABSORPTION (SA), ORAL (O)	NIOSH CHIEF HEALTH EFFECTS CONSIDERED
Ketones [i.e., acetone $(CH_3)_2CO$]	General solvents, chemical and pharmaceutical manufacturing	Irritation; liver, kidney and nervous system effects
Lead, inorganic Pb	Batteries; pigments in paints, inks and ceramics; explosives; alloying and making other compounds (I), (O)	Kidney, blood and nervous system effects
Malathion	Insecticide (I), (SA), (O)	Nervous system effects
Mercury, inorganic Hg	In electrical equipment such as rectifiers; instruments, both laboratory and industrial; in thermometer making; in fungicides; paint making (I), (SA), (O)	Central nervous system and mental effects

CURRENT OSHA OCCUPATIONAL ENVIRONMENTAL STANDARD	NIOSH RECOMMENDATION FOR OCCUPATIONAL ENVIRONMENTAL EXPOSURE LIMIT	SPECIAL COMMENTS; CLINICAL TESTS, IF AVAILABLE
Acetone 2400 mg/m^3 Methyl ethyl ketone 590 mg/m^3 Methyl *n*-propyl ketone 700 mg/m^3 Methyl *n*-butyl ketone 410 mg/m^3 Methyl *n*-amyl ketone 465 mg/m^3 Methyl isoamyl ketone—none Diisobutyl ketone 290 mg/m^3 Cyclohexanone 200 mg/m^3 Mesityl oxide 100 mg/m^3 Diacetone alcohol 240 mg/m^3 Isophorone 140 mg/m^3 All values 8-hr TWA	590 mg/m^3 TWA 590 mg/m^3 TWA 530 mg/m^3 TWA 4 mg/m^3 TWA 465 mg/m^3 TWA 230 mg/m^3 TWA 140 mg/m^3 TWA 100 mg/m^3 TWA 40 mg/m^3 TWA 240 mg/m^3 TWA 23 mg/m^3 TWA	Urinalysis required; warning of nervous system effects in workers exposed to methyl *n*-butyl ketone
50 µg/m^3, 8-hr TWA; over 8-hr exposure to be determined by formula	Less than 100 µg/m^3	Air levels to be maintained so that worker blood lead remains at or below 69µ/100 ml; blood monitoring required. Federal standard promulgated November 14, 1978 Blood—Preserved whole blood must be submitted. Commercial tubes with anticoagulant that have been specially prepared to eliminate contamination are available. Heparinized tubes are preferred; 3 ml of whole blood is a sufficient sample. *Do not* send serum or plasma for lead analysis Normal range: See Chapter 3 Urine—Urine must be collected in a container that has been washed in nitric acid and rinsed with double-distilled water to avoid contamination. At least 50 ml of urine should be submitted in specially prepared containers
15 mg/m^3, 8-hr TWA	15 mg/m^3 TWA	Skin contact to be prevented; blood monitoring required (see Chapter 3)
0.1 mg/m^3 ceiling	0.05 mg/m^3 TWA	Submit at least 50 ml of urine. Urine is the specimen of choice for screening for exposure. Blood (10 ml) should be preserved with heparin or EDTA Normal range—0–30 µg/24 hr—urine; 6–12 µg/liter—blood

SUBSTANCE, AGENT OR ENVIRONMENTAL FACTORS	MAIN USES, SOURCES AND POTENTIAL OCCUPATIONAL EXPOSURES, I.E., INHALATION (I), SKIN CONTACT (S), SKIN ABSORPTION (SA), ORAL (O)	NIOSH CHIEF HEALTH EFFECTS CONSIDERED
Methyl alcohol	Formaldehyde production; found in inks, dyes and in varnishes (I), (SA)	Blindness; metabolic acidosis
4,4″-Methylenebis	Curing agent in isocyanide polymers (I), (SA)	Cancer
Methylene chloride CH_2Cl_2	As an insecticide and fumigant; in paint and varnish removers; as a general solvent for cleaning and found in fire extinguishers (I), (SA)	Central nervous system effects; carbon monoxide toxicity
Methyl parathion	Insecticide (I), (SA), (O)	Nervous system effects
Nickel carbonyl $Ni(CO)_4$	In nickel refining; as a catalyst in making certain petroleum, plastic and rubber products (I)	Cancer
Nickel, inorganic and compounds $NiCl_2$, $Ni(NO_3)_2$, $NiSO_4$	In alloying for stainless steel making and plating; as a catalyst and in batteries (I), (S)	Skin effects; lung and nasal cancer
Nitric acid HNO_3	Manufacturing fertilizers and explosives; in laboratories (I), (S)	Dental erosion; nasal and lung irritation
Nitriles	Widespread uses, including plastics, dyestuffs, synthetic intermediates, pharmaceuticals; some as lubricating oil additive, gasoline additive; some as solvents (I), (SA)	Hepatic, renal, respiratory, cardiovascular, gastrointestinal and nervous system effects
Nitrogen oxides	As an intermediate in nitric and sulfuric acid making; nitration of organic compounds and in making explosives (I)	Airway effects
Nitroglycerin: ethylene glycol dinitrate	Mainly to manufacture dynamite (I), (SA)	Circulatory system effects

CURRENT OSHA OCCUPATIONAL ENVIRONMENTAL STANDARD	NIOSH RECOMMENDATION FOR OCCUPATIONAL ENVIRONMENTAL EXPOSURE LIMIT	SPECIAL COMMENTS; CLINICAL TESTS, IF AVAILABLE
200 ppm TWA	200 ppm TWA (262 mg/m^3); 800 ppm ceiling (1048 mg/m^3) (15-minute)	
None—standard remanded by court	3 μg/m^3 TWA; skin contact to be avoided	Chest x-ray, blood and urine testing required
500 ppm, 8-hr TWA; 1000 ppm acceptable ceiling; 2000 ppm maximal ceiling (5 minutes in 2 hours)	75 ppm TWA (261 mg/m^3); 500 ppm ceiling (1740 mg/m^3) to be lowered in presence of carbon monoxide	Blood monitoring required (see Chapters 3 and 14)
None	0.2 mg/m^3 TWA	Skin contact to be prevented; blood monitoring required for cholinesterase activity. Whole blood should be collected using heparin as the anticoagulant. The plasma should be separated after centrifuging and a sample of the packed red cells should also be submitted. Normal ranges: See Chapter 13
7 μg/m^3 (1 ppb), 8-hr TWA	7 μg/m^3 (1 ppb) TWA	Recommendations for chest x-ray, pulmonary function testing and urine monitoring
1 mg/m^3, 8-hr TWA	15 μg Ni/m^3 TWA	Chest x-ray and pulmonary function testing required
2 ppm, 8-hr TWA	2 ppm TWA (5 mg/m^3)	Hazardous liquid, eyes and skin; chest x-ray required (See Chapter 14).
70 mg/m^3 (40 ppm), 8-hr TWA (acetonitrile); 3 mg/m^3 (0.5 ppm), 8-hr TWA (skin) (tetramethyl succinonitrile)	To be TWA values: acetonitrile: 34 mg/m^3 (20 ppm); *n*-butyronitrile: 22 mg/m^3 (8 ppm); propionitrile: 14 mg/m^3 (6 ppm); malononitrile: 8 mg/m^3 (3 ppm); adiponitrile: 18 mg/m^3 (4 ppm); succinonitrile: 20 mg/m^3 (6 ppm) To be ceiling values (15-minute): acetone cyanohydrin: 4 mg/m^3 (1 ppm); glycolonitrile: 5 mg/m^3 (2 ppm); tetramethyl succinonitrile: 6 mg/m^3 (1 ppm). When present as mixtures or with sources of cyanide, exposure to be considered additive and environmental limit to be calculated	Chest x-ray and pulmonary function testing required. Trained personnel and first-aid kits to be available
NO_2: 5 ppm, 8-hr TWA NO: 25 ppm, 8-hr TWA	NO_2: 1 ppm (1.8 mg/m^3) ceiling (15-minute) NO_2: 25 ppm TWA (30 mg/m^3)	Pulmonary function testing required (See Chapter 14)
2 mg/m^3 (skin), 8-hr TWA (nitroglycerin); 1 mg/m^3 (skin) ceiling (EDGN)	0.1 mg/m^3 ceiling (20-minute)	Skin contact to be prevented; recommended limit for either substance alone or mixtures

SUBSTANCE, AGENT OR ENVIRONMENTAL FACTORS	MAIN USES, SOURCES AND POTENTIAL OCCUPATIONAL EXPOSURES, I.E., INHALATION (I), SKIN CONTACT (S), SKIN ABSORPTION (SA), ORAL (O)	NIOSH CHIEF HEALTH EFFECTS CONSIDERED
Organotin compounds	Stabilizers in polymers, in biocides and as catalysts (I), (SA)	Eye, skin, liver, nervous system and heart effects
Parathion	Insecticide (I), (SA), (O)	Nervous system effects
Phenol	In making aromatic compounds; disinfectants; reagent and chemical analyses (I), (S), (SA)	Skin, eye, central nervous system, liver and kidney effects
Phosgene	An intermediate in chemical making by chlorination of the oxides; phosgene may occur as a by-product of combustion or multichlorine compounds with contact heat or flame (I)	Airway effects
Polychlorinated biphenyls	Electrical insulation in certain condensers; in transformers as a coolant ("transformer oil"); as a heat transfer agent (SA)	Cancer; skin, liver and reproductive effects
Refined petroleum solvents	Varied solvent use (I), (S)	Skin, lung and nerve irritation
Silica, crystalline SiO_2	In manufacturing glass, porcelain and pottery; in making molds and cores for metal casting. Encountered during blasting in granite, in tunneling, mining; cutting stone and granite; making refractory bricks; in grinding and polishing compounds (I)	Chronic lung disease (silicosis)

CURRENT OSHA OCCUPATIONAL ENVIRONMENTAL STANDARD	NIOSH RECOMMENDATION FOR OCCUPATIONAL ENVIRONMENTAL EXPOSURE LIMIT	SPECIAL COMMENTS; CLINICAL TESTS, IF AVAILABLE
0.1 mg tin/m^3, 8-hr TWA	0.1 mg tin/m^3 TWA	Chest x-ray, blood and urine monitoring, eye tests, heart examination and nervous system testing required; hazardous liquid, skin and eyes (See Chapter 14)
0.11 mg/m^3 TWA	0.05 mg/m^3 TWA	Skin contact to be prevented. Blood monitoring required for cholinesterase activity. Whole blood should be collected using heparin as the anticoagulant. The plasma should be separated after centrifuging and a sample of the packed red cells should also be submitted Normal ranges: See Chapter 13
5 ppm, 8-hr TWA (skin)	20 mg/m^3 TWA (5.2 ppm); 60 mg/m^3 ceiling (15.6 ppm) (15-minute)	Hazardous substance, skin and eyes
0.1 ppm, 8-hr TWA	0.1 ppm TWA (0.4 mg/m^3); 0.2 ppm ceiling (0.8 mg/m^3) (15-minute)	Pulmonary function testing and chest x-ray required
1 mg/m^3, 8-hr TWA (42% chlorine); 0.5 mg/m^3, 8-hr TWA (54% chlorine)	1 μg/m^3 TWA	Blood testing required. Medical warning of adverse effects to be given to women workers of childbearing age and nursing mothers (see Chapter 3)
500 ppm, 8-hr TWA (2950 mg/m^3)	350 mg/m^3 TWA; 1800 mg/m^3 ceiling (15-minute)	Blood and urine monitoring required. Action level for petroleum ether, rubber solvent, naphtha to be 200 mg/m^3 TWA; action level for mineral spirits and Stoddard solvent to be 350 mg/m^3 TWA; action level for kerosene to be 100 mg/m^3. Hazardous substance, skin (See Chapter 14)
250/% SiO + in mppcf or 10 mg/m^3/% SiO + 2	50 μg/m^3 TWA, respirable free silica	Chest x-ray, pulmonary function testing required

SUBSTANCE, AGENT OR ENVIRONMENTAL FACTORS	MAIN USES, SOURCES AND POTENTIAL OCCUPATIONAL EXPOSURES, I.E., INHALATION (I), SKIN CONTACT (S), SKIN ABSORPTION (SA), ORAL (O)	NIOSH CHIEF HEALTH EFFECTS CONSIDERED
Sodium hydroxide NaOH	In laundering and bleaching materials; making cotton products, soaps, paper and petroleum and making mercerized cotton and in the electrolytic extraction of zinc in tin plating and oxide coatings (I), (S)	Airway irritation
Sulfur dioxide SO_2	Sulfuric acid making; in bleaching, food processing and making sodium sulfite (I), (S)	Respiratory effects
Sulfuric acid H_2SO_4	In fertilizer making; cleaning metals; making chemicals such as explosives; plastics; petroleum refining; cleaning of metals (I), (S)	Pulmonary irritation
1,1,2,2-Tetrachloroethane	A solvent in making artificial pearls (I), (SA)	Liver, gastrointestinal and nervous system effects
Tetrachloroethylene	Solvent and in dry cleaning (I)	Nervous system, heart, respiratory and liver effects
Thiols	Wide use as intermediates in synthesis of pharmaceuticals and pesticides; as warning agents in gases; as stabilizers in plastics and rubber; in certain flotation processes for some ores; hide depilatory; antioxidant in sheet steel pickling (I), (SA)	Irritation; eye, skin, blood and nervous system effects
o-Tolidine	In making dyes, as an intermediate (I), (SA)	Nasal irritation; cancer
Toluene $C_5H_5CH_3$	A solvent in paints and other coatings; found in some gasolines and making chemicals (I), (SA)	Central nervous system depressant
Toluene diisocyanate	Making polyurethane foams and plastics (I)	Airway effects

CURRENT OSHA OCCUPATIONAL ENVIRONMENTAL STANDARD	NIOSH RECOMMENDATION FOR OCCUPATIONAL ENVIRONMENTAL EXPOSURE LIMIT	SPECIAL COMMENTS; CLINICAL TESTS, IF AVAILABLE
2 mg/m^3, 8-hr TWA	2 mg/m^3 ceiling (15-minute)	Hazardous liquid, eyes and skin
5 ppm, 8-hr TWA	0.5 ppm TWA (1.3 mg/m^3)	Pulmonary function testing required
1 mg/m^3, 8-hr TWA	1 mg/m^3 TWA	Hazardous liquid, eyes and skin
5 ppm, 8-hr TWA (skin)	1 ppm TWA (6.87 mg/m^3)	Skin contact to be prevented. Blood monitoring required
100 ppm, 8-hr TWA; 200 ppm acceptable maximal ceiling; 300 ppm maximal ceiling (5 minutes in 3 hours)	50 ppm TWA (339 mg/m^3; 100 ppm ceiling (678 mg/m^3) (15-minute)	Medical warning of possible congenital abnormalities required
10 ppm, 8-hr TWA (butymercaptan); 10 ppm ceiling (methyl and ethyl mercaptan)	Ceilings (15-minute): benzenethiol: 0.5 mg/m^3 (0.1 ppm); 1-methanethiol: 1.0 mg/m^3 (0.5 ppm); 1-ethanethiol: 1.3 mg/m^3 (0.5 ppm); 1-propanethiol: 1.6 mg/m^3 (0.5 ppm); 1-butanethiol: 1.8 mg/m^3 (0.5 ppm); 1-pentanethiol: 2.1 mg/m^3 (0.5 ppm); 1-hexanethiol: 2.4 mg/m^3 (0.5 ppm); 1-hepthanethiol: 2.7 mg/m^3 (0.5 ppm); 1-octanethiol: 3.0 mg/m^3 (0.5 ppm); 1-nonanethiol: 3.3 mg/m^3 (0.5 ppm); 1-decanethiol: 3.6 mg/m^3 (0.5 ppm); 1-undecanethiol: 3.9 mg/m^3 (0.5 ppm); 1-dodecanethiol: 4.1 mg/m^3 (0.5 ppm); 1-hexadecanethiol: 5.3 mg/m^3 (0.5 ppm); 1-octadecanethiol: 5.9 mg/m^3 (0.5 ppm); cyclohexanethiol: 2.4 mg/m^3 (0.5 ppm); mixtures of thiols to be controlled by calculation of equivalent concentrations	Hazardous substance, skin. Blood and urine monitoring required
None	20 μg/m^3 ceiling skin contact	Urine testing required: quarterly urine monitoring recommended
200 ppm, 8-hr TWA; 300 ppm acceptable ceiling; 500 ppm maximal ceiling (10-minute)	100 ppm TWA (375 mg/m^3); 200 ppm ceiling (750 mg/m^3) (10-minute)	
0.02 ppm ceiling	0.005 ppm TWA (0.035 mg/m^3); 0.02 ppm ceiling (0.14 mg/m^3) (20-minute)	Chest x-rays, blood tests, pulmonary function testing required. Recommendations revised. See Diisocyanates (See Chapter 14)

SUBSTANCE, AGENT OR ENVIRONMENTAL FACTORS	MAIN USES, SOURCES AND POTENTIAL OCCUPATIONAL EXPOSURES, I.E., INHALATION (I), SKIN CONTACT (S), SKIN ABSORPTION (SA), ORAL (O)	NIOSH CHIEF HEALTH EFFECTS CONSIDERED
1,1,1-Trichloroethane CH_3CCl_3	A solvent in cleaning (I), (SA)	Nervous system, liver and heart effects
Trichloroethylene $Cl_2C=CHCl$	Degreasing, dry cleaning and extracting other chemicals; intermediate in chemical making (I)	Central nervous system depressant; cancer
Tungsten and cemented tungsten carbide	Alloying iron and steel for cutting tools (I)	Lung and skin effects
Ultraviolet radiation	Welding; certain sterilizers (S)	Skin and eye effects
Vanadium (oxides) V_2O_5 Ferrovanadium—FeV	In alloying steels; as a catalyst in chemical and petroleum industries, glass pigmentation and in ceramic glazing (I), (S) Ferrovanadium used in alloying steel and for tools (I), (S)	Eye, skin and lung effects
Vinyl acetate $CH_3COOCH=CH_2$	Plastic production (I), (S)	Irritation
Vinyl chloride $H_2C=CClH$	In making polyvinyl resins, in methylchloroform manufacturing and in certain propellents (I)	Liver cancer
Vinyl halides	Plastic production (I), (S)	Cancer
Waste anesthetic gases and vapors	Hospital operating and recovery room personnel; allied health workers (I)	Reproductive effects; motor and audio-visual performance decrements
Xylene $C_6H_4(CH_3)_2$	A solvent in the manufacture of other organic compounds (I), (SA)	Central nervous system depressant; airway irritation
Zinc oxide ZnO	In zinc processing or making zinc alloys (I)	Metal fume fever

CURRENT OSHA OCCUPATIONAL ENVIRONMENTAL STANDARD	NIOSH RECOMMENDATION FOR OCCUPATIONAL ENVIRONMENTAL EXPOSURE LIMIT	SPECIAL COMMENTS; CLINICAL TESTS, IF AVAILABLE
350 ppm 8-hr TWA	350 ppm ceiling (1910 mg/m^3) (15-minute)	Action level set at 200 ppm TWA; medical warning of possible congenital abnormalities required (See Chapter 3)
100 ppm	25 ppm (134 mg/m^3) TWA	Workers to be warned of hazards
100 ppm, 8-hr TWA; 200 ppm acceptable ceiling; 300 ppm maximal ceiling (5 minutes in any 2 hours). None	Insoluble tungsten: 5 mg/m^3, TWA soluble tungsten; 1 mg/m^3 TWA. Dust of cemented tungsten carbide (& 2% cobalt); 0.1 mg cobalt/m^3 TWA. Dust of cemented tungsten carbide (& 0.3% nickel); 15 mg/m^3 TWA	Pulmonary function testing and chest x-ray required (See Chapter 14)
10 mW/cm averaged over any 1-hr period	1.0 mW/cm for over 1000 sec; 100 mW sec/cm for periods under 1000 sec	
Vanadium pentoxide (dust) 0.5 mg/m^3 ceiling; (fume) 0.1 mg/m^3 ceiling. Ferrovanadium: 1 mg/m^3, 8-hr TWA	Vanadium compounds: 0.05 mg/m^3 ceiling (15-minute); metallic vanadium and vanadium carbide: 1 mg/m^3 TWA	Pulmonary function testing and chest x-ray required
None	15 mg/m^3 (4 ppm) ceiling (15-minute)	
1 ppm, 8-hr TWA; 5 ppm ceiling (15-minute)	Minimal detectable level; 1 ppm ceiling (2.55 mg/m^3) (15-minute)	Standard promulgated October 4, 1974. Liver function testing required (see Chapter 3)
1 ppm, 8-hr TWA; 5 ppm ceiling (15-minute)	As promulgated for vinyl chloride in 29 CFR 1910.1017 with eventual goal of zero exposure	Document includes vinyl chloride, vinylidene chloride, vinyl bromide vinyl fluoride and vinylidene fluoride monomers
None for substance when used as anesthetic agent	2 ppm ceiling (halogenated anesthetic agents) (1-hour); 25 ppm TWA during periods of use (nitrous oxide)	Employees to be advised of potential effects; abnormal outcome of pregnancies of employees and spouse to be documented (see Chapter 3)
100 ppm, 8-hr TWA	100 ppm TWA (434 mg/m^3); 200 ppm ceiling (868 mg/m^3) (10-minute)	
5 mg/m^3, 8-hr TWA	5 mg/m^3 TWA; 15 mg/m^3 ceiling (15-minute)	At least 10 ml of urine or 2 ml serum should be submitted according to restrictions given under urine lead Normal range: Serum—0.5–1.55 ppm (50–155 μg/100 ml). Urine—mean 600 μg/24 hr or less than 1 ppm. Range —(0.15–1 mg/24 hr)

Index

M

O

P

Q

R